ANNUAL REVIEW OF PHARMACOLOGY

HENRY W. ELLIOTT, *Editor*
California College of Medicine, University of California, Irvine

RONALD OKUN, *Associate Editor*
California College of Medicine, University of California, Irvine

ROBERT GEORGE, *Associate Editor*
University of California School of Medicine, Los Angeles

VOLUME 14

1974

ANNUAL REVIEWS INC.   4139 EL CAMINO WAY   PALO ALTO, CALIFORNIA 94306

ANNUAL REVIEWS INC.
Palo Alto, California, USA

International Standard Book Number: 0-8243-0414-4
Library of Congress Catalog Number: 61-5649

Assistant Editors	Toni Haskell
	Virginia Hoyle
Indexers	Mary Glass
	Susan Tinker
Subject Indexer	Dorothy Read

PRINTED AND BOUND IN THE UNITED STATES OF AMERICA

PREFACE

Pharmacology has always been a bridge discipline with one foot in the laboratory and the other in the clinic. Today the scope of the field has enlarged to encompass the entire environment as the need increases to determine the effects of industrial and agricultural chemicals and pollutants on all life forms. The new drugs, potent and usually multi-actioned, also demand careful evaluation as we realize the importance of drug interactions and drug-tissue interactions which may have delayed effects extending to future generations. There is plenty for pharmacologists and toxicologists of all persuasions to do. Very few ultimate mechanisms of either therapeutic or toxic actions of drugs and chemicals have been nailed down and benefit-risk (or is it risk-benefit?) ratios must be determined not only for therapeutic agents but for many chemicals and pollutants which have either contributed to or are a result of our unprecedented standard of living. An item for serious consideration is the fact that the cost in money and manpower of safety and efficacy studies for a new drug is so great that fundamental work on the drug is often delayed or neglected to the detriment of rational drug therapy and the science of pharmacology.

All these factors point out that this volume is an epitome of Pharmacology 1974. Between a fascinating reminder of the early days of our science and the familiar "review of reviews" are chapters on mechanisms of drug action, pharmacokinetics, pharmacodynamics, comparative pharmacology, clinical pharmacology, toxicology, mutagenesis, and chemotherapy. A record 31 articles reflect the many faces of pharmacology and the responsibilities of pharmacologists to their fellow passengers on planet earth.

We note with regret the retirement of Assistant Editor Virginia Hoyle, who always managed to turn a problem into a game and a frown into a smile. We welcome her replacement, Toni Haskell, who has already proven her talents by her work on this volume, and we thank our Indexers, Dorothy Read, Mary Glass, and Susan Tinker for their help in bringing Volume 14 to you.

THE EDITORIAL COMMITTEE

CONTENTS

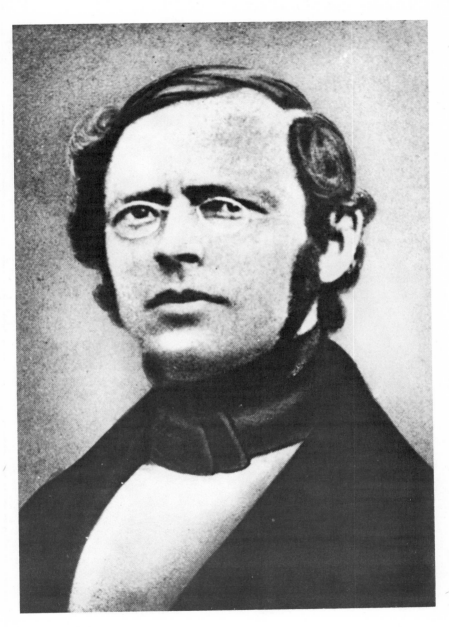

Rudolf Buchheim

1820—1879

RUDOLF BUCHHEIM AND THE BEGINNING OF PHARMACOLOGY AS A SCIENCE

✦6576

Ernst R. Habermann

Pharmakologisches Institut der Justus Liebig-Universität Giessen, West Germany

Birthday celebrations, academic plaudits, and obituary notices comprise, with regularity, a sequence of ornamenting attributes. The top award that an investigator can receive is to be honored as the founder of a new science or at least of a new branch of science. However, as always in history, since the number of praiseworthy researchers by far outweighs the maximal number of individual fields of science, it has proven unavoidable that more than one person has been credited with founding "their" science. Pharmacology is no exception. The mindful, regular reader of *Annual Review of Pharmacology* may find many examples from introductory chapters containing personal, historical, or regional backgrounds of various people.

My view of science and history is different. Research and researchers are embedded in the sociological conditions of their respective times. Scientific growth needs well-prepared soil. The seed that is first to find a favorable environment will overgrow the others. In this sense, scientific greatness is a kind of not earned but "inborn merit" (Goethe).

1. BIOGRAPHICAL DATA

Origin and Development

Reference is made mainly to the descriptions given by Buchheim's student and successor Schmiedeberg (1), to the obituary notices of his colleague Rossbach (2) and his friend Hirsch (3), and to information collected by Oelssner (4) and myself (11).

Rudolf Buchheim was born on March 1, 1820 in Bautzen, which at that time was part of the kingdom of Saxony. His father, Christian Friedrich Buchheim, was a physician and a district medical officer there. Rudolf Buchheim lost his parents early. His father died when he was 4, and his mother when he was 14 years of age (10). In 1838 he left the high school (Gymnasium) in Bautzen to enroll in the

1

Medical Academy (Chirurgisch-Medizinische Akademie) in Dresden, the capital of Saxony. Three years later, in the fall of 1841, he continued his studies at the University of Leipzig, where, as a student, he started scientific work. He became an assistant in the "Anatomisch-Physiologische Anstalt" under E. H. Weber. Here a physiological chemist introduced him to the chemical aspects of medicine, which profoundly influenced his later activities. On January 7, 1845, he took his doctor's degree with an inaugural dissertation on the behavior of egg white, pepsin, and mucin against various reagents, and the resorption and elimination of ferrous sulfate when mixed with protein.

Publicistic Activities

It is doubtful that Buchheim's subsequent activities from 1845 to 1847 resulted from genuine interest only. As a "Privatgelehrter in Leipzig" he had to earn his and his family's livelihood. In 1845 he had married Minna Peschek, daughter of a minister in Zittau. They had six children.

From 1845 to 1847 Buchheim edited the *Pharmazeutisches Zentralblatt*. The journal covered a much more extensive area of chemistry than its title indicated. Later on, it was transformed into the still existing *Chemisches Zentralblatt*. In addition, Buchheim wrote the sections on physiological chemistry for Schmidt's *Jahrbücher der Medizin*. His third and most important task was the edition and adaptation of Jonathan Pereira's *The Elements of Materia Medica*. The book, translated into German, was widely distributed. The first volume of Buchheim's edition with 844 pages appeared in 1846 and the second with 929 pages in 1848. Thus, before having done any specific laboratory research himself, Buchheim tried to evaluate critically the bulk of pharmacological knowledge and views of his time. Today, this sequence is occasionally reversed. The importance of his publicistic activities can hardly be overestimated. In his editions of *Elements of Materia Medica* he dealt with the mode of drug action. By that, he at least intended to replace the descriptive, empirical *Materia Medica* by a science based on logical connections. Schmiedeberg (1) believed that Buchheim's "literary period" was the time of his apprenticeship. Under such circumstances, Buchheim had no other teacher than himself.

His Best Time at Dorpat

More than a century later, the Buchheim of 1847 appears to us as an especially active, talented young man. His exceptional and somewhat dominating personality had not yet become apparent. However, the young Buchheim must already have impressed university administrators as having one of the best brains available in his field. Less than one year after he had received his doctor's degree, he was offered the position of professor ("Außerordentlicher Professor für Arzneimittellehre, Diätetik, Geschichte und Enzyklopädie der Medizin") at the University of Dorpat (Esthonia). He accepted this position in 1847. In 1849 he was promoted to full professor ("Ordentlicher Professor"), after having had to declare that "he did not belong to a freemason's lodge, nor to a secret society neither within or outside the empire, nor intend to join such an organization in the future" (10). At that time (up to 1891), the lectures at the University of Dorpat were given in German, although Dorpat was under Russian administration. The university, despite being located in a cultural fringeland, attracted many outstanding individuals in science and medicine, including Friedrich Bidder and Carl Schmidt. Buchheim completed the triumvirate.

Carl Schmidt, at this time, was able to demonstrate free hydrochloric acid in gastric secretions, and the unequal distribution of potassium and sodium between blood plasma and erythrocytes. Later, also in Dorpat, Alexander Schmidt described thrombin as the principal factor of blood coagulation. Thus, his 20 years in Dorpat brought Buchheim into the main stream of the rapidly developing fields of science and medicine and became his most productive period. He also gained the confidence of his faculty, which twice elected him dean. Shortly after his establishment, he converted part of his home into a laboratory for pharmacological work and financed the scientific endeavors himself. As Schmiedeberg expressed it, "Buchheim was the promoter of the first pharmacological laboratory, and he kept that glory for an unusually long time." The spirit and the equipment of this laboratory were well known to Schmiedeberg, who worked in it for his doctoral thesis in medicine: "Über die quantitative Bestimmung des Chloroforms im Blut und sein Verhalten gegen dasselbe." He noted and reported the relatively high standards to be met by the doctoral candidates: At least one year was devoted to research which could only be done after graduation from medical school. In addition a rigorous examination had to be passed before the doctor's degree was finally awarded. Graduates with such doctoral degrees enjoyed considerable esteem and financial benefit. Over the years, enough qualified people were interested in doing research in pharmacology for their thesis to keep the laboratory active. Buchheim often participated in the laboratory investigations himself. Some self-experiments were reported, which resulted in self-intoxications. A total of almost 100 papers appeared during that time, most of them written in Latin as doctoral theses, and only a few published in journals.

Until 1851 the pharmacological laboratory remained in Buchheim's home. It is not known where it was located between 1851 and 1860, but from 1856 to 1860 a pharmacological institute was founded as part of the "Alte Anatomicum." Impatiently, Buchheim moved into it before it was finished, and this caused some difficulties. The main laboratory of the institute had at least one bench for the professor and two benches for independent co-workers (10).

Dissatisfaction and Death at Giessen

Even the very favorable working conditions—for that time—did not keep Buchheim at Dorpat. He wished to return to Central Europe, especially because of his children, whom he wanted to educate in Germany. Nevertheless, in 1863 he refused a position at the University of Breslau, because the working conditions there were not satisfactory. At the end of 1866 he received simultaneous offers from the medical faculties in the Hessian Giessen and the Prussian Bonn. Buchheim went to Giessen, because Hesse, not Prussia, prescribed a thorough examination of therapeutics. Schmiedeberg became Buchheim's successor at Dorpat and stayed there until 1872, when he went to Strassbourg to establish his famous laboratory.

For Buchheim, facilities and contacts with congenial friends were significantly fewer in Giessen than they had been in Dorpat. There were only a few rooms which his predecessor in Giessen, Philipp Phoebus, had considered a pharmacological institute. In reality, there was merely a collection of illustrative, often curious material for teaching materia medica. However, students liked those rooms very much, especially during the winter. This was evident from warnings written by Phoebus to restrain the vandalism of his pupils, who apparently cleaned their long pipes there. Laboratory rooms were in a distant future. So Buchheim set up working facilities in his home again. It seemed, however, that he won only a few co-workers, not more than four of whom are known by name. As at the beginning of Buchheim's scientific career, literary activity prevailed at its end. After 1874, he became progressively ill. A retinal disease confined him to darkened rooms for long periods of time during the winter of 1874–1875. On June 30, 1879 a stroke paralyzed him. He did not recover from a second stroke and died on December 25, 1879, survived by his wife. The pharmacological institute he had designed was still not completed.

2. HIS CONTRIBUTION TO THE DEVELOPMENT OF PHARMACOLOGY AS A SCIENCE

Rudolf Buchheim was born into a time that could be called the "Gründerzeit" of medicine. Appreciation of scientific methods and thinking replaced the speculative medicine of the Romanticism. During those few decades, the fundamentals of modern medicine were established: Pasteur opened the ways to microbiology; Darwin developed the theory of descendence; Virchow published the cellular pathology; two physicians, Helmholtz and Mayer, formulated the law of conservation of energy; many diseases of man were morphologically and functionally defined. Chemistry and physiology advanced rapidly. The time was ripe also for the scientific foundation of therapeutics. Buchheim introduced two principles, which appear self-evident to us. Each alone would have had a considerable bearing on our field, but both were interdependent, and Buchheim's greatness rests upon their combination.

The Natural System of Drugs

The first and most important achievement was the concept of a "natural system" for the classification of drugs, based on their mode of action. This concept must have been quite revolutionary at that time, as a considerable nonacceptance of it indicated. Until then the materia medica was a collection of therapeutic material in the word's narrowest sense. Its classification was cursory, for example, by origin or by chemistry. No wonder critical physicians questioned whether such museal knowledge should be transmitted to students. The "Oudenotherapie" of the Vienna school expressed the complete rejection of materia medica: Since causally acting drugs were not available anyway, physicians could only confine themselves to descriptive nosology, as the botanist registers growth and withering of a plant.

Buchheim's concept pointed in another direction. The mode of action should be elucidated by scientific means: this, once achieved, should eventually lead to a more rational therapy. He wanted pharmacology to be "a theoretical, i.e., elucidating science, which should provide all the information on drugs necessary for the precise understanding of their therapeutic values." On the basis of this postulate he arranged the contents of his *Lehrbuch der Arzneimittellehre* (6), the first edition of which appeared between 1853–1856. Of course, not many drugs of that time would have survived when subjected to Buchheim's postulates. The same would apply to many of today's drugs too. The understanding of the mode of action of drugs is like the truth in general: it is the asymptote of cognition. Buchheim's critique at least opened the eyes of his contemporaries. They became aware of the scantiness of their pharmacological knowledge and of their crude therapeutic empiricism. Buchheim postulated a new science, and did not hesitate to project its ultimate goal when he wrote (5):

> If we translate our often obscure ideas about drug actions into an exact physiological language, this should, without doubt, be a considerable achievement. However, scientific cognition of the action of a given drug would imply our ability to deduce each of its actions from its chemical formula.

This incredibly bold statement was written at a time when chemical formulation was at its very beginning. It is to be remembered that the benzol nucleus had just been introduced by Kékulé. Buchheim also drew attention to the relevance of statistical methods and to metabolism for understanding drug effects (6). He formulated pharmacology as an independent science, both from its philosophy and from its methodological approach (7):

> The new era of pharmacology will bear its date not from the discovery of chloral hydrate, but from that time when pharmacology will cease to ornate itself by the waste of other disciplines; when pharmacology with its own area and aided by related sciences, will become equivalent to its sisters, chemistry and physiology.

When Buchheim tried to classify drugs according to their mode of action, many "white areas" became apparent. He realized how insufficient present knowledge was for his task, and he fully understood the preliminary character of his system. In a paper on irritant substances, he wrote:

> We are used to deleting drugs from the series of irritants, as soon as we have gained some insight into their mode of action. Therefore, it is to be expected that, with increasing knowledge, the number of irritants will decrease until the term will fade eventually from pharmacology.

Towards an Experimental Pharmacology

For those reasons, the institution of experimental pharmacology appeared inevitable to him. Of course, the action of drugs had already been studied in man and animals, but mostly in a physiological or a biochemical connection, seldom to achieve a rational therapy (9). Buchheim may have been inspired by the great French physiologist Francois Magendie (1783–1855), whose work was undoubtedly known to him (9). Buchheim's determination carried him on. As soon as he had a firm footing in Dorpat or in Giessen, he founded pharmacological laboratories and trained co-workers. He conducted his investigations under considerable financial sacrifice without much government support.

What about Buchheim's own achievements in the experimental sector? Before answering this question, it must be stated that Buchheim published astonishingly few papers presenting experimental material. Most results were buried in dissertations, often written in Latin. Sometimes, when he tried to disprove a supposedly wrong hypothesis given in the literature, he just reverted to his Fort Knox of facts.

Buchheim preferred the chemical and physicochemical way of thinking. The mode of action of drugs could not yet be analyzed with complicated substrates, for instance, the central nervous system, whose function and structure were still obscure. Simple biological systems were needed, approximated as far as possible to chemical or physical models. It may be more than a merely historical parallel that the molecular biology of today has taken the same successful path. Buchheim made use of the possibilities of the just-emerging organic chemistry by purifying and characterizing active ingredients of drugs and by studying their metabolic fate. While working with chloral hydrate, Buchheim detected its hypnotic effects for the first time. He was convinced—as at that time everyone was—of its metabolic transformation into chloroform and formic acid, although he realized that the body is a physiological-chemical, not a chemical laboratory. Nevertheless, he tried to introduce acid equivalents into the body in that manner. He regarded the sleep-promoting action as a side effect, and omitted publishing this finding, as he often did. A few years later, Liebreich started from the same wrong assumption of chloral hydrate metabolism and introduced it into therapy as the first hypnotic. Buchheim was too late when, pushed to a reply, he mentioned his Dorpat protocols.

His preference for physicochemical explanations became apparent when he tried to elucidate the mechanism of acidification of gastric juice and the changes in urinary pH values. He asked the modern question for transport processes and believed, in this respect, in a specific reaction between ions and proteins. He studied water movements in the damaged web of the frog and related them to diffusion and water binding capacities of the surrounding media. For model experiments in vitro, he made use of the collodium membrane. He devoted much effort, though with varying success, to the analysis of the structure and mode of action of laxants.

The multiplicity of the problems dealt with in Buchheim's laboratories can be grouped roughly as follows (1):

   I. Diffusion; endosmosis; mode of action of laxant salts; resorption and elimination of alkali and earth alkali ions and acids.
  II. Heavy metals, arsenic, phosphorus, potassium iodide.
 III. Anthelminthics, organic laxants, irritants.
 IV. Fate of various organic substances in the body.
  V. Drugs and digestion, nutrition and metabolism.
 VI. Pharmacology and chemistry of alkaloids.
VII. Ethanol, chloroform and blood gases.

I cannot help concluding that no great discovery was connected specifically with Buchheim's name. However, he introduced into pharmacology the methods that were essential for later achievements.

3. RESIGNATION AND POSTHUMOUS FAME

During the last years of his life, resignation grew within him to a considerable degree. It is true that pharmacological departments were erected at most German universities during the 1870s. But in an essay written in 1876, dealing with the task and the significance of pharmacology within German universities, Buchheim deplored many drawbacks. Medical students had only a minimal interest in pharmacological facts. Drugs were often used irrationally. There was no bedside pharmacology. The field was in low esteem by clinicians, for instance by the great surgeon Billroth. Some of Buchheim's remarks on the academic career should be underlined today:

> Not seldom the duties of a professor of pharmacology were conferred to a lecturer who had been omitted on other occasions, and who was, after long perseverance, designed to sail into the port of the faculty under that flag. Therefore, the position of the pharmacologist was mainly taken by a home-made man and endowed with the lowest salary. The duties of the pharmacologist were admittedly not too difficult. At first, he bought a textbook of chemistry and one of botany and told his audience what was written in those books about preparation and properties of chemicals or about geography, genealogy and botanical properties of drugs. Then the diseases were enumerated, against which single remedies had been tried at any time. . . . Excellent chemists or physiologists, needed for the development of pharmacology, will be offered much better opportunities in their own fields. Which goal can be reached by a man having devoted himself with all his abilities and efforts to pharmacological research? A professorship with a minimum salary and an empty auditorium! (8)

One hundred and fifty years now have passed since Buchheim's birth. Each honor bestowed on him during his lifetime would have appeared to his clearheaded, calm character, as inadequate; the modest number of posthumous honors would not have annoyed him. His home in Giessen, which had served also as his laboratory, survived the war nearly undamaged, while the city was destroyed. About 50 years ago, a memorial tablet was installed in it—by whom and on what occasion cannot be ascertained. His birthplace in Bautzen was marked by a similar tablet, on the occasion of the ninth annual meeting of the *Pharmakologische Gesellschaft der DDR*. I shall not forget the scene at the romantic "Schloβstrasse" in Bautzen where a small group of pharmacologists, tired from the meeting and feeling chilly in the December air, honored their grand man before his native house while the present inhabitants watched with the curtains pulled aside. The street in Giessen, where the Pharmakologisches Institut was located, bears his name and medical students risk being examined about the main features of Buchheim's work.

However, the most affectionate and instructive memory stems from his sole congenial follower, Oswald Schmiedeberg. Without the biography and bibliography from his pen (1), many details would have been forgotten. It was also Schmiedeberg who introduced Buchheim's thoughts and working methods, which were conceived in the more provincial university cities of Dorpat and Giessen, into pharmacological research all over the world. In this way, Buchheim became indeed one of the founders of pharmacology as a science.

Literature Cited

1. Schmiedeberg, O. 1912. *Arch. Exp. Pathol. Pharmakol.* 67:1–54
2. Rossbach, M. J. 1880. *Berlin Klin. Wochenschr.* 477–79
3. Hirsch, B. 1880. *Arch. Pharm.* 13:161–69
4. Oelssner, W. 1969. *Verh. Deut. Ges. Exp. Med.* 22:364–70
5. Buchheim, R. 1872. *Uber die "scharfen" Stoffe. Arch. Heilk.* 1
6. Buchheim, R. 1853–56. *Lehrbuch der Arzneimittellehre.* Leipzig: Aufl. Voss
7. Buchheim, R. 1872. *Virchow's Arch.* 56:1
8. Buchheim, R. 1876. *Arch. Exp. Pathol. Pharmakol.* 5:261
9. Holmstedt, B., Liljestrand, G. 1963. *Readings on Pharmacology,* 76–80. Oxford: Pergamon
10. Loewe, S. 1924. *Arch. Exp. Pathol. Pharmakol.* 104:1
11. Habermann, E. 1969. *Verh. Deut. Ges. Exp. Med.* 22:371–77

RELATIONSHIPS BETWEEN THE CHEMICAL STRUCTURE AND BIOLOGICAL ACTIVITY OF CONVULSANTS[1]

❖6577

J. R. Smythies
Department of Psychiatry, University of Alabama Medical Center, Birmingham, Alabama

Introduction

A large part of classical pharmacology consists of experimental determinations of the relationship between chemical structure and biological activity. This study of structure-activity relationships (SAR) has proceeded by the random syntheses of a large number of chemical relatives of known agonists or antagonists of a particular transmitter or hormone and testing their activity on the appropriate isolated tissues. Another approach is to synthesize some quite novel chemical structure and then test it on a wide variety of biological systems in the hope that this trial-and-error approach has on this occasion achieved a hit. The "lock-and-key" model of transmitter-receptor and hormone-receptor interactions introduced by Fischer presupposes that a close complementarity exists between the molecular structure of the active drug and the molecular structure of the receptor. However, as nothing was known about the molecular structure of receptors, the SAR data could not be interpreted except in the vaguest and most general terms. It is clear that, if only we knew the precise molecular structure of a particular receptor, it would be possible to explain just why certain drugs were agonists, and others antagonists, at this receptor and also to design new drugs on a rational basis (Martin-Smith 1). It is still true that we have no certain knowledge about the structure of any receptor, owing to the formidable technical difficulties involved in isolating the receptor protein and determining its amino acid sequence and tertiary conformation. However, it has proven possible to deduce a general theory of the molecular structure of protein-based receptors based on a search for complementarity between drugs known to act at these receptors and the range of possibilities of protein structures that could be

[1]A contribution of the Neuroscience Program, University of Alabama. This communication was aided in part by NIMH Grant No. MH 21437-01.

9

involved (Smythies 2). This general theory has been successful in explaining the bulk of the SAR data and a detailed specification has been made in the case of the following receptors: acetylcholine (neuromuscular junction, ganglionic, and muscarinic); GABA, glutamate, and glycine; α- and β-adrenergic and dopamine; and various prostaglandins. A partial specification has been made for the serotonin receptor. The same technique has been used to specify the molecular structure of the sodium channel with explanations for the mechanism of action of tetrodotoxin, saxitoxin, batrachotoxin, aconitine, veratridine, and the local anesthetics of the procaine class (Smythies 2). It has also been applied to presynaptic storage and release mechanisms for acetylcholine and adrenaline, carrying explanations for the mechanism of action of morphine, scorpion neurotoxin, and reserpine (Smythies 2, Smythies et al 3). The general hypothesis has given rise to a number of specific predictions which are currently under experimental test in a number of centers. This review will concentrate on an aspect of the general theory most amenable to such crucial tests, namely the GABA and glycine receptors.

Brief Statement of the General Theory

My hypothesis is based on a combination of the Kusnetsov & Ghokov (4), Gill (5), and Barlow (6) hypotheses. The former suggested that the most likely form of the receptor protein was parallel β chains cross-linked by their opposing amino acids by hydrogen or ionic bonding. Gill (5) suggested that the most likely mode of action of agonists like acetylcholine and the amino acid transmitters with their strongly charged groups was to disrupt an ionic link between two amino acids bearing opposite charges. Barlow (6) suggested that the ACh receptor in the neuromuscular junction contained a grid of anionic sites some 14 Å apart. Investigations using Corey–Pauling–Kaltun (CPK) molecular models suggested that a Kusnetsov–Ghokov–Barlow–Gill grid could be constructed if the receptor was based on four rungs of such a ladder composed of ionically bonded Arg and Glu moieties (Figure 1). The SAR data further indicated that such a flat, two-dimensional grid could be converted into a three-dimensional receptor cup by the addition of two further segments of protein chain (secondary chains) to the two (primary) chains of the grid. Each secondary chain forms in part a formal β-pleated sheet with the primary chain and in part runs over one outer rung of the ladder. The receptors for different transmitters may now be specified by the Arg-Glu vs Glu-Arg sequence of the primary chains, and by differences in the amino acid sequence of the secondary chains [there are three main types of secondary chain: F, E, and DN (see below)] and by the direction the protein chains run, as detailed in my book (2).

TESTING THE HYPOTHESIS   In the case of certain receptors such as the cholinergic neuromuscular junction or muscarinic receptor a wide variety of compounds are known that block them. CPK molecular models of any of these may be placed in a CPK model of the postulated receptor and derivatives can be designed that should either be inactive or more active depending on the strategic placement of additional lipophilic, hydrogen bonding, or ionic groups. Work along these lines is proceeding in a number of centers. However, in the case of other receptors much less is known in the SAR field and so a new strategy becomes possible as outlined in the next section.

Convulsant Drugs and the GABA and Glycine Receptors

Although there are a large number of convulsant poisons known, the mechanism of action of only a few of these has been worked out—e.g. strychnine, which blocks the glycine receptor, and picrotoxin and bicuculline, which block the GABA receptor. Of course not all convulsants act by blocking one or other of these receptors. Some, such as allylglycine,[1] block the enzyme glutamate decarboxylase and thus lower brain GABA levels. Others act by other mechanisms. However, a study of the molecular structure of a number of known convulsants has enabled me to predict with confidence which will have anti-GABA and which will have antiglycine properties.

The specification of the GABA receptor was based on the molecular structure of GABA, picrotoxin (Figure 5b), and bicuculline (Figure 5a) and that of the glycine receptor on glycine and strychnine. The primary structure of the GABA receptor is Glu-Arg; Arg-Glu; Glu-Arg; Glu-Arg; and the secondary chains have the sequence (*right*) -x-*His-x-Val* (or Ile)-Pro-Gly-x-Gly- (an E chain) and (*left*) -x-Gly-x-Gly-Pro-*x-Ile-x-Asp-x* (an F chain) with the italic portion forming the β-pleated sheet structure with the underlying primary chain in each case (Figure 2). The glycine receptor has only 3 rungs instead of 4: primary structure Arg-Glu; Glu-Arg; Glu-Arg and secondary chains (both DN) have the sequences -Gly-x-Gly-Pro-x-*Asp*-x and -Gly-x-Gly-Pro-x-*His*-x.

The GABA Receptor

GABA binds in its model receptor with its carboxyl group caught between three protons (2 from Arg of rung 3 and 1 from His), its amino group binds to the Glu of rung 2 (repelling Arg of rung 2), and its α-methylene group binds lipophilically to the adjacent Ile.

The molecule of bicuculline forms a lid over the receptor cup binding as diagrammed in Figure 3 and picrotoxin binds as suggested in Figure 4. Its square upper section slots into the rectangular "inside" of the F secondary chain with extensive lipophilic interactions and a hydrogen bond from OH to His. The two carboxyl oxygens now jut down with the correct locations and bond angles to receive hydrogen bonds from the two spare protons on the two Args (of rungs 2 and 3) in the floor of the receptor.

Based on this molecular structure it has been possible to predict that the following convulsant poisons act by competitive inhibition (blockade) of the GABA receptor. In each case an outline of the molecular complementarity between drug and receptor is given. A perusal of Figures 5–9 will emphasize the remarkable range of chemical structures involved. Nevertheless the molecular models indicate that they are all complementary to the simple protein structure specified.

[1] The action of allylglycine in inhibiting GAD (32) has been challenged by Roper (33).

1. Cicutoxin (Figure 5e). This remarkable molecule may be considered as a dense π cloud bent in the middle through some 40° with a lipophilic "tail" at each end, to each of which is attached an hydroxyl group. Figure 6 indicates how this is related to the model receptor. The π cloud contributed to by the ethylene and acetylene π electrons crosses the 2 spare protons of both arginines in the floor of the receptor (thus forming 4 hydrogen bonds: for this the 40° bend is required). One hydroxyl binds to His (N:) and the other to Asp (O:) and both propylene chains make extensive lipophilic contacts. The related molecules of oenanthotoxin (Figure 5f) and cunaniol make similar contacts.

2. Tetramethylenedisulphotetramine (Figure 7a). This small compact molecule is totally different in form from cicutoxin yet it is also most closely related to the model receptor. It sits in the middle (Figure 8) caught between His, Asp, Val, Ile, and the two Args with 3 hydrogen bonds, 1 ionic bond, and 3 lipophilic contacts with all these as shown in the figure.

3. Kopsine (Figure 7b) is of particular interest, as the line diagram suggests it has a resemblance to strychnine and therefore might be expected to block glycine receptors. However, the molecular models indicate it is too large to fit the smaller glycine receptor and is adapted to fit the larger GABA receptor instead. The ring carbonyl O receives a hydrogen bond from the Arg NH in the floor of the receptor, the protonated amino group binds to Asp, and the other carbonyl O receives a hydrogen bond from His. The hydroxyl forms an internal hydrogen bond to the methoxy O so as to orient the adjacent carbonyl O correctly. There are also extensive lipophilic contacts. The molecule thus combines the attributes of both picrotoxin and bicuculline.

4. Figure 7c shows the formula of the synthetic convulsant dicetol and also predicts which out of the 16 possible stereoisomers will be most active. Each carbonyl O binds to Arg NHs in the floor of the receptor, one hydroxyl binds to His and one to Asp, and there are extensive lipophilic contacts to Ile and Val on each side.

5. Two bicuculline-like structures are the synthetic compounds 3-methyl-7-methoxy-8-(dimethylaminomethyl)-flavone (Figure 7d) and the equivalent chromone (Figure 7e).

6. Yet another way of achieving the same effect is illustrated by dregamine (Figure 7f) based on an indole ring.

7. The skin of European fire and Alpine salamanders is chemically most interesting as it contains two convulsant poisons: one, samandarine (Figure 9a), is complementary to the GABA model receptor and the other, cycloneosamandione (Figure 9b), is complementary to the glycine receptor.

8. The latest convulsant alkaloid shown to be a GABA antagonist (Curtis 7) is Shikimin (Figure 5d). The molecular model shows it to be a homograph of picrotoxin but with more extensive binding to elements in the receptor. Each carbonyl O receives a hydrogen bond from an Arg NH underneath. The two hydroxyls on the five-carbon ring can now both bind electrostatically to the same O of Asp, and the hydroxyl on the six-carbon ring forms an electrostatic link to the O: of Glu of rung 2 and the fourth hydroxyl binds to His N:. The hydrocarbon ring system plus

one attached methyl group (that on the six-carbon ring) form lipophilic bonds with Val and Ile (Figure 4b).

9. The convulsant compound benzyl penicillin (Figure 5g) cannot be made by the CPK models available, owing to its four-carbon ring. However, an approximation to this made out of plasticine indicates that it has the essential square form plus two carbonyl pseudopods to be a picrotoxin-like GABA antagonist.

10. A GABA antagonist based on the steroid ring may be represented by 3β-acetoxy-5α-hydroxy-6β-morpholino-5α-pregnan-20-one (Figure 9c).

The Glycine Receptor

Glycine (Figure 12a) binds to its model receptor with its amino group caught between Asp and Glu, its carboxyl group between His and Arg, and there is a lipophilic contact between its single methylene group and an adjacent Gly moiety in the receptor protein in addition (Figure 10). The squat squarish molecule of strychnine fills the receptor cup almost completely with an ionic bond from its protonated amino N to Asp and a hydrogen bond from His to its carbonyl O, as indicated in Figure 11a. The molecules of lordanosine (Figure 12b), thebaine (Figure 12c), and dendrobine (Figure 12d), which are also known to act by blocking the glycine receptor, are all complementary to this model receptor in different ways (see Figure 11b,c).

Antiglycine Compounds

The model predicts that the following compounds owe their convulsant properties to blockade of the glycine receptor.

1. Akuammine (Figure 13a). This is not surprising since it is a close chemical relative of strychnine; however, superficially it also resembles kopsine (Figure 7b), which as we have seen fits my GABA receptor and not the glycine receptor model.

2. Securenine (Figure 13b). This resembles picrotoxin adapted to fit the glycine receptor with a single pseudopod (the carbonyl O), making contact with the Arg NH in the floor of the receptor cup and the NH group binding to Asp.

3. Dioscorine (Figure 13c). It achieves a similar result using a different chemical structure.

4. Calycanthine (Figure 13d). This fits the receptor cup quite differently. The molecule has a right-angled bracket shape (as does thebaine). One benzene ring intercalates between the rungs of the primary "ladder" structure and the other forms a "lid." One amino N binds to Asp ionically and the other forms a hydrogen bond to His.

5. 5,7-Diphenyl-1,3-diazadamantan-6-ol (Figure 13e). In the case of this compact molecule both benzene rings intercalate into the inter-rung space: one between rungs 1 and 2 and the other between rungs 2 and 3. One amino group binds to Asp and the hydroxyl to His.

New Compounds

A perusal of recent copies of *Chemical Abstracts* reveals a wealth of activity in the chemical identification of new alkaloids. In fact this process has outstripped the pharmacological estimate of what biological action, if any, these new compounds might have. A comparison of molecular models of a wide range of these new compounds suggests that a small number may have convulsant properties, to wit:

PREDICTED ANTI-GABA COMPOUNDS

1. Secodaphniphylline (Figure 14a). This achieves a remarkably close fit to the entire cavity of the model receptor cup with bonds to Asp (NH) and His (carbonyl O) as well.

2. Taspine (Figure 14b) and Thaliglucinone (Figure 14c). These resemble the convulsant chromone listed above (Figure 7e).

PREDICTED ANTI-GLYCINE COMPOUNDS

1. 4-Hydroxydendroxine (Figure 14c).

2. Elegantine (Figure 14d). This fills the glycine receptor cup much as secodaphniphylline fills the GABA receptor cup.

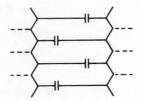

Figure 1 An Arg-Glu grid. The short apposed amino acid is Glu and the long one is Arg.

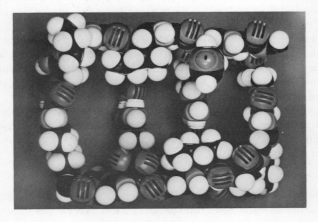

Figure 2 A CPK model of the postulated GABA receptor.

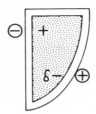

Figure 3 A diagram of how the trapezoid-shaped molecule of bicuculline fills the trapezoid-shaped GABA receptor cup with two complementary electrostatic bonds to His (+) and Asp (−) in the receptor protein.

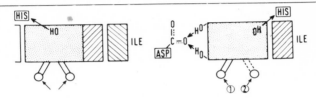

Figure 4 Diagram of suggested mode of binding of *a.* picrotoxin and *b.* shikimin in the GABA receptor. The arrows indicate correct hydrogen bonds from Arg NHs to Carbonyl Os.

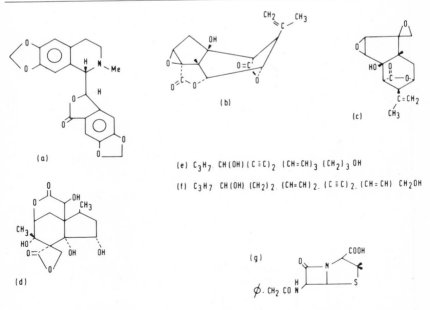

(e) $C_3H_7 \cdot CH(OH)(C\equiv C)_2 (CH=CH)_3 (CH_2)_3 OH$

(f) $C_3H_7 \cdot CH(OH)(CH_2)_2 (CH=CH)_2 (C\equiv C)_2 (CH=CH) CH_2OH$

Figure 5 *a.* Bicuculline; *b.* picrotoxin; *c.* coryamertin; *d.* shikimin; *e.* cicutoxin; *f.* oenanthotoxin; *g.* benzyl penicillin.

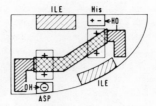

Figure 6 Diagram of interaction between cicutoxin and the model GABA receptor.

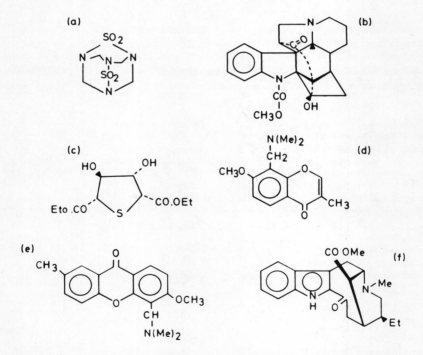

Figure 7 *a.* Tetramethylenedisulphotetramine; *b.* kopsine; *c.* dicetol; *d.* 3-methyl-7-methoxy-8 (dimethylaminomethyl)-flavone; *e.* the equivalent chromone; *f.* dregamine.

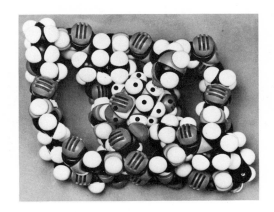

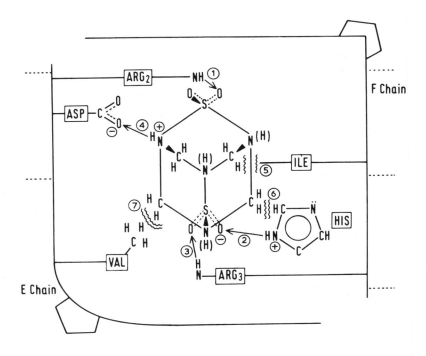

Figure 8 a. CPK model (*top*) and *b.* diagram of tetramethylenedisulfotetramine bound in the model receptor (*bottom*).

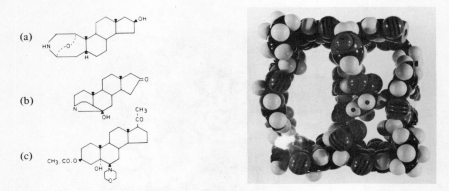

Figure 9 (*left*) *a.* samandarine; *b.* cycloneosamandione; *c.* 3β-acetoxy-5α-hydroxy-6β-morpholino-5α-pregnan-20-one.

Figure 10 (*right*) CPK model of glycine bound in its model receptor.

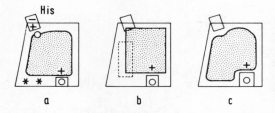

Figure 11 Diagram of how various convulsants fill the glycine receptor. *a.* strychnine: the two stars indicate where the two methoxy groups of brucine fit; *b.* lordanosine; *c.* dendrobine: the circle in the square represents Asp.

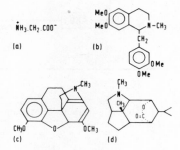

Figure 12 *a.* Glycine; *b.* lordanosine; *c.* thebaine; *d.* dendrobine.

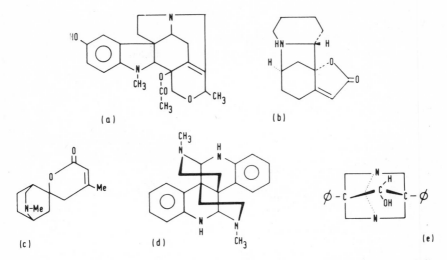

Figure 13 a. Akuammine; *b.* securenine; *c.* dioscorine; *d.* calycanthine; *e.* 5,7-di-phenyl-1,3-diazadamantan-6-ol.

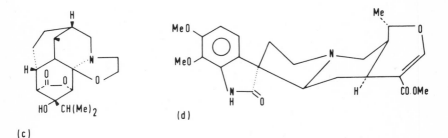

Figure 14 a. Secodaphniphylline; *b.* taspine; *c.* 4-hydroxydendroxine; *d.* elegantine.

ACKNOWLEDGMENTS

I am grateful to Professor David Curtis for the benefit of many helpful discussions and to Professor Sir John Eccles, FRS, for the interest he has kindly shown in these ideas.

APPENDIX   Further information about the compounds cited.

1. Cicutoxin. Source: *Cicuta virosa* L. *Umbelliferae* (Water Hemlock) *Ref.* (8)
2. Oenanthotoxin.   Source: *Oenanthe crocata Umbelliferae* (Hemlock Water Dropwort) (W. Europe) *Ref.* (9)
3. Cunaniol. Source: *Clibadium Sylvestre* (Aubl.) *Baill.* (Brazil) *Ref.* (10)
4. Tetramethylenedisulphotetramine. Source: Synthetic. *Ref.* (11, 12)
5. Kopsine. Source: *Kopsia fructicosa* A.D. *Apocynaceae* (Java) *Ref.* (13, 14)
6. 2,5 - dicarbethoxy - 3,4 - dihydroxy - thiophane (dicetol). Source: Synthetic. *Ref.* (15, 16)
7. 3-methyl-7-methoxy-8-(dimethylaminomethyl)-flavone (and equivalent chromone). Source: Synthetic.   *Ref.* (17, 18)
8. 3β-acetoxy-5α-hydroxy-6β-morpholino -5α-pregnan-20-one. Source: Synthetic. *Ref.* (19)
9. Samandarine and cycloneosamandione. Source: Skin of European Fire and Alpine Salamander. *Ref.* (20)
10. Dregamine. Source: *Voacanga dregei Apocynaceae* and *Tabernae montana*

Sp. *Apocynaceae* (Madagascar). *Ref.* (21)
11. Securenine. Source: *Securinega suffructicasa* Rehder, *Euphorbiaceae* (Ussuri region, USSR) *Ref.* (22)
12. Akuammine. Source: *Picralima klaineana,* also *Vinca major* (L) *Ref.* (23)
13. Calycanthine.   Source: *Calycanthus floridus* L. *Calycanthaceae* (S.E. United States) *Ref.* (24)
14. Dioscorine. Source: *Dioscorea hispida* Deunst. *Ref.* (25)
15. 5,7-diphenyl-1,3-diazadamantan-6-ol. Source: Synthetic. *Ref.* (26)
16. Secodaphniphylline. Source: *Daphniphyllum macropodum Ref.* (27)
17. Taspine. Source: *Leontice eversmanii.* Bunge, *Berberidaceae Ref.* (28)
18. Thaliglucinone.   Source: *Thalictrum rugosum Ref.* (29)
19. 4-hydroxydendroxine. Source: *Dendrobium nobile* (*Orchidaceae*) *Ref.* (30)
20. Elegantine. Source: *Vinca elegantissima* Hort. N. O. *Apocynaceae* (rare herb growing in Nilgiri Hills Assam). *Ref.* (31)

Literature Cited

1. Martin-Smith, M. 1971. *Drug Design,* ed. E. J. Ariëns, 2:454–530. New York: Academic. 645 pp.
2. Smythies, J. R. 1973. *The Molecular Structure of Receptor Mechanisms,* In preparation and a communication to the VIth Winter Conference for Brain Research, Vail, Colorado, January 1973
3. Smythies, J. R., Antun, F., Yank, G. R., Yorke, C. 1971. *Nature* 231:185–88
4. Kusnetsov, S. G., Ghokov, S. N. 1962. *"Synthetic Atropine-like Substances."* Leningrad: State Publicity House of Medical Literature. English Transl.: U. S. Dept. Comm.J.P.R.S. 19757
5. Gill, E. W. 1965. Drug receptor interactions In *Progress in Medicinal Chemistry,* ed. G. P. Ellis, G. B. West, 4:39–85. London: Butterworth
6. Barlow, R. B. 1964. *Introduction to Chemical Pharmacology.* London: Butterworth. 451 pp.
7. Curtis, D. 1972. Personal communication
8. Hill, B. E., Lythgoe, B., Mirvish, S., Trippett, S. 1955. *J. Chem. Soc.* (II), 1770–75
9. Grundy, H. F., Howarth, F. 1956. *Brit. J. Pharmacol.* 11:225–30
10. Quillam, J. P., Stables, P. R. 1969. *Pharm. Res. Commun.* 1:7–14
11. Haskell, A. R., Voss, E. 1957. *J. Am. Pharm. Assoc. Sci. Ed.* 45:239–42
12. Hagen, J. 1950. *Deutsch. Med. Wochschr.* 75:183–84
13. Bhattacharya, A., Chatterjee, A., Bose, P. K. 1949. *J. Am. Chem. Soc.,* 71:3370–72

14. Govindachari, T. R. et al 1962. *Helv. Chem. Acta.* 45:1146–52; 1963. 46:572–77
15. Dadkar, N. K., Damle, S. K., Gaitonde, B. B. 1968. *Jap. J. Pharmacol.* 18:436–44
16. Sahasrabudhe, M. B. et al 1959. *Nature* 184:201–2
17. Da Re, P., Mancini, V., Toth, E., Cima, L. 1968. *Arzneim. Forsch.* 18:718–20
18. Da Re, P. et al 1959. *Nature* 184:362–63
19. Hewett, C. L., Savage, D. S., Lewis, J. J., Sugrue, M. F. 1964. *J. Pharm. Pharmacol.* 16:765–67
20. Alauddin, M., Martin-Smith, M. 1962. *J. Pharm. Pharmacol.,* 14:469–95
21. Albert, O., Dupont, M., Quirin, M. 1970. *Ann. Pharm. Fr.* 28:697–706
22. Saito, S. et al 1966. *Chem. Pharm. Bull.* 14:313–14
23. Joule, J. A., Smith, G. F. 1962. *J. Chem. Soc.* (I), 312–23
24. Hendrickson, J. H., Göschke, R., Rees, R. 1964. *Tetrahedron* 20:565–79
25. Bevan, C. W. L., Hirst, J. 1958. *Chem. Ind.* 36:103
26. Longo, V. G., Silvestrini, B., Bovet, D. 1959. *J. Pharm. Exp. Ther.* 126:41–49
27. Toda, M., Hirata, Y., Yananura, S. 1972. *Tetrahedron* 28:1477–84
28. Shamma, M., Moniot, J. L., 1971. *J. Chem. Soc. D* 1065–66
29. Mollov, N. M. , Thuan, L. N., Panov. P. P. 1972. *Chem. Abst.* 76:85970h
30. Okamoto, T. 1972. *Chem. Pharm. Bull.* 20:418–21
31. Bhattacharyya, J., Pakrashi, S. C. 1972. *Tetrahedron Lett.* (2):159–62
32. Alberici, M., Rodriguez de Lores Arna, De Robertis, E. 1969. *Biochem. Pharmacol.* 18:137–44
33. Roper, S. 1970. *Nature* 226:373–74

CYCLIC AMP AND CYCLIC GMP[1]

❖6578

Theodore Posternak

Institute of Biological Chemistry, University of Geneva, Geneva, Switzerland

A chapter on "Cyclic AMP and Drug Action" has already been published in *Annual Review of Pharmacology* (1). In spite of its restrictive title, this paper covered most of the knowledge about the biochemical and biological effects of cAMP that was available in 1969. During the last four years, investigations of cAMP and cGMP have continued at an accelerated rate. Due to the restriction in the number of pages, the present review had to be selective and not exhaustive. We wanted to avoid a mere compilation of bibliographic references. The bibliography is therefore incomplete and only certain areas, which seemed to the author of special interest, have been described.

EFFECT OF cAMP ON SOME ENZYMES

Muscle phosphorylase has been most extensively studied. It exists in a form *b* (mol wt 185,000) that requires AMP for an allosteric activation and in a form *a* (mol wt 370,000) that is active without AMP. Activation is also effected by phosphorylation of some serine residues in phosphorylase b by a phosphorylase kinase which converts it to the a form (2). The phosphorylase kinase itself exists in a nonphosphorylated, inactive form, which is converted to a phosphorylated active form by the action of a cAMP-dependent protein kinase which might be called phosphorylase kinase kinase (3). This enzyme can also use as substrates other proteins like casein and protamine. The role of cAMP has been recently elucidated (4–7). cAMP-dependent protein kinases are composed of a catalytic subunit C and of a regulatory subunit

---

[1] Abbreviations: cAMP (adenosine 3',5'-monophosphate); db-cAMP (N⁶,2'-O-dibutyryl adenosine 3',5'-monophosphate); N⁶-mb-cAMP (N⁶-monobutyryl adenosine 3',5'-monophosphate); 2'-O-mb-cAMP (2'-O-monobutyryl adenosine 3',5'-monophosphate); cGMP (guanosine 3',5'-monophosphate); db-cGMP (N²,2'-O-dibutyryl guanosine 3',5'-monophosphate); RO-201724 [4-(3-butoxy-4-methoxybenzyl)-2-imidazolidone]; SC-2964 (1-methyl-3-isobutyl-xanthine); SO-20009 [1-ethyl-4-(isopropylidenehydrazine-1H-pyrazolo-3,4)-pyridine-5-carboxylic acid ethyl ester]; GH (growth hormone); TSH (thyroid stimulating hormone); mRNA (messenger ribonucleic acid); tRNA (transfer ribonucleic acid); UDPG (uridine diphosphoglucose).

23

R. cAMP binds to R; this promotes the dissociation of the enzyme according to the equation

$$cAMP \; + \; C\text{–}R \; \rightleftharpoons \; R\text{–}cAMP \; + \; C$$

$$\text{inactive} \qquad\qquad\qquad \text{active}$$
$$\text{complex} \qquad\qquad\qquad\quad \text{form}$$

In addition, a protein inhibitor I of these enzymes has been discovered in a wide range of mammalian tissues (8, 9). It lowers the initial velocities; the interaction of I is noncompetitive with ATP and casein. The factor I does not catalyze the dephosphorylation of the phosphoprotein produced and its action is independent of the nature of some of the protein substrates. Among several possible modes of action, the following one could be demonstrated (10):

$$R\text{–}C \; + \; cAMP \; \rightleftharpoons \; C \; + \; R\text{–}cAMP$$
$$C \; + \; I \qquad \rightleftharpoons \; C\text{–}I$$
$$\qquad\qquad\qquad\quad \text{inactive}$$
$$\qquad\qquad\qquad\quad \text{form}$$

The catalytic unit C must therefore be free before the reaction with I that leads to its inactivation. In other tissues (liver, adrenal cortical tissue, and brain), the mechanism of activation of phosphorylase may be different.

Glycogen synthetase (UDPG-glycogen transglucosidase) exists in the skeletal muscle in two forms: I and D. The former is independent of glucose-6-P for activity, while the latter is dependent on this cofactor (11). The conversion of I to D involves a phosphorylation by a cAMP-dependent synthetase kinase (12–14). On the other hand, the conversion of D to I (activation) is a dephosphorylation catalyzed by a relatively specific phosphatase (12, 15). More recently, phosphorylase kinase kinase and synthetase kinase were shown to be the same enzyme (16, 17). cAMP activates the breakdown of glycogen by stimulating phosphorylase, but inhibits the synthesis of the polysaccharide by inactivating glycogen synthetase.

Similar cAMP-dependent protein kinases were found in many other tissues. In certain cases, cAMP, 5'-AMP, and 5'-ADP activate phosphofructokinases; how-ever, the existence of a cAMP-dependent kinase that would convert the enzyme to an active form by phosphorylation is uncertain. An allosteric effect has not been ruled out; it has been suggested that cAMP, AMP, and ADP compete with ATP, which is inhibitory, for an allosteric site of phosphofructokinase (18). Triglyceride lipase is stimulated by cAMP, which actually activates a kinase that phosphorylates the lipase and converts it to a so-called active hormone-sensitive lipase. This explains the lipolytic effect of epinephrine and its antagonism by insulin and prostaglandins which decrease cAMP levels in fat pads (19).

One general theory proposed regarding the mechanism of action of cAMP in-volves modifications of Ca^{2+} levels and an increase in the permeability of cell membranes to Ca^{2+} (20). Another theory involves activation of protein kinases by cAMP (21). Although the second representation rests, in certain cases, on a firm experimental basis, it seems premature to reduce to this common denominator the multitude of effects of cAMP.

CYCLIC GMP

cGMP is the only cyclic nucleotide besides cAMP that is known with certitude to occur in nature. This compound was discovered in urine as radioactive phosphoorganic compound after injection of inorganic ^{32}P into rats (22). Assay methods have been worked out (23–26) that allow a more detailed study of cGMP, which has been detected in all mammalian tissues investigated so far, as well as in several lower phyla. In most tissues the concentrations of cGMP are generally at least tenfold lower than those of cAMP. For instance, in various rat tissues, the amounts of cGMP are between 10^{-8} and 10^{-7} mol/kg of wet tissue (24–26). Hormones that increase cAMP levels do not elevate cGMP levels; theophylline does, however, increase these levels in some tissues. In plasma, and especially in urine, large amounts of cGMP and cAMP are excreted; in rat urine the daily excretion is several times higher than the amounts of cyclic nucleotides contained in a given time in the whole body. The excretions of cAMP and cGMP are generally controlled independently by hormonal effects. This fact suggests the existence of a specific enzyme system, guanyl cyclase, which catalyzes the synthesis of cGMP and uses GTP as substrate. In contrast to adenyl cyclase, it is soluble in most tissues of the rat and has been partially purified from lung and liver (27, 28); it appears to be mostly particulate in the rat small intestine (29). The richest source has been found in the sperm of the sea urchin, where the levels are up to 1000 times higher than in rat tissues; there the enzyme is entirely particulate (30). Detergents like 1% Triton solubilized or dispersed the particulate form and enhanced its apparent activity (29, 30). The question of the formation of pyrophosphate in addition to cGMP from GTP, and the question of the reversibility of the reaction, are still open. Guanyl cyclase is almost absolutely dependent on Mn^{2+}, which cannot be replaced by Mg^{2+} or by Ca^{2+}. However, in the presence of low amounts of Mn^{2+}, Ca^{2+} produces a strong stimulation. In contrast to adenyl cyclase, guanyl cyclase is not activated by fluoride in broken cell preparations, and the activity in cell free systems from liver and heart is unaffected by the hormones so far tested: glucagon (27), insulin (27), epinephrine (27), ACTH (31), thyroxine, and cortisol.

In broken cell preparations, cGMP is generally inactive or much less active than cAMP (32). Concerning the activation of kinases, cGMP in high amounts produces in some cases the same maximum stimulation as cAMP. However, half maximal activation of the enzymes required concentration of cGMP about 100 times higher with respect to rat liver glycogen synthetase kinase (33) or to the synthetase activity of a protein kinase from rabbit skeletal muscle (17). cGMP has been found virtually without effect on a cAMP-dependent protein kinase from adipose tissue (34) or from heart and skeletal muscle (35). An interesting exception was seen with a preparation of protein kinase from lobster muscle, where cGMP was as effective as cAMP (36). Subsequently, two fractions of protein kinase activity could be separated from lobster muscle, which had quite different affinities for cGMP and cAMP. The approximate K_m values of one fraction were 0.08 μM and 4 μM respectively, while the K_m values of the other fraction were 1.2 μM and 0.02 μM respectively (37).[2] cGMP does not seem to inhibit the formation of cAMP or to alter the effect of cAMP in liver phosphorylase activation.

In intact cell systems, on the other hand, the two cyclic nucleotides produced similar effects when applied in high concentration, that is, under unphysiological conditions, for instance in fat cells (38). In the perfused rat liver, cGMP was ⅓–½ as potent as cAMP in stimulating net glycogenolysis, glucose neogenesis, and release of K^+ (39). Insulin antagonized the effect of exogenous cAMP, but not of exogenous cGMP, on glucose release. The effectiveness of cGMP was explained by its accumulation in liver to a much greater extent than cAMP. In addition, high concentrations of exogenous cGMP can produce an elevation of intracellular cAMP in some tissues, perhaps by inhibiting phosphodiesterase. These results have been partially contested in a recent paper (40). In isolated fat cells incubated in Krebs-Ringer phosphate buffer with Ca^{2+} and Mg^{2+} without K^+, cGMP produced lipolysis but to a much lower degree than cAMP (41). There are contradictory statements concerning the activity of cGMP in stimulating steroidogenesis in intact adrenal cells in vitro (31, 42). The physiological significance in vivo of cGMP seemed therefore doubtful, but more recently some interesting observations were reported. The cGMP levels in the isolated perfused rat heart were elevated by acetylcholine (43). In addition, treatment of mice with oxotremorine increased cGMP in cerebral cortex and in cerebellum (44); later, it has been stated that in mouse cerebellum slices cGMP is not directly involved in cholinergic neurotransmission mechanism (45). These changes both in heart and brain were, however, prevented by the anticholinergic agent atropine. In the presence of high concentration of KCl (125 mM) and of SC-2964, acetylcholine increases the levels of cGMP two- to threefold in some tissues in the presence, but not in the absence, of 1.8 mM Ca^{2+} (46). Db-cGMP as well as carbachol, an acetylcholine analog, decreased the rate of rhythmic beating of culture rat heart cells, while epinephrine and db-cAMP accelerate this rate (47). The conclusion might therefore be drawn that cGMP is involved in some way in cholinergic transmission.

cAMP AND cGMP PHOSPHODIESTERASES

These enzymes, which by hydrolysis of the 3'-O-phosphate bond convert the cyclic nucleotides to 5'-AMP and 5'-GMP respectively, appear as regulatory factors that control the levels of cAMP and cGMP. By Agarose and Sephadex gel filtration, the presence of three fractions could be shown in the brain cortex, the kidney, and the adipose tissues of rats (48, 49). One of these fractions (I) is particulate, the other two (II and III) are soluble and have mol wt of 400,000 and 200,000 respectively, according to gel filtration. The higher mol wt fraction II has for cAMP an apparent K_m of about $1.10^{-4} M$ and for cGMP a K_m of about $1.10^{-5} M$. The hydrolysis of both substrates appears to take place competitively. The lower mol wt fraction III does

[2]cAMP and cGMP-dependent protein kinases have similar components and are inhibited and activated respectively by a protein which is present in lobster tail muscle and has been called "modulator." This factor is similar to the protein inhibitor I (see above) and alters in some cases the substrate specificity of the protein kinases.

not catalyze the hydrolysis of cGMP under normal assay conditions and has for cAMP a K_m of $5.10^{-6}M$ or lower; cGMP is a noncompetitive inhibitor. The particulate fraction I has kinetic properties similar to those of the lower mol wt fraction and is perhaps a membrane bound form of the latter. It was found that the ratio of the high K_m to the low K_m cAMP phosphodiesterases was markedly different in the various areas of the rat brain (50). In rat heart, only fractions similar to II and III could be detected (48). Several authors found in bovine heart two fractions, but their K_m values varied with the methods of separation: e.g. after acrylamide gel electrophoresis and ultracentrifugation, the main fraction (mol wt 125,000 as estimated by analytic ultracentrifugation) had apparent K_m values of 5.10^{-5} and $2.10^{-4}M$ for cGMP and cAMP respectively (51). In rat liver (52) three fractions were separated by DEAE chromatography: two soluble fractions of mol wt 400,000, as determined by gel filtration, and a particulate fraction. One of the soluble fractions hydrolyses cGMP (K_m from 3.10 to $6.10^{-6}M$), and this fraction seems to be a specific cGMP phosphodiesterase whose activity is unaffected by cAMP. The second soluble fraction hydrolyses both cAMP and cGMP (K_m 4.10 and $2.10^{-5}M$ respectively); each substrate acts as a competitive inhibitor of the hydrolysis of the other substrate. cGMP at 1 μM concentration is, however, an activator of cAMP hydrolysis. The particulate fraction has a high affinity for cAMP (K_m $6.10^{-6}M$) and is a cAMP phosphodiesterase, which is inhibited by cGMP in a hyperbolic fashion. More recently, the soluble supernatant fraction of rat cerebellar homogenate was subjected to electrophoresis on a polyacrylamide gel column and six peaks of cAMP phosphodiesterase activity were found (53). The substrate specificities of these peaks are, however, still unknown; the low and high mol wt fractions mentioned above are thus probably mixtures of isoenzymes.

In earlier studies, it was found that the brain cAMP enzyme required Mg^{2+}; Mn^{2+} could completely replace Mg^{2+} while Co^{2+} and Ni^{2+} could only partially replace Mg^{2+}. A soluble fraction of the rat brain enzyme was stimulated by $10^{-6}M$ Ca^{2+} in the presence of $3.10^{-3}M$ Mg^{2+} (54). It has been reported that the activity of cAMP phosphodiesterase from brain was completely dependent on the addition of another brain protein (55).[3] However, this activator stimulated only two of the six peaks obtained by polyacrylamide electrophoresis (53); Ca^{2+} increases the activity of only one of these two peaks.

In summary, phosphodiesterases appear as complex mixtures of different forms hydrolizing cAMP and/or cGMP. Their activity may be regulated by interaction between cAMP and cGMP, and by protein interaction.

Imidazole was reported to stimulate a phosphodiesterase preparation from brain but only at high concentration; this stimulation is therefore not of physiological significance. Methylxanthines (theophylline, caffein) are the classical inhibitors of cAMP phosphodiesterases. Many authors have emphasized the fact that methylxanthines may display numerous pharmacological effects that do not directly involve

---

[3]Similar protein activators have been found in several mammalian tissues. The bovine heart activator enhances the V_{max} of the cAMP-dependent bovine heart phosphodiesterase and decreases the K_m for cAMP.

phosphodiesterase inhibition. SC-2964 is a more potent xanthine derivative. Several other inhibitors have been discovered: puromycin, triiodothyronine, ATP, diazoxide, chlorpropamide, tolbutamide, and papaverine. Imidazole derivatives may be strong inhibitors; among them, RO-201724 is the most potent compound and has been reported to inhibit selectively the hydrolysis of cAMP as compared to cGMP. SO-20009 is a pyridine derivative. Certain analogs of cAMP are also potent inhibitors.[4] The differences of the chemical structure of all these phosphodiesterase inhibitors is quite remarkable.

SOME ANALOGS OF cAMP

cAMP has in general a weak effect in intact cells, due to the impermeability of cell membranes to phosphorylated compounds and to the destruction by phosphodiesterases. The preparation of synthetic analogs of cAMP started with the idea of obtaining substances endowed with either a better penetration through cell membranes or with a better resistance to the action of phosphodiesterases. The first synthetic analog contained in acyl group, most frequently a butyryl group, in N^6 and/or 2'-O (56, 57). These lipophilic fatty acid residues were introduced in the hope that they might facilitate passage across cell membranes; in a similar way, db-cGMP was prepared. The 2'-OH group has been blocked (56–58), not only by acylation, but also, for instance, by methylation; it is replaced by hydrogen in 2'-deoxy-cAMP. The ribose moiety in cAMP has been replaced by D-arabinose or D-xylose. The phosphodiester group has been modified by replacement of one of the two oxidic O atoms by S (cyclic phosphorothiotate) or by a CH_2 group. 5'-amido analogs were obtained by replacing 5'-O with NH or NCH_3 (59). Substituted amides (cyclic phosphoramidates) (60) and the methyl ester of cAMP were also prepared (56). Another type of analog contains the ribose moiety attached to the 3-position instead of the 9-position of adenine (cyclic iso-AMP) (61). A series of analogs were prepared that involved modifications of the adenine skeleton: cAMP N^1-oxide (56, 57); C–2, C–6 (62–64), and C–8 (65, 66) substituted compounds. The C–6 NH_2 group and the C–8 hydrogen have thus been replaced by halogens or by NHR, NR_1R_2, OH, OR, SH, and SR groups. Finally, in tubercidine-3',5'-phosphate N–7 is replaced by a CH group (67).

The effects of some of these analogs have been investigated on enzyme preparations. The unblocked 2'-OH in the ribo-configuration was found to be necessary for the activation of cAMP dependent protein kinases (58). 2'-O-substituted analogs were attacked somewhat more slowly than cAMP by several phosphodiesterases, and they inhibit moderately the action of these enzymes on cAMP, this effect being dependent on the nature of the substituent and on the origin of the enzymes. Among the 8-substituted analogs, the 8-thio, the 8-hydroxy, and the 8-amino derivatives were more active in decreasing order than cAMP towards bovine, brain, or liver protein kinases (58, 68). They were relatively resistant to rabbit kidney and rat brain phosphodiesterases and were good inhibitors of these enzymes, the 8-thio-derivative being especially active (58, 67). Db-8-thio-cAMP and 8-thio-cAMP at fivefold

---

[4]Other phosphodiesterase inhibitors occur in nature, e.g. a protein factor in amoebae and cytokinesins in higher plants.

higher concentration than cAMP produced a 80% and 30% inhibition respectively of the action of rat brain phosphodiesterase; on the other hand, at much lower concentration, both derivatives produced a 30% activation (69). The 6-substituted analogs were more readily cleaved than the 8-substituted ones by pig and rat brain phosphodiesterase, with the exception of N^6-mb-cAMP, which is quite resistant. Some 6-alkylthio-derivatives were more effective than cAMP as activators of cAMP-dependent bovine brain protein kinases. The 6-thio-derivative was 70% more active than cGMP towards the cGMP-dependent lobster kinase (64). Tubercidine-3',5'-phosphate was as effective as cAMP as an activator of dog heart and liver phosphorylase kinase kinase (67).

The study of the effects on intact cells gave the following results. While cAMP was practically inactive, db-cAMP, N^6-mb-cAMP, and 2'-O-mb-cAMP activated the phosphorylase in rat (68) and dog (70) liver slices and produced hyperglycemia in the intact dog (56); cAMP, db-cAMP, and several 8-substituted derivatives were examined for their ability to activate steroidogenesis in the isolated rat adrenal cells and lipolysis in the rat epididymal lipocytes (71). The maximal activation of most of these compounds was similar, but the concentrations required to produce half maximal activities were different; according to this criterion, the 8-methylthio, the 8-bromo, the 8-hydroxy cAMP, dbc-cAMP, and cAMP displayed activities in decreasing order. Extensive investigations were carried out on the release in vitro of hormones from rat anterior pituitaries. N^6-alkyl derivatives (with the exception of N^6-t-butyl cAMP where the substituent is too bulky) and iso-cAMP were more effective than cAMP in increasing TSH release (62). The same derivatives and also 8-bromo-cAMP and 8-thio-cAMP increased more effectively than cAMP the release of GH, but not the release of prolactin. The effect of 8-thio-cAMP was considerably enhanced by dibutyrylation (65). Iso-cAMP, which is quite active on TSH release, was far less potent on GH release (72). It has been found that cAMP and the potent analogs, which produce in vitro significant release of GH from pituitaries, are more active on male rats than on female or castrated male rats. On the other hand, 3–6 $\times 10^{-3}$ cGMP produced an essentially opposite pattern (69).

Db-cAMP is now a very popular compound, which has been used in a multitude of biological experiments that cannot be reported here. Its action on intact cells is generally better than the action of cAMP, although a number of exceptions have been reported. According to a recent publication (73), db-cAMP is taken up by HeLa cells to a much higher degree than cAMP; by the action of an esterase, it is converted to N^6-mb-cAMP, which accumulates inside the cells. This monobutyrate is bound by the R unit of kinases as well as cAMP itself and represents perhaps the active form. Other authors working with thyroid cells (74) found a considerable uptake of exogenous cAMP and they suggested that the high levels of intracellular cAMP may generate the production of a cAMP inhibitor (75) which has been detected in a variety of tissues. The formation of this inhibitor was reported to be prevented by N^6-mb-cAMP.

The mechanism of action of biologically active analogs that do not contain acyl groups involves perhaps again a better penetration through cell membranes; their resistance to phosphoesterases and, in some cases, their inhibitory effects on these enzymes, may also play a role, as in the case of the acyl derivatives.

cAMP AND GENE TRANSCRIPTION OR TRANSLATION

cAMP stimulates the synthesis and induction of a number of enzymes. The role of a cAMP dependent histone kinase has been suggested in higher organisms (76). A stimulation of DNA synthesis occurs in the parotid gland in response to iso-proterenol, a potent β-agonist that enhances the level of cAMP (77). At the molecular level, the most penetrating investigations are concerned with the synthesis of inducible enzymes in bacteria, especially in *Escherichia coli.* The presence of cAMP in this microorganism was detected a few years ago; its concentration inside the cells was lowered by glucose (78); in addition, the formation of enzymes induced by a new substrate is repressed by glucose. It was then discovered that exogenous cAMP overcame this repression of the synthesis of β-galactosidase and of other inducible enzymes (79). At the level of DNA, the lac operon, which effects the synthesis of β-galactosidase, is composed in sequence of three regulatory genes (i, p, and o) and of three structural genes (z, y, and a). The latter code for β-galactosidase, galacto-side permease, and thiogalactoside transacetylase respectively. The i gene codes for a repressor, which binds to the operator gene o, thereby preventing the transcription, that is the synthesis of mRNA. The new substrate (inducer), for instance isopropyl-β-thiogalactoside (IPTG), stimulates lac mRNA synthesis by binding to the repressor and reduces its affinity for the o gene. The p or promotor gene controls the maximum rate of the lac operon expression. Mutants of *E. coli* were isolated that were unable to metabolize various substrates even in the presence of cAMP. These mutants were subsequently found to lack a protein that could bind cAMP and that has been named the cAMP receptor protein (CRP) (80) or the catabolic gene activator protein (CAP) (81). Purified CRP has a mol wt of 45,000; it is composed of two identical subunits and is very basic; it has no detectable protein kinase activity (82). When lac DNA, RNA polymerase, CRP, and cAMP are incubated together in vitro in the absence of the nucleoside triphosphates, which are the substrates of RNA polymerase, a rifamycin resistant complex is formed. As rifamycin rapidly inactivates free RNA polymerase, the latter is contained in the complex in a protected form. Upon addition of nucleoside triphosphates, lac mRNA is formed (83). It seems likely that RNA polymerase binds at the promotor, for when DNA containing a defective promotor is used in vitro, no RNA is made. A hypothetic model involves first the formation of the complex cAMP-CPR which, due to an allosteric change of CPR, binds to the promotor site close to the lac operator. A conformational modification of DNA takes place so that RNA polymerase can bind to p. In the presence of nucleoside triphosphates, the transcription ensues. The formation of gal mRNA is supposed to take place in a similar way; this mRNA is involved in the synthesis of one of the enzymes of galactose metabolism. These models do not involve any phosphorylation.

The effect of cAMP seems thus to occur at the transcriptional level. Another mechanism is, however, probably involved in the synthesis of another inducible enzyme, tryptophanase. cAMP stimulates this synthesis when it is added after mRNA synthesis has been arrested either by the removal of the inducer (trypto-phane) or by treatment with actinomycin D or proflavin. This suggests that cAMP was acting in this case at the translational level to increase the peptide chain elongation (84).

A possible mechanism of the action of cAMP at the translational level is suggested by the following work. cAMP is bound in the presence of GTP and Mg^{2+} to a second protein, the G translocation factor, in addition to the CPR factor required for β-galactosidase synthesis. The G factor functions as or with a ribosome-dependent GTPase in the process by which the tRNA molecules are shifted on the ribosome as it moves along mRNA (85). cAMP would thus be involved in the GTP conversion to GDP, which releases the energy required for translocation. Another example of action at the translational level is afforded by a work on liver tyrosine transaminase, where cAMP releases the enzyme from polysomes bound to membranes; in addition, a soluble factor is required (86).

CELL PROLIFERATION

Contradictory reports can be found concerning the effect of cAMP on cell mitosis, especially in cancerous tissues. High levels of cAMP have been considered as a stimulating factor, e.g. in parotid gland (77, 87); however, other investigations point to a defect in cAMP formation as a concomitant of abnormal cell proliferation. The exogenous cAMP was reported to inhibit the growth of two virus-transformed derivatives of a line of hamster kidney fibroblast, in tissue culture (88). Cells transformed by a polyoma virus contained lower adenyl cyclase activity than control cells or cells transformed by Rous sarcoma virus (89). The growth of HeLa cells and of a line of chick fibroblast was inhibited by exogenous cAMP (90). These tissue culture studies were extended with similar results to other cell lines. It was reported that Rous sarcoma virus-induced hamster tumor cells, when treated with cAMP or with db-cAMP, regain some morphological and growth characteristics of normal fibroblasts (91). Db-cAMP slows growth and decreases saturation density of cell lines like 3T3, which present contact inhibition. In the skin disease called psoriasis, a four- to twelvefold accelerated epidermal cell division occurs as well as an accumulation of glycogen. cAMP concentrations and adenyl cyclase contents are lower in psoriatic skin than in normal skin; in addition, db-cAMP inhibited epidermal cell division (92–94). It has even been reported that derivatives of cAMP could suppress the growth of tumors in experimental animals (95, 96).

Lymphocytes are cells whose proliferation is stimulated by antigenes. Two mitogenic agents, phytohemagglutinin and concanavaline A at optimal concentration produce a ten- to fiftyfold increase in the concentration of lymphocyte cGMP within the first 20 min of exposure. On the other hand, no change was seen in the concentration of cAMP (97).

The conclusion has been drawn that an increase of the level of cellular cGMP may represent one of the active signals that induce cell division, while the elevation of the cAMP level may limit or inhibit mitosis. Many other experiments will be necessary in order to confirm these considerations, which are still partially hypothetic.

Literature Cited

1. Breckenridge, B. M. 1970. *Ann. Rev. Pharmacol.* 10:19–33
2. Fischer, E. H., Krebs, E. G. 1966. *Fed. Proc.* 25:1511 (Abstr.)
3. Walsh, D. A., Perkins, J. P., Krebs, E. G. 1968. *J. Biol. Chem.* 243:3763–65
4. Gill, G. N., Garren, L. D. 1970. *Biochem. Biophys. Res. Commun.* 39: 335–43
5. Tao, M., Salas, M. L., Lipmann, F. 1970. *Proc. Nat. Acad. Sci. USA* 67:408–14
6. Reimann, E. M., Brostrom, C. O., Corbin, J. D., King, C. A., Krebs, E. G. 1971. *Biochem. Biophys. Res. Commun.* 42:187–94
7. Rubin, C. S., Erlichman, J., Rosen, O. M. 1972. *J. Biol. Chem.* 247:36–44
8. Walsh, D. A. et al 1971. *J. Biol. Chem.* 246:1977–85
9. Ashby, C. D., Walsh, D. A. 1972. *J. Biol. Chem.* 247:6637–42
10. Ashby, C. D., Walsh, D. A. 1973. *J. Biol. Chem.* 248:1255–66
11. Rosell-Perez, M., Villar-Palasi, C., Larner, J. 1962. *Biochemistry* 1:763–68
12. Friedman, D. L., Larner, J. 1963. *Biochemistry* 2:669–75
13. Larner, J. 1966. *Trans. N.Y. Acad. Sci.* 29:192
14. Appleman, M. M., Birnbaumer L., Torres, H. N. 1966. *Arch. Biochem. Biophys.* 116:39–43
15. Larner, J. et al. 1968. *Advan. Enzyme Regul.* 6:409
16. Schlender, K. K., Wei, S. H., Villar-Palasi, C. 1969. *Biochim. Biophys. Acta* 191:272–78
17. Soderling, T. R. et al. 1970. *J. Biol. Chem.* 245:6317–28
18. Stone, D. B., Mansour, T. E. 1967. *Mol. Pharmacol.* 3:177
19. Steinberg, D., Huttunen, J. K. 1972. *Advan. Cycl. Nucleot. Res.* 1:47–62
20. Rasmussen, H. 1970. *Science* 170: 404–12
21. Kuo, J. F., Greengard, P. 1969. *J. Biol. Chem.* 244:3417–19
22. Ashman, D. F., Lipton, R., Melicow, M. M., Price, T. D. 1963. *Biochem. Biophys. Res. Commun.* 11:330–34
23. Kuo, J. F., Greengard, P. 1972. *Advan. Cycl. Nucleot. Res.* 2:41–50
24. Ishikawa, E., Ishikawa, S., Davis, J. W., Sutherland, E. W. 1969. *J. Biol. Chem.* 244:6371–76
25. Goldberg, N. D., Dietz, S. B., O'Toole, A. G. 1969. *J. Biol. Chem.* 244:4458–66
26. Steiner, A. L., Parker, C. W., Kipnis, D. M. 1970. *J. Clin. Invest.* 49:43a
27. Hardman, J. G., Sutherland, E. W. 1969. *J. Biol. Chem.* 244:6363–70
28. White, A. A., Aurbach, G. D. 1969. *Biochim. Biophys. Acta* 191:686–97
29. Schultz, G., Bohme, E., Munske, K. 1969. *Life Sci.* 8:1323
30. Gray, J. P., Hardman, J. G., Bibring, T. W., Sutherland, E. W. 1970. *Fed. Proc.* 29:608 (Abstr.)
31. Mahaffee, D., Watson, B., Ney, R. L. 1970. *Clin. Res.* 18:73
32. Rall, T. W., Sutherland, E. W. 1962. *J. Biol. Chem.* 237:1228–32
33. Glinsmann, W. H., Hern, E. P. 1969. *Biochem. Biophys. Res. Commun.* 36: 931–36
34. Corbin, J. D., Krebs, E. G. 1969. *Biochem. Biophys. Res. Commun.* 36: 328–36
35. Krebs, E. G., unpublished observations
36. Kuo, J. F., Greengard, P. 1969. *Proc. Nat. Acad. Sci. USA* 64:1349–55
37. Kuo, J. F., Greengard, P. 1970. *J. Biol. Chem.* 245:2493–98
38. Murad, F., Manganiello, V., Vaughan, M. 1970. *J. Biol. Chem.* 245:3352–60
39. Exton, J. H., Hardman, J. G., Williams, T. F., Sutherland, E. W., Park, C. R. 1971. *J. Biol. Chem.* 246:2658–64
40. Helderman, J. H., Wilson, D. F., Levine, R. A. 1972. *Arch. Int. Pharmacodyn. Ther.* 199:389–93
41. Braun, T., Hechter, O., Bär, H. P. 1969. *Proc. Soc. Exp. Biol. Med.* 132:233
42. Glinsmann, W. H., Hern, E. P., Linarelli, L. G., Faresi, R. V. 1969. *Endocrinology* 85:711
43. George, W. J., Polson, J. B., O'Toole, A. G., Goldberg, N. D. 1970. *Proc. Nat. Acad. Sci. USA* 66:398–403
44. Ferrendelli, J. A., Steiner, A. L., McDougal, D. B., Kipnis, D. M. 1970. *Biochem. Biophys. Res. Commun.* 41: 1061–67
45. Ferrendelli, J. A., Kinscherf, D. A., Chang, M. M. 1973. *Fed. Proc.* 32:680 (Abstr.)
46. Schultz, G., Hardman, J. G., Hurwitz, L., Sutherland, E. W. 1973. *Fed. Proc.* 32:773 (Abstr.)
47. Krause, E. G., Halle, W., Wollenberg, A. 1972. *Advan. Cycl. Nucleot. Res.* 1: 301–05
48. Thompson, W. J., Appleman, M. M. 1971. *J. Biol. Chem.* 246:3145–50
49. Thompson, W. J., Appleman, M. M. 1971. *Biochemistry* 10:311–16
50. Weiss, B., Strada, S. J. 1972. *Advan. Cycl. Nucleot. Res.* 1:357–74

51. Goren, E. W., Rosen, O. M. 1972. *Arch. Biochem. Biophys.* 153:384
52. Russell, T. R., Terasaki, W. L., Appleman, M. M. 1973. *J. Biol. Chem.* 248: 1334–40
53. Uzunov, P., Weiss, B. 1972. *Biochim. Biophys. Acta* 284:220–26
54. Kakiuchi, S., Yamazaki, R., Theshima, Y. 1972. *Advan. Cycl. Nucleot. Res.* 1: 455–77
55. Cheung, W. Y. 1971. *J. Biol. Chem.* 246:2859–69
56. Posternak, T., Sutherland, E. W., Henion, W. F. 1962. *Biochim. Biophys. Acta* 65:558–60
57. Falbriard, J. G., Posternak, T., Sutherland, E. W. 1967. *Biochim. Biophys. Acta* 148:99–105
58. Miller, J. P. et al. 1973. *Biochemistry* 12:1010–16
59. Murayama, A., Jastorff, B., Hettler, H. 1970. *Angew. Chem. Int. Ed.* 9:640–41
60. Meyer, R. B., Shuman, D. A., Robins, R. K. 1973. *Tetrahedron Lett.* 269–72
61. Cehovic, G., Marcus, I., Vengadabady, S., Posternak, T. 1968. *C.R. Soc. Phys. Hist. Nat. Genève* 3:135–39
62. Posternak, T., Marcus, I., Gabbai, A., Cehovic, G. 1969. *C.R. Acad. Sci. Sér. D* 269:2408–12
63. Michal, G., DuPlooy, M., Woschee, M., Nelböck, M., Weimann, G. 1970. *Z. Anal. Chem.* 252:183–88
64. Meyer, R. B. et al. 1972. *Biochemistry* 11:2704–09
65. Posternak, T., Marcus, I., Cehovic, G. 1971. *C.R. Acad. Sci. Sér. D* 272:622–25
66. Muneyama, K., Bauer, R. J., Shuman, D. A., Robins, R. K., Simon, L. N. 1971. *Biochemistry* 10:2390–95
67. Hanze, A. R. 1968. *Biochemistry* 7: 932–39
68. Bauer, R. J., Swiatek, K. R., Robins, R. K., Simon, L. N. 1971. *Biochem. Biophys. Res. Commun.* 45:526–31
69. Cehovic, G., Posternak, T., Charollais, E. 1972. *Advan. Cycl. Nucl. Res.* 1: 521–40
70. Henion, W. F., Sutherland, E. W., Posternak, T. 1967. *Biophys. Biochim. Acta* 148:106–13
71. Free, C. A., Chasin, M., Paik, V. S., Hess, S. M. 1971. *Biochemistry* 10: 3785–89
72. Cehovic, G., Marcus, I., Gabbai, A., Posternak, T. 1970. *C.R. Acad. Sci. Sér. D* 271:1399–1401

73. Kaukel, E., Mundhenk, K., Hilz, H. 1972. *Eur. J. Biochem.* 27:197–200
74. Szabo, M., Burke, G. 1972. *Biochim. Biophys. Acta* 264:289–99
75. Murad, F., Rall, T. W., Vaughan, M. 1969. *Biochim. Biophys. Acta* 192: 430–45
76. Langan, T. A. 1968. *Science* 162:579–80
77. Malamud, D. 1969. *Biochem. Biophys. Res. Commun.* 35:754–58
78. Makman, R. S., Sutherland, E. W. 1965. *J. Biol. Chem.* 240:1309–14
79. Perlman, R. L., Pastan, I. 1969. *Biochem. Biophys. Res. Commun.* 37: 151–57
80. Emmer, M., de Crombrugghe, B., Pastan, I., Perlman, R. L. 1970. *Proc. Nat. Acad. Sci. USA* 66:480–87
81. Zubay, G., Schwartz, D., Beckwith, J. 1970. *Proc. Nat. Acad. Sci. USA* 66: 104–10
82. Anderson, W. B., Schneider, A. B., Emmer, M., Perlman, R. L., Pastan, I. 1971. *J. Biol. Chem.* 246:5929–37
83. Nissley, S. P., Anderson, W. B., Gottesman, M., Perlman, R. L., Pastan, I. 1971. *J. Biol. Chem.* 246:4671–78
84. Pastan, I., Perlman, R. L. 1969. *J. Biol. Chem.* 244:2226–32
85. Kuwano, M., Schlessinger, D. 1970. *Proc. Nat. Acad. Sci. USA* 66:146–52
86. Chuah, C. C., Oliver, I. T. 1971. *Biochemistry* 10:2990–3001
87. MacManus, J. P., Whitfield, J. F. 1970. *Endocrinology* 86:934
88. Ryan, W. L., Heidrick, M. L. 1968. *Science* 162:1484–85
89. Burk, R. R. 1968. *Nature* 219:1272–75
90. Heidrick, M. L., Ryan, W. L. 1970. *Cancer Res.* 30:376
91. Johnson, G. S., Friedman, R. M., Pastan, I. 1971. *Proc. Nat. Acad. Sci. USA* 68: 425–29
92. Voorhees, J. J., Duell, E. A., Bass, L. J., Powell, J. A., Harrell, E. R. 1972. *Arch. Dermatol.* 105:695–701
93. Wright, R. K., Mandy, S. H., Halprin, K. M., Hsia, S. L. 1973. *Arch. Dermatol.* 107:47–58
94. Voorhees, J. J., Duell, E. A., Kelsey, W. H. 1972. *Arch. Dermatol.* 105:384–86
95. Chandra, P., Gericke, D. 1972. *Naturwissenschaften* 59:205
96. Keller, R. 1972. *Life Sci. Part II.* 11:485
97. Hadden, J. W., Hadden, E. M., Haddox, M. K., Goldberg, N. D. 1972. *Proc. Nat. Acad. Sci. USA* 69:3024–27

BIOAVAILABILITY OF DRUGS   ❖6579
FROM FORMULATIONS AFTER
ORAL ADMINISTRATION

L. F. Chasseaud and T. Taylor

Department of Metabolism and Pharmacokinetics, Huntingdon Research Centre,
Huntingdon, England

An administered drug can elicit only the pharmacologic response for which it was developed, provided that sufficient concentrations of drug reach and are available to the receptors. Determination of the likely availability of the active drug to the receptors is the basis of bioavailability testing. Drugs that are chemically equivalent may not be therapeutically equivalent because of differences in dosage form. Certainly, the more potent the pharmacologic action of the drug, the more imperative is the need for bioavailability testing (1), but only recently has such testing gained acceptance as a worthwhile and necessary adjunct (2–4) to the gamut of tests to which new and existing drugs are subjected.

Among the multiplicity of terms coined in recent years, that of bioavailability has been the subject of much discussion and considerable misunderstanding. Bioavailability, or biologic availability, has been usefully reviewed or discussed by several authors (5–16). Confusion has arisen, however, over interchange of the terms biologic availability (bioavailability), physiologic availability, generic equivalence, and therapeutic equivalence, all of which have been used to define essentially the same events. Bioavailability, which in this decade has become the preferred term, describes the extent to which and the rate at which the active drug reaches the systemic circulation, and ultimately the receptors or sites of action at concentrations that are effective, and thereby defines the efficiency of the dosage formulation as an extravascular drug delivery system. Because it is generally impossible to measure receptor drug concentrations, these are measured in the circulation, venous or arterial, from which the receptors receive their supply. Alternatively, urinary concentrations of the active drug or a characteristic metabolite can be measured (13, 17, 18). There is no guarantee, however, that a drug reaching the systemic circulation will also reach the receptors in adequate concentrations. Sometimes the response of the receptors to the drug may be quantified in controlled clinical trials, for example, the

35

lowering of blood sugar by hypoglycemics (19, 20), the excretion of electrolytes after administration of diuretics (21), or the anticoagulant effects of certain coumarins (22), but it is important to know whether the intensity of the pharmacologic effect in a particular case is a function of drug concentration in the body.

VARIATIONS IN BIOAVAILABILITY

In reality, because the drug has to cross several membranes, exist in numerous physiologic environments, and be subjected to tissue uptake, biotransformation, and excretion (18, 23–26), much of an administered dose never reaches the receptors. So that patients are provided with drug formulations that are physically and chemically stable, pharmaceutically reliable, and aesthetically acceptable, drugs are prepared in various physical forms with a number of other ingredients which may influence their bioavailability. To be absorbed from the gastrointestinal tract, the drug must be presented in a soluble form to the site of absorption; for example, an administered tablet must disintegrate and the particles must dissolve in the gastrointestinal milieu before absorption can occur. Different dosage forms of drugs may thus provide varying amounts of the drug for absorption and thereby cause differences in the onset, extent, and duration of pharmacologic effect. These differences may derive from physiologically modified bioavailability and be due to the physiology or pathology of the patient and/or his genetic makeup (27), or alternatively from dosage form-modified bioavailability and be due to the methods of manufacture or to the physicochemical properties of the drug (13) (Table 1). This review is mainly concerned with the latter category. For these reasons (Table 1), in vitro tests which do not take into account some of these factors cannot be presumed to predict in vivo drug availability. The in vitro system must be compared against the in vivo case (28) for every formulation type, and in vitro systems are generally only useful for quality control or for the selection of suitable formulations for in vivo testing.

Table 1 Factors affecting bioavailability (13)

Dosage form	Physiologic
Particle size, Polymorphic form, Solvation, Hydration, Chemical form, pH, Solubility characteristics, Formulation adjuvants, Manufacturing method	Age, Sex, Physical state of patient, Time of administration, Stomach emptying, Intestinal motility, Food, Other drugs, Disease

PARAMETERS OF BIOAVAILABILITY

The bioavailability of a drug is characterized by two important parameters: the area under the blood concentration-time relationship and the peak height of this relationship together with its time of occurrence. Figure 1 illustrates the plasma concentration-time relationships for a hypothetical drug which needs to attain a minimum concentration in the plasma to be pharmacologically active. Above the maximum safe concentration, a drug such as digoxin (29) causes toxicity. Inspection of the relationships shows that a formulation producing curve I is ineffective, that producing curve II is active and the preferred dosage form, and that producing curve III is active but also leads to toxicity. Similarity of the areas under all three curves in Figure 1 does not necessarily indicate that the drug will be therapeutically effective in all cases. As a criteria of bioavailability, therefore, both parameters should be considered. Rates of bioavailability are likely to be important for drugs with a low therapeutic index, sparingly soluble drugs, drugs that are destroyed in the gastrointestinal tract or are actively absorbed, or when adequate drug concentrations are required rapidly, as with antibiotics, analgesics, coronary vasodilators, and hypoglycemics. Differences in bioavailability are, however, equivalent to differences in dosage. Suitable reduction in dosage for formulation III and increase in dosage for formulation I should produce a therapeutic and nontoxic response (Figure 1). If bioavailability is estimated from urinary excretion data, suitable parameters are the cumulative excretion of drug (or metabolite) in the urine and the maximum excretion rate and time of its occurrence.

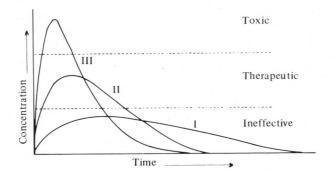

ESTIMATION OF BIOAVAILABILITY

Earlier methods of estimating bioavailability were qualitative, such as monitoring the disintegration of formulations in the gastrointestinal tract (30–32). Disintegration of a formulation or indeed the dissolution of its contents does not provide absolute proof of absorption. The concept of bioavailability was introduced in 1945 (33) during studies of the relative absorption of vitamins from pharmaceutical preparations and was estimated by comparing the fraction of a dose from a test formulation, and that from an aqueous solution, excreted in the urine during a fixed time. An aqueous solution was considered to present the drug in an ideal form for absorption. More generally, bioavailability may be measured as the ratio

$$\text{Bioavailability} = \frac{\text{amount of drug absorbed from test formulation}}{\text{amount of drug absorbed from reference formulation}} \times 100\%$$

where the reference formulation is one from which the drug is readily absorbed, or, preferably, is known to be clinically effective. So measured, bioavailability is a statement of *relative* absorption, not of amount absorbed.

For bioavailability studies, healthy volunteers are preferred to patients because disease states may influence drug bioavailability (34) or elimination (35). Subjects should be selected on the basis of a satisfactory medical examination, normal renal and hepatic function, and freedom from a history of renal, hepatic, gastrointestinal, and endocrine disorders or from a known sensitivity to drugs. Female subjects should be selected only if they are unlikely to be pregnant during or for some time after the studies. The very thin or obese should be excluded so that wide intersubject variations in apparent volumes of distribution are avoided. The use of subjects aged between 18 and 50 years reduces anomalous age-dependent responses (36, 37). Since large intra- and intersubject variations in absorption commonly occur, a sufficient number of subjects, usually 6 to 20, should be used to permit a satisfactory statistical analysis of the data (18, 38–40), and to demonstrate equivalence, a larger number may be necessary. The subjects should give their informed consent and should not be taking other drugs. Equal doses of test and reference formulations should be administered, as plasma concentrations or clearances may not be linearly related to the dose (41, 42). Experimental designs (43) are commonly of a complete crossover type, where every subject receives each formulation according to a random treatment schedule (38). The intensity of the pharmacologic effect of a drug is often nonlinearly related to the logarithm of the administered dose (23) and the therapeutic consequences of changes in dose due to modification of bioavailability may be more serious at lower doses. For this reason acceptable limits of bioavailability must be established for each drug at or near the expected therapeutic dose (13).

Bioavailability is usually estimated from a statistical comparison of either average drug concentrations in the blood (18) or areas to infinite time under the drug concentration-time relationships in the blood after administration of single doses of both test and reference formulations. The duration of sampling is relatively short and improvements in methodology allow accurate determinations of very low drug concentrations. In single-dose studies, sufficient blood samples should be withdrawn to describe adequately the critical phases of the concentration-time relationship: (*a*) absorption which allows at least a qualitative comparison of the rates of availability, (*b*) time of occurrence of maximal concentrations, and (*c*) the decline of concentrations during the elimination phase. During the latter phase, drug concentrations may fall to very low levels, and inadequate analytical procedures could introduce errors into the calculation of areas to infinite time. The precision of the analytical method should be known and the level of sensitivity should exceed the expected peak blood concentration by at least twentyfold. Total areas under the concentration-time curves are usually measured by the trapezoidal rule (44) up to the last sampling time, and the remaining area to infinite time is calculated from the concentration at that time and the observed rate constant for drug elimination from plasma (45). The calculated areas may be normalized (13, 18, 45, 46) to correct for intra- and intersubject variations in dose, body weight, and the apparent elimination (biological) half-life of the drug. This allows bioavailabilities estimated in studies performed at different times with different subject panels to be validly compared.

Under some circumstances it may be preferable to estimate bioavailability during a sequence of multiple doses, so that experimental conditions resemble the clinical situation (13, 18). After multiple dosing, blood concentrations are greater and more easily measured, but experimental control is more complex. In multiple dose studies, bioavailability can be estimated, after attainment of steady state conditions, by comparison of the areas under the blood concentration-time curves during a complete dosage interval or by comparison of maximal and minimal concentrations reached during the dosage interval. This obviates the need for calculation of areas to infinite time, which may be a prime source of error in single-dose studies.

Estimates of bioavailability from urinary excretion data require complete collection of the urine for at least seven drug half-lives, and control of urinary pH may be necessary for certain drugs, such as weak bases (47). Loss of a single sample could invalidate the estimation of bioavailability from measurement of cumulative excretion data, and rates of urinary excretion may not correspond to rates of gastrointestinal absorption. This method is advantageous because the subjects need not undergo numerous venepunctures for blood withdrawal, and drug analysis is simpler, but it should not be used when the drug is extensively biotransformed and less than 20% is excreted in the urine unchanged or as a characteristic metabolite.

All the experimental data obtained should be analyzed by the appropriate statistical procedures (40) with due regard for the methodology used. It should be estimated what differences need to occur between formulations before these are statistically significant.

Seven methods of estimating bioavailability have been described by Wagner & Nelson (48), some of which differ only in the mathematical treatment of the experimental data. Wagner (18) has critically appraised the assumptions involved.

FACTORS AFFECTING BIOAVAILABILITY

Since absorption occurs only after the drug is in solution, orally administered drugs in solid form must first dissolve in the gastrointestinal fluids. The rate at which dissolution occurs is an important determinant of bioavailability and is dependent on several factors. Drugs administered in solid form as capsules or tablets need to disaggregate so that dissolution may occur more readily.

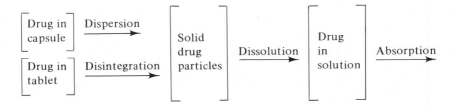

Particle Size

The greater the surface area of drug in contact with the gastrointestinal fluids, the more rapid the dissolution rate. Thus with decrease in particle size, there is an increase in dissolution rate (49, 50). The bioavailabilities of spironolactone (51) and phenacetin (52) are improved by a reduction in particle size. However, particle size reduction provides more opportunity for particle interaction, which may sometimes lead to aggregation. Nitrofurantoin, in high concentrations, causes gastric irritation and nausea when taken orally and it is thus preferable to present this drug to the gastrointestinal tract as larger, slower-dissolving crystals (53, 54).

Diffusion from the Dosage Form

The rate of bioavailability of a drug is enhanced if the rate of diffusion from the dosage form is increased either by use of a more soluble drug form or by alteration of the microenvironment surrounding the drug particle (8, 12). Administration of soluble salts of penicillin V resulted in higher blood levels of antibiotic than were obtained with the less soluble free acid (55, 56). The rates of absorption of different aspirin formulations correlated with their solubility characteristics (57).

Crystalline Form

Some drugs such as barbiturates (58) exist in several crystalline forms of differing solubilities and other physical properties (59, 60) with resultant differences in bioavailability (61). The amorphous is more soluble than the crystalline form.

Hydration

The hydration state of a drug influences its solubility, and the anhydrous form is usually more soluble. Anhydrous ampicillin has a greater extent of bioavailability in dogs and man than the less soluble trihydrate (62).

Formulation Ingredients

Some of the agents added to formulations which can influence the bioavailability of the drug include fillers, binders, disintegration aids, lubricants, surfactants, and suspending agents. Hydrophobic lubricants such as magnesium stearate prevented adequate contact between the gastrointestinal fluids and the drug solids, thereby slowing dissolution, whereas the hydrophilic sodium laurylsulfate produced the opposite effect (63). Surfactants may alter the rate and extent of absorption of certain drugs (64). Absorption of phenacetin was apparently enhanced by Tween 80 (52).

Pharmaceutical or Dosage Form

The compressed tablet provides a low surface area for dissolution and must first disintegrate (65). Coated tablets, particularly enteric coated types, may release the drug unevenly. The rate of dispersion of drug particles from a capsule influences the bioavailability of the drug, but in general a capsule is considered a reliable dosage form. Drugs with a short biological half-life are sometimes formulated as sustained- or timed-release products (44), but care is necessary since failure of the formulation could result in toxic levels of drug (66). The expected relative bioavailabilities from various dosage forms are shown in Table 2.

Table 2   Dosage forms for oral administration (8)

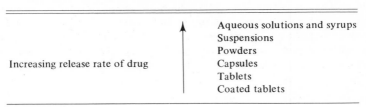

Increasing release rate of drug ↑	Aqueous solutions and syrups Suspensions Powders Capsules Tablets Coated tablets

Compressed tablets are the most widely used form of oral medication, and an accepted laboratory standard measurement of drug release from the tablet has been the disintegration test which merely measures physical breakup of the tablet. This test does not predict drug bioavailability in vivo (65, 67, 68) although it can be assumed that a tablet formulation failing to disintegrate within about 30 min would provide only slowly available drug.

The dissolution rate test provides a means of ranking various solid dosage forms in vitro and, although the results may correlate with in vivo bioavailability (18, 69–72), measured dissolution rates can be affected by test conditions (73, 74). Levy (67) compared various commercial aspirin tablets and found that absorption from the gastrointestinal tract correlated with dissolution but not disintegration rate data. In vitro techniques must always be suspect because they do not compensate for the nervous and circulatory systems that charactize the biological case.

Gastrointestinal Conditions

Absorption of drugs may be affected by the physiologic status (disease, pH, peristalsis) of the gastrointestinal tract. Administration of laxatives, such as $MgSO_4$, may cause dilution of the intestinal contents and enhance intestinal motility, thereby reducing the time available for drug absorption. A pH-dependent dissolution stage precedes tetracycline absorption in man (75), and simultaneous administration with antacids or milk reduces absorption, because these contain divalent metal ions which form a poorly absorbed chelate with tetracycline (76–78). Administration of drugs with food usually reduces or delays absorption (79). Aspirin (80), dicloxacillin (81), and penicillin V (56) were absorbed best by fasting subjects. However, absorption of griseofulvin was least in fasting subjects and was enhanced by meals with a high fat content (82). Dietary components influence the absorption of paracetamol (83) and acetaminophen (84). Drugs that are unstable in acid media are formulated for safe passage through the stomach with an enteric coating (18, 85). Such coatings are pH sensitive and may prematurely disintegrate in the stomach if antacids are taken simultaneously. The action of sustained- or timed-release products formulated with organic solvent-sensitive coatings may be undesirably enhanced by concomitant intake of alcoholic beverages (12).

Drug Interactions

·Drug interactions occurring in the gastrointestinal tract, such as lincomycin and kaolin-pectin (38), may be considered as pharmaceutical incompatabilities and avoided by consideration of the relevant physicochemical properties of the formulation ingredients. Drug interactions in the body or during absorption, however, occur by modification of absorption, distribution, biotransformation, excretion, and action at receptor sites (86–92) and are a consequence of polypharmacy. Examples include displacement of protein-bound drugs by other drugs (12, 25, 93–97) and enzyme induction (88, 98, 99). Age, nutrition, and pathological states are other important determinants of drug interactions (100).

Influence of Route of Administration

Most orally administered drugs are absorbed into the hepatic portal system where extensive biotransformation may result in only a small proportion of the original drug reaching the peripheral circulation. Attempts to estimate the extent of absorption by comparison of the areas under plasma concentration-time curves obtained after oral and intravenous administration are thus invalidated by this "pass effect" of the liver (101–104), as plasma clearances vary according to the route of administration. Extensive biotransformation during passage through the gastrointestinal epithelium may also reduce the bioavailability of an orally administered drug (105). Despite some intersubject variations, an increase in dosage in the ratio 1:1.5: 2–3:3–4:3–5 was thought necessary to obtain similar blood concentrations of pentazocine after intravenous, intramuscular, oral (solution), rectal, and oral (tablet) administration respectively (106). Plasma concentrations were erratic after rectal administration of aspirin (107) when absorption would be limited by the rate of drug diffusion through a viscous medium. The nature of the suppository base would strongly influence bioavailability.

GENERIC PRODUCTS

Nonproprietary preparations are chemically equivalent if they contain the same active drug and they would be therapeutically equivalent if they produced the same biological response. Chemically equivalent formulations from different manufacturers, referred to as generic products, often differ widely in their methods of manufacture and content of pharmacologically inert ingredients. In recent years, controversy has arisen over the possible extent to which such generic products may or may not be therapeutically equivalent. The problem is one of bioavailability (5, 11, 16, 18). Controlled studies in man on twelve commercial drug products showed inequivalence in ten cases (18) in either the rate or extent of bioavailability. Differences in the therapeutic equivalence of some formulations has been noted in clinical practice (11, 108, 109), but it is not entirely clear that formulation effects are alone responsible, especially in cases where therapeutic efficacy is not directly related to drug concentrations in the blood (110) or where the clinical response is subjective. Prescott & Nimmo (11) ranked normal individuals as fast and slow absorbers of paracetamol and showed that plasma concentrations were similar after ingestion of a suspension, effervescent tablet, and plain tablet by the former but not the latter subjects, which suggests that the inequivalence of some products may only arise in certain subjects.

Maximal plasma concentrations and rates of absorption of chloramphenicol differed after administrations of four different formulations to human subjects (111). Less pronounced differences were observed in another study (112) when fourteen different formulations as capsules, tablets, and suspensions were administered orally. These differences were unlikely to have been caused by intersubject variations in rates of absorption or biotransformation. In both studies the rate of bioavailability was related to the in vitro dissolution time; those preparations providing the lowest plasma concentrations showed the slowest dissolution rates. Differences in either rate or extent of bioavailability of generic products have been shown for digoxin (113, 114), ampicillin (115), phenylbutazone (116), warfarin (117), a combination of trimethoprim-sulfamethoxazole (118), sulfonamides (119, 120), and tetracyclines (121–124), although no differences were found between several products containing phenylbutazone (125) and sulfamethizole (126). Six preparations of isoniazid were shown to be therapeutically equivalent (127) and in vivo bioavailability paralleled in vitro tests. The bioavailability of triple sulfa from 20 generic products was similar (128), although the drugs were more slowly absorbed from the formulations than from aqueous solutions, and there was no in vivo correlation with widely varying dissolution rates. Of generic products, digoxin formulations continue to attract much interest (136–139).

While in vitro tests provide a means of ranking formulations, the available evidence (18) challenges the usefulness of tests in vitro to predict bioavailability in vivo (73, 129–132). Efforts are being made to design in vitro tests capable of predicting the in vivo performance of generic products (73, 133–135), but in vivo studies are currently the only reliable way of ascertaining whether drugs are available from their formulations for absorption and production of a therapeutic response. Although drug formulation has been studied extensively in vitro, the extent of generic inequivalence and its clinical significance is at present unknown but may be expected to have more relevance to drugs of poor water solubility, as known examples of inequivalence seem to reflect the dissolution rather than the disintegration rates of the products. The relative importance of equivalence is also linked to the disease being treated. A criticism of most bioavailability studies that detect differences between generic products is that these studies do not define the extent (if any) to which a particular inequivalence endangers the well being of the patient.

Literature Cited

1. Castle, W. B., Astwood, E. B., Finland, M., Keefer, C. S. 1969. *J. Am. Med Assoc.* 208:1171–72
2. *Drug Res. Rep.* September 2, 1970. p. 11
3. *Food Drug Cosmetic Law Rep.* January 15, 1973. No. 518
4. Hayes, T. A. 1971. *Drug Cosmet. Ind.* 109:44ff
5. *Pharmacology* 1973. 8:17–215
6. Barr, W. H. 1969. *Drug Inf. Bull.* 3: 27–45
7. Academy of Pharmaceutical Sciences. 1970. *J. Am. Pharm. Assoc.* NS10:107–116
8. Levy, G. 1970. In *Prescription Pharmacy,* ed. J. B. Sprowls Jr., 36–102. Philadelphia:Lippincott. 2nd ed. 662 pp.

9. Schneller, G. H. 1970. *Am. J. Hosp. Pharm.* 27:487–88
10. Wagner, J. G. 1971. *Drug Intell. Clin. Pharm.* 5:115–28
11. Prescott, L. F., Nimmo, J. 1971. *Acta Pharmacol. Toxicol.* 39, Suppl. 3:288–303
12. Cadwallader, D. E. 1971. *Biopharmaceutics and Drug Interactions.* New Jersey: Roche Lab. 140 pp.
13. Ritschel, W. A. 1972. *Drug Intell. Clin. Pharm.* 6:246–56
14. Kaplan, S. A. 1972. *Drug Metab. Rev.* 1:15–34
15. Smith, R. N. 1972. *Lancet* ii:528–30
16. Florence, A. T. May 20, 1972. *Pharm. J.*, 456–63
17. Baldridge, J. L. 1969. *Bull. Parenteral Drug Assoc.* 23:40–47
18. Wagner, J. G. 1971. *Biopharmaceutics and Relevant Pharmacokinetics.* Hamilton, Ill.: Drug Intell. Publ. 357 pp.
19. Nelson, E., Knoechel, E. L., Hamlin, W. E., Wagner, J. G. 1962. *J. Pharm. Sci.* 51:509–14
20. Varley, A. B. 1968. *J. Am. Med. Assoc.* 206:1745–48
21. Tannenbaum, P. J., Rosen, E., Flanagan, T., Crosley A. P. Jr. 1968. *Clin. Pharmacol. Therap.* 9:598–604
22. Nagashima, R., O'Reilly, R. A., Levy, G. 1969. *Clin. Pharmacol. Therap.* 10:22–35
23. Barr, W. H. 1968. *Am. J. Pharm. Ed.* 32:958–81
24. Goldstein, A., Aronow, L., Kalman, S. M. 1968. *Principles of Drug Action.* New York:Harper & Row. 848 pp.
25. Chasseaud, L. F. 1970. *Foreign Compound Metabolism in Mammals,* 1:1–33. London: Chem. Soc.
26. Rowland, M. In *Clinical Pharmacology, Basic Principles in Therapeutics,* ed. K. L. Melmon, H. F. Morrelli, 21–60. New York:Macmillan. 686 pp.
27. Vesell, E. S. 1972. *Fed. Proc.* 31:1253–69
28. Morrison, A. B., Campbell, J. A. 1965. *J. Pharm. Sci.* 54:1–8
29. Smith, T. W., Haber, E. 1970. *J. Clin. Invest.* 49:2377–86
30. Wruble, M. S. 1930. *Am. J. Pharm.* 102:318–28
31. Maney, P. V., Kuever, R. A. 1941. *J. Am. Pharm. Assoc.* 30:276–82
32. Abbott, A. H. A., Allport, N. L. 1943. *Quart. J. Pharm.* 16:183–96
33. Oser, B. L., Melnick, D., Hochberg, M. 1945. *Ind. Eng. Chem. Anal. Ed.* 17:401–11

34. Bates, J. H., Schultz, J. C., Abernathy, R. S. 1965. *Clin. Res.* 13:77
35. Dettli, L., Spring, P., Ryter, S. 1971. *Acta. Pharmacol. Toxicol.* 29, Suppl. 3:211–24
36. Bender, A. D. 1964. *J. Am. Geriat. Soc.* 12:114–34
37. Mann, Jr., D. E. 1965. *J. Pharm. Sci.* 54:499–510
38. Wagner, J. G. 1966. *Can. J. Pharm. Sci.* 1:55–68
39. Harris, L. E. 1971. *Drug Cosmet. Ind.* 109:48ff
40. Roberts, C. D., Sloboda, W. 1971. *Drug Cosmet. Ind.* 109:50ff
41. Levy, G. 1968. In *Importance of Fundamental Principles in Drug Evaluation,* ed. D. H. Tedeschi, R. E. Tedeschi, 141–72. New York:Raven. 480 pp.
42. Gibaldi, M. 1971. *Ann. NY Acad. Sci.* 179:19–31
43. Cochran, W. G., Cox, G. M. 1957. *Experimental Designs.* New York: Wiley. 2nd ed. 611 pp.
44. Notari, R. E. 1971. *Biopharmaceutics and Pharmacokinetics.* New York: Dekker. 307 pp.
45. Wagner, J. G. 1967. *J. Pharm. Sci.* 56:652–53
46. Ritschel, W. A. 1970. *Drug Intell. Clin. Pharm.* 4:332–47
47. Beckett, A. H. 1966. *Dansk. Tidsskr. Farm.* 40:197–203
48. Wagner, J. G., Nelson, E. 1964. *J. Pharm. Sci.* 53:1392–1403
49. Wagner, J. G. 1962. *Antibiotica et Chemotherapia.* 12:53–84
50. Fincher, J. H. 1968. *J. Pharm. Sci.* 57:1825–35
51. Bauer, G., Rieckmann, P., Schaumann, W. 1962. *Arzneim.-Forsch.* 12:487–89
52. Prescott, L. F., Steel, R. F., Ferrier, W. R. 1970. *Clin. Pharmacol. Therap.* 11:496–504
53. Paul, H. E., Hayes, K. J., Paul, M. F., Borgmann, A. R. 1967. *J. Pharm. Sci.* 56:882–85
54. Conklin, J. D., Hailey, F. J. 1969. *Clin. Pharmacol. Therap.* 10:534–39
55. Kaipainen, W. J., Härkönen, P. 1956. *Scand. J. Clin. Lab. Invest.* 8:18–20
56. Juncher, H., Raaschou, F. 1957. *Antibiot. Med. Clin. Therap.* 4:497–507
57. Leonards, J. R. 1963. *Clin. Pharmacol. Therap.* 4:476–79
58. Speiser, P. 1971. *Pharm. Int.* 5:5–16
59. Haleblian, J., McCrone, W. 1969. *J. Pharm. Sci.* 59:911–29
60. Aguiar, A. J. 1969. *Drug Inf. Bull.* 3:17–26

61. Khalil, S. A., Moustafa, M. A., Ebian, A. R., Motawi, M. M. 1972. *J. Pharm. Sci.* 61:1615–17

62. Poole, J. W., Owen, G., Silverio, J., Freyhof, J. N., Rosenman, S. B. 1968. *Curr. Therap. Res.* 10:292–303

63. Levy, G., Gumtow, R. H. 1963. *J. Pharm. Sci.* 52:1139–44

64. Gibaldi, M., Feldman, S. 1970. *J. Pharm. Sci.* 59:579–89

65. Lowenthal, W. 1972. *J. Pharm. Sci.* 61:1695–1711

66. Ritschel, W. A. 1971. *J. Pharm. Sci.* 60:1683–85

67. Levy, G. 1961. *J. Pharm. Sci.* 50:388–92

68. Levy, G., Hollister, L. E. 1964. *NY J. Med.* 64:3002–05

69. Katchen, B., Symchowicz, S. 1969. *J. Pharm. Sci.* 58:1108–11

70. Poole, J. W. 1969. *Drug Inf. Bull.* 3:8–16

71. Weintraub, H., Gibaldi, M. 1970. *J. Pharm. Sci.* 59:1792–96

72. Giles, A. R., Gumma, A. 1973. *Arzneim.-Forsch.* 23:98–100

73. Levy, G. 1963. *J. Pharm. Sci.* 52:1039–46

74. Arnold, K., Gerber, N., Levy, G. 1970. *Can. J. Pharm. Sci.* 5:89–92

75. Barr, W. H., Adir, J., Garrettson, L. 1971. *Clin. Pharmacol. Therap.* 12:779–84

76. Kirby, W. M. M., Roberts, C. E., Burdick, R. E. 1961. *Antimicrob. Agents Chemotherap.*, 286–92

77. Rosenblatt, J. E., Barrett, J. E., Brodie, J. L., Kirby, W. M. M. 1966. *Antimicrob. Agents Chemotherap.*, 134–41

78. Neuvonen, P. J., Gothoni, G., Hackman, R., Björksten, K. 1970. *Brit. Med. J.* 4:532–34

79. Peterson, O. L., Finland, M. 1942. *Am. J. Med. Sci.* 204:581–88

80. Wood, J. H. 1969. *Lancet* ii:212

81. Doluisio, J. T., LaPiana, J. C., Wilkinson, G. R., Dittert, L. W. 1969. *Antimicrob. Agents Chemotherap.* 49–55

82. Crounse, R. G. 1961. *J. Invest. Dermatol.* 37:529–33

83. McGilveray, I. J., Mattok, G. L. 1972. *J. Pharm. Pharmacol.* 24:615–19

84. Jaffe, J. M., Colaizzi, J. L., Barry, H. 1971. *J. Pharm. Sci.* 60:1646–50

85. Parrott, E. L. 1970. In *Prescription Pharmacy*, ed. J. B. Sprowls Jr., 103–62. Philadelphia:Lippincott. 2nd ed. 662 pp.

86. Prescott, L. F. 1969. *Lancet* ii:1239–43

87. Ariëns, E. J. 1969. *J. Mond. Pharm.* 3:263–79

88. Vesell, E. S., Passananti, G. T., Greene, F. E., Page, J. G. 1971. *Ann. NY Acad. Sci.* 179:752–73

89. Larry, P. P., Kitler, M. E. 1971. *Dis. Nerv. Syst.* 32:105–14

90. Dayton, P. G., Perel, J. M. 1971. *Ann. NY Acad. Sci.* 179:67–87

91. Brown, S. S. 1972. *Foreign Compound Metabolism in Mammals*, 2:456–74. London: Chem. Soc.

92. Morrelli, H. F., Melmon, K. L. 1968. *Calif. Med.* 109:380–89

93. Eisen, M. J. 1964. *J. Am. Med. Assoc.* 189:64–65

94. Brodie, B. B. 1965. *Proc. Roy. Soc. Med.* 58:946–55

95. Aggeler, P. M., O'Reilly, R. A., Leong, L., Kowitz, P. E. 1967. *New Engl. J. Med.* 276:496–501

96. Hartshorn, E. A. 1968. *Drug Intell. Clin. Pharm.* 2:58–66

97. Sellers, E. M., Koch-Weser, J. 1971. *Ann. NY Acad. Sci.* 179:212–25

98. Conney, A. H. 1967. *Pharmacol. Rev.* 19:317–66

99. Breckenridge, A., Orme, M. 1971. *Ann. NY Acad. Sci.* 179:421–31

100. Hartshorn, E. A. 1968. *Drug Intell. Clin. Pharm.* 2:174–80

101. Gibaldi, M., Feldman, S. 1969. *J. Pharm. Sci.* 58:1477–80

102. Gibaldi, M., Boyes, R. N., Feldman, S. 1971. *J. Pharm. Sci.* 60:1338–40

103. Gibaldi, M., Feldman, S. 1972. *Eur. J. Pharmacol.* 19:323–29

104. Rowland, M. 1972. *J. Pharm. Sci.* 61:70–74

105. Dollery, C. T., Davies, D. S., Conolly, M. E. 1971. *Ann. NY Acad. Sci.* 179:108–14

106. Beckett, A. H., Kourounakis, P., Vaughan, D. P., Mitchard, M. 1970. *J. Pharm. Pharmacol.* Suppl. 22:169–74

107. Coldwell, B. B., Boyd, E. M. 1966. *Can. J. Physiol. Pharmacol.* 44: 909–18

108. Campagna, F. A., Cureton, G., Mirigian, R. A., Nelson, E. 1963. *J. Pharm. Sci.* 52:605–6

109. Lozinski, E. 1960. *Can. Med. Assoc. J.* 83:177–78

110. Freestone, D. S. 1969. *Lancet* ii:98–99

111. Glazko, A. J., Kinkel, A. W., Alegnani, W. C., Holmes, E. L. 1968. *Clin. Pharmacol. Therap.* 9:472–83

112. Bell, H. et al 1971. *Pharmacology* 5:108–20

113. Lindenbaum, J., Mellow, M. H., Blackstone, M. O., Butler, V. P. Jr. 1971. *New Engl. J. Med.* 285:1344–47

114. *Lancet* 1972. ii:311–12

115. MacLeod, C. et al 1972. *Can. Med. Assoc. J.* 107:203–9
116. Searl, R. O., Pernarowski, M. 1967. *Can. Med. Assoc. J.* 96:1513–20
117. Wagner, J. G., Welling, P. G., Lee, K. P., Walker, J. E. 1971. *J. Pharm. Sci.* 60:666–77
118. Langlois, Y., Gagnon, M. A., Tétreault, L. 1972. *J. Clin. Pharmacol.* 12:196–200
119. Van Petten, G. R., Becking, G. C., Withey, R. J., Lettau, H. F. 1971. *J. Clin. Pharmacol.* 11:27–34
120. Van Petten, G. R., Becking, G. C., Withey, R. J., Lettau, H. F. 1971. *J. Clin. Pharmacol.* 11:35–41
121. Brice, G. W., Hammer, H. F. 1969. *J. Am. Med. Assoc.* 308:1189–90
122. MacDonald, H., Pisano, F., Burger, J., Dornbush, A., Pelcak, E. 1969. *Drug Inf. Bull.* 3:76–81
123. Blair, D. C., Barnes, R. W., Wildner, E. L., Murray, W. J. 1971. *J. Am. Med. Assoc.* 215:251–54
124. Barr, W. H., Gerbracht, L. M., Letcher, K., Plaut, M., Strahl, N. 1972. *Clin. Pharmacol. Therap.* 13: 97–108
125. Van Petten, G. R., Feng, H., Withey, R. J., Lettau, H. F. 1971. *J. Clin. Pharmacol.* 11:177–86
126. Mattok, G. L., McGilveray, I. J. 1972. *J. Pharm. Sci.* 61:746–49
127. Gelber, R., Jacobsen, P., Levy, L. 1969. *Clin. Pharmacol. Therap.* 10:841–48
128. Withey, R. J., Van Petten, G. R., Lettau, H. F. 1972. *J. Clin. Pharmacol.* 12:190–95
129. Hamlin, W. E., Nelson, E., Ballard, B. E., Wagner, J. G. 1962. *J. Pharm. Sci.* 51:432–35
130. Levy, G., Leonards, J. R., Procknal, J. A. 1967. *J. Pharm. Sci.* 56:1365–67
131. Garrett, E. R. 1971. *Acta Pharmacol. Toxicol.* 29, Suppl. 3:1–29
132. Mattok, G. L., Hossie, R. D., McGilveray, I. J. 1972. *Can. J. Pharm. Sci.* 7:84–87
133. Smolen, V. F. 1969. *Hosp. Pharm.* 4: 14–16
134. Ipsen, J. 1971. *Curr. Therap. Res.* 13: 193–208
135. Withey, R. J., Feng, H., Cook, D., Van Petten, G. R., Lettau, H. F., 1971. *J. Clin. Pharmacol.* 11:187–95
136. Falch, D., Teien, A., Bjerkelund, C. J. 1973. *Brit. Med. J.* 1:695–97
137. Sorby, D. L., Tozer, T. N. 1973. *Drug Intell. Clin. Pharm.* 7:78–83
138. Lindenbaum, J., Butler, V. P. Jr., Murphy, J. E., Cresswell, R. M. 1973. *Lancet* ii:1215–17
139. Wagner, J. G. et al 1973. *J. Am. Med. Assoc.* 224:199–204

MOVEMENT OF DRUGS ❖6580
ACROSS THE GILLS OF FISHES

Joseph B. Hunn and John L. Allen
Fish Control Laboratory, La Crosse, Wisconsin

INTRODUCTION

The physiochemical properties of drugs that influence their movement across biological membranes are fairly well established and include lipid solubility, water solubility, degree of ionization, chemical stability, and molecular weight. In general, any substance that is distinctly charged, or is otherwise fat-insoluble, and has a molecular weight in excess of 100 is almost certain to be virtually excluded from entering cells from the outside unless the particular cell is equipped with a specific transport system for this class of substance (Le Fevre 1).

Historically, much of our knowledge about drug absorption was developed using plant and animal cells. Experimentation on whole animals has mainly been centered on homeotherms with little work on poikilotherms, especially the fishes. The available literature on fishes deals essentially with the influence of lipid solubility on movement of drugs across the gills. Much of the work we reveiw was not performed to study drug dynamics in fishes per se but to evaluate chemicals for use in fisheries. With these limitations in mind, we attempt to use data on toxicity, efficacy, and residues of three chemicals—a weak base (MS-222), a base (quinaldine), and an acid (TFM)—to show that both lipid solubility and degree of ionization play a significant role in the movement of these compounds across the gills of fishes.

FISH: THE EXPERIMENTAL ANIMAL

Fish have been used as experimental animals since the eighteenth century (Nigrelli 2). More recently, fish and goldfish *(Carassius auratus)* in particular have been used in testing the toxicity and pharmacologic properties of drugs (Powers 3, Cutting et al 4, Levy & Gucinski 5, Levy & Miller 6, Gibaldi & Nightingale 7, Nightingale & Gibaldi 8).

One of the major difficulties in using fish as test animals is quality control, especially when they are taken directly from the wild. One normally has to assume a fish is healthy if it shows no overt symptoms of disease and if its behavior is "normal" under the circumstances in which it is held (Hunn et al 9). In working

47

with goldfish, many authors equate size of fish with age. This does not, however, assure that the fish are the same chronological age, because they may be stunted intentionally during culture to keep them of marketable size over various periods of time.

Wild fish are inadvertently exposed to various xenobiotics in their environment that can influence the level of drug-metabolizing enzymes (De Waide 10). On the other hand, species raised under intensive culture may be deliberately exposed to various chemicals such as therapeutic agents, used to control parasites or bacterial infections, and herbicides used to control algae, etc. Many times it is difficult, if not impossible, to get information concerning chemical treatments the fish have been subjected to during their life.

Blood flow through the gills of fishes is variable and can be influenced by the pharmacologic action of the drug being taken up. In vitro studies by Steen & Kruysse (11) and Richards & Fromm (12) have demonstrated a variable shunt system with regulation of filamental and lamellar flow by vasoconstriction and vasodilation. Fromm et al (13) showed that the rate of fluid flow in isolated-perfused gill of rainbow trout *(Salmo gairdneri)* could be reduced as much as 24% by the commonly used anesthetic tricane methanesulfonate (MS-222). Indeed, various studies including those of Houston et al (14) indicate that MS-222 does influence the cardiovascular and respiratory system to the extent that the uptake of the drugs would be affected through reduced blood flow and movement of water across the gills. The movement of the drug across the gills, therefore, should be studied with the possibility in mind that its pharmacological action may well influence the rate of uptake.

A disturbing aspect of the methods used in testing drugs against fish is the use of distilled water as a test medium. Most fish, especially goldfish, are held in tap water or well water that is similar in chemical composition to the water in which they were cultured. Although the fish are hyperosmotic to this medium, it does not impart the osmotic stress that transfer to distilled water does. The use of reconstituted water of known composition that can be buffered to a desired pH is certainly more desirable than distilled water (Marking 15).

LIPID-SOLUBLE DRUGS

Since the turn of the century, investigators have shown that many drugs appeared to penetrate cells by diffusion at rates that could be correlated with their solubility in fat solvents. In addition, evidence has accumulated that indicates that the unionized form of most drugs is the form which penetrates the cell membranes most readily. Despite some well-documented exceptions (Keberle 16), the passage of drugs across cell membranes is governed mainly by physical processes and is predictable from the pK_a and lipid solubility of the drug.

MS-222: A Weak Base

The methanesulfonate of *meta*-aminobenzoic acid ethyl ester has been used to anesthetize poikilothermic vertebrates for over 40 years (Schoettger 17). But only recently have there been attempts to understand the pharmacodynamics of this drug. In the 1960s the toxicity of MS-222 was defined under controlled conditions for four freshwater salmonids and an ictalurid (Marking 18, Schoettger et al 19). Residues of free and acetylated MS-222 were measured in these species following anesthesia using a modified Bratton-Marshall method (Walker & Schoettger 20). This method of analysis did not distinguish whether or not the residue was an acid or an ester. The residue studies indicated that the drug was eliminated rapidly by these fish, after transfer to fresh water.

In 1968 a study on the marine dogfish, *Squalus acanthias,* established some interesting concepts about the physical properties of MS-222 as well as the routes of excretion following injection (Maren et al 21). The pK_a of MS-222 was determined to be 3.5, and the partition coefficient using chloroform:water buffered to pH 7.4 was 312, a very high lipid solubility.

A divided box technique was used to separate gill excretion from urinary excretion in dogfish injected intraperitoneally (ip) with MS-222 at the rate of 21 mg/kg. During a 170 min postinjection period, 26,000 μg were excreted across the gills compared to 10 μg in the urine, thus indicating that the gills were the major route of excretion. Using data from the divided-box experiment, the authors calculated a plasma half-life of the drug of 4 hr. This calculation assumed excretion only via the gill, as their data had shown that the renal contribution was negligible. The actual plasma half-life in free-swimming fish was found to be about 1.5 hr, suggesting that excretory mechanisms other than gill or renal function were involved. Biotransformation, biliary excretion, and/or increased blood flow through the gills during swimming could not be ruled out, as they were not investigated. This study did establish, however, that diffusion across the gill, not renal excretion, was the major route of elimination of MS-222 following ip injection. Passage of the lipid-soluble free base through the gill could be expected, as only 0.01% of the MS-222 would be ionized at body pH.

Hunn et al (22) using rainbow trout, *Salmo gairdneri,* found that MS-222 does indeed cross the gills of fishes in either direction. Trout were anesthetized in a 100-mg/liter solution of MS-222, and the excretion of the drug was followed for 24 hr. Whole blood concentrations of the free drug in trout, after 2.0–2.5 min in the anesthetic bath, reached about 74% of the bath concentration. Blood concentrations of MS-222 declined rapidly during the postanesthesia period in fresh water and reached background levels in 8 hr. In trout given ip injections of MS-222 (10 mg/kg), only 15–21% of the dose was excreted via the kidney during 24 hr, postinjection. Injection of 10 to 100 mg/kg ip had no anesthetizing action on the trout. Using data from these studies, the authors indicated that the major route of elimination was extrarenal, presumabaly via the gills. Thus, MS-222 moves rapidly across the gills during the short anesthetization period and given ip in doses as great as 100 mg/kg, it did not induce anesthesia.

The rapid movement of MS-222 across the gills of channel catfish *(Ictalurus punctatus)* was observed during experiments designed to measure brain concentrations of the drug necessary to induce anesthesia (Hunn 23). Catfish were exposed to a 200 mg/liter solution of MS-222 at 17°C for up to 11 min. These fish exhibited loss of equilibrium after 1 min, loss of reflex in 3 min, and were approaching medullary collapse in 11 min. Whole blood concentrations of free drug were 35% of that of the anesthetic bath in 0.5 min and 50% in 1 min. At loss of reflex, the concentration averaged about 70% of that of the anesthetic solution. Brain tissue at loss of reflex contained the highest average concentration of all brain samples taken during the 11 min exposure. Catfish placed into fresh water after 3 min of exposure to a 200 mg/liter solution of MS-222 righted themselves in 2–3 min and were actively swimming in 8 min. The estimated whole blood half-life of free MS-222 in those fish was 6 min. This study again shows the rapid rate of movement of this drug across the gills of fishes. Further studies on nine other species of freshwater fishes confirmed the observations made on the uptake of the drug by channel catfish (Hunn 24).

Studies on anesthesia of brook trout, *Salvelinus fontinalis,* also revealed rapid movement of MS-222 into the blood following immersion in an anesthetic bath at temperatures as low as 3.5°C. Clearance of the anesthetic from the blood was estimated to be 90% in 55 min at 5°C (Houston & Woods 25).

Investigation of the pharmacology of MS-222 in *Squalus acanthias* confirms that the drug can move across the gills of fishes in either direction with great facility (Stenger & Maren 26). This study also shows that the time course of anesthesia is best correlated with the level of free drug in arterial blood. The authors also conclude that MS-222 has a local anesthetic action.

These studies on MS-222 revealed that the drug probably moves across the gills of fishes by diffusion. The rate of diffusion is rapid and apparently associated with high lipid solubility of the free base and the concentration gradient. Other factors influencing the movement of the drug and ultimate equilibration are biotransformation, tissue distribution, plasma protein binding, and renal and biliary excretion. Biotransformation of MS-222 is evident in the appearance in blood and tissues of the hydrolysis product (free acid) as well as in the acetylated amino congener. Preliminary work in this laboratory indicates that the gallbladder may be a site of accumulation of the acid metabolite(s). Species differences in ability to cleave the ester bond of MS-222 also are evident (Luhning 27). Apparently renal excretion of MS-222 or its acetylated derivative is minor; however, the kidney is the major route for elimination of acid metabolites. This deserves further study as most evidence is still circumstantial. In addition, the dymamics of the drug and its metabolites in bile need illumination.

Quinaldine: A Base

The potential of quinaldine (2-methylquinoline) as a fish anesthetic was first reported by Muench (28) in 1958. Greenough (29) patented a fish transport medium containing a buffer, an antibiotic, and quinaldine. Schoettger & Julin (30) evaluated the efficacy of quinaldine as an anesthetic for seven species of fish. In their report they cited a survey of chemicals used at national fish hatcheries that indicated quinaldine had been used as an anesthetic for a wide variety of fish. They reported that quinaldine concentrations of 15 or 16 mg/liter rapidly induced loss of equilibrium in trout and that 15 to 30 mg/liter are effective on channel catfish, bluegill

(Lepomis macrochirus), and largemouth bass *(Micropterus salmoides)*. They reported that its major assets include rapid action and prolonged maintenance of anesthesia. However, fish retain a degree of reflex responsiveness.

Baldridge (31) reported in 1969 that quinaldine produced rapid anesthesia in young lemon sharks, *Negaprion brevirostris,* and that recovery was rapid. The following year Trams & Brown (32) found that quinaldine tended to be more concentrated in shark tissues of high lipid content than in muscle or whole blood. Their studies also showed fast uptake of quinaldine from bath solutions and rapid recovery of the sharks from anesthesia following withdrawal from the drug. Brown et al (33) reported rapid uptake of quinaldine by sharks with the highest concentrations found in the brain. They also reported that routes of entrance of quinaldine other than the gill cannot be excluded. They found that an electric eel exposed to 0.5 mmol/liter of quinaldine absorbed the drug at a rate of 4.3 μmol/min. The authors (33) suggest that the gills of this species would not function in the drug absorption process; they therefore concluded that drug uptake proceeded through the integument.

Sills & Harman (34) reported that quinaldine produced rapid anesthesia in striped bass, *Morone saxatilis.* Concentrations of 25 to 55 mg/liter of quinaldine produced loss of equilibrium within 2–5 min. Striped bass exposed to 40 mg/liter of quinaldine for 10 min were analyzed by gas chromatography and were found to contain muscle residues of 2.13 mg/kg. The fish recovered rapidly from anesthesia, and the half-life of the quinaldine residue in muscle was approximately 1 hr. Sills et al (35) found that muscle residues of quinaldine in ten species of coldwater and warmwater fish followed the same general pattern as that found in striped bass.

Unpublished work at our laboratory demonstrates that largemouth bass exposed to 30 mg/liter of quinaldine for 15 min accumulate the highest concentrations (25.4 μg/g) of quinaldine residue in the brain. Brain concentrations of quinaldine after 15 min of withdrawal of fresh water were 4.8 μg/g. Rainbow trout exposed to 1 mg/liter of quinaldine for 12 hr had plasma concentration of 3.1 μg/ml. The plasma concentrations decreased to 0.4 μg/ml after 4 hr of withdrawal from the anesthetic. Two channel catfish were catheterized and exposed to 25 mg/liter of quinaldine sulfate in a metabolism chamber with a flow of 1200 ml/min for 1 hr. Urine collected during 3 hr after termination of the exposure contained 2.7 and 1.8 μg of quinaldine/ml, while those collected 8 hr after termination of exposure contained 1.7 and 0.4 μg of quinaldine/ml. No quinaldine was detected in the urine collected 11 and 24 hr after termination of the exposure. When rainbow trout were exposed to 15 mg/liter of quinaldine sulfate for 30 min, the bile contained 25.7 μg/ml quinaldine residue, which was approximately twice the plasma concentration. The small amount of quinaldine excreted in the urine indicates this is not a major route of excretion of quinaldine. Also, no large concentration of quinaldine has been found in the gallbladder bile. These samples were analyzed by the gas chromatographic and ultraviolet spectrophotometric methods of Allen & Sills (36, 37). Some metabolites would not be detected by these methods. These studies indicate that quinaldine probably moves outward across the gills of fishes by diffusion. Other possible routes of elimination of the drug include renal excretion and biotransformation, although renal excretion of quinaldine appears to be a minor route of elimination of the drug and no metabolites of quinaldine have been found as yet. The drug appears to be excreted in its original form. However, this should be investigated further with ^{14}C-labeled quinaldine.

Schoettger & Julin (30) reported an effect of pH on the efficacy of the anesthetic in 1969. The drug was completely ineffective as an anesthetic on seven species of fish tested at pH 5.0. Also, when smallmouth bass, *Micropterus dolomieui,* were anesthetized with 20 mg/liter of quinaldine at pH 7.0, they recovered from anesthesia within 20 to 25 min after the pH was lowered to 5.0. Channel catfish were not affected by exposure to 50 or 60 mg/liter of quinaldine for 1 hr at pH 5.0. However, when the pH of the former solution was raised to 7.0 and that of the latter to 10.3, the fish were narcotized in 3 to 10 min. Marking (38) noted that quinaldine is more toxic to fish in soft water than in hard water and that the soft water used had a lower pH than hard water. Sills & Allen (39) in 1971 correlated the effect of pH on the efficacy and residues of quinaldine with the ionization constant of quinaldine ($pK_a = 5.42$). Quinaldine was partitioned between hexane and aqueous solutions at pH 4, 5, 6, 7, and 8. The percent of quinaldine found in the hexane at each pH compared very closely with the percent quinaldine existing in the free base form as calculated from the pK_a.

Sills & Allen (39) also demonstrated that the muscle residue of quinaldine in largemouth bass exposed to 35 mg/liter of quinaldine for 15 min was lower at pH 5 (2.15 μg/g) than at pH 7 (5.37 μg/g) or pH 8 (4.89 μg/g). Calculating the amount of quinaldine-free base available in aqueous solutions at pH 5.0, they were able to anesthetize largemouth bass using 125 mg/liter quinaldine (34.4 mg/liter of quinaldine-free base). The residue of quinaldine found in the muscle of these fish (3.91 μg/g) was comparable with the quinaldine residue found in the muscle of those fish exposed to the anesthetic at pH 7 and 8. At the lower pH, 72.5% of the quinaldine is protonated and exists as the lipid-insoluble quinaldinium ion that does not readily cross the gill membrane. At pH 7, 97.4% of the quinaldine is in the lipid-soluble free base form. The biological activity of this compound in fish is altered drastically by the pH of the media in which they are exposed. The effect of the ionic equilibrium of the molecule does not, however, affect efficacy of the compound in most situations where it is used. The efficacy, toxicity, and residues of the chemical all indicate that the lipid-soluble free base of quinaldine is the form that passes across the gills of fishes.

TFM: An Acid

The selective larval lampricide 3-trifluormethyl-4-nitrophenol (TFM) is used to control the sea lamprey *(Petromyzon marinus)* in the Great Lakes (Schnick 40). Work at this laboratory to retain the registered use of this compound has involved studies on the toxicity to and residues in nontarget fishes. The toxicity of TFM to chinook salmon *(Oncorhynchus tshawytscha)* is greater in soft water than in hard water, and is pH dependent (Table 1). Similar results were obtained with six other freshwater species of fish (Marking & Olson, unpublished). Safety of the compound to fish can be predicted knowing the pK_a (TFM—6.07) and the LC50 at a particular

Table 1 Toxicity of TFM (35.7%) to fingerling chinook salmon at selected temperatures, hardnesses, and pH's in reconstituted water

Temp. (°C)	Water hardness	pH	LC50 and 95% confidence interval (μl/l) at	
			24 hr	96 hr
7	soft	7.5	6.22 5.51–7.03	4.27 3.89–4.69
12	soft	7.5	5.98 5.09–7.03	4.20 3.52–5.02
17	soft	7.5	5.38 4.83–5.99	3.54 3.19–3.92
12	very soft	6.6	3.68 3.20–4.23	1.94 1.62–2.33
12	hard	7.8	16.0 15.2–18.7	10.0 8.98–11.1
12	very hard	8.2	41.5 36.0–47.8	19.0 16.2–22.2
12	soft[a]	6.5	3.12 2.77–3.52	2.45 2.16–2.77
12	soft[a]	8.5	33.4 28.9–38.6	18.0 15.4–21.0
12	soft[a]	9.5	254 215–300	171 154–190

[a]Buffered reconstituted water after Marking (15).

pH. The effect of pH on the toxicity of TFM, therefore, appears correlated with the concentration of lipid-soluble free phenol. This observation is supported further by the partitioning of TFM between an organic solvent, chloroform or hexane, and aqueous buffers between pH's 4 and 9. The amount of TFM in the organic phase followed closely the amounts of free phenol at various pH's.

Residues of TFM in the muscle tissue of fish exposed to the lampricide at various pH's also reflect the unavailability of free phenol at high pH's (Figure 1). For example, when channel catfish were exposed to a 1 mg/liter solution of TFM (18.5°C) for 12 hr at pH's 6, 7, 8, and 9, the free TFM residues in muscle were 3.21, 1.5, 0.33, and 0.03 μg/g, respectively.

Biotransformation probably also plays a role in the movement of TFM across the gills of trout. Lech & Costrini (41) and Lech (42) demonstrated that the major metabolite of TFM in rainbow trout is the glucuronide conjugate which is excreted largely in the bile. Hunn & Allen (unpublished) exposed rainbow trout to a 5 mg/liter solution of TFM in well water at 12°C for 15, 30, 45, 60, and 120 min.

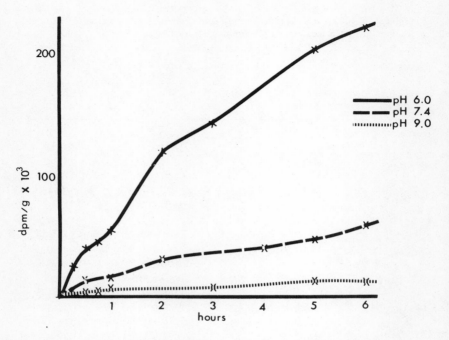

Figure 1 The uptake of ^{3}H-labeled TFM by rainbow trout at three pH's on a whole fish basis.

The concentration of free TFM in the gallbladder bile was 4.12 μg/ml after 120 min while the concentration of TFM glucuronide rose to 196 μg/ml during the same period. The plasma concentration of free TFM was 2.73 μg/ml after 120 min while the glucuronide concentration was 0.87 μg/ml. The rapid rise in accumulation of glucuronide in the bile started between 45 and 60 min of exposure (14 μg/ml to 55 μg/ml). Biotransformation of TFM to the water-soluble glucuronide would reduce its passage across the gills.

No attempts have been made to measure the movement of TFM back across the gills following exposure to the lampricide, although one might predict that outward diffusion may be slower than with the basic compounds discussed previously, because TFM exists mostly as the phenolate ion at the pH of blood. In spite of this, TFM is promptly cleared from fish muscle during 24 hr of recovery in fresh water, and the half-time of free TFM in blood of rainbow trout injected with 2.5 mg/kg TFM ip was shown to be 0.78 hr (Lech et al 43). It is interesting to note that during the rapid decline in free TFM blood levels of ip-injected trout, a large percentage of the injected dose is recovered in bile as the glucuronide conjugate (Lech et al 43). This phenomenon may be related to the lack of rapid gill diffusion due to the presence of high levels of the phenolate ion in blood with subsequent presentation of relatively large amounts of TFM to the kidney and liver for conjugation and excretion via the biliary and urinary routes.

TFM, then, is an example of a phenolic compound whose movement across the gills is influenced both by the pH of the medium the fish is exposed in as well as by the biotransformation and excretion of a metabolite of the parent compound.

ACKNOWLEDGMENTS

The authors wish to thank Dr. John J. Lech of the Medical College of Wisconsin for his encouragement and use of unpublished data.

Literature Cited

1. Le Fevre, P. G. 1972. *Absorption, Distribution, Transformation and Excretion of Drugs*, ed. P. K. Knoefel, 5–38. Springfield: Thomas. 210 pp.
2. Nigrelli, R. F. 1953. *Trans. NY Acad. Sci.* 15:183–86
3. Powers, E. B. 1917. *Ill. Biol. Monogr.* 2:7–73
4. Cutting, W., Baslow, M., Read, D., Furst, A. 1959. *J. Clin. Exp. Psychopathol.* 20:26–32
5. Levy, G., Gucinski, S. P. 1964. *J. Pharmacol. Exp. Ther.* 146:80–86
6. Levy, G., Miller, K. E. 1965. *J. Pharm. Sci.* 54:1319–24
7. Gibaldi, M., Nightingale, C. H. 1968. *J. Pharm. Sci.* 57:226–30
8. Nightingale, C. H., Gibaldi, M. 1971. *J. Pharm. Sci.* 60:1360–63
9. Hunn, J. B., Schoettger, R. A., Whealdon, E. W. 1968. *Prog. Fish Cult.* 30:164–67
10. De Waide, J. H. 1971. *Metabolism of Xenobiotics.* Drukkerij Leijn: Nijmegen. 164 pp.
11. Steen, J. B., Kruysse, A. 1974. *Comp. Biochem. Physiol.* 12:127–42
12. Richards, B. D., Fromm, P. O. 1969. *Comp. Biochem. Physiol.* 29:1063–70
13. Fromm, P. O., Richards, B. D., Hunter, R. C. 1971. *Prog. Fish Cult.* 33:138–40
14. Houston, A. H., Madden, J. A., Woods, R. J., Miles, H. M. 1971. *J. Fish. Res. Bd. Can.* 28:625–33
15. Marking, L. L. 1969. *Bull. Wildlife Disease Assoc.* 5:291–94
16. Keberle, H. 1971. *Acta Pharmacol. Toxicol.* 29:30–47
17. Schoettger, R. A. 1967. *US Bur. Sport Fish. Wildl. Invest. Fish Contr.* 16:1–15
18. Marking, L. L. 1967. *US Bur. Sport Fish. Wildl. Invest. Fish Contr.* 12:1–10
19. Schoettger, R. A., Walker, C. R., Marking, L. L. 1967. *US Bur. Sport Fish. Wildl. Invest. Fish Contr.* 17:1–14
20. Walker, C. R., Schoettger, R. A. 1967. *US Bur. Sport Fish. Wildl. Invest. Fish Contr.* 14:1–10
21. Maren, T. H., Embry, R., Broder, L. E. 1968. *Comp. Biochem. Physiol.* 26:853–64
22. Hunn, J. B., Schoettger, R. A., Willford, W. A. 1968. *J. Fish. Res. Bd. Can.* 25:25–31
23. Hunn, J. B. 1968. *US Bur. Sport Fish. Wildl. Resour. Publ.* 64:119–20
24. Hunn, J. B. 1970. *US Bur. Sport Fish. Wildl. Invest. Fish Contr.* 42:1–8
25. Houston, A. H., Woods, R. J. 1972. *J. Fish. Res. Bd. Can.* 29:1344–46
26. Stenger, V. G., Maren, T. H. 1973. In press
27. Luhning, C. W. In press
28. Muench, B. 1958. *Prog. Fish Cult.* 20:42–44
29. Greenough, E. E. 1963. Patent No. 3,110,285
30. Schoettger, R. A., Julin, A. M. 1969. *US Bur. Sport Fish. Wildl. Invest. Fish Contr.* 22:1–10
31. Baldridge, D. H. Jr. 1969. *Bull. Mar. Sci.* 19:880–96
32. Trams, E. G., Brown, E. A. B. 1970. *Life Sci.* 9:27–35
33. Brown, E. A. B., Franklin, J. E., Pratt, E., Trams, E. G. 1972. *Comp. Biochem. Physiol.* 42A:223–31
34. Sills, J. B., Harman, P. D. 1970. *Proc. Southeast. Assoc. Game Fish Comm.* 24:546–49
35. Sills, J. B., Allen, J. L., Harman, P. D., Luhning, C. W. In press
36. Allen, J. L., Sills, J. B. 1970. *JAOAC* 53:20–23
37. Allen, J. L., Sills, J. B. 1970. *JAOAC* 53:1170–71
38. Marking, L. L. 1969. *US Bur. Sport Fish. Wildl. Invest. Fish Contr.* 23:1–10
39. Sills, J. B., Allen, J. L. 1971. *Trans. Am. Fish. Soc.* 100:544–45
40. Schnick, R. A. 1972. *U.S. Bur. Sport Fish. Wildl. Invest. Fish Contr.* 44:1–31
41. Lech, J. J., Costrini, N. V. 1972. *Comp. Gen. Pharmacol.* 3:160–66
42. Lech, J. J. 1973. *Toxicol. Appl. Pharmacol.* 24:114–24
43. Lech, J. J., Pepple, S., Anderson, J. 1973. *Toxicol. Appl. Pharmacol.* 25:542–52

NEW ASPECTS OF THE MODE OF ACTION OF NONSTEROID ANTI-INFLAMMATORY DRUGS

❖6581

S. H. Ferreira[1] *and J. R. Vane*[1]

Department of Pharmacology, Royal College of Surgeons, London, England

This review surveys recent work on the possible mode of action and on the effects of that group of drugs variously known as non-narcotic analgesics, nonsteroidal anti-inflammatory drugs, aspirin-like drugs, antiphlogistic acids, and so on. These drugs show, to a greater or lesser degree, the therapeutic properties of reducing pain, inflammation, and fever and the side effects of causing gastrointestinal irritation and renal pathology. Some aspects of the pharmacology of these drugs have previously been reviewed in this series (1, 2).

MECHANISM OF ACTION

Several different hypotheses have been advanced to explain the actions of aspirin-like drugs. These include an interference with oxidative phosphorylation (3), the displacement of an endogenous anti-inflammatory peptide from plasma protein (4–6), interference with the migration of leucocytes (7, 8), inhibition of leucocytic-phagocytosis (9), stabilization of lysosomal membranes (10), inhibition of the generation of lipoperoxides (11), and hyperpolarization of neuronal membranes (12–14). Recently, interest in this field was stimulated enormously by the discovery (15–17) that aspirin-like drugs inhibit the synthesis of prostaglandins. This discovery disclosed a mechanism of action of aspirin-like drugs and coincidentally provided a valuable way of exploring the involvement of prostaglandins in other pathological and physiological processes. In the first of the three papers Vane (15) tested aspirin-like drugs as direct inhibitors of prostaglandin synthetase, using a cell-free preparation of prostaglandin synthetase that synthesized radioactive prostaglandin E_2 and $F_{2\alpha}$ from tritium-labelled arachidonic acid (18). Indomethacin, aspirin, and salicy-

[1]Present address: Wellcome Research Laboratories, Langley Court, Beckenham, Kent, England.

late strongly inhibited the synthesis of prostaglandins. Concurrently, Smith & Willis (16), using human platelets, tested their own hypothesis that aspirin-like drugs interfere with prostaglandin production, perhaps by inhibiting phospholipase. Aspirin had no effect on platelet phospholipase activity but reduced prostaglandin release, as did indomethacin. Since prostaglandins cannot be detected in platelets before thrombin treatment, they deduced that aspirin was interfering with prostaglandin production. Ferreira et al (17) confirmed the results in a more complex system, the dog perfused spleen, which released prostaglandins when contracted by either catecholamines or nerve stimulation. This release, also due to fresh synthesis of prostaglandins, was abolished by indomethacin.

POTENCY OF ASPIRIN-LIKE DRUGS AGAINST PROSTAGLANDIN PRODUCTION

Since those three pioneering papers, the inhibitory action of aspirin-like drugs on prostaglandin production has been amply confirmed and demonstrated in almost all laboratory species and many other biological preparations (Table 1), using a variety of assay techniques ranging from bioassay through radiometric, spectrophotometric, polarographic, chromatographic, to mass-spectrometric. Several interesting points have emerged, associated both with the absolute and relative potencies of the aspirin-like drugs.

Absolute Potencies

The absolute potency of the anti-inflammatory drugs against prostaglandin synthetase varies with the enzyme preparation used and the experimental conditions. On enzyme from bovine seminal vesicles (51, 52) ID_{50} concentrations for indomethacin were 10–100 times greater than those on synthetase from dog spleen or guinea pig lung. But the concentrations of arachidonic acid substrate used were also 15–30 times higher and the ID_{50} of indomethacin against sheep seminal vesicle enzyme varies directly with the substrate concentration (52). Since prostaglandin generation can be detected at much lower concentrations by bioassay than by chemical or physicochemical assay, absolute potency of aspirin-like drugs may also appear to vary with the type of assay used. Another factor that seems to influence activity is the way in which the enzyme is prepared. For instance, fluorindomethacin (38) and indomethacin (41) competitively inhibit microsomal enzyme preparations from sheep and bovine seminal vesicles; in contrast, on acetone-dried powder preparation of sheep vesicular glands, the inhibitory effect was irreversible and increased by pre-incubation (39)

Relative Potencies

The potencies of aspirin-like drugs as prostaglandin synthetase inhibitors, calculated on a molar basis relative to aspirin $= 1$, are presented in Table 2. In general, the overall rank order of potency is independent of the enzyme preparation, although there are some minor variations (even when the same preparation is used). However, there is a tremendous variation in the relative activities of aspirin and indomethacin

Table 1 Preparations in which aspirin or indomethacin have been shown to inhibit prostaglandin synthesis or release

Species	Tissue	Preparation	Reference
Guinea pig	lungs	cell-free homogenates	15
		perfused	19
	whole body	in vivo	20
	uterus	in vitro	21
Dog	spleen	microsomal fraction	22
		chopped	23
		perfused	17
	kidney	in situ	24–26
	brain	cell-free homogenates	27
	platelets	in vivo and in vitro	28
Cat	spleen	perfused	29, 30
	kidney	in vivo	31
	CNS	in vivo	32
Rabbit	jejunum	isolated smooth muscle	33, 34
	brain	cell-free homogenates	27
	kidney	in vivo	35
	eye	in vivo	36
	spleen, kidney, iris-ciliary body, retina	cell-free homogenates	37
Ram	seminal vesicles	microsomal fraction	38
		acetone powder	39
Human	platelets	in vitro	16
		in vivo	16
	semen	in vivo	40
	whole body	in vivo	41
	skin	in vitro	42
	stomach	in vitro	43
Bull	seminal vesicles	microsomal fraction	44
Rat	pregnant uterus	in vitro	45–47
	skin inflammatory exudate	in vivo, in vitro	48
	kidney	in vivo	31
Mouse	tumors	homogenates	49
		tissue culture	50
	brain	freeze dried powder	47
Gerbil	brain	freeze dried powder	47

(the two substances most often studied) from preparation to preparation. On rabbit brain synthetase, for instance, the ratio is 19:1 whereas on bovine seminal vesicles it is 2140:1.

Table 2 Relative potencies of aspirin-like drugs against different preparations of prostaglandin synthetase[a]

Tissue	Guinea pig lung (15)	Dog Spleen (22)	Rabbit brain (27)	Bovine Seminal Vesicles (BSV) (44)	BSV (51)	BSV (52)	Sheep Seminal Vesicles (SSV) (38)	SSV (39)
Drug								
Aspirin[b]	1 [35]	1 [37]	1 [61]	1 [15,000]	1 [820]	1 [9000]	1 [83]	1 [9000]
Ibuprofen					0.7	4.5	55	
Phenylbutazone		5			1.9	6.4	6.6	
Naproxen				150	3.7	24	14	
Pluflenamic acid					17		33	
Mefenamic acid		52			54		40	
Indomethacin	47	217	17	2140	410	236	185	900
Niflumic acid		336				76	68	
Meclofenamic acid		370				692		

[a]Reference numbers are given in parentheses.
[b]For aspirin, the ID_{50} concentrations (μM) are given in brackets.

Despite these variations in potency, inhibition of prostaglandin biosynthesis is clearly a general characteristic of aspirin-like drugs. It also seems to be a unique characteristic, for compounds representing many other types of pharmacological activity were inactive (<10% inhibition at 100 $\mu g/ml$); these included chloroquine, morphine, mepyramine, probenecid, azathioprine, *para*- and *meta*-hydroxybenzoic acid, promethazine, atropine, methysergide, phenoxybenzamine, propranolol, iproniazid, droperidol, chlorpromazine, and disodium cromoglycate. Tetrahydrocannabinol is said to be a prostaglandin synthetase inhibitor in concentrations as low as 10 μM, but the dose/response curve is very flat and the ID_{50} concentration (by extrapolation) is some 500 times higher (53).

ANTI-INFLAMMATORY ACTIVITY

Orally administered drugs have many hazards to face before circulating to a microsomal enzyme and it is therefore surprising to find any relationship between in vitro inhibition of prostaglandin synthetase and the anti-inflammatory activity. Yet for drugs where activities have been compared, the rank order was the same against carrageenin rat paw oedema as against spleen synthetase, except that indomethacin was out of order for the rat paw test (22). An even more striking correlation is shown by studying optical isomers of naproxen and indomethacin analogs. In each instance, the isomer with anti-inflammatory activity also strongly inhibited prostaglandin synthetase, whereas the one with weak anti-inflammatory activity was also weak against the synthetase (38, 44).

Sodium salicylate has only weak activity against prostaglandin synthetase in vitro (15) whereas it is as strong as aspirin in anti-inflammatory tests in vivo (54). A possible explanation of this anomaly was provided by Willis et al (48), who found the prostaglandin content of an inflammatory exudate in the rat was equally reduced by aspirin and sodium salicylate in vivo. However, when a broken cell preparation of the exudate was incubated in vitro, even though aspirin was still effective, salicylate had no action. They suggested (48) that salicylate may be converted in vivo to an active metabolite. Hamberg (41) also found salicylate to be as effective as aspirin against prostaglandin synthetase in man.

The antipyretic drug 4-acetamidophenol (acetaminophen or paracetamol), which is 10 times less effective than aspirin on the dog spleen synthetase, has almost the same potency as aspirin on the brain enzymes (27, 48). Thus, the fact that paracetamol has antipyretic activity without anti-inflammatory activity can be explained by the differential sensitivity of the prostaglandin synthetases from different tissues. There are other examples of differential enzyme inhibition. Fenclozic acid inhibited guinea pig lung prostaglandin synthetase but appeared to stimulate prostaglandin synthesis by mouse ascites tumour homogenates (49). Bhattacherjee & Eakins (37) found a thousandfold variation in the ID_{50} of indomethacin against prostaglandin synthetases from different tissues of the rabbit. One enzyme from the spleen, ID_{50} was $0.05\,\mu g/ml$, from kidney $5.0\ \mu g/ml$, from the iris-ciliary body, $18.5\ \mu g/ml$, and from the retina, $50\ \mu g/ml$. Also of interest is the demonstration of species variation; a much higher dose (per kg) of indomethacin was needed to inhibit total prostaglandin production in guinea pigs (20) than in man (41).

For inhibition of prostaglandin biosynthesis to account for the anti-inflammatory action of aspirin-like drugs, normal therapeutic doses should lead to effective plasma concentrations. Certainly, free plasma concentrations during therapy with several aspirin-like drugs often exceed those needed to inhibit prostaglandin synthetase from dog spleen. Taking indomethacin as an example, the plasma concentration in man reaches $2\ \mu g/ml$. Because of protein binding (which is a property common to many of these drugs) the free plasma concentration would be $0.2\ \mu g/ml$. However, the ID_{50} for indomethacin in dog spleen synthetase is only $0.05\ \mu g/ml$ (22).

That free plasma concentrations are more than sufficient to explain the anti-inflammatory activity by prostaglandin synthetase inhibition has also been shown in man. Therapeutic doses of indomethacin (200 mg daily), aspirin (3 g daily) or salicylate (3 g daily) reduced by 77–98% the output of prostaglandin metabolite in urine (41).

Comparison with Other Proposed Mechanisms of Action of Aspirin-Like Drugs

Inhibition of prostaglandin biosynthesis is clearly achieved by therapeutic doses of aspirin-like drugs. This contrasts with the much higher concentrations (15–$60\ \mu M$) of salicylate needed to uncouple oxidate phosphorylation (55). Similarly, indomethacin gave a 50% inhibition of prostaglandin synthetase at a concentration of $0.17\ \mu M$, whereas as much as $250\ \mu M$ was required to produce 50% inhibition of oxidative phosphorylation in mitochondria (3). In fact, no convincing evidence relating uncoupling potency to anti-inflammatory activity has been obtained (55).

Inhibition of leucocyte phagocytosis (9) also occurs only with high concentrations of these drugs.

Another possible mechanism of action for aspirin-like drugs is the stabilization of lysosomal membranes. However, there is an inverse correlation between potency as anti-inflammatory agents and as stabilizers of lysosomal membranes (10). Furthermore, at doses that inhibit inflammation, some stabilization of the lysosomes might be expected, but in carrageenin exudates there was no consistent change in the content of free β-glucuronidase at a time when prostaglandin synthesis was inhibited by salicylates (48).

Smith and his colleagues (4–6) have shown that L-tryptophan is displaced from serum protein binding sites by anti-inflammatory drugs. They proposed that such drugs act by displacing peptides from their binding sites on serum proteins and that the free form of the peptide protects connective tissues from the effects of inflammatory insults. Confirmation of this hypothesis will depend upon isolating an anti-inflammatory peptide from serum. Thomas & West (56) have shown that crysteine (also an anti-oxidant) reduced an experimental inflammation but obtained no effect with serine or phenylalanyl-phenylalanine.

Interference with migration of leucocytes is no longer a tenable hypothesis, for aspirin and indomethacin affect only migration of monocytes (8, 57) and not of polymorphonuclear cells.

The remaining alternative hypotheses are interference with generation of lipoperoxides (11) and hyperpolarization of neuronal membranes (12, 13). Both of these could be explained by inhibition of prostaglandin synthetase.

Salicylates and other nonsteroid anti-inflammatory drugs inhibit protein biosynthesis in toxic amounts only and at these high plasma concentrations many cellular enzyme systems are blocked. Thus, the symptoms of salicylate intoxication may be the result of inhibition of many important enzymic activities (55).

The release of rabbit aorta contracting substance (RCS) (58) from guinea pig lungs during anaphylaxis is blocked by aspirin and its congeners at concentrations as low as those required to inhibit prostaglandin generation. Several indications, including RCS formation from arachidonic acid (59, 60), its appearance always with prostaglandins (61), its instability (59), and the inhibition of its release by aspirin-like drugs suggested to Gryglewski & Vane (23, 62) that RCS is the cyclic endoperoxide postulated as an unstable intermediate in the biosynthesis of prostaglandins. Recently Hamberg & Samuelsson have isolated the cyclic endoperoxide intermediate and shown that it contracts rabbit aorta (63). These results indicate an interference by aspirin-like drugs at an early stage in the synthesis of prostaglandins. The work of Takeguchi & Sih (51) points in the same direction. Oxidation of the co-factor epinephrine occurs during the transformation of the hydroperoxide to the endoperoxide. This oxidation was inhibited by several aspirin-like drugs. Recently, Flower et al (52) studied the effect of several nonsteroid anti-inflammatory agents on the generation of prostaglandin E_2, $F_{2\alpha}$, D_2, and malondialdehyde by prostaglandin synthetase from bovine seminal vesicles. The ID_{50} concentrations of aspirin-like drugs were mostly similar for all the products, suggesting that they acted prior to formation of the endoperoxide intermediate. An exception was phenylbutazone; at the ID_{50} concentration for prostaglandins E_2 and $F_{2\alpha}$ it had no effect on the formation of either prostaglandin D_2 or malondialdehyde, suggesting that phenylbutazone interferes with the enzymes that convert the cyclic endoperoxide to prostaglandins E_2 and $F_{2\alpha}$.

The Contribution of Prostaglandins to Inflammation

How can we fit the release of prostaglandins into the overall inflammatory process? Certainly we cannot ignore the roles of other known and established mediators, such as histamine, 5-hydroxytryptamine, bradykinin, and slow-reacting substances in anaphylaxis (SRS-A); nor can we adequately review their roles in the space available. For such a review, the reader is referred to Spector & Willoughby (64) and Rocha e Silva & Garcia-Leme (65). Perhaps the most practical way is to outline in general terms the sequence of events, but to concentrate on evidence for the involvement of the prostaglandins. In doing so, we shall develop the idea, propounded by Ferreira (66), that low concentrations of prostaglandins sensitize pain receptors to stimulation by other inflammatory mediators. Such a sensitization may also hold for the other facets of the inflammatory response, such as oedema (67). If it does, the inhibition of prostaglandin biosynthesis by aspirin-like drugs will also seemingly decrease the actions of histamine, bradykinin, and the other mediators.

Release of Chemical Mediators

In different types of inflammation, some mediators may have more prominent roles than others because of the relative sensitivities of the tissues in which they are released. The sequence of mediator release may also be important. For instance, in anaphylactic shock in the lung there is an explosive and simultaneous release of histamine, SRS-A, RCS, and prostaglandins E_2 and $F_{2\alpha}$ (see 19). However, in the inflammatory response to subcutaneous injection of carrageenin in the rat, there is a sequential release (67a). At first there is an output of histamine, which then declines, perhaps because the preformed stores in mast cells have been exhausted. This is followed by bradykinin formation. There is little prostaglandin activity (< 5 ng/ml) until 3 hr after the carrageenin injection but then the concentration gradually rises to an average plateau of 80 ng/ml between 18–24 hr. As the concentration of prostaglandins rose, so did that of histamine, once more reaching more than 1 μg/ml at 24 hr. This secondary release of histamine may be associated with fresh synthesis, for in many situations (68) "nascent histamine" formation has been described, due to increased activity of histidine decarboxylase.

Di Rosa et al (7) used depleting agents or antagonists to study the role of different mediators in rat foot-paw oedema induced by carrageenin. To abolish the first phase of the response, they had to use a combination of antagonists of histamine and 5-hydroxytryptamine or deplete both agents with compound 48/80. A kininogen-depleting agent (cellulose sulfate), presumably preventing formation of bradykinin, depressed the 1.5–2.5 hr oedema. They agreed that prostaglandins were released thereafter and also noted (8) that the "prostaglandin phase" of the oedema (which coincided with the arrival of PMN leucocytes in large numbers) was most susceptible to aspirin-like drugs. Other results (7) suggested that the early phase of turpentine-induced pleurisy in the rat was mainly histamine-mediated and that 5-HT and kinins were much less important in this type of inflammation.

Prostaglandin generation occurs in many forms of damage to the skin, including contact dermatitis (69), inflammation due to ultraviolet light (70), and scalding (71).

The invasion of the inflamed area by PMN cells may also be important for the maintenance of prostaglandin generation (and thereby of the inflammation). Higgs & Youlten (72) showed that phagocytosis was accompanied by prostaglandin release and suggested that this could constitute a control mechanism for further influx of phagocytes, since prostaglandin E_1 is leucotactic (73, 74). Phagocytosis (and therefore leucotaxis) would continue as long as the injurious agent or tissue debris was present.

As in peripheral inflammatory responses, there is a generation of prostaglandin E-like substance in the central nervous system during fever (75).

The Inflammatory Effects of Prostaglandins

ERYTHEMA   Prostaglandins of the E and F series (the ones likely to be generated in inflammation) cause erythema and prostaglandin E_1 is effective at doses as low as 1 ng; for $F_{1\alpha}$ 1 μg is needed (76, 77). There are, however, two features of the vascular effects of prostaglandins not shared by other putative mediators of inflammation. The first is a sustained action and the second is the ability to counteract the vasoconstriction caused by substances such as norepinephrine and angiotensin. The erythema induced by intradermal injection or subdermal infusions (66) illustrates well the long-lasting action of prostaglandins (sometimes up to 10 hr). This long-lasting action confers an important property upon the prostaglandins, in that the appearance and the magnitude of their effects not only depend on the actual concentration but also upon the duration of their release or infusion (66).

In contrast to the long-lasting effects upon cutaneous vessels and superficial veins, the vasodilator actions of prostaglandins on other vascualr beds vanish within a few minutes. However, sometimes, there then remains a long-lasting reduction in response to vasoconstrictor substances (78). It could be that the long duration of prostaglandin erythema in man is partially due to a reduced local reactivity to the sympathetic mediator. In addition to this direct effect on the skin vessels, prostaglandins may also be causing vasodilatation by blockade of the sympathetic control mechanism since prostaglandins are known to inhibit the release of the adrenergic mediator (79). Such a mechanism, however, has not yet been proved to operate in vivo.

OEDEMA   Prostaglandins, like bradykinin, histamine, and 5-hydroxytryptamine, cause increased vascular permeability by inducing vascular leakage at the postcapillary and collecting venules (74). Although most active substances exhibit a general relationship between ability to increase vascular permeability and erythema formation, these effects result from actions on different components of the vessel. Erythema represents a local pooling of blood due to a relaxation of the smooth muscles of the walls of the arterioles and venules, whereas increased vascular permeability is thought to result from the contraction of the venular endothelial cells (80). In fact, prostaglandins, produce vasodilatation more effectively than oedema. Prostaglandin E_1, when compared with histamine in the guinea pig skin, produces a similar degree of erythema (but much longer-lasting) and a smaller wheal (76). Similarly, in man histamine, bradykinin, and prostaglandin E_1 each cause erythema and oedema when injected intradermally. However, prostaglandin E_1 induces long-lasting erythema and a much less pronounced oedema (66). There is no difference in the duration of the increased vascular permeability induced by histamine or prostaglandin (81).

Prostaglandins E_1, E_2, and A_2, but not $F_{2\alpha}$ caused oedema when injected into the hind paws of rats (82). Prostaglandin E_1 (on a weight basis) was as effective as bradykinin, though higher doses (40–80 μg), instead of causing increased effects like bradykinin, produces erythema without oedema. When prostaglandin E_1 was given together with histamine or 5-hydroxytryptamine, it elicited an additive effect rather than a synergistic one. We reinvestigated this problem and found that the rat paw oedema caused by mixtures of prostaglandin E_1 with histamine or bradykinin was substantially greater than that expected by simple addition. Moreover, histamine-bradykinin mixtures produced effects no greater than histamine alone (67).

If a prostaglandin is sensitizing blood vessels to the permeability effects of other mediators (as happens with pain receptors: see later), then the actions of anti-inflammatory drugs on oedema can be explained by removal of this sensitization. Thus, the contribution that prostaglandins make to the oedema of inflammation is by increasing the effects of the other known mediators, such as histamine and bradykinin. To test this idea, carrageenin-induced paw swelling was measured in rats treated with indomethacin. Low concentrations of prostaglandin E_1 or E_2 added to the carrageenin injection strikingly increased oedema formation. Clearly, prostaglandin E can sensitize the blood vessels to the permeability-increasing effects of the other mediators locally released by carrageenin, and removal of endogenous prostaglandin generation (and therefore of the sensitization) explains the anti-oedema effects of aspirin-like drugs (67).

PAIN   In man, prostaglandins cause headache and pain along the veins into which they are infused (83, 84). When given intradermally (66) or intramuscularly (85) in concentrations higher than those expected to occur in inflammation (67a, 70), prostaglandin E_1 causes long-lasting pain. However, induction of hyperalgesia (i.e. a state in which pain can be elicited by normally painless mechanical or chemical stimulation) seems to be a typical effect of prostaglandins. Prostaglandins injected into dog knee joints produce incapacitation (86). Prostaglandin E_1 was 10 times more potent than prostaglandin E_2; the reactions to both began within 15 min and lasted for several hours. With prostaglandin $F_{2\alpha}$ there was an initial brief effect followed by a delayed gradual increase over 4 hr.

A long-lasting hyperalgesia occurred when minute amounts of prostaglandin E_1 were given intradermally (77) or infused subdermally (66). Ferreira's (66) subdermal infusion experiments, which were carried out in order to mimic the continuous release of mediators at the site of an injury, showed that the hyperalgesic effects of prostaglandins were cumulative, since they depended not only on concentration, but also on duration of the infusions. This cumulative sensitizing activity of the pain receptors was later also observed in dog spleen (87, 88) and rat paw (89). In Ferreira's experiments, during separate subdermal infusions of prostaglandin E_1, bradykinin, or histamine (or a mixture of bradykinin and histamine) there was no overt pain; but when prostaglandin E_1 was added to bradykinin or histamine (or a mixture of both), strong pain occurred.

Another important observation concerned pruritus (66). Neither histamine, bradykinin, nor prostaglandin E_1 infusions by themselves caused itch. However, when prostaglandin E_1 was infused along with histamine, itching was always recorded. This role of prostaglandins in potentiating the effects of histamine has recently been confirmed (89a). When prostaglandin E_1 was infused with bradykinin, there was pain rather than itch.

When applied to a blister base, prostaglandins do not cause pain (90). This may be because a blister base is already an inflamed site, made hyperalgesic by the local release of prostaglandins. Thus, in an area already saturated with prostaglandins, a further application will not elicit a further response. Presumably, endogenous prostaglandin production in the blister base enhances the pain-producing properties of added substances. This sensitizing action of prostaglandins to pain induced by bradykinin has recently been shown to occur in dog spleen also, a preparation used by Lim and his colleagues (91–93) to show that aspirin-like drugs act peripherally as analgesics. Injection of bradykinin or epinephrine released prostaglandins from dog spleen in similar amounts, both in vitro and in vivo (87, 88, 94). As epinephrine is a much weaker pain-producing substance than bradykinin in this system, a prostaglandin could not be the *mediator* of the pain-producing activity of bradykinin.

The reflex rise in blood pressure induced by intra-arterial bradykinin injections into the spleen of lightly anaesthetized dogs was also used as an indication of sensory stimulation (93). Doses of bradykinin that released prostaglandin from the spleen caused reflex increases in blood pressure in proportion to the dose used and these were reduced by indomethacin. When prostaglandin E_1 was given with the bradykinin in the indomethacin-treated dogs, the reflex increase in blood pressure was restored, sometimes to greater than control values (87, 89).

An explanation of the analgesic action of aspirin-like drugs is shown diagramatically in Figure 1. It is generally agreed that the analgesic action of morphine occurs centrally, whereas the work of Lim et al (91–93) clearly showed that aspirin had a peripheral effect. By preventing prostaglandin release in inflammation, aspirin prevents the sensitization of the pain receptors to mechanical stimulation or to the other chemicals. This hypothesis also explains why aspirin is ineffective as an analgesic in uninflamed tissues, as shown by the Randall-Selito test (95). Presumably, aspirin is only effective as an analgesic in tissues in which prostaglandin formation is taking place.

Fatty acid hydroperoxides can also cause pain in man (66). Intensity of the pain produced by intradermal injections of hydroperoxides of arachidonic, linoleic, and linolenic acids was greater than that induced by either the parent fatty acids or acetylcholine, bradykinin, histamine, or prostaglandin E_1. Thus lipoperoxides formed during prostaglandin biosynthesis may also be important as pain-producing

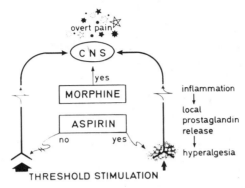

Figure 1   The role of prostaglandins in pain production.

substances. Certainly RCS, which may be the cyclic endoperoxide precursor of prostaglandins (63), has strong pharmacological activity in that it contracts rabbit aorta and many other arterial muscle strips (58, 96), as do the lipoperoxides generated by lipoxidase acting on unsaturated fatty acids such as arachidonic, linoleic, and linolenic acid (23, 28).

It is worth noting that aspirin-like drugs do not affect the hyperalgesia or the pain caused by direct action of prostaglandins. Aspirin, phenylbutazone, or indomethacin were ineffective against the incapacitation induced by prostaglandins in the dog knee joint (86). Indomethacin diminished the nociceptive effect of many agents injected intraperitoneally in mice (97) or intra-arterially in dog spleen (93), but it did not abolish either the writhing response in mice or the sensitization of dog splenic sensory nerves induced by prostaglandins (87, 97).

Thus, the anti-inflammatory acids do not reduce the effects of prostaglandins but reduce those effects caused by substances that induce generation of prostaglandins. A possible exception to this is the action of *fenamates,* which have some antagonist action at receptors for prostaglandins (98) as well as potent antisynthetase activity.

FEVER   Fever is often associated with an inflammatory process. Prostaglandin E_1 is the most powerful pyretic agent known, when injected either into cerebral ventricles, or directly into the anterior hypothalmus (99, 100). The hyperthermic effect is dose-dependent, almost immediate, and lasts for about 3 hr. Prostaglandin E_1 or E_2 causes fever by an action on the same region as that on which monoamines and pyrogens act to affect temperature.

Fever always occurs during induction of human abortion with prostaglandin $F_{2\alpha}$ (101); however, prostaglandin $F_{2\alpha}$ is a rather ineffective pyretic agent in cats and rabbits (99). The pyrogenic action of prostaglandin E_2 is greater than that of $F_{2\alpha}$ in animals, but when used for induction of abortion, it is infused at one tenth the rate used for prostaglandin $F_{2\alpha}$ and only 15% of the patients showed an increase in temperature (102). In the human studies, elevation of temperature showed better correlation with the infusion rate than with the time course of the abortion. Thus, the generation of prostaglandins in some areas of the central nervous system or its presence in the general circulation may induce fever in animals, including man. In man, the remission of pain and fever is often the first indication of the effectiveness of therapeutic doses of aspirin-like drugs.

Generation of a prostaglandin E-like substance in the central nervous system has been measured during fever (75) and the concentrations in the CSF rise after intravenous pyrogen by 2.5–4 times, sometimes to as much as 35 ng/ml.

Aspirin-like drugs do not abolish either the formation of endogenous pyrogen by leucocytes (103) or the pyretic action of prostaglandins injected into the third ventricle of cats (99). However, they inhibit both the generation of prostaglandins in the central nervous system and the fever caused by pyrogens or 5-hydroxytryptamine given into the cerebral ventricles (32).

MIGRATION OF LEUCOCYTES AND GRANULOMA FORMATION   There is no conclusive evidence that prostaglandins are leucotactic in an inflammatory process. In vitro only prostanglandin E_1 in a concentration at least 10 times higher than that found in inflammatory exudates produces a modest migration of polymorphonuclear leucocytes when compared with activated plasma (73, 74). In man, with a skin window technique, prostaglandin E_1 and prostaglandin $F_{1\alpha}$ did not alter the cellular sequence and number of cells of the exudate of a cutaneous inflammation (104). Arora et al (105) found no increased leucocytic emigration into a skin area previously treated (1–4 hr) by local injection of prostaglandin E_1.

One important aspect of an inflammatory reaction is the granuloma formation associated with an increased production of collagen. Local prostaglandin E_1 enhances the granuloma formation by cotton pellets (105) and increases collagen synthesis in chick embryo tibiae (106). However, in rats when prostaglandin E_1 was inoculated locally into air pouches at high dosages (50–100 μg), it did not elicit a granulomatous reaction (82). Aspirin-like drugs diminished granuloma formation by cotton pellets (107). However, emigration of PMN cells in an acute inflammatory reaction was not modified by indomethacin or phenylbutazone although monocyte emigration was greatly reduced (8, 57). This observation indicates that prostaglandins may be the leucotactic factor responsible for the accumulation of monocytes, one of the aspects of the conversion of an acute inflammatory reaction into a chronic one.

SIDE EFFECTS

Some of the toxic effects of large doses of aspirin-like drugs may be due to inhibition of other enzyme systems, as discussed earlier. However, inhibition of prostaglandin biosynthesis may also lead to unwanted side effects in organs that depend upon prostaglandins for normal physiological function.

The aspirin-like drugs all induce gastrointestinal irritation, which may lead to ulceration. Prostaglandin synthesis and release can be provoked by many different forms of mechanical stimulation, including gentle massage (19, 108). Thus, mechanical stimulation of the mucosa associated with gastrointestinal contractions, may lead to synthesis intramurally of a prostaglandin that in some way protects the mucosa from damage.

There are several possible protective mechanisms. Prostaglandin E_1 inhibits gastric acid secretion (109) so a locally released prostaglandin may be a braking mechanism to prevent hyperacidity, which can lead to mucosal damage. Such a mechanism is supported by the fact that indomethacin increased a submaximal secretion of acid induced by pentagastrin in rats (110). However, Bennett et al (111) found that submaximal gastric secretion in man, also induced by pentagastrin, was generally decreased slightly by indomethacin. They suggested that the function of locally released prostaglandins in the stomach may be to increase bloodflow to the mucosa and that the vasoconstriction consequent upon removal of this effect by aspirin-like drugs may lead to ischaemia, tissue death, and bleeding.

Another possibility might be that inhibition of prostaglandin biosynthesis in the stomach leads to a local accumulation of a prostaglandin precursor, such as arachidonic acid, and that this causes the irritation.

The anti-inflammatory acids also cause varying degrees of nephrotoxicity, with some incidence of papillary necrosis. Some, like phenylbutazone, lead to retention of sodium chloride and water. The prostaglandins are natruiretic (112, 113) and are found in renal medulla (114–116), together with prostaglandin synthetase (117), which is located in cells forming the collecting tubules (118). Thus, some of the renal side effects of anti-inflammatory drugs may depend upon their interaction with prostaglandin synthetase in the kidney.

Recently, indomethacin has been shown to be slightly more potent than theophylline as a phosphodiesterase inhibitor (119). If other aspirin-like drugs have a similar effect, this may also account for some of their side effects.

The major concern in the current research for new drugs is to minimize their side effects. To minimize the side effects commonly associated with broad-spectrum, nonspecific, anti-inflammatory drugs, Shen (120) suggested a cocktail mixture consisting of several narrow spectrum agents, each acting specifically at one of the many facets of complex inflammatory reactions, such as lysosomal enzymes, inflammatory mediators, etc. Considering the differential sensitivity of the prostaglandin synthetases, it may also be possible to develop specific inhibitors for the synthetase of each tissue, or group of tissues. If such a search could include the requirement that the synthetase of stomach and kidney were *not* inhibited, the common side effects may be eliminated.

CONCLUSIONS

Nonsteroid anti-inflammatory drugs inhibit prostaglandin biosynthesis in concentrations likely to be found in body fluids during therapy. The evidence that we have assembled, together with the actions of prostaglandins (erythema, pyresis, sensitization of vascular tissue to increased permeability, and sensitization of pain receptors), overwhelmingly supports our theory that this antienzyme effect is the mechanism of action of aspirin-like drugs. Intermediates in prostaglandin biosynthesis may also play a part in the inflammatory process. Prostaglandin synthetases prepared from different tissues show different sensitivities to aspirin-like drugs. This property, which may reflect a series of isoenzymes, can explain the variations in activity within the group of compounds.

Inhibition of prostaglandin biosynthesis by aspirin-like drugs, especially indomethacin (as one of the most potent) can also be used to explore the involvement of prostaglandins in pathological and physiological processes. Already, it has demonstrated the involvement of prostaglandins in the maintenance of tone of isolated smooth muscle preparations (33, 34, 121), in the control of uterine activity in vivo and in vitro (45, 46, 122–125), in normal ovary function (126–129), in modulation of lipolysis in isolated fat cells (130), in modulation of sympathetic nervous activity in vitro (30, 79), and in regulation of blood flow in the kidney (25, 26, 130a), adipose tissue (131), and during haemodynamic shock (132).

The fact that aspirin is a relatively nontoxic drug, consumed in enormous quantities throughout the world, suggests that prostaglandin synthetase is not an enzyme vital for the existence of the organism. This fits with the concept that prostaglandins are modulators of the activity of the body, perhaps mainly involved in local communication between cells, especially in defensive reactions induced by damage or stress.

This review covers literature available to us in England before June 1973. Other reviews that discuss the general relationship between prostaglandins and aspirin-like drugs are references 48 and 133–139.

Literature Cited

1. Kuzell, W. 1968. *Ann. Rev. Pharmacol.* 8:357–76
2. Weiner, M., Piliero, S. J. 1970. *Ann. Rev. Pharmacol.* 10:171–98
3. Whitehouse, M. W., Haslam, J. M. 1962. *Nature* 196:1323–24
4. McArthur, J. N., Dawkins, P. D., Smith, M. J. H., Hamilton, E. B. D. 1971. *Brit. Med. J.* 2:677–79
5. McArthur, J. N., Dawkins, P. D., Smith, M. J. H. 1971. *J. Pharm. Pharmacol.* 23:393–98
6. Smith, M. J. H., Dawkins, P. D., McArthur, J. N. 1971. *J. Pharm. Pharmacol.* 23:451
7. Di Rosa, M., Giroud, J. P., Willoughby, D. A. 1971. *J. Pathol. Bacteriol.* 104:15–29
8. Di Rosa, M., Papadimitriou, J. M., Willoughby, D. A. 1971. *J. Pathol. Bacteriol.* 105:239–56
9. Chang, Yi-Han, 1972. *J. Pharmacol. Exp. Ther.* 183:235–44
10. Ignarro, J. L., Colombo, C. 1972. *Nature New Biol.* 239:155–57
11. Sharma, S. C., Mukhtar, H., Sharma, S. K., Murt, C. R. K. 1972. *Biochem. Pharmacol.* 21:1210–14
12. Barker, J. L., Levitan, H. 1971. *Science* 172:1245–47
13. Levitan, H., Barker, J. L. 1972. *Science* 176:1423–25
14. Levitan, H., Barker, J. L. 1972. *Nature New Biol.* 239:55–57
15. Vane, J. R. 1971. *Nature New Biol.* 231:232–35
16. Smith, J. B., Willis, A. L. 1971. *Nature New Biol.* 231:235–37
17. Ferreira, S. H., Moncada, S., Vane, J. R. 1971. *Nature New Biol.* 231:237–39
18. Ånggard, E., Samuelsson, B. 1965. *J. Biol. Chem.* 240:3518–21
19. Piper, P. J., Vane, J. R. 1971. *Ann. NY Acad. Sci.* 180:363–85
20. Hamberg, M., Samuelsson, B. 1972. *J. Biol. Chem.* 247:3495–3502
21. Poyser, N. L. 1973. *Advances in the Biosciences 9,* ed. S. Bergström, S. Bernhard, 631–34. Vieweg, Braunschweig: Pergamon. 887 pp.
22. Flower, R. J., Gryglewski, R., Herbaczynska-Cedro, K., Vane, J. R. 1972. *Nature New Biol.* 238:104–6
23. Gryglewski, R., Vane, J. R. 1972. *Brit. J. Pharmacol.* 45:37–47
24. Aiken, J. W., Vane, J. R. 1972. *Pharmacologist* 13:564
25. Aiken, J. W., Vane, J. R. 1973. *J. Pharmacol. Exp. Ther.* 184:678–87
26. Herbaczynska-Cedro, K., Vane, J. R. 1972. *Supplement to Advances in the Biosciences 9,* ed. S. Bergström, S.

Bernhard, Abstr. 945. Vieweg, Braunschweig: Pergamon

27. Flower, R. J., Vane, J. R. 1972. *Nature* 240:410–11

28. Ferreira, S. H., Vargaftig, B. 1973. *Biorheology.* 10:288–89

29. Ferreira, S. H., Moncada, S. 1971. *Brit. J. Pharmacol.* 43:491P

30. Ferreira, S. H., Moncada, S., Vane, J. R. 1973. *Brit. J. Pharmacol.* 47:48–58

31. Somova, L. See Ref. 21, 335–40

32. Milton, A. S. See Ref. 21, 495–500

33. Ferreira, S. H., Herman A. G., Vane, J. R. 1972. *Brit. J. Pharmacol.* 44:328P

34. Herman, A. G., Eckenfels, A., Ferreira, S. H., Vane, J. R. 1972. *V Int. Congr. Pharmacol. San Francisco,* Abstr. 597

35. Davis, H., Horton, E. W. 1972. *Brit. J. Pharmacol.* 46:658–75

36. Eakins, K. E., Whitelocke, R. I. F., Perkins, E. S., Bennett, A., Ungar, W. G. 1972. *Nature New Biol.* 239: 248–49

37. Bhattacherjee, P., Eakins, K. E. 1973. *Pharmacologist* 15:298 (Abstr.)

38. Ham, E. A., Cirillo, V. J., Zanetti, M., Shen, T. Y., Kuehl, F. A. Jr. 1972. *Prostaglandins in Cellular Biology,* ed. P. W. Ramwell, B. B. Pharris, 343–52. New York-London: Plenum. 526 pp.

39. Smith, W. L., Lands, W. E. M. 1971. *J. Biol. Chem.* 246:6700–2

40. Collier, J. G., Flower, R. J. 1971. *Lancet* ii:852–53

41. Hamberg, M. 1972. *Biochem. Biophys. Res. Commun.* 49:720–26

42. Ziboh, V. A., McElligott, T., Hsia, S. L. See Ref. 21, 457–60

43. Bennett, I. S., Stamford, I. F., Ungar, W. G. See Ref. 21, 265–69

44. Tomlinson, R. V., Ringold, H. J., Qureshi, M. C., Forchielli, E. 1972. *Biochem. Biophys. Res. Commun.* 46:552–59

45. Aiken, J. W. 1972. *Nature* 240:21–25

46. Vane, J. R., Williams, K. I. 1973. *Brit. J. Pharmacol.* 48:629–39

47. Williams, K. I. 1973. *Brit. J. Pharmacol.* 47:628P

48. Willis, A. L., Davison, P., Ramwell, P. W., Brocklehurst, W. E., Smith, B. See Ref. 38, 227–59

49. Sykes, J. A. C., Maddox, I. S. 1972. *Nature New Biol.* 237:59–61

50. Levine, L. 1972. *Biochem. Biophys. Res. Commun.* 47:888–96

51. Takeguchi, C., Sih, C. J. 1972. *Prostaglandins* 2:169–84

52. Flower, R. J., Cheung, H. S., Cushman, D. W. 1973. *Prostaglandins* 4:325–41

53. Burstein, S., Raz, A. 1972. *Prostaglandins* 2:369–74

54. Collier, H. O. J. 1969. *Advan. Pharmacol. Chemother.* 7:333–405

55. Smith, M. J. H., Dawkins, P. D. 1971. *J. Pharm. Pharmacol.* 23:729–44

56. Thomas, G., West, G. B. 1973. *Brit. J. Pharmacol.* 47:662P

57. van Arman, C. G., Carlson, R. P., Risley, E. A., Thomas, R. H., Nuss, G. W. 1970. *J. Pharmacol. Exp. Ther.* 175: 459–65

58. Piper, P. J., Vane, J. R. 1969. *Nature* 223:29–35

59. Vargaftig, B. P., Dao, N. 1971. *Pharmacology* 6:99–108

60. Palmer, M. A., Piper, P. J., Vane, J. R. *Brit. J. Pharmacol.* In press

61. Piper, P. J., Vane, J. R. 1969. *Prostaglandins, Peptides and Amines,* ed. P. Mantegazza, E. W. Horton, 15–19. New York-London: Academic. 191 pp.

62. Gryglewski, R., Vane, J. R. 1971. *Brit. J. Pharmacol.* 43:420–21

63. Hamberg, M., Samuelsson, B. 1973. *Proc. Nat. Acad. Sci. USA* 70:899–903

64. Spector, W. G., Willoughby, D. A. 1968. *The Pharmacology of Inflammation.* London: Engl. Univ. Press. 123 pp.

65. Rocha e Silva, M., Garcia-Leme, J. 1972. *Chemical Mediators of the Acute Inflammatory Reaction.* Oxford-New York: Pergamon. 263 pp.

66. Ferreira, S. H. 1972. *Nature New Biol.* 240:200–3

67. Moncada, S., Ferreira, S. H., Vane, J. R. *Nature New Biol.* In press

67a. Willis, A. L. See Ref. 61, 31–38

68. Schayer, R. W. 1960. *Am. J. Physiol.* 198:1187–92

69. Greaves, M. W., Sondergaard, J., McDonald-Gibson, W. 1971. *Brit. Med. J.* 2:258–60

70. Greaves, M. W., Sondergaard, J. 1970. *J. Invest. Dermatol.* 54:365–67

71. Änggård, E., Jonsson, C. E. 1971. *Acta Physiol. Scand.* 81:440–47

72. Higgs, G. A., Youlten, L. J. F. 1972. *Brit. J. Pharmacol.* 44:330P

73. Kaley, G., Weiner, R. 1971. *Nature New Biol.* 234:114–15

74. Kaley, G., Weiner, R. 1971. *Ann. NY Acad. Sci.* 180:338–50

75. Feldberg, W., Gupta, K. P. 1973. *J. Physiol. Lond.* 228:41–53

76. Solomon, L. M., Juhlin, L., Kirschbaum, M. B. 1968. *J. Invest. Dermatol.* 51:280–82
77. Juhlin, S., Michaelsson, G. 1969. *Acta Dermatol. Venereol. Stockholm* 49:251–61
78. Weiner, R., Kaley, G. 1969. *Am. J. Physiol.* 217:563–70
79. Hedqvist, P. See Ref. 21, 461–73
80. Majno, G. et al 1972. *Inflammation Mechanism and Control,* ed. I. A. Lepow, P. A. Ward, 13–20. New York-London: Academic. 409 pp.
81. Crunkhorn, P., Willis, A. L. 1971. *Brit. J. Pharmacol.* 41:49–56
82. Glenn, E. M., Bowman, B. J., Rohloff, N. A. See Ref. 38, 329–43
83. Bergström, S., Duner, H., Von Euler, U. S., Pernow, B., Sjovall, J. 1959. *Acta Physiol. Scand.* 45:145–51
84. Collier, J. G., Karim, S. M. M., Robinson, B., Somers, K. 1972. *Brit. J. Pharmacol.* 3:474P
85. Karim, S. M. M. 1971. *Ann. NY Acad. Sci.* 180:483–98
86. Rosenthale, M. E., Dervina, A., Kassarich, J., Singer, S. 1972. *J. Pharm. Pharmacol.* 24:149–50
87. Ferreira, S. H., Moncada, S., Vane, J. R. 1973. *Brit. J. Pharmacol.* 47:629
88. Ferreira, S. H., Moncada, S., Vane, J. R. 1973c. *Brit. J. Pharmacol.* 49:86–97
89. Willis, A. L., Cornelsen, M. 1973. *Prostaglandins* 3:353–58
89a. Greaves, M. W., McDonald-Gibson, W. 1973. *Brit. Med. J.* 3:608–9
90. Horton, E. W. 1973. *Nature* 200:892–93
91. Guzman, F., Braun, C., Lim, R. K. S. 1962. *Arch. Int. Pharmacodyn. Ther.* 136:353–84
92. Guzman, F., Braun, C., Lim, R. K. S., Potter, G. D., Rodgers, D. W. 1964. *Arch. Int. Pharmacodyn. Ther.* 149:571–88
93. Lim, R. K. S. et al 1964. *Arch. Int. Pharmacodyn. Ther.* 152:25–58
94. Moncada, S., Ferreira, S. H., Vane, J. R. 1972. *V Int. Congr. Pharmacol., San Francisco,* Abstr. 959
95. Randall, L. O., Selitto, J. J. 1957. *Arch. Int. Pharmacodyn. Ther.* 111:409–19
96. Palmer, M. A., Piper, P. J., Vane, J. R. 1970. *Brit. J. Pharmacol.* 40:547P
97. Collier, H. O. J., Schneider, C. 1972. *Nature New Biol.* 236:141–43
98. Collier, H. O. J., Sweatman, W. J. F. 1968. *Nature* 219:864–65
99. Milton, A. S., Wendlandt, S. 1971. *J. Physiol.* 218:325–36
100. Feldberg, W., Saxena, P. N. 1971. *J. Physiol.* 217:547–56
101. Hendricks, C. H., Brenner, W. E., Ekbladh, L., Brotanek, V., Fishburne, J. I. 1971. *Am. J. Obstet. Gynecol.* 3:564–78
102. Filshie, G. 1971. *Ann. NY Acad. Sci.* 180:552–57
103. Clark, W. G., Moyer, S. G. 1972. *J. Pharmacol. Exp. Ther.* 181:183–91
104. Sondergaard, J., Wolff-Jurgensen, P. 1972. *Acta Dermatol. Venereol. Stockholm* 52:361–64
105. Arora, S., Lahiri, P. K., Sanyal, R. K. 1970. *Int. Arch. Allergy Appl. Immunol.* 39:186–91
106. Blumenkrantz, N., Sondergaard, J. 1972. *Nature New Biol.* 239–46
107. Winter, A. C., Risley, A. E., Nuss, G. W. 1963. *J. Pharmacol. Exp. Ther.* 141:369–76
108. Ferreira, S. H., Vane, J. R. 1967. *Nature* 216:868–73
109. Shaw, J. E., Ramwell, P. W. 1968. *Prostaglandin,* ed. P. W. Ramwell, J. E. Shaw, 55–56. New York-London: Wiley. 402 pp.
110. Main, I. H., Whittle, B. J. R. 1972. *Brit. J. Pharmacol.* 44:331P
111. Bennett, A., Stamford, I. F., Ungar, W. G. 1973. *J. Physiol. Lond.* 229:349–60
112. Lee, J. B. 1972. *Prostaglandins* 1:55–70
113. McGiff, J. C. et al. 1970. *Circ. Res.* 28:765–82
114. Crowshaw, K., McGiff, J. C., Strand, J. C., Lonigro, A. J., Terragno, N. A. 1970. *J. Pharm. Pharmacol.* 22:302–4
115. Daniels, E. G., Hinman, J. W., Leach, B. E., Muirhead, E. E. 1967. *Nature, Lond.* 215:1298–99
116. Lee, J. B., Crowshaw, K., Takman, B. H., Attrep, K. A., Gougoutas, J. Z. *Biochem. J.* 105:1251–60
117. Crowshaw, K. 1971. *Nature New Biol.* 231:240–42
118. Janszen, F. H. A., Nugteren, D. H. 1971. *Histochemie* 27:159–64
119. Flores, A. G. A., Sharp. G. 1972. *Am. J. Physiol.* 233:1392–97
120. Shen, T. Y. 1972. *Angew. Chem.* 11:460–72
121. Eckenfels A., Vane J. R. 1972. *Brit. J. Pharmacol.* 45:451–62
122. Chester, R., Dukes, M., Slater, S. R., Walpole, A. L. 1972. *Nature* 240:37–38
123. Waltman, R., Tricomi, V., Palav, A. 1973. *Prostaglandins* 3:47–58
124. Harper, M. J. K., Skarnes, R. C. 1972. *Prostaglandins* 2:295–309

125. Harper, M. J. K., Skarnes, R. C. See Ref. 21, 789–93
126. Armstrong, D. T., Grimwich, D. L. 1972. *Prostaglandins* 1:21–28
127. Behrman, H. R., Orczyk, G. P., Creep, R. O. 1972. *Prostanglandins* 1:245–58
128. O'Grady, J. P., Caldwell, B. J., Auletta, J. F., Speroff, L. 1972. *Prostaglandins* 1:97–106
129. Tsafriri, A., Lindner, H. R., Zor, H., Lamprecht, S. A. 1972. *Prostaglandins* 2:1–10
130. Illiano, G., Cuatrecasas, P. 1971. *Nature New Biol.* 234:72–74
130a. Lonigro, A. J., Itskovitz, H. D., Crowshaw, K., McGiff, J. C. 1973. *Circ. Res.* 32:712–17

131. Bowery, B., Lewis, G. P. 1973. *Brit. J. Pharmacol.* 47:305–14
132. Collier, J. G., Herman, A. G., Vane, J. R. 1973. *J. Physiol.* 230:19P
133. Vane, J. R. 1972. *Hospital Practice* 7:61–67
134. Vane, J. R. See Ref. 80, 261–75
135. Vane, J. R. See Ref. 21, 395–411
136. Vane, J. R. 1973. *Proc. V Int. Congr. Pharmacol., San Francisco.* 5:352–78. Basel: Karger
137. Ferreira, S. H., Vane, J. R. *The Prostaglandins II,* ed. P. W. Ramwell. New York-London: Plenum. In press
138. Ferreira, S. H., Vane, J. R. *Int. Meet. Future Trends Inflammation.* In press
139. Flower, R. J. *Pharmacol. Rev.* In press

RENAL PHARMACOLOGY: ❖6582
COMPARATIVE, DEVELOPMENTAL,
AND CELLULAR ASPECTS

Yu. V. Natochin

Sechenov Institute of Evolutionary Physiology and Biochemistry, Leningrad, USSR

Understanding the mechanism of action of drugs requires a penetrating insight into the functioning not only of the organ itself but also each of its cells. Therefore, in this review the findings of biochemical and biophysical investigations as well as the results of studies on the ultrastructure of nephron cells and their functional analogs have been used. The data on the kidney comparative pharmacology and physiology are of primary importance for comprehending tendencies in the development of the renal transport systems and evolution of the kidney.

The comparative approach, in the broad sense, suggests a comparison of the kidney function in animals at different evolutionary stages, work of cells from various nephron parts and other organs specially adapted for ion transport (amphibian skin and urinary bladder, gills, etc). Comparison of the data on the function of kidneys in phylogenesis, with the results of study of changes in the renal activity in ontogenesis, permits discussion of principles of development of various renal functions.

This review is confined to an analysis of the effect of diuretics and some hormones on kidneys in various classes of vertebrates, in animals in postnatal ontogenesis, and on isolated biological membranes, the functional analogs of renal tubules. In this connection interesting reviews and monographs have appeared in the last few years (1–5).

NEW DATA ON VERTEBRATE NEPHRON STRUCTURE

Morphological investigations of recent years have made alterations in classical concepts of the vertebrate kidney structure (6, 7). In nephrons of the lampreys *Lampetra fluviatilis* (8, 9) and *Petromyzon marinus* (10) there are not only proximal tubules and collecting ducts, as has been previously suggested, but also intermediate and distal tubules. Cytochemical characteristics (enzymes, mucopolysaccharides) of

75

lamprey renal tubules are similar to respective parts in kidneys of other vertebrates (8, 11). Distal tubules have been found in kidneys of a few marine teleosts *Spicara smaris* L., *Mugil cephalus* L., *Myoxocephalus scorpius* L. (12, 13). A short distal tubule has been detected even in the aglomerular *Nerophis ophidion* (14) but is absent in kidneys of *Pleuronectes platessa* (15) and *Lophius piscatorius* (16). Such features of the kidney anatomy (and involved functional properties) as the medulla in birds and mammals, and the renoportal system in fishes, amphibians, reptiles, and birds, are of great importance for assessing the action of various drugs on the kidney.

ELEMENTS OF TRANSPORT SYSTEM IN KIDNEY CELL

Studies of the kidney of mammals and amphibians, and the skin and urinary bladder of amphibians are aimed at elucidating functional organization of the ion transport system and especially that of Na in the cell. Filtered Na enters the nephron lumen. Cells of the proximal tubule reabsorb Na against a small gradient: in *Necturus* at a concentration over 66 meq/liter, in rats, over 95 meq/liter (17). The essential difference between lower and higher vertebrates is the volume of their proximal reabsorption. At the proximal convoluted tubule sites accessible to micropuncture, (TF/P) in [(tubular fluid/plasma) inulin] makes up 2.61 (18) and 2.53 (19) in rats and 1.75 (20) in dogs, whereas in the frog *Rana temporaria* even in final urine (u/p) in equals 1.3 (21). The lower level of filtration and the lesser volume of proximal reabsorption are typical of cold-blooded vertebrates (22).

During reabsorption Na enters the cell from the lumen through the apical membrane, passes across the cell, and discharges to blood with the aid of pumps located in the lateral and basal plasmatic membranes. Analysis of properties of various elements of the Na transport system is of particular significance for renal pharmacology, because their difference enables us to choose appropriate drugs for each element.

In accord with widespread opinion, Na entrance into the cell from lumen is a passive process (23). The same explanation is offered for Na entrance through the apical cell membrane of amphibian urinary bladder and skin (24). However, there are different points of view as to how this occurs (25, 26). Thus it is suggested that the apical membrane of the active layer of frog skin cells contains a sodium pump (27). According to another hypothesis, Na moves along the outer membrane through the intercellular junction (28). The latter hypothesis is at variance with the data presented on the half-period of Na wash-out from the transport pool at the action of ouabain (29). These evidences show that Na is transferred to the cell cytoplasm.

It is believed (23, 24, 30) that in the renal tubule cell and its functional analogs, Na channels and ion pumps are spatially separated. This is also evidenced by the difference in chemical properties of the apical and basal plasmatic membranes (31, 32) and the tubular cell ultrastructure. These findings corroborate the assumption that Na channels localize in the apical membrane and ion pumps in the basal plasmatic membrane. There are many infoldings and a great number of mitochondria at the base of the nephron proximal tubule cell of mammals (33), in the distal segment of fishes (7), amphibians (22), and mammals (34). The basal infoldings and mitochondria in the proximal tubule are not numerous in lamprey and frogs, which show a low level of proximal reabsorption, but are abundant in the nephron proximal and distal tubules of animals with intensive Na transport (22). The ultrastructure of mitochondria depends not only on the amount of Na reabsorbed but also on the gradient against which Na is transferred. In the cells of the distal tubles of lamprey (9), frogs, and rats (22), where Na is transferred in lesser amount but against a larger gradient, each mitochondria contains more crysts than the proximal tubule cell. The ultrastructure of the nephron cell correlates with the Na transport level, this fact speaking in favor of transcellular rather than paracellular Na transport in the kidney. The high permeability of tubular walls, however, must affect the activity of the nephron. In this context, the paracellular transport of substances from the tubular lumen to the peritubular space and in the opposite direction is discussed (23, 35, 36).

The question of the size and meaning of the Na transport pool is open to argument. The Na transport pool constitutes a lesser portion of the total amount of Na in the cell (26, 29, 37). Cell Na content changes at the action of hormones and diuretics. As shown by X-ray microanalysis, the intracellular content of Na, Cl (but not K) increases in both limbs of the loop of Henle from the cortex to the medulla. The Na intracellular content is higher in the thin descending limb than in the thick ascending one. This difference disappears during furosemide diuresis (38).

Nephron cells have several types of sodium pumps, among them an Na/K exchange pump and an electrogenic pump (39). It is also suggested that Na reabsorption is provided by the neutral NaCl pump rather than by the electrically coupled Cl^- transport following Na^+ (40). Bicarbonate plays the important part in Na reabsorption (41), as in its absence NaCl reabsorption is nearly as small as that after kidney poisoning with ouabain (42).

The K transport mechanism in the tubules differs from that of Na. There are considerable specific variations of K reabsorption in the proximal tubules of various animals. The use of selective liquid ion-exchange microelectrodes shows that TF/P_k in the last convolution of the proximal tubule is 0.8 ± 0.01 in rat (43) and 1.9 ± 0.2 in *Necturus maculosis* (44). In *Amphiuma,* filtered K does not reabsorb in the proximal tubule (45), as it does in rats.

Cells of the distal tubule play a decisive role in K excretion. The interrelations between K active transport to the cell on the luminal and peritubular membrane and K passive secretion through the apical membrane determine the amounts of K excreted (39, 44, 46). The K transport pool of the distal tubule cell makes up a smaller portion of the cellular K. The K transport pool is enhanced significantly upon transition from K reabsorption to secretion (45). A considerable K secretion is observed at the action of acetazolamide or after the maintenance of *Amphiuma* (45) and *Rana temporaria* (47) in a medium with high K concentration. Under K load the activity of the ion in the distal tubule cell of the rat kidney increases from 46.5 ± 9.6 mM to 60.5 ± 2.1 mM (48).

The transport systems of organic acids are probably similar in kidneys of most vertebrates. PAH is secreted by the kidneys in lamprey (49), cartilaginous (50) and bony (51) fishes, and amphibians (52). Probenecid decreases PAH transport in kidneys of rabbits (53, 54) and that of mercurial diuretics in kidneys of mammals and fishes (55). Probenecid inhibits the effect of arginine vasotocin in the kidneys of water snakes and frogs as well as the transport of organic acids. It fails to inhibit the hydroosmotic effect of theophylline on the frog urinary bladder, affecting it probably at the level of the tissue receptors of neurohypophyseal peptides (56). In the chick kidney PAH transport may be blocked with novobiocin. Its action is similar (though not identical) to that of probenecid (57).

COMPARATIVE STUDY OF DIURETIC ACTION

Ethacrynic acid decreases Na reabsorption with kidneys of rats (58), dogs (59, 60), chickens (61), frogs (21), marine fishes (62), and lampreys (63). In rabbit, ethacrynic acid affects both kidney and intestine (64), and influences the ionic content of the inner ear endolymph (65).

Furosemide inhibits Na reabsorbtion in the kidneys of various mammals (66), birds (63), amphibians (21, 67), fishes (62, 68), and cyclostomes (63). Hydrochlorothiazide, mercaptomerin, aminophylline, and ouabain decrease ion excretion by the chick kidney (61). The natriuretic effect of hydrochlorothiazide in rats is much higher than in hens (69). Brinaldix induces Na excretion in rats (70), dogs (71), *Oncorhynchus nerka, Salvelinus malma,* and *M. scorpius* (72). After the 1–10 mg/kg brinaldix injection the Na excretion fraction (EF_{Na}) increases from 1.6 to 5.1% in rat and from 9 to 24% in *S. malma* (72). Acetazolamide inhibits Na reabsorption in the kidneys of mammals, birds, alligators, frogs, some fishes, and lampreys (3, 73, 74), in the gills of fishes (75, 76), and in the turtle urinary bladder (77).

Amiloride enhances Na excretion by the kidneys of rat (78), dog (79), and man (80), and inhibits Na transport in the colon of amphibians (81), in erythrocytes (82), and in cells of salivary gland ducts (83). At the same time amiloride does not produce any effect on Na transport in the gills of goldfish, while in eel Na leakage is increased (84). Triamterene induces natriuresis and decreases K excretion in man (85, 86), the water snake *Natrix cyclopion* (87), and others.

Thus components of the Na reabsorption system sensitive to the action of various types of modern diuretics are found in representatives of all classes of vertebrates. As a rule diuretics increase EF_{Na} in lower vertebrates more sharply than in mammals, despite the fact that Na excretion is lower when counted by weight or body surface. This is caused by a lesser glomerular filtration rate (GFR) and consequently a lesser load on the nephron.

Experiments on amphibian skin and urinary bladder membranes are of particular interest for studying cellular action mechanisms of diuretics. The response of cells of these organs and the nephron cells to hormones is similar (88), whereas their reaction to diuretics may vary. As demonstrated in experiments with frog skin, hydrochlorothiazide, furosemide, and salyrgan increase short circuit current (SCC) (89). In skin of the toad *Bufo bufo,* furosemide and salyrgan decrease SCC (90). In the skin of *Rana temporaria,* furosemide does not affect SCC while mercusal and ethacrynic acid inhibit it (91). In toad skin ethacrynic acid enhances but furosemide decreases Na transport (81). Mercurial diuretics increase Na transport in the frog skin (89, 92) and reduce it in the toad urinary bladder (93). Furosemide and ethacrynic acid diminish SCC and increase dc resistance of membrane in the toad urinary bladder (94). As the effects of furosemide and ouabain are not additive (95) it is supposed that their action mechanisms are similar. One cannot admit it without reserve, because in the skin of *Rana temporaria* SCC is inhibited by various cardiac glycosides (96) but is not changed upon addition of furosemide (91, 97). In the frog cornea, furosemide inhibits SCC. The effect of furosemide is probably determined by its action on Cl transport (97). Brinaldix inhibits SCC of the frog skin (98) by increasing the osmolarity induced by polyethylenglycol 400, which has been used as a clopamide solvent in the ampule with brinaldix.

SODIUM PERMEABILITY: ITS ACTIVATION AND INHIBITION

Among saluretics, amiloride and triamterene differ qualitatively by the sites of their action on the cell (99). They inhibit Na transport when added to the solution at the outer surface of the skin and urinary bladder cells. They begin to act immediately and Na transport is restored after the washout (100, 101). The same degree of inhibition is observed after the addition of $4 \cdot 10^{-7}$ M amiloride and 10^{-4} M triamterene (100). Amiloride interacts with a certain component in the cell apical membrane characterized by saturation kinetics (102). As a result Na influx to the cell is decreased (103, 104). Pumps, however, continue discharging Na from the cell so long as the transport pool is exhausted (105). The percentage of Na transport inhibition induced by amiloride is not dependent on the original level of SCC (106) being observed at any Na concentration in the mucosal solution (107). As has been demonstrated on erythrocytes, amiloride inhibits passive influx of Na to the cell without affecting the efflux (82). After amiloride is added, the lowering O_2 consumption is mainly caused by the decrease of Na transport (108, 109). Amiloride itself does not influence O_2 consumption in concentrations required for Na transport inhibition (110). It appears that amiloride prevents Na entrance to the Na transport compartment without affecting the pump (37). The interaction of amiloride with the membrane receptor increases in the presence of bivalent ions in solution near the outer surface of the frog skin and decreases in a solution without Ca. It is probable that amiloride, Ca, and membrane receptor make up a complex preventing Na entrance to the cell (111). In the toad urinary bladder the membrane component to which amiloride is bound is removed with amphotericin B (112).

In the presence of amiloride, hormones (aldosterone, insulin, vasopressin) enhance Na and water transport through the wall of the toad urinary bladder and skin (112). The action of vasopressin (104) and other hormones is connected with the increase of Na permeability of the cell apical membrane. Amphotericin (113) and nistatine (114) also increase K permeability of the cell membrane of the frog skin. The distinguishing feature of amiloride and triamterene effects is their ability to enhance natriuresis at the same or diminished level of K excretion (85, 115). These drugs reduce Na reabsorption in the distal tubule (116) and K secretion (117).

Amiloride decreases the potential difference in the distal tubule. This blocks K passive secretion to the nephron lumen. Guignard & Peters (115) suggest that amiloride and triamterene exert two independent effects, one of which is displayed as K sparing, and the second as natriuresis and H^+ inhibition of secretion.

ACTION OF DRUGS ON CELL METABOLISM AND ION PUMPS

This section is of particular importance for investigation of the action mechanisms of diuretics. Despite numerous works on the topic, the achievements are not great. Studies of the action of diuretics on key enzymes of the Na transport system and cell energy metabolism have shown that these drugs affect a number of metabolic processes. As has been established with certainty, the effect of acetazolamide is produced by carbonic anhydrase inhibition (118). The problem of the biochemical action mechanism of many diuretics is more complicated. Changes in the enzymatic activity from the action of diuretics are not the same in different parts of the kidney. The activity of malic dehydrogenase decreases notably in the rat kidney cortex after polythiazide and furosemide administration. The latter reduces while ethacrynic acid enhances the activity of this enzyme in the kidney medulla. Furosemide increases the succinic dehydrogenase activity in the cortex and decreases it in the medulla (119). In guinea pigs furosemide lowers the activity of acid phosphatase, succinic dehydrogenase, and leucinaminopeptidase in the nephron cell which involves changes in the mitochondrial structure (120). By contrast, in rats, at a maximum of furosemide diuresis, no sharp changes occur in the structure of mitochondria from the cells of the proximal and distal tubules (121). According to Schmidt & Dubach (122) furosemide inhibits Na,K-ATPase in the cells of the distal segment. Nechay et al claim that in the kidneys of dogs and rats Na,K-ATPase are the receptors of ethacrynic acid (123) and mercurial diuretics (124). The inhibition of Na,K-ATPase has been found in microsomes of the kidney cortex cells of guinea pigs (125, 126). Landon & Fitzpatrick, however, hold a contrary opinion (127). These authors have shown that in rabbits and rats, both in vivo and in vitro, the diuretic effect of ethacrynic acid does not involve changes in the mitochondrial O_2 consumption and inhibition of Na,K-ATPase. Ethacrynic acid and furosemide have no effect on the Na,K-ATPase activity of plasmatic membranes of the rat kidney, but amiloride decreases it (128).

It would be not reasonable to cite here numerous data on alteration in the activity of various enzymes after diuretic administration. The diversity of effects does not permit the suggestion that changes in activity are determined by the key role of a given enzyme in reaction to the test diuretic.

To sum up the literature concerning the change of the Na,K-ATPase activity from natriuretic effects of various drugs (1, 128–130) we may conclude that only the effect of cardiac glycosides is completely determined by inhibition of the enzyme (131, 132). At least on the strength of the available data, the effect of a great number of other substances on Na transport cannot be directly related to the level of Na,K-ATPase activity measured in the kidney.

In the kidney cortex and urinary bladder cells there is an ouabain-insensitive transport of electrolytes (133, 134). It depends on the energy metabolism and is completely blocked by uncouplers or anaerobiosis (135, 136). This transport system responsible for regulation of the cell volume is related to pH and Ca concentration in the external solution (133). Experiments with kidneys of toads (137), guinea pigs (136), and dogs (138) show that nephron cells contain two pumps. One is Na/K and is inhibited by ouabain; the other provides Na and Cl transport and is inhibited by ethacrynic acid. In the nephron cells Na and Cl transport proceeds in the presence of high concentrations of ouabain when Na,K-ATPase is completely inhibited (139, 140). Na reabsorption may be independent of K entrance to the cell from peritubular fluid (141). The relative role of each pump in Na reabsorption in vivo in cells from different nephron parts is still uncertain. Both pumps seem to be localized in one cell but not in different cell populations (142). However, the hypothesis of ethacrynic acid inhibition of the second Na pump is not shared by all authors, since ethacrynic acid affects various metabolic processes and possibly reduces the energy supply of the Na pump (133). In the light of the hypothesis about the existence in kidney of a Na reabsorption mechanism independent of Na,K-ATPase, of primary importance are the data of Kessler suggesting that the election transport system provides energetically the reabsorption of Na without participation of ATP as an intermediate agent (143).

Ethacrynic acid and furosemide increase natriuresis but do not change the kidney O_2 consumption (144). Consequently, the effect of some diuretics does not depend on the inhibition of cell energy metabolism but may be due to other causes. It has been assumed that furosemide increases Na permeability of the basal plasma membrane; Na passive transport to the cell from peritubular fluid increases and, although the total amount of transported Na (and O_2 consumption involved) does not change, the intensity of Na reabsorption from the tubule is diminished (145).

According to another hypothesis the above saluretics enhance inner membrane resistance, which increases the expenditure of energy for Na reabsorption. As O_2 consumption remains unchanged at the action of furosemide, Na reabsorption decreases (145). Moreover, it may be suggested that saluretics influence membranes, disturbing their interaction with cell energy systems. Ethacrynic acid inhibits renal membrane stimulation of mitochondrial respiration, and mercurial diuretics decrease membrane stimulation of glycolysis. Cellular effects of some diuretics may be caused by uncoupling the oxydative metabolism from ion transport systems (1, 146).

One of the most important problems in the study of the diuretics action mechanism is to answer the question whether drugs reduce reabsorption of all ions or affect only Na transport. In the latter case the enhancement of excretion of other ions must depend on the degree of their transport coupling with Na transfer. In man and higher vertebrates, after administration of furosemide, chlorothiazide, acetazolamide, and metolazone, the excretion of Na and of Ca, Mg phosphates increases. This may be due to the reduction of proximal reabsorption (147–149). In amphibians brinaldix does not affect diuresis. It inhibits Na reabsorption and increases K excretion but does not influence Ca and Mg excretion (98). Unlike the kidneys of mammals, birds (150), and amphibians (151), those of hagfishes (152) and marine cartilaginous and bony fish kidneys are capable of secreting magnesium after $MgCl_2$ injection (7, 153–158). A direct correlation has been found between Mg secretion and Na reabsorption in *O. nerka* (159). In the marine teleosts *Scorpaena porcus* there is a reverse correlation between Na and Mg concentration in urine (158). In *O. kisutch*, after injections of brinaldix and $MgCl_2$, Mg secretion and Na reabsorption decreases equivalently (159). Injections of furosemide, ethacrynic acid, and brinaldix in the partially aglomerular fish *M. scorpius* enhance Na concentration in urine and lower its Mg content at a stable level of diuresis (62). It is necessary to consider the formation mechanism of "primary urine" in aglomerular fishes since it has become known that at the action of floridzine glucose concentration in the urine of *Lophius americanus* increases from 1.31 to 16.7 mg% (160). Thus in the case of coupled cation transport (for instance, Mg secretion) diuretics cease to transfer ions to the lumen as a result of Na reabsorption inhibition. In the case of independent reabsorption of each cation the Na reabsorption decreases mainly under the effect of diuretics. This conclusion is true for instances of saluretic administration when no sharp changes occur in diuresis. This is observed in lower vertebrates, which show comparatively low fluid reabsorption and whose kidneys are not capable of accomplishing osmotic diuresis (22) and NaCl excretion after the injection of NaCl hypertonic solutions (161).

The Na reabsorption system plays an essential role in the transport of various substances in the renal tubule cell (162). Na transport in the nephron cell is related to the transport of K (46), Mg (158), PAH, and glucose (163, 164). In the isolated kidneys of *Rana ridibunda*, furosemide, convallotoxin, and mersalyl inhibit Na and glucose reabsorption as well as PAH secretion (67). In the kidneys of *Rana temporaria*, furosemide, ethacrynic acid, brinaldix, etc inhibit fluorescein secretion without affecting its storage in the proximal tubule cell (21). Dissociation of the ouabain effect on Na and PAH transports has been noted. In dogs this inhibitor causes prolonged inhibition of Na reabsorption and gradual return of PAH secretion to the control level (165).

REGULATION OF KIDNEY FUNCTION

We consider here only data on cellular action mechanisms of hormones and drugs that either activate or inhibit hormonal effects. The question of hormonal regulation of water-salt metabolism and kidney function in vertebrates is reviewed in a few recent publications (2, 3, 166–172). The findings of comparative endocrinology are of exceptional interest for studying regulation principles of cellular processes in animals at different developmental levels.

The system of Na balance regulation is different in lower and higher vertebrates. In lampreys aldosterone does not influence the kidney electrolyte excretion (73). The kidneys of cyclostomes and cartilaginous fishes contain no renin (173, 174). The appearance of the renin-angiotensin system and aldosterone as factors of Na balance regulation by the kidneys (2) is likely to be followed by the formation of some natriuretic factors, at least in higher vertebrates. Substances with natriuretic activity can be secreted to mammalian blood (175–178). By now peptides of high natriuretic activity have been synthesized (175). The prostaglandins PGA_2 and PGE_2 are considered to play a role in regulation of Na excretion (179, 180).

Changes in Na reabsorption are regulated in the cell in at least two ways: via protein synthesis de novo (e.g. in the aldosterone case) and via formation of 3',5'-AMP from ATP. Vasopressin enhances water permeability and Na transport in the urinary bladder cells stimulating adenylcyclase (181–183). 3',5'-AMP and theophylline, which inhibits the phosphodiesterase that degrades 3',5'-AMP, act like vasopressin. Dopamine (184) and epinephrine inhibit the effect of vasopressin on water permeability; epinephrine does not change cellular reactions to 3',5'-AMP. The inhibiting effect of epinephrine is probably localized at an adenylcyclase level (181). It is eliminated by phenoxybenzamine (α-adrenergic blocking agent) (181). Small doses of noradrenalin increase water permeability and Na transport in the isolated frog skin epithelium. Both these effects disappear after the skin has been treated with the β-blocking agent propranolol (185). It is conceivable that β-receptors contribute to the increase of the 3',5'-AMP level; α-receptors produce the opposite effect (186). Administration of epinephrine to man blocks the antidiuretic effect of vasopressin (187). Another factor regulating adenylcyclase activity is prostaglandin E_1. This substance inhibits the vasopressin effect reducing the intracellular 3',5'-AMP content (188). Prostaglandin E_1 does not affect adenylcyclase isolated from the urinary bladder. It appears that prostaglandins are natural regulators of cell function (182). Indomethacin blocks prostaglandin synthesis and release and enhances response of the toad urinary bladder cells to vasopressin (189). Cu^{2+} lowers the effects of oxytocin and theophylline on osmotic permeability (190).

The question of mechanisms increasing permeability to water and Na transport at the action of 3',5'-AMP is still to be answered. The increase of Na transport under the influence of neurohypophyseal hormone is ascribed both to the increase of permeability of the apical plasmatic membrane (191–193) and to Na pump stimulation (194). Most convincing is the hypothesis of double vasopressin effect on Na permeability of the membrane and Na pump (194, 195).

The question of mechanisms increasing permeability to water is even more arguable. According to one hypothesis vasopressin increases the diameter of pores in the apical membrane through which water flows along the osmotic gradient (191, 196). The hypothesis of Hays (197) is that vasopressin increases the number but not the size of the pores. Eggena claims that under the influence of vasopressin the osmotic water flow occurs through narrow nonpolar channels in the membrane (198). A third hypothesis states that vasopressin increases permeability to intercellular space water (199–201). The antidiuretic reaction is observed only when the renal artery is injected with large amounts of hyaluronidase (199). Small amounts, however, lead to antidiuresis when the enzyme is introduced from ureter to collecting ducts (202).

In rats, aldosterone increases Na reabsorption in the proximal and distal tubules (203, 204); in aquatic snakes it is mainly in the proximal segment (205). Aldosterone penetrates the cell nucleus where it is bound by chromatine stereospecific for mineralcorticoids (206). Spirolactone blocks the binding of ^{3}H-aldosterone with chromatine in the rat kidney (207). The primary aldosterone binding seems to be with 4S nonhistone chromosomal protein. About 600 aldosterone molecules are bound by the kidney cell nucleus (207). Aldosterone stimulates synthesis in the RNA nucleus (208), as well as protein synthesis, providing the increase of Na transport (209). It is likely that aldosterone influences the synthesis of two types of proteins that increase *(a)* Na permeability of the apical membrane of amphibian urinary bladder and skin cells (210, 211) and *(b)* work of the Na pump (212). Aldosterone enhances the action of vasopressin, p ssibly decreasing the decay rate of 3',5'-AMP (213). An aldosterone antagonist, SC 19886, inhibits the aldosterone-stimulated Na transport through the frog urinary bladder (214). The spirolactone SC 14266 can inhibit Na transport in the frog skin even in the absence of aldosterone in solution (215).

Angiotensin II enhances permeability to the urinary bladder water in the toads *Bufo parachemis* and *B. arenarum,* and potentiates the 3',5'-AMP effect (216). In toad kidneys, angiotensin II induces antinatriuresis and antidiuresis (217). In rats, small doses reduce Na excretion while large doses lead to natriuresis (218). The vasoconstrictory effect of angiotensin may account for its diuretic action in rats (219). Na and K reabsorption in the isolated dog kidney increases at the action of insulin (220). The effect of this hormone seems to be caused by Na pump activation (221, 222).

The effect of methylxanthines is partly due to alteration in the response of cells to hormones and mediators. Theophylline is an inhibitor of phosphodiesterase and in its presence 3',5'-AMP inactivation decreases and vasopressin action becomes more durable (181). In the case of moderate dehydration in man, aminophylline increases reabsorption of osmotically free water. In patients with diabetes insipidus, aminophylline produces no effect on water and Na excretion by the kidney (223). The aminophylline inhibition of Na reabsorption is increased during hydration or after vasopressin injection and is diminished during hyperhydration (224). Theophylline also affects proximal reabsorption (225). It must be taken into account that the action of theophylline on epithelial cells may differ from their reaction to 3',5'-AMP and neurohypophyseal hormones (226, 227).

ONTOGENESIS

The kidneys of newborn mammals (199, 200, 228) and birds immediately after hatching (229) are functionally immature, indicated by the lower GFR (222–230), less effective secretory ability (PAH, phenolred, excretion) (199, 231), reduced effectiveness of amino acid reabsorption (232), and decreased ability of osmotic concentration (200). Salt loads, such as NaCl (233), KCl (234), $CaCl_2$ and $MgCl_2$ (235) are discharged more slowly.

In postnatal ontogenesis along with functional (236), morphological (237) and biochemical maturation of the kidney occurs (238). In the kidneys of newborn rats during the first month the activity of alkaline phosphatase, carbonic anhydrase (239) succinic, α-ketoglutaric, and glutamic dehydrogenase (8) increases and the content of acid mucopolysaccharides in the medulla also increases (199). Mitochondria of adult rat kidneys show much higher activity of cytochromoxidase and succinic cytochromreductase as compared with the 10 day old rats (240). This indicates qualitative changes of the kidney membrane system in the course of development. In 3 week old rats the activity of Na,K-ATPase of the microsomal fraction does not differ from that of adult rats (241). The kidneys of newborn babies and animals differ considerably from adult kidneys in their response to various drugs. In early ontogenesis of rats and dogs the reaction of the kidneys to vasopressin is lowered (242, 243) and there is no response to epinephrine (243). In newborn rats aldosterone does not decrease Na concentration in urine and spirolactone does not influence the ratio Na/K in urine (244). The inability of ontogenetically immature kidneys to develop osmotic diuresis after administration of Na_2SO_4, urea, glucose, and NaCl is typical (233). Due to the low secretory ability of the renal cell, diuretics (cyclopenthiazide, acetazolamide) are excreted more slowly by young rat kidneys (245). This probably explains the more prolonged action of some diuretics in young rats (246). In newborn rats theophylline increases GFR after the fifth day, whereas cyclopenthiazide, acetazolamide, mersalyl, etc do not affect GFR. In rats T_{mPAH} decreases after acetazolamide administration and increases at the action of mersalyl. The other drugs are not effective (247). After aminophylline administration the maximum value of EF_{Na} is 3.9% in young calves and 15.2% in cattle; for hydrochlorothiazide it is 4.2 and 3.9% respectively (248).

Furosemide, triamterene, and other diuretics exert a natriuretic effect on the kidneys of newborn children (249) and animals (246, 250). After the injection of 1 mg/kg furosemide to 8 and 90 day old babies Na excretion increases during the first hour 39- and 131-fold respectively (249). This may be a result not so much of a lower effectiveness of the cellular action as of a still smaller loading of nephrons due to reduced GFR.

The available data does not permit as yet a quantitative estimation of changes in some of the transport systems of nephron cells in phylogenesis and ontogenesis. Since saluretics (furosemide, ethacrynic acid, etc) are efficient in all classes of vertebrates and even in early postnatal ontogenesis of mammals, this is evidence for the presence of the main cellular systems of Na transport. By contrast, the response to some hormones differs in lower and higher vertebrates and develops gradually during postnatal ontogenesis. A considerable increase of GFR and proximal reabsorption levels is characteristic of the kidney development in ontogenesis. The GFR and the proximal reabsorption are higher in warm-blooded animals. These factors provide more efficient excretion of substances and create a possibility for vigorous osmotic diuresis.

Literature Cited

1. Landon, E. J., Forte, L. R. 1971. *Ann. Rev. Pharmacol.* 11:171–88
2. Bentley, P. J. 1971. *Endocrines and Osmoregulation.* Berlin: Springer
3. Heller, H., La Pointe, J. *Comparative Pharmacology,* ed. M. Michelson, Vol. 2. Oxford: Pergamon. In press
4. Suki, W. N., Eknoyan, G., Martinez-Maldonado, M. 1973. *Ann. Rev. Pharmacol.* 13:91–106
5. Dirks, J. H., Seely, J. F. 1969. *Ann. Rev. Pharmacol.* 9:73–84
6. Smith, H. W. 1961. *From Fish to Philosopher.* New York: Doubleday
7. Hickman, C. P. Jr., Trump, B. F. 1969. *Fish Physiology,* ed. W. S. Hoar, D. J. Randall, 1:91–240. New York: Academic

8. Natochin, Yu. V. 1964. *Proc. 2nd Int. Congr. Nephrol.* 1963:657–60
9. Vinnichenko, L. N. 1966. *Electron Microscopy of Animal Cells,* ed. E. M. Cheisin, 5–25. Leningrad: Nauka
10. Youson, J. H., McMillan, D. B. 1971. *Am. J. Anat.* 130:281–303
11. Helmy, F. M., Hack, M. H. 1967. *Comp. Biochem. Physiol.* 20:55–63
12. Krestinskaya, T. V., Manusova, N. B. *Arkh. Anat. Gistol. Embriol.* In press
13. Krestinskaya, T. V., Manusova, N. B., Natochin, Yu. V. 1973. *Vopr. Ikhtiol.* 13:676–83
14. Olsen, S., Ericsson, J. 1968. *Z. Zellforsch.* 87:17–30
15. Olsen, S. 1970. *Acta Pathol. Microbiol. Scand. Suppl.* 212:81–96
16. Ericsson, J. L. E., Olsen, S. 1970. *Z. Zellforsch.* 104:240–58
17. Windhager, E. E. 1968. *Micropuncture Techniques and Nephron Function.* London: Butterworths
18. Heller, J. 1971. *Physiol. Bohemoslov.* 20:139–45
19. Kuschinsky, W., Wahl, M., Wunderlich, P., Thurau, K. 1970. *Pfluegers Arch.* 321:102–20
20. Knox, F. G., Schneider, E. G., Dresser, T. P., Lynch, R. E. 1970. *Am. J. Physiol.* 219:904–10
21. Bresler, V. M., Natochin, Yu. V. 1973. *Biull. Eksp. Biol. Med.* N 6:67–69
22. Natochin, Yu. V. 1972. *Zh. Evol. Biokhimii Fiziol.* 8:289–97
23. Giebisch, G. 1969. *Nephron* 6:260–81
24. Ussing, H. H. 1971. *Phil. Trans. Roy. Soc. B* 262:85–90
25. Lyttkens, L. 1972. *Upsala J. Med. Sci. Suppl.* 11:1–12
26. Moreno, J. H., Reisin, I. L., Boulan, E. R., Rotunno, C. A., Cereijido, M. 1973. *J. Memb. Biol.* 11:99–115
27. Leblanc, G. 1972. *Pfluegers Arch.* 337:1–18
28. Cereijido, M., Rotunno, C. A. 1968. *J. Gen. Physiol.* 51:280S–89S
29. Dörge, A., Nagel, W. *Pfluegers Arch.* 337:285–97
30. Ussing, H. H. 1971. *Electrophysiology of Epithelial Cells,* ed. G. Giebisch, 3–16. Stuttgart: Schattauer
31. Schmidt, U., Dubach, U. C. 1972. *Experientia* 28:385–86
32. Silverman, M. 1973. *Fed. Proc.* 32:257 (Abstr.)
33. Thoenes, W., Langer, K. H. 1969. *Renal Transport and Diuretics,* ed. K. Thurau, H. Jahrmärker, 37–64. Berlin: Springer
34. Ericsson, L. E., Trump, B. F. 1969. *The Kidney,* ed. C. Rouiller, F. Muller, 1: 351–440. New York: Academic
35. Whittembury, G., Rawlins, F. A. 1971. *Pfluegers Arch.* 330:302–9
36. Walser, M. 1971. See Ref. 34, 3:127–207
37. Dörge, A., Nagel, W. 1970. *Pfluegers Arch.* 321:91–101
38. Kriz, W., Schnermann, J., Höhling, H. J., Von Rosenstiel, A. P., Hall, T. A. 1972. *Rec. Advan. Renal Physiol.,* 162–71
39. Giebisch, G., Boulpaep, E. L., Whittembury, G. 1971. *Phil. Trans. Roy. Soc. B* 262:175–96
40. Maude, D. L. 1970. *Am. J. Physiol.* 218:1590–95
41. Ullrich, K. J., Radtke, H. W., Rumrich, G. 1971. *Pfluegers Arch.* 330:149–61
42. Rumrich, G., Ullrich, K. J. 1969. *J. Physiol.* 197:69P–70P
43. Khuri, R. N., Agulian, S. K., Wise, W. M. 1971. *Pfluegers Arch.* 322:39–46
44. Khuri, R. et al 1972. *Pfluegers Arch.* 338:73–80
45. Wiederholt, M., Sullivan, W. J., Giebisch, G. 1971. *J. Gen. Physiol.* 57: 495–525
46. Giebisch, G. 1971. See Ref. 34, 3: 329–82
47. Sokolova, M. M., Bakhteeva, V. T. 1972. *6th Orbeli Conf. Evol. Physiol. Leningrad,* 200
48. Khuri, R. N., Agulian, S. K., Kalloghlian, A. 1972. *Pfluegers Arch.* 335:297–308
49. Malvin, R. L., Carlson, E., Legan, S., Churchill, P. 1970. *Am. J. Physiol.* 218:1506–9
50. Forster, R. P., Goldstein, L., Rosen, J. K. 1972. *Comp. Biochem. Physiol.* 42A:3–12
51. Hickman, C. P. Jr. 1965. *Roy. Soc. Can.,* Sect. III, 3:213–36
52. Tanner, G. A., Kinter, W. B. 1966. *Am. J. Physiol.* 210:221–31
53. Sheikh, I. 1972. *J. Physiol.* 227:565–90
54. Grantham, J., Qualizza, P., Irwin, R. 1973. *Fed. Proc.* 32:381 (Abstr.)
55. Cafruny, E. J., Cho, K. C., Gussin, R. Z. 1966. *Ann. NY Acad. Sci.* 139: 362–74
56. Dantzler, W. H., Shaffner, D. P., Chiu, P. J. S. 1970. *Am. J. Physiol.* 218: 929–36
57. Fujimoto, J. M., Lech, J. J., Zamiatowski, R. 1973. *Biochem. Pharmacol.* 22: 971–79
58. Deetjen, P., Büntig, W. E., Hardt, K., Rohde, R. 1969. *Progr. Nephrol,* ed. G.

Peters, F. Roch-Ramel, 255–61. Berlin: Springer
59. Wolf, K., Bieg, A., Fülgraff, G. 1969. *Eur. J. Pharmacol.* 7:342–44
60. Imbs, J. L., Desaulles, E., Velly, J., Bloch, R., Schwartz, J. 1972. *Pfluegers Arch.* 331:294–306
61. Nechay, B. R. 1967. *J. Pharmacol. Exp. Ther.* 158:471–74
62. Natochin, Yu. V., Gusev, G. P., Goncharevskaya, O. A., Lavrova, E. A., Shakhmatova, E. I. 1972. *Comp. Biochem. Physiol.* 43A:253–58
63. Shakhmatova, E. I. 1973. *Natriuretic function of the vertebrate kidney.* Thesis. Inst. Evol. Physiol. Leningrad
64. Chez, R. A., Horger, E. O., Schultz, G. 1969. *J. Pharmacol. Exp. Ther.* 168:1–5
65. Cohn, E. S., Gordes, E. H., Brusilow, S. W. 1971. *Science* 171:910–11
66. Peters, G., Roch-Ramel, F. 1969. *Handb. Exp. Pharm.* 24:386–405
67. Vogel, G., Stoeckert, I., Tervooren, U. 1966. *Arch. Pharmakol. Exp. Pathol.* 255:245–53
68. Schmidt-Nielsen, B. 1973. *Fed. Proc.* 32:382 (Abstr.)
69. Dicker, S. E., Eggleton, M. G., Haslam, J. 1966. *J. Physiol.* 187:247–55
70. Flückiger, E., Schalch, W., Taeschler, M. 1963. *Schweiz. Med. Wschr.* 93:1232–37
71. Terry, B., Hook, J. B. 1968. *J. Pharmacol. Exp. Ther.* 160:367–74
72. Natochin, Yu. V. 1969. *Zh. Evol. Biokhimii Fiziol.* 5:333–35
73. Bentley, P. J., Follett, B. K. 1963. *J. Physiol.* 169:902–18
74. Sakai, F., Enomoto, Y. 1964. *Arch. Int. Pharmacodyn.* 151:358–64
75. Maetz, J. 1971. *Phil. Trans. Roy. Soc. B* 262:209–49
76. Motais, R., Garcia-Romeu, F. 1972. *Ann. Rev. Physiol.* 34:141–76
77. Kotchabhakdi, N., Leitch, G. 1972. *Comp. Biochem. Physiol.* 43A:143–53
78. Frati, L., Mozzi, R., Rossi, R., Covelli, I. 1971. *Farmaco Ed. Prat.* 26:626–31
79. Baer, J. E., Jones, C. B., Spitzer, S. A., Russo, H. F. 1967. *J. Pharmacol. Exp. Ther.* 157:472–85
80. Pozet, N., Lech, P., Traeger, J. 1972. *J. Méd. Lyon* 53:1233–37
81. Eigler, J., Crabbé, J. See Ref. 33, 195–207
82. Aceves, J., Cereijido, M. 1973. *J. Physiol.* 229:709–18
83. Schneyer, L. H., Young, J. A., Schneyer, C. A. 1972. *Physiol. Rev.* 52:720–77
84. Cuthbert, A. W., Maetz, J. 1972. *Comp. Biochem. Physiol.* 43A:227–32
85. Wilkinson, W. H. See Ref. 33, 255–66
86. Sidorenko, B. A., Kharchenko, V. I., Tolstykh, A. N., Melnichenko, G. A. 1971. *Cardiologia* 11:20–30
87. Elizondo, R. S., LeBrie, S. J. 1969. *Am. J. Physiol.* 217:419–25
88. Dicker, S. E. 1970. *Hormones* 1:352–63
89. Herms, W., Hofmann, K. E. 1965. *Arch. Exp. Pathol. Pharmak.* 251:355–74
90. Eigler, J., Carl, H., Edel, H. H. 1966. *Klin. Wschr.* 44:417–24
91. Natochin, Yu. V., Lavrova, E. A. *Biull. Eksp. Biol. Med.* In press
92. Lebedev, A. A. 1971. *Kardiologia* N1:89–94
93. Jamison, R. L. 1961. *J. Pharmacol. Exp. Ther.* 133:1–6
94. Lipson, S., Hays, R. M. 1966. *J. Clin. Invest.* 45:1042
95. Sullivan, L. P., Tucker, J. M., Scherbenske, M. J. 1971. *Am. J. Physiol.* 220:1316–24
96. Natochin, Yu. V., Lavrova, E. A. 1972. *Experientia* 28:942–43
97. Candia, O. A. 1973. *Fed. Proc.* 32:245 (Abstr.)
98. Natochin, Yu. V. 1972. *Farmakol. Toksikol.* N1:49–52
99. Baer, J. E., Beyer, K. H. 1972. *Progr. Biochem. Pharm.* 7:59–93
100. Crabbé, J. 1968. *Arch. Int. Pharmacodyn.* 173:474–77
101. Bentley, P. J. 1968. *J. Physiol.* 195:317–30
102. Biber, T. U. L. 1971. *J. Gen. Physiol.* 58:131–44
103. Ferguson, D. R., Smith, M. W. 1972. *J. Endocrinol.* 55:195–201
104. Yonath, J., Civan, M. M. 1971. *J. Membrane Biol.* 5:366–85
105. Nagel, W., Dörge, A. 1970. *Pfluegers Arch.* 317:84–92
106. Nielsen, R., Tomilson, R. W. S. 1970. *Acta Physiol. Scand.* 79:238–43
107. Salako, L. A., Smith, A. J. 1970. *Brit. J. Pharmacol.* 39:99–109
108. Parisi, M., Bentley, P. J. 1970. *Biochim. Biophys. Acta* 219:234–37
109. Cuthbert, A. W., Wong, P. Y. D. 1971. *Biochim. Biophys. Acta* 241:713–15
110. Salako, L. A., Smith, A. J. 1970. *Brit. J. Pharmacol.* 38:702–18
111. Cuthbert, A. W., Wong, P. Y. D. 1972. *Mol. Pharmacol.* 8:222–29
112. Ehrlich, E. N., Crabbé, J. 1968. *Pfluegers Arch.* 302:79–96
113. Nielsen, R. 1971. *Acta Physiol. Scand.* 83:106–14

114. Natochin, Yu. V., Bakhteeva, V. T., Lavrova, E. A. 1973. *Biophysics of membrane,* 484–89. Kaunas: Med. Inst.
115. Guignard, J. P., Peters, G. 1970. *Eur. J. Pharmacol.* 10:255–67
116. Deetjen, P. See Ref. 33, 215–26
117. Duarte, C. G., Chomety, F., Giebisch, G. 1971. *Am. J. Physiol.* 221:632–40
118. Maren, T. H. 1969. *Handb. Exp. Pharmacol.* 24:195–256
119. Janata, V., Schück, O. 1971. *Int. J. Clin. Pharmacol.* 4:200–3
120. Mohr, H. J. See Ref. 58, 281–89
121. Vinnichenko, L. N., Natochin, Yu. V., Sabinin, G. V., Shakhmatova, E. I. 1973. *Arkh. Anat. Gistol. Embriol.* N8:61–68
122. Schmidt, U., Dubach, U. C. 1970. *Nephron* 7:447–58
123. Nechay, B. R., Contreras, R. R. 1972. *J. Pharmacol. Exp. Ther.* 183:127–36
124. Nechay, B. R., Palmer, R. F., Chinoy, D. A., Posey, V. A. 1967. *J. Pharmacol. Exp. Ther.* 157:599–617
125. Charnock, J. S., Potter, H. A., McKee, D. 1970. *Biochem. Pharmacol.* 19:1637–41
126. Davis, P. W. 1970. *Biochem. Pharmacol.* 19:1983–89
127. Landon, E. J., Fitzpatrick, D. F. 1972. *Biochem. Pharmacol.* 21:1561–68
128. Ebel, H., Ehrich, J., De Santo, N. G., Doerken, U. 1972. *Pfluegers Arch.* 335:224–34
129. Williamson, H. E. 1970. *Proc. 4th Int. Congr. Nephrol.* 2:144–52
130. Nechay, B. R., Nelson, J. A. 1970. *J. Pharmacol. Exp. Ther.* 175:717–26
131. Martinez-Maldonado, M., Allen, J. C., Inagaki, C., Tsaparas, N., Schwartz, A. 1972. *J. Clin. Invest.* 51:2544–51
132. Allen, J. C., Martinez-Maldonado, M., Eknoyan, G., Suki, W. N., Schwartz, A. 1971. *Biochem. Pharmacol.* 20:73–80
133. Kleinzeller, A. 1972. *Metabolic Pathways,* 6:91–131. New York: Academic
134. Janaček, K., Rybová, R., Slavíková, M. 1972. *Biochim. Biophys. Acta* 288:221–24
135. Kleinzeller, A., Knotkova, A. 1964. *J. Physiol.* 175:172–92
136. Whittembury, G., Proverbio, F. 1970. *Pfluegers Arch.* 316:1–25
137. Whittembury, G., Fishman, J. 1969. *Pfluegers Arch.* 307:138–53
138. Weinschelbaum, de J. S., Vieyra, A., MacLaughlin, M. 1972. *Biochim. Biophys. Acta* 279:320–30
139. Proverbio, F., Robinson, J. W. L., Whittembury, G. 1970. *Biochim. Biophys. Acta* 211:327–36
140. Torretti, J., Hendler, E., Weinstein, E., Longnecker, R. E., Epstein, F. H. 1972. *Am. J. Physiol.* 222:1398–1405
141. Giebisch, G., Sullivan, L. P., Whittembury, G. 1973. *J. Physiol.* 230:51–74
142. Whittembury, G. See Ref. 30, 153–78
143. Kessler, R. H. 1966. *Ann. NY Acad. Sci.* 139:356–61
144. Fülgraff, G., Wolf, K., Adelmann, J., Krieger, A. K. 1969. *Arch. Pharmacol. Exp. Pathol.* 263:485–95
145. Fülgraff, G. 1970. *Proc. 4th Int. Congr. Nephrol.* 2:119–26
146. Landon, E. J., Fitzpatrick, D. F. 1970. *Proc. 4th Int. Congr. Nephrol.* 2:127–36
147. Suki, W. N., Dawoud, F., Eknoyan, G., Martinez-Maldonado, M. 1972. *J. Pharmacol. Exp. Ther.* 180:6–12
148. Eknoyan, G., Suki, W. N., Martinez-Maldonado, M. 1970. *J. Lab. Clin. Med.* 76:257–66
149. Nielsen, S. P., Andersen, O., Steven, K. E. 1969. *Acta Pharmacol. Toxicol.* 27:469–79
150. Robinson, R., Portwood, R. 1962. *Am. J. Physiol.* 202:309–12
151. Gusev, G. P., Manusova, N. B. 1971. *Zh. Evol. Biokhimii Fiziol.* 7:478–83
152. Munz, F. W., McFarland, W. N. 1964. *Comp. Biochem. Physiol.* 13:381–400
153. Bieter, R. N. 1933. *J. Pharmacol. Exp. Ther.* 49:250–56
154. Berglund, F., Forster, R. P. 1958. *J. Gen. Physiol.* 41:429–40
155. Gusev, G. P., Vasilieva, V. F., Natochin, Yu. V., Shakhmatova, E. I. 1969. *Zh. Evol. Biokhimii Fiziol.* 5:30–37
156. Vasilieva, V. F., Gusev, G. P., Natochin, Yu. V., Shakhmatova, E. I. 1969. *Vopt. Ikhtiol.* 9:546–55
157. Miles, H. M. 1971. *Comp. Biochem. Physiol.* 38A:787–826
158. Natochin, Yu. V., Gusev, G. P. 1970. *Comp. Biochem. Physiol.* 37:107–11
159. Natochin, Yu. V., Sokolova, M. M., Gusev, G. P., Shakhmatova, E. I., Lavrova, E. A. 1969. *Dokl. Akad. Nauk SSSR* 186:732–35
160. Malvin, R. L., Cafruni, E. J., Kutchai, H. 1965. *J. Cell. Comp. Physiol.* 65:381–84
161. Dantzler, W. H. 1966. *Am. J. Physiol.* 210:640–46
162. Deetjen, P. 1969. *Kardiologia* 9(11):12–17
163. Vogel, G., Kröger, W. 1965. *Pfluegers Arch.* 286:317–22

164. Vogel, G., Stoeckert, I. 1966. *Pfluegers Arch.* 292:309–15
165. Nechay, B. R., Chinoy, D. A. 1968. *Eur. J. Pharmacol.* 3:322–29
166. Sawyer, W. H. 1968. *Handb. Exp. Pharmakol.* 24:717–47
167. Morel, F., Jard, S. 1968. *Handb. Exp. Pharmakol.* 24:655–716
168. Sawyer, W. H. 1972. *Fed. Proc.* 31: 1609–14
169. Olivereau, M., Ball, J. N. 1970. *Mem. Soc. Endocrinol.* 18:57–85
170. Hanke, W. 1970. *Fortschr. Zool.* 20: 112–380
171. Ball, J. N. 1969. *Gen. Comp. Endocrinol.* suppl. 2:10–25
172. Payan, P., Maetz, J. 1971. *Gen. Comp. Endocrinol.* 16:535–54
173. Nishimura, H., Oguri, M., Ogawa, M., Sokabe, H., Imai, M. 1970. *Am. J. Physiol.* 218:911–13
174. Capelli, J. P., Wesson, L. G. Jr., Aponte, G. E. 1970. *Am. J. Physiol.* 218:1171–78
175. Cort, J. H., Lichardus, D., Eds. 1970. *Regulation of Body Fluid Volumes by the Kidney.* Basel: Karger
176. Berliner R. W., Brenner, B., Falchuk, K., Keimowitz, R. 1970. *Proc. 4th Int. Congr. Nephrol.* 2:99–106
177. Blythe, W. B., D'Avila, D., Gitelman, H. J., Welt, L. G. 1971. *Circ. Res.* 28, Suppl. 11:21–31
178. Lichardus, B., Poneč, J. 1972. *Experientia* 28:471–72
179. Lee, J. B. 1972. *Prostaglandins* 1:55–70
180. Strandhoy, J. W. 1973. *Fed. Proc.* 32: 398 (Abstr.)
181. Handler, J. S., Orloff, J. 1971. *Proc. Symp. Cell. Processes Growth, Development, Differentiation,* 301–18
182. Bär, H. P., Hechter, O., Schwartz, I. L., Walter, R. 1970. *Proc. Nat. Acad. Sci. USA* 67:7–12
183. Hynie, S., Sharp, G. W. G. 1971. *Biochim. Biophys. Acta* 230:40–51
184. Bentley, P. J. 1972. *J. Pharmacol. Exp. Ther.* 181:155–60
185. Rajerison, R. M., Montegut, M., Jard, S., Morel, F. 1972. *Pfluegers Arch.* 332:313–31
186. Robison, A., Sutherland, E. W. 1970. *Circ. Res.* 26, Suppl. 1:147–61
187. Fisher, D. A. 1968. *J. Clin. Invest.* 47: 540–47
188. Orloff, J., Handler, J. S., Bergström, S. 1965. *Nature* 205:397–98
189. Flores, A. G. A., Sharp, G. W. G. 1972. *Am. J. Physiol.* 223:1392–97
190. Parisi, M., Piccinni, Z. F. 1972. *J. Endocrinol.* 55:1–9
191. Leaf, A. 1967. *Am. J. Med.* 42:745–56
192. Macknight, A. D. C., Leaf, A., Civan, M. M. 1971. *J. Membrane Biol.* 6: 127–37
193. Handler, J. S., Preston, A. S., Orloff, J. 1972. *Am. J. Physiol.* 222:1071–74
194. Janáček, K., Rybova, R. 1970. *Pfluegers Arch.* 318:294–304
195. Finn, A. L. 1971. *J. Gen. Physiol.* 57: 349–62
196. Andersen, B., Ussing, H. 1957. *Acta Physiol. Scand.* 39:228–39
197. Hays, R. M. 1972. *Curr. Top. Membranes Transp.* 3:339–66
198. Eggena, P. 1972. *J. Gen. Physiol.* 59: 519–33
199. Ginetzinsky, A. G. 1964. *Physiological Mechanisms of Water and Salt Homeostasis.* Leningrad: Nauka
200. Dicker, S. E. 1970. *Mechanisms of Urine Concentration and Dilution in Mammals.* London: Arnold
201. Natochin, Yu. V. 1972. *Physiology of the Kidney,* 206–15. Leningrad: Nauka
202. Ivanova, L. N., Perechvalskaya, T. V. 1968. *Dokl. Acad. Nauk SSSR* 181: 1013–16
203. Hierholzer, K., Stolte, H. 1969. *Nephron* 6:188–204
204. Wiederholt, M., Behn, C., Schoormans, W., Hansen, L. 1972. *J. Steroid Biochem.* 3:151–58
205. LeBrie, S. J. 1972. *Fed. Proc.* 31:1599–1608
206. Edelman, I. S. 1972. *J. Steroid Biochem.* 3:167–71
207. Swaneck, G. E., Chu, L., Edelman, I. S. 1970. *J. Biol. Chem.* 245:5382–89
208. Rousseau, G., Crabbé, J. 1972. *Eur. J. Biochem.* 25:550–59
209. Fimognari, G. M., Fanestil, D. D., Edelman, I. S. 1967. *Am. J. Physiol.* 213:954–62
210. Crabbé, J. 1972. *J. Steroid Biochem.* 3: 557–66
211. Leaf, A., Macknight, A. D. C. 1972. *J. Steroid Biochem.* 3:237–45
212. Janáček, K., Rybová, R., Slavíkova, M. 1971. *Pfluegers Arch.* 326:316–23
213. Stoff, J. S., Handler, J. S., Orloff, J. 1972. *Proc. Nat. Acad. Sci. USA* 69: 805–8
214. Porter, G. A., Kimsey, J. 1972. *J. Steroid Biochem.* 3:201–8
215. Nutbourne, D. M., Howes, J. D., Ferguson, N. E. 1971. *25th Int. Congr. Physiol. Sci.,* Munich, 422
216. Coviello, A. 1971. *Int. Conf. Physiol. Pharmacol. Cyclic AMP,* Milan, 83
217. Coviello, A. 1969. *Acta Physiol. Lat. Am.* 19:73–82

218. Malvin, R. L., Vander, A. J. 1967. *Am. J. Physiol.* 213:1205–8
219. Finberg, J. P. M., Peart, W. S. 1972. *J. Physiol.* 220:229–42
220. Nizet, A., Lefebvre, P., Crabbé, J. 1971. *Pfluegers Arch.* 323:11–20
221. Herrera, F. C. 1965. *Am. J. Physiol.* 209:819–24
222. Crabbé, J. 1972. *J. Steroid Biochem.* 3:229–35
223. Natochin, Yu. V., Golod, G. M., Natochina, T. M. 1965. *Ter. Arkh.* 37:57–64
224. Nechay, B. R. 1971. *J. Pharmacol. Exp. Ther.* 176:377–82
225. Stribrna, J., Schück, O. 1968. *Int. J. Clin. Pharmacol.* 1:504–13
226. Cuthbert, A. W., Painter, E. 1968. *J. Physiol.* 199:593–612
227. Rajerison, R. M., Montegut, M., Jard, S., Morel, F. 1972. *Pfluegers Arch.* 332:302–12
228. McCance, R. A. 1972. *J. Roy. Coll. Phys.* 6:235–45
229. Cooke, H. J., Young, J. A. 1970. *Pfluegers Arch.* 318:315–24
230. Heller, J., Čapek, K. 1965. *Physiol. Bohemoslov.* 14:433–38
231. Bräunlich, H. 1970. *Acta Biol. Med. Germ.* 24:327–38
232. Young, J. A., Freedman, B. S. 1971. *Clin. Chem.* 17:245–66
233. Norina, O. A. 1957. *Rep. Evol. Physiol. Leningrad* 2:172–80
234. Bräunlich, H., Puschmann, R. 1972. *Acta Biol. Med. Germ.* 28:89–98
235. Vasilieva, V. F., Vorobéva, K. P., Gusev, G. P. 1971. *Evolution of Vegeta-tive Functions,* ed. E. M. Kreps, 77–86. Leningrad: Nauka
236. Edelman, C. M. Jr., Spitzer, A. 1969. *J. Pediat.* 75:509–19
237. Boss, J. M. N., Dlouha, H., Kraus, M., Kreček, J. 1963. *J. Physiol.* 168:196–204
238. Dicker, S. E., Shirley, D. G. 1971. *J. Physiol.* 212:235–43
239. Wacker, G. R., Zarkowsky, H. S., Burch, H. B. 1961. *Am. J. Physiol.* 200:367–69
240. Brabcová, J., Jelinek, J., Drahota, Z. 1971. *Physiol. Bohemoslov.* 20:467–72
241. Potter, D., Jarrah, A., Sakai, T., Harrah, J., Holliday, M. A. 1969. *Pediat. Res.* 3:51–59
242. Vasilieva, V. F. 1960. *Rep. Evol. Physiol. Leningrad* 4:220–23
243. Dlouhá H., Kreček, J., Krečková, J. 1963. *Physiol. Bohemoslov.* 12:443–52
244. Bentley, P. J. 1963. *J. Endocrinol.* 26:361–65
245. Bräunlich, H., Ankermann, H. 1970. *Acta Biol. Med. Germ.* 25:325–36
246. Mohr, C., Kersten, L., Bräunlich, H. 1971. *Acta Biol. Med. Germ.* 26:361–69
247. Bräunlich, H. 1970. *Acta Biol. Med. Germ.* 25:315–23
248. Aronson, A. L., Scoville, D., Nechay, B. R. 1969. *4th Int. Congr. Pharmacol.,* 119
249. Chroma, M., Janovsky, M., Popp, M., Martinek, J. 1969. *Mschr. Kinderheilk.* 117:369–70
250. Čapek, K., Dlouhá, H., Kraus, M. 1969. *Pfluegers Arch.* 307:61R

DRUGS AFFECTING MOVEMENT DISORDERS

❖6583

André Barbeau

Department of Neurobiology, Clinical Research Institute of Montreal, Montreal, Canada

INTRODUCTION

Movement is one of the fundamental properties of life. Without movement, it is almost impossible for humans to communicate with the outside world. To the neurologist, movement disorders can include equally well the restrictions caused by paralysis or atrophy and the addition of abnormal involuntary movements. These changes can be due to biochemical or organic lesions anywhere along the neuraxis, from the cortex to the neuromuscular junction. It would be impossible, within the scope of the present review, to study all these possibilities. We will therefore understand the term "movement disorders" as referring to modifications in motor behavior involving disturbances within the so-called "Extrapyramidal System" (1).

This system, however, is not yet clearly defined and could conceivably include disorders affecting all regions not strictly "pyramidal," such as the cerebellum and parts of the spinal cord. For example, ataxia, myoclonus, and spinal spasticity are truly movement disorders but will not be discussed in the present review. The disorders we will study all involve, in whole or in part, damage to the following centers (the so-called basal ganglia): striatum (caudate, putamen), globus pallidus, thalamus, subthalamic nucleus, substantia nigra. The lesions may be limited to such centers or they may also involve other systems (pyramidal, cerebellar, spinal, cortical) but, at least at some moment in time, symptoms related to damage of the above nuclei are clinically evident.

We could approach the problem of drugs upon movement disorder by listing all "extrapyramidal diseases" and their treatment. Besides the cumbersome enumeration so involved, as exemplified by the list of more than 130 entities in a recent nosography of extrapyramidal disorders (2), no functional analysis would be possible. Thus instead of diseases we have decided to center our discussion around *symptoms*. We will not detail the treatment of Parkinson's disease, a subject well covered recently by many authors (4–13, 34), but will concentrate on the clinical pharmacology of tremor, of rigidity, and of akinesia.

Symptoms of basal ganglia diseases have conveniently been classified by Martin (3) as either negative or positive. The only true negative symptom of basal gangliar disorder is akinesia (or more exactly hypokinesia). Since it is now the one sign best corrected by L-dopa (L-3,4-dihydroxyphenylalanine) and similar drugs, we will study it in detail. The positive symptoms most usually seen are tremor, rigidity, dystonia, chorea, athetosis, and tics. All can to some extent be modified by drugs already on the market, or being tried experimentally. These modifications, and the rationale behind them, will form the basis of the present chapter.

Finally, drugs could affect movement disorders by *causing* them, experimentally (tremorine) or clinically (phenothiazines). The best example of this phenomenon is the production of a parkinsonian syndrome including akinesia, rigidity, and tremor by the chronic use of a number of phenothiazines or butyrophenones, which all act upon central dopamine receptors (14–25). The same drugs can produce abnormal involuntary movements as an acute reaction or a strange chorea-like syndrome when withdrawn after long use: the so-called tardive dyskinesias (17, 26–33). Although this latter subject could be of considerable interest, we will not include its study in the present review limited to drugs that modify *existing non-drug-induced* movement disorders.

THE PHARMACOTHERAPY OF AKINESIA

The problem of akinesia is one of the most fascinating aspects of the physiology of the extrapyramidal system, although its very existence has been recognized clearly only since the introduction of stereotaxic surgery, when separation from rigidity was finally permitted. Early biochemical studies in parkinsonism (35–42) indicated that the phenomenon of bradykinesia was the symptom best correlated with the deficit in dopamine. This was subsequently confirmed by studies that related the presence of akinesia with low dopamine and homovanillic acid (HVA) in the urine (38, 39, 43), the cerebrospinal fluid (39, 44, 45), and the brain (46). The introduction of L-dopa to the therapy of Parkinson's disease (37, 47–49) has confirmed clearly that akinesia is the first symptom responsive to correction (8, 50).

1. Definition of Akinesia

In clinical terms, akinesia as seen in Parkinson's disease is a symptom complex, manifested by a number of phenomena just recently better identified (51, 52). From a study of nearly 100 cases of parkinsonism with almost pure akinesia, we have been able to delineate the following important components of this syndrome (53, 54):

(*a*) A defect in *motor initiative* including slow initiation of movements and a decreased motivation to move, leading to conservation of kinetic energy through the loss of associated movements.

(*b*) A defect in the *kinetic melody,* i.e. the ability to change rapidly from one motor pattern to the next in a smooth flow of movement as dictated by circumstances or willful decisions.

(*c*) A defect in the *strategy of learning.* The patient is unable to perform the Goldstein Sorting Test, in which he is asked to separate a number of common objects in conceptual groups based for example on size, consistency, color, or other physical or utilitarian characteristics. Unless new possibilities are specifically pointed out to him, the parkinsonian akinetic patient, like the frontal lobe patient (55), is unable to *shift* to a new grouping.

(*d*) A *rapid fatiguability,* first studied by Schwab and collaborators (51) and since confirmed by many others (56).

It is within the scope of this syndrome, as here defined, that the best overall results have been obtained since the introduction of L-dopa. It is extremely important to remember this point because, unfortunately, other symptoms of parkinsonism such as tremor will not respond equally well to the specific replacement therapy. Moreover, misdiagnosis of tremor syndromes as Parkinson's disease has led to the unwarranted prescription of L-dopa, often with alarming complications. The rationale behind the use of L-dopa has been reviewed by many authors (4–11, 37, 39, 41, 42, 57–63, 65, 73, 74) and the actual results compiled and analyzed repeatedly (8, 37, 50, 64–72). We shall limit our discussion to the salient features of the neuropharmacology of akinesia, and emphasize the problems still to be solved.

2. Rationale for L-dopa Treatment of Akinesia

For a number of years it had been known that reserpine could produce a parkinsonian syndrome. The reason for this became clearer when Bertler & Rosengren (75) and Sano and collaborators (76) demonstrated that dopamine had a characteristic distribution within the brain different from that of noradrenaline, and that it was depleted by reserpine (80). A specific role for dopamine in the extrapyramidal system was soon postulated by Carlsson (77) and Barbeau (36). In quick succession it was shown that there existed in Parkinson's disease: (*a*) a decrease in dopamine content in the basal ganglia (40, 41), more evident on one side in hemiparkinsonism (78), and correlated with the damage to the substantia nigra (79); (*b*) a decreased dopamine and HVA content in the striatum and substantia nigra (81, 82), the latter being the starting point for a newly identified nigro-striatal dopaminergic pathway (83–86) which, when experimentally destroyed in monkeys or rats, results in significant decreases in the concentrations of dopamine, HVA, tyrosine-hydroxylase and dopa-decarboxylase in the striatum (83, 86–89); (*c*) a decrease in dopa-decarboxylase and glutamic acid decarboxylase in human parkinsonian brain (46, 90, 91); (*d*) a decrease in urinary dopamine excretion (43), and in cerebrospinal fluid (CSF) HVA concentration (for review see 39); (*e*) an increased dopamine turnover rate towards HVA rather than noradrenaline (92–94), indicative of a more generalized defect in dopamine binding or storage, perhaps related to some deficiency in magnesium (38, 39, 95–98, 155).

All of these observations led Hornykiewicz (99, 158) to define a dopamine-deficiency syndrome, which we (53, 54, 58, 59) equate with clinical akinesia as outlined above. The evidence to date (5, 8, 39) indicates that L-dopa is the drug of choice to correct this dopamine deficiency and akinesia, probably through the formation of dopamine by the remaining functional nigro-striatal dopaminergic neurons (41, 42, 73, 79, 99), although some authors still question this conclusion (70, 100). The development of carefully controlled methodology for the study of the minor pathways of catecholamine metabolism in man (101–111, 156) should soon permit clarification of this problem, especially if plasma levels of dopamine could be measured, perhaps by radioimmunological assays. Thus the rationale for the treatment of akinesia, as opposed to Parkinson's disease *in toto,* involves the design of methods primarily for restoring striatal dopamine function. L-dopa is now clearly established as the leading contender for this role. We will see later that other drugs can be added to decrease the side effects or to substitute for L-dopa, at least in part. However, it is important to remember that akinesia is not the only symptom of Parkinson's disease, and that a dopamine deficiency in the brain is not the only biochemical defect isolated or postulated. Indeed most other symptoms seen in this disease (tremor, rigidity, etc) are probably the result of an imbalance of neurotransmitters within the striatum. The concept of a dopaminergic-cholinergic imbalance was first proposed by McGeer (112) and Barbeau (37, 58) and expanded upon by Duvoisin, Klawans, Steg, and many others (74, 113–115). It now involves complex interrelationships between dopamine, acetylcholine, serotonin, histamine, noradrenaline, and γ-aminobutyric acid (GABA) in various parts of the brain (53, 54, 58, 116) but particularly the extrapyramidal system. We will later draw upon the conclusions of these studies to explain the rationale for the treatment of tremor, rigidity, chorea, and dystonia (see below), such treatment being essentially based on restoration of the disturbed balance (59).

3. Problems With L-dopa Therapy of Akinesia

Slow gradual increments of L-dopa have permitted marked improvement in most of the symptoms of Parkinson's disease, and particularly the reversal of akinesia, in approximately 70% of the patients so treated. The results are almost identical from one center to the next (4–13, 49, 50, 117). However, as has been repeatedly stated, this success was not reached without major and important problems which have been thoroughly discussed by many authors (4, 7, 8, 11, 50, 53, 63, 65, 117–119). A short review of these problems will serve to indicate that, despite evident benefits, L-dopa therapy is not yet a panacea, but that some solutions are already being proposed, based on a wealth of laboratory experiments and clinical observations.

(a) *Diagnosis.* The most common cause of therapeutic failures, in our experience, has been the misdiagnosis of Parkinson's disease, particularly with other tremor syndromes. Moreover, encouraged by the initial success of L-dopa, many neurologists have assessed the therapeutic potential of this drug in other disorders, including more than 20 neurological conditions with some akinesia, such as chronic manganese poisoning, progressive supranuclear palsy, the Parkinson-dementia complex of Guam, Wilson's disease (for review see 72, 120). Except in a few rare instances, the results have been uniformly disappointing. The exceptions will be discussed further in this chapter.

(b) *Peripheral side effects.* Side effects were encountered to an important degree during the early days of this experimental approach. Better understanding of the necessity of increasing very slowly the daily dosage of L-dopa has permitted some reduction in the incidence of nausea, vomiting, and postural hypotension (8, 50).

The real advance, however, took place when it was realized that because dopamine itself does not cross the blood-brain barrier, the degree of conversion of dopa to dopamine by systemic decarboxylase is of paramount importance in determining the percentage of orally administered dopa available for penetration into the brain and its subsequent action there. The enzymatic barrier for L-dopa has been the subject of detailed experimental studies in animals (121–123). The increase of cerebral dopamine induced by L-dopa is markedly enhanced by inhibitors of dopa-decarboxylase (124–130), and such compounds have been extensively studied in the laboratory and in clinical trials following the initial observation in humans by Birkmayer & Mentasti in 1967 (131). Ro4-4602[1] has been tested in Europe (132–134) and in Canada (135, 136), and its use over the last five years has recently been extensively reviewed (137). MK-485[2] or MK-486 (Methyl-dopa-hydrazine) has been studied mainly in England (138, 139) and the USA (140, 141). α-Methyl-dopa, a drug used for the treatment of hypertension, also possesses some dopa decarboxylase inhibitory capacity and has been partially successful in the same context (142, 143); in fact a recent note (144) claims that it is as powerful as methyl-dopa-hydrazine in potentiating the effects of L-dopa and alleviating undesirable peripheral side effects. All these trials present essentially similar results, indicating that the combination is indeed preferable to L-dopa alone (157). The incidence of nausea and vomiting is considerably reduced or abolished (130, 137). Dopamine is known to possess a number of cardiovascular and renal actions (for review see 145). It could have been expected that L-dopa would also produce some cardiovascular effects. This has indeed been the case with ventricular arrythmias and occasional drops in blood pressure (146). Combined therapy (L-dopa plus a dopa-decarboxylase inhibitor) has considerably reduced or abolished the incidence of arrythmias (136, 137).

Another advantage of combined therapy, besides the marked reduction in L-dopa dosage, has been the possibility of using pyridoxine in patients treated with L-dopa. Since pyridoxine is important in many brain enzymatic processes, such as dopa-decarboxylation, it was feared that large doses of L-dopa would induce a deficiency state, with subsequent complications, and therefore pyridoxine supplements were given to patients to enhance the dopa effect. However, Duvoisin and collaborators (147) reported that such a regimen could negate all beneficial effects in some patients, prompting a number of studies on the mechanism of action behind this phenomenon (148–151). The negative action of pyridoxine in patients with L-dopa can be blocked when peripheral dopa-decarboxylase inhibitors are used, thus slowing down the peripheral degradation of L-dopa (152, 153). The present state of the art concerning dopa-decarboxylase inhibitors has been summarized in a recent Symposium (154).

(c) *Psychiatric side effects.* For many years it has been known that a decrease in intellectual ability can be observed in a fair proportion of patients with Parkinson's disease, occasionally leading to actual dementia (159–162). There is also evidence that this mental deterioration in highest integrative functions is more closely asso-

[1][N'-(DL-seryl)-N²-(2,3,4-Trihydroxybenzyl)-hydrazine] HCl; Hoffmann-LaRoche.
[2]β-(3,4-dihydroxyphenyl)-α-hydrazino-α-methyl-DL-proprionic acid; Merck Sharp & Dohme.

ciated with the symptom akinesia (163, 164). Studies from our laboratory (52, 53, 165) have attempted a quantification of psychomotor components of akinesia and have delineated a significant impairment in the ability to elaborate a motor pattern or plan of action. This impairment was more evident with progressive complexity of the puzzle test utilized. The presence of akinesia is probably the single most important factor in a rapid progression of the illness. Indeed, Hoehn & Yahr (166) demonstrated that 40% of the akineto-rigid patients are invalid within five years, while fewer than 10% of those whose first symptom was tremor reached this stage after the same period. With this background, it was of great interest that along with a more or less specific anti-akinetic effect (8), L-dopa therapy has been observed to produce intellectual awakening or alerting (50, 167–169) and occasionally ameliorated thinking capacity. Some authors have even reported actual improvement in learning ability, auditory perception, and intermediate memory functions (169), as measured by verbal IQ and performance IQ scores (167, 170–173). This improvement appeared to be greatest in tests measuring perceptual organization, such as block designs and object assembly (165, 174), although Klaiber and collaborators (175) noted that even within this test specialization only the simple tasks were modified and the more complex procedures involving a sequence of actions, or making a decision, remained essentially unchanged. Riklan (176), however, still maintains that an increase in behavioral activation or arousal is responsible for the observed increments in test scores of intellectual functions following short- and long-range L-dopa therapy, while Garron and collaborators (177) confirm that late onset of Parkinson's disease and the symptom akinesia tend to be associated with intellectual deterioration.

Short-term results with L-dopa not only showed some evidence of improved intellectual function, but were often accompanied by a vast array of psychiatric disturbances. These have been the subject of a number of reviews (68, 119, 178–181) and even two recent books (182, 183). The reader is referred to these papers, to which there is very little to add. It is evident that the above observations have led many authors to use L-dopa as a research tool in mental disease and to strengthen the arguments in favor of the role of catecholamines, and particularly dopamine, in mental function (184–186).

With more long-term use of L-dopa, many physicians (187–189) are becoming aware of a subtle mental change occurring in some patients on chronic L-dopa therapy, but apparently not correlated to the degree of physical impairment. This motor/psychological dissociation is potentially very important. Patients outwardly intellectually bright, mobile, well oriented, and not depressed, perform at a definitely low level on tasks involving constructive and perceptual organization. In studies using the Kohs block design tests (165) it was shown that, despite the initial improvement within the first few months of L-dopa therapy, there is an inexorable gradual decrease in performance in all groups of parkinsonian patients, with a slow return to pretreatment levels. The slope of this progression is identical to that observed in patients not receiving L-dopa. It was concluded that L-dopa does not stop the underlying progression of the disease, even while correcting the motor performance for long periods of time. Moreover we could also conclude that L-dopa per se does not appear to be responsible for the progressive loss in intellectual performance, at least as measured with the Kohs block design test. It is thus probable that, as time goes on, we will see more and more of the dementias associated with the advanced state of Parkinson's disease.

(d) *Oscillations in performance.* After a certain time on high doses of L-dopa therapy, there appears with progressively increasing frequency in some patients a variation in the level of performance during the day. These diurnal changes were first reported by Cotzias and collaborators (50) and studied in detail by us (8, 53, 137, 190). The patients experienced a bimodal pattern of performance during the day, with good periods usually in the morning and early evening, and bad periods during which akinesia reappeared in the afternoon and late evening. Despite numerous modifications in diet, drug regimen, or dosage, the oscillations became more pronounced. They were made worse by independent patterns of abnormal involuntary movements (AIM) and there appeared, again with increasing frequency, a strange phenomenon marked by a rapid change-over from the "free" to the "rigid" conditions, or inversely. This switch effect has received the name "on and off phenomenon" because of its occasional very rapid unfolding (37). Some clinical characteristics of the patients during the bad periods made them different from the pre-dopa experience and led us and others to use the term "akinesia paradoxica" (137, 191, 193). We have described four types of diurnal oscillations, which are in fact four stages in a continuous process (for complete description see 137, 190). The early (Stage 1) oscillations are the result of a variable deficiency in effective dopamine, as shown through determinations of plasma dopa (156). The more severe oscillations (Stages 2 to 4) are the result of additive phenomena due to L-dopa overdosage, where too much dopamine displaces serotonin and noradrenaline (54, 253). These phenomena involve the simultaneous production of AIM and of a hypotonic akinesia. Clinical experiments designed to accomplish a slow, gradual reduction in L-dopa dosage over a 10 month period (190) conclusively demonstrated a marked reduction in the incidence and severity of these two side effects, without loss of motor performance in almost all subjects. We concluded that in many patients manifesting AIM and hypotonic akinesia we were unnecessarily giving between 1 and 1.5 L-dopa *in excess* of the minimum requirements. This conclusion was supported by the results of plasma dopa determinations in some of these patients (192). From these observations we proposed two L-dopa schedules in the therapy of Parkinson's disease: an *induction* dosage usually fairly high, and a *maintenance* regimen, which required much lower levels of L-dopa.

In the previous paragraphs we have reviewed some of the problems (diagnosis, peripheral, and psychiatric side effects, oscillations in performance) inherent to the long-term pharmacotherapy of akinesia with L-dopa. The other well-known problem, of course, is the development of abnormal involuntary movements. Because this subject is germane to the physiopathology of the "positive" symptoms which will be described later, we will omit a discussion of AIM at this point.

4. L-Dopa Analogs or Substitutes in the Treatment of Akinesia

As seen above, the treatment of akinesia is based essentially upon the replacement of effective brain dopamine. It was thus to be expected that a variety of other approaches would be tried to achieve the same goal. Although, to date, none of the other drugs studied have equalled L-dopa in range of efficacy, it may be worthwhile to summarize these findings:

(a) *m-Tyrosine.* Like dopa, *m*-tyrosine penetrates into the brain and is subsequently converted to *m*-tyramine, an amine capable of stimulating dopamine receptors, as demonstrated by its awakening effect in reserpine-treated mice (194) and in preliminary human trials (37, 195). In animal studies, Andén and collaborators (196) and Ungerstedt and collaborators (197) demonstrated that *m*-tyrosine can mimic the behavioral effect of L-dopa treatment after depletion of endogenous monoamine stores. In rats with a unilateral 6-OH-dopamine-induced lesion of the nigro-neostriatal dopamine pathway, the administration of 1-*m*-tyrosine in combination with an extracerebral dopa-decarboxylase inhibitor caused marked turning of the rat towards the intact side and mimicked the action of L-dopa in this model (197). Similarly in monkeys with unilateral ventromedial tegmental lesions, the same combination caused a transient relief of the tremor of the ipsilateral extremities (197). Unfortunately recent clinical trials in human parkinsonian patients failed to confirm similar actions in man (198).

(b) *γ-Hydroxybutyrate.* γ-Hydroxybutyrate, a natural metabolite of the mammalian brain (199), possesses sedative, hypnotic, and anesthetic properties and has been introduced clinically as an hypnotic agent (200). This compound can produce a selective, dose-dependent increase in brain dopamine in different species, particularly within the basal ganglia (201-204). It appears to stimulate dopamine synthesis without inhibiting either monoamine oxidase or catechol-O-methyl transferase (205). Some preliminary favorable results in man (206) have not been confirmed by others (207).

(c) *3-O-Methyl-dopa.* 3-Methyl-4-hydroxyphenylalanine (3-O-methyl-dopa) is an important metabolite of L-dopa in animals and man (208). It has now been demonstrated that this compound, through demethylation, can serve as a precursor to dopamine (209). This property, coupled with a relatively long half-life and its long persistence in the blood was the basis for initial optimistic therapeutic trials (210) which, unfortunately, could not be confirmed, even by the same authors (211–213).

(d) *Enzyme inhibitors.* Dopamine is metabolized mainly through three enzymatic systems: dopamine-β-hydroxylase, monoamine oxidase, and catechol-O-methyl transferase (COMT) (for review see 61, 62). Attempts to enhance brain dopamine levels through inhibition of each of these enzymes have been carried out with variable results. In animals disulfiram, a dopamine-β-hydroxylase inhibitor, has been found to be a potent agent in increasing the brain dopamine concentration (214). In man it has not been very useful, mainly because it enhances nausea (215). Another such agent, fusaric acid, had been claimed to be a useful adjuvant by Hidaka (216), but Mena and collaborators (217) could demonstrate no clear-cut effect, except a reduction in L-dopa-induced involuntary movements.

Monoamine-oxidase inhibitors can be useful when used alone in Parkinson's disease (218), but simultaneous use with L-dopa can be dangerous, often producing marked elevations in blood pressure (37, 219). They are not recommended as standard therapy at this stage, except in the presence of idiopathic hypotension (220).

Finally, inhibition of COMT could probably be of some use, especially to help reduce adventitious movements. The best known inhibitor, pyrogallol, is too toxic for human use. Ericsson (221) has initiated preliminary clinical trials with N-butylgallate (GPA-1714) with some potentiation of L-dopa effects and reduction in nausea, vomiting, and involuntary movements. These results have not yet been confirmed by others.

The use of peripheral dopa-decarboxylase inhibitors (Ro4-4602, MK-485, MK-486, α-methyl-dopa) has been discussed above in relation to L-dopa peripheral side effects.

(e) *Amantadine.* In 1969, Schwab and collaborators (222) made the fortuitous, but important, discovery that amantadine hydrochloride, used as an antiviral agent on A-2 Asian influenza, also possessed some activity in controlling the symptoms of parkinsonism. This observation created great interest because the structure of the compound was totally unlike that of other known antiparkinson agents (223). These results were soon confirmed by many authors from all parts of the world (224–232). A number of well-controlled double-blind studies (224, 226, 228, 229, 231, 233, 234) leave no doubt that amantadine has a place in the management of Parkinson's disease (235, 236). Recently it has also been used in combination with L-dopa (237–240) with debatable additive results, unless the dosage of L-dopa was not optimal because of side effects. Again the best results were obtained against akinesia, but modifications in rigidity and tremor could be observed in a significant number of cases.

The mechanism of action of amantadine has not yet been clearly delineated. Studies on experimental animals have shown that there exists some interrelationship between amantadine and catecholamines. Amantadine releases catecholamines from neuronal stores in the peripheral nervous system (241–252). It also causes release of dopamine within the brain (242–245). However, amantadine does not clearly modify the CSF concentrations of the metabolites HVA or 5-HIAA (246). High concentration of amantadine inhibits the uptake of dopamine and noradrenaline by rat brain homogenates (245), but this action is weak or inexistent (247–250) at physiological concentrations. The main effect of amantadine appears to be stimulation of dopaminergic structures in the presence of normal neurotransmission in noradrenergic neurons (233, 251). Indeed amantadine antagonized spiroperidol-induced catalepsy and this effect was not abolished by α-methyl-p-tyrosine (an inhibitor of catecholamine biosynthesis).

(f) *Apomorphine.* Analogs of dopamine have been developed and tried in Parkinson's disease. Surprisingly, their effect has been more important upon the symptom tremor than upon akinesia. They will therefore be discussed in more detail under the appropriate heading.

THE PHARMACOTHERAPY OF TREMOR

1. Classification of Tremor Syndromes and Rationale for Treatment

Tremor is a rhythmic involuntary oscillation of a limb around its position of equilibrium (10). *Physiological tremor* is that form normally present during the initiation of any motor activity and is usually of little apparent clinical significance except when exaggerated. It varies from 5 to 15 cycles per second (254–257). *Postural tremor* is usually present in an extremity during sustained motor activity and is identified most readily in the upper extremity upon resisting gravity. Rarely present at rest, its most common form, benign essential tremor, is usually inherited as a mendelian dominant trait (257–261). It can be limited to the extremities or also involve head, chin, tongue, and speech. *Intention tremor* is seen primarily during movement and usually indicates some involvement of the cerebellum or of the cerebellar outflow system (brachium conjunctivum, red nucleus, and related structures). It can be associated with both resting or postural tremor. It is more an instability of movement than a true tremor. Finally a very common form of tremor is *resting (or static) tremor,* which is present primarily at rest and often disappears upon initiation of movement, to reappear during sustained posture. Its frequency varies from 3–8 cyles per second. This form of tremor is the most frequent in Parkinson's disease, where its mechanism has been thoroughly studied. Parkinsonian tremor is characterized by alternating excitation of flexion and extension muscles. It is not our purpose in this chapter to review these important studies on the mechanism of tremor or on the tremorigenic center, for this has been done by many authors (262–268). Suffice it to recall that normal extrapyramidal function may depend upon a sensitive balance between inhibitory dopaminergic neurons and excitatory cholinergic fibers in the basal ganglia (37, 112). When studying the pathophysiology and treatment of akinesia, we stressed the importance of the nigrostriatal dopaminergic pathways. The other pole of this balance system appears to be involved in the causation of tremor. Indeed neuroleptics, central anticholinesterases, and central muscarinic agents produce tremor in the normal human, while reserpine, tetrabenazine, physostigmine, and acetylcholine all exacerbate parkinsonian tremor by an action that is reversed by central anticholinergic drugs (for review see 4). Finally there is some evidence that serotonin may be involved in the pathophysiology of tremor (87–89).

2. New Antitremor Agents

From the above considerations we see that a number of therapeutic approaches have been used to control tremor in humans, be it of the resting type, as in Parkinson's disease or of the postural type, as in benign essential tremor. We will review only some of the newer compounds, which have recently been experimentally studied.

(a) *Anticholinergic and antihistaminic drugs.* These agents have been extensively used for nearly a century, in the form of naturally occurring alkaloids or, since 1940, as synthetic compounds. They are still useful for the partial relief of tremor and rigidity, but not in all patients, if used carefully with a gradual upward titration. Side effects (dryness of mouth, diplopia, confusion, constipation) are frequent. Complete reviews have recently reassessed these substances in the light of present L-dopa therapy (4, 11, 13) and further data will be found in the paragraph on the treatment of rigidity. The only new drug of promise in this class of which we are aware is a dihydromorphanthridine derivative called EX 10-029[3] (269).

(b) *Propranolol.* The β-adrenergic blocker propranolol, which is best known in cardiology, has been used against parkinsonian tremor after the stimulation of β-adrenergic receptors was shown to increase tremor (270–272). The first studies, with pronethalol, propranolol, or oxprenolol alone, indicated clear-cut improvement of the action component of parkinsonian tremor, but less so of the resting tremor (273–277). Combined treatment with L-dopa was also evaluated and a significant additive therapeutic action on tremor was seen with this combination (278). There was no further additive improvement on rigidity or akinesia. Propranolol actually proved to be of even more use against essential tremor. The first observation along this line was made by Winkler & Young in 1971 (279) and has since been amply confirmed (280–283). Our own results (283) indicate that 75% of essential tremor patients can benefit from the addition of propanolol.

(c) *Apomorphine and pyribedil.* More specific stimulation of dopamine receptors in the brain can be obtained with drugs such as apomorphine (284, 285). Some effect of apomorphine upon parkinsonian symptomatology had been noted as early as 1951 by Schwab and collaborators (286), but it was Cotzias' group that clearly demonstrated this effect, alone or in combination with L-dopa (287–290). This was later confirmed by others (291, 292). With or without L-dopa, apomorphine diminished tremor and rigidity. It decreased bradykinesia mainly in patients receiving L-dopa. Düby and collaborators (290) explained this dual action by the molecule of apomorphine, part resembling dopamine and part resembling phenylethylamine, which can displace neurotransmitters from cellular sites.

In 1971, Corrodi and collaborators (293) described a new type of dopamine receptor stimulating agent which has since been named Trivastal® (ET-155, Pyribedil[4]). Tested upon surgically induced tremor in monkeys, it relieved these tremors while concomitantly evoking involuntary movements (294). Preliminary clinical studies with Trivastal (D. B. Calne, C. Fieschi, T. N. Chase, A. Barbeau, personal communications) indicate that this drug is indeed useful against Parkinson tremor in a certain number of cases. Although its action against dopamine receptors is uncontested, there also appears to be some effect upon the cholinergic system (S. Garrattini, J. Minnich, A. Barbeau, unpublished results). Further studies are needed to elucidate the mode of action of this interesting compound.

(d) *Agents modifying brain serotonin.* As indicated above, there is some evidence that serotonin may be involved in Parkinson's disease, particularly in tremor mechanisms (97, 295–297). L-dopa, in some cases, can reduce the resting tremor of parkinsonian patients (8). It also decreases the brain content of serotonin (298), possibly through some displacement or release mechanism. In tremorine-induced

[3]EX 10-029: 11-(3-dimethylaminopropylidene)-5-methyl-5,6-dihydromorphanthridine dicyclohexylsulfamate; Lakeside Laboratories.

[4]Trivastal: 1-(2"-pyrimidyl)-4-piperonylpiperazine; Servier, France.

tremor in mice, 5-hydroxytryptophan and a serotonin-like agent quipazine[5] were found to antagonize the tremor (299). It was thus justified to attempt some modifications of serotonin's metabolism in parkinsonian patients. Van Woert and co-workers (300) first attempted to lower brain serotonin content further with the serotonin depletor D,L-*para*-chlorophenylalanine (*p*-CPA). This depletion was not therapeutically useful in patients with Parkinson's disease and did not consistently produce adverse effects similar to those seen with L-dopa therapy. On the other hand, imipramine and desmethylimipramine, tricyclic antidepressants that inhibit the uptake of serotonin into neural tissue, reportedly ameliorate parkinsonian rigidity and tremor (301, 302). Attempts to increase brain serotonin further with L-5-hydroxytryptophan (5-HTP), or tryptophan with pyridoxine, indicate a rapid exacerbation of both rigidity and tremor (303–305). The mechanism underlying this exacerbation of symptom has not yet been elucidated.

THE PHARMACOTHERAPY OF RIGIDITY

1. Physiopathology and Rationale for Treatment

Rigidity is detected clinically as resistance to passive movement. It differs from spasticity of corticospinal origin in that it affects agonists and antagonists equally, and it is uniform throughout the whole range of passive movement being tested. It is exacerbated by mental concentration or by active movement of another limb.

The central nervous system controls the muscles through two sets of coordinated efferent systems, the α- and γ-motoneurons (306). Two types of experimental rigidity are apparent: α- rigidity is regarded as resulting from direct α-motoneuron drive, while γ- rigidity is attributed to excessive fusimotor activity. It is not yet clear which type of rigidity is predominant in Parkinson's disease. Studies by Steg (307) demonstrate that reserpine treatment of rats with unilateral lesions of the nigro-striatal dopaminergic neurons produce rigidity only on the unoperated side and a marked increase in the α- and decrease in the γ-motoneuron excitability on the contralateral rather than the ipsilateral side. Thus, according to Steg, rigidity is attributed to striatal cholinergic dominance producing α-motoneuronal dominance of efferent muscle control. Similarly γ-deficit is related to akinesia. On the basis of this rationale, it is evident that anticholinergic drugs should be the best approach to the treatment of parkinsonian rigidity. The belladonna alkaloids and synthetic anticholinergic drugs have long been recognized as beneficial in this disease. Their use has been reviewed by many authors (4–13) and will not be further discussed here, except to say that even since the advent of L-dopa, it has still been necessary to resort to combined treatment (308). Recent evidence tends to incriminate chronic anticholinergic drug therapy in the pathophysiology of some adventitious movements in man.

2. Experimental Drugs

In 1969, Coyle & Snyder (309) demonstrated that certain drugs used for the treatment of Parkinson's disease blocked dopamine uptake in striatal synaptosomes from

[5]Quipazine: 2-(1-piperazinyl) quinoline.

rats treated with reserpine, and proposed that this was their main mechanism of action. On the basis of this hypothesis a search for new compounds was undertaken by many laboratories. For example Ohashi, Hitomi & collaborators (310–312) studied Piroheptine,[6] a drug that proved to have some effects in drug-induced tremor (tremorine, oxotremorine, and pilocarpine) and catatonia. It potentiated the L-dopa effect in motor activity and the methamphetamine effect in conditioned avoidance response. However, it should be mentioned that in vivo studies indicate that not all antiparkinson drugs act by blocking dopamine uptake (313, 314). Thus benztropine, ethybenztropine, diphenylpyraline, brompheniramine, chlorphenira- mine, and methixene caused a clear-cut but not marked reduction of catecholamine accumulation in the dopamine neurons following intraventricular α-methyl-nor- adrenaline injections or dopa administration to reserpine-nialamide pretreated rats. Other anticholinergic drugs such as atropine, scopolamine, and benzhexol, and antihistamine compounds such as diphenhydramine and orphenadrine did not cause any certain blockade of catecholamine uptake into the dopamine neurons (314).

Molina-Negro & Illingworth (315) firmly believe that postural rigidity in Parkin- son's disease is due to hyperactivity of the γ-system. Based on this hypothesis, the same authors (316) claim good results against the symptom of rigidity with cy- clobenzaprine (MK-130). Our own experience with this drug (A. Barbeau, unpub- lished results) is far from conclusive. We were able to reduce tremor and rigidity only by producing marked somnolence.

In mammals the predominant control over melanocyte-stimulating hormone (MSH) release from the pituitary is exerted by a hypothalamic factor, MSH release- inhibitory hormone or MIF (317). This factor has been isolated from bovine hypo- thalamic tissue and its structure determined, thereby permitting synthesis of the compound (318). The structure of MIF was shown to be that of a tripeptide: L- prolyl-L-leucyl-glycine amide (Pro-Leu-Gly-NH$_2$). Melanocyte stimulating hor- mone will increase skin pigmentation in frogs and parkinsonian symptoms in man, while MIF and dopamine can lighten frogs previously darkened by destruction of the hypothalamus when the substances are applied directly to the pituitary gland (319). This dichotomy was noticed several years ago to offer some justification for the trial of MIF as an antiparkinson agent (320). Recent pharmacological studies have indicated that Pro-Leu-Gly-NH$_2$ can potentiate the behavioral effects of L- dopa and reduce the tremor induced in mice by administration of oxotremorine. These effects of MIF were shown to be independent of MSH since they occurred in hypophysectomized animals (321, 322). We have now demonstrated that L- prolyl-L-leucyl-glycine amide possesses some antiparkinsonian activity in man and that it can reduce some drug-induced dyskinesias (323). The principal effect of this substance was a clear-cut and significant reduction in rigidity. The mechanism of action of MIF upon catecholamines in the brain is not yet elucidated, but recently Carman (324) has proposed that it may be acting by inhibiting catechol-O-methyl transferase (COMT).

[6]Piroheptine: 3-(10, 11-dihydro-5H-dibenzo-[a, d]-cyclohepten-5-ylidene)-1-ethyl-2-methyl- pyrrolidine.

THE PHARMACOTHERAPY OF OTHER DYSKINESIAS

1. Specific Experimental Approaches

Many other dyskinesias are known to occur in humans. The interest in the biochemistry of Parkinson's disease has revived research into the understanding of such entities as Huntington's chorea, dystonia musculorum deformans, and even congenital athetosis. Many studies are still being carried out on the metabolism of copper, penicillamine, and ceruloplasmin in Wilson's disease (325–328) and L-dopa has even been tried with variable results (329, 330). However, this subject will not be covered in the present review, nor will other uses of L-dopa in a number of other extrapyramidal disorders (for review see 331).

(a) *Chorea and tics.* There is a considerable wealth of information from human and animal pharmacological studies indicating that the metabolism of cerebral monoamines must be involved in the pathophysiology of the choreic syndrome. These studies illustrate that the abnormal movements of Huntington's chorea are improved by a variety of agents, such as reserpine, tetrabenazine, α-methyl-paratyrosine, α-methyl-dopa, phenothiazines, and butyrophenones, all of which act by interferring with normal dopamine metabolism either by depleting the amine, by substituting for it, or by blocking the specific receptors on which it acts (116, 333). Conversely L-dopa will make choreic symptoms worse and has even been used as an experimental predictive test (334, 335). This would seem to indicate increased concentration, or at least increased utilization, of dopamine within the extrapyramidal centers of the brain and has led to some therapeutic approaches in order to block this activity (336). This and other aspects of the pathophysiology of Huntington's chorea have been thoroughly reviewed in a recent monograph edited by Barbeau, Chase & Paulson (337). It now appears that more emphasis should be placed on the state of basal ganglia receptor responsiveness than on the absolute concentrations of amines (338). In this context (116) we feel that Huntington's chorea should be considered as a state of dopaminergic dominance, in the same way Parkinson's disease is a state of cholinergic dominance.

An article by the MRC Brain Metabolism Unit of Great Britain (343) has suggested that lithium may stabilize the sensitivity of amine-containing systems in the central nervous system. In view of the reported hypersensitivity of dopamine receptors in Huntington's chorea (341), it is of interest that Dalén (344) has suggested the use of lithium carbonate in this illness, with encouraging results in six patients. This has now been confirmed by others (345, 346) and the approach merits a thorough investigation, especially if lithium proves to be able to reduce receptor hypersensitivity (347).

The important factor for the clinical symptoms may involve the relative degree of stimulation of striatal dopamine and serotonin receptors. It has indeed been shown that 5-hydroxytryptophan, a precursor of serotonin, worsens choreiform movements in patients with Huntington's chorea (339, 340). However, methysergide, a serotonin antagonist, when used chronically did not produce improvement in Huntington's chorea patients (341), thus indicating that serotonin alone has a limited role in the production of chorea. This conclusion is confirmed by recent studies where D,L-parachlorophenylalanine, a potent inhibitor of serotonin synthesis, was ineffective in modifying motor behavior in Huntington's chorea (342).

Recent developments regarding the role of γ-aminobutyric acid (GABA) as a putative neurotransmitter in the nervous system are of direct import on the understanding and treatment of Huntington's chorea (350). Indeed high levels of GABA and glutamic acid decarboxylase (GAD) have been noted in structures associated with the globus pallidus and substantia nigra (348, 349). Recently some evidence has been obtained to show that the inhibitory influence from the caudate to the substantia nigra is mediated by GABA (351). Thus it is likely that a GABA-ergic pathway exists between the caudate and the substantia nigra on the one hand and the globus pallidus on the other, and that it may be involved in the pathophysiology of the symptoms in Huntington's chorea (350). Such a postulate has now received important experimental evidence through the demonstration of a deficiency in GABA in the brain of Huntington's chorea patients (352) and of a similar deficiency in GAD (353). This important discovery should lead to trials of a number of agents that may increase GABA levels in the brain. Unfortunately this avenue is not easy, for GABA itself does not cross the blood-brain barrier.

A similar rationale could be used for the treatment of tics, particularly those seen in Gilles de la Tourette's disease. To date there is evidence that butyrophenones, and particularly haloperidol, are the best available drugs (354–356).

(b) *Dystonia and spasmodic torticollis.* The torsion dystonias have been studied in detail in an excellent review by Eldridge (357) and the rationale for the use of L-dopa in these disorders outlined at the same symposium by Barbeau (358). Some biochemical modifications in CSF were also reviewed by Chase (359). Recently Wooten and collaborators (364) have demonstrated an elevated plasma dopamine-β-hydroxylase activity in patients with autosomal dominant torsion dystonia, but not in the recessive form. Based on these studies Coleman & Barnet (360) first reported some improvement in dystonia musculorum deformans with L-dopa, and in other patients with 5-hydroxytryptophan (361). However Mandell (362) and Barrett and collaborators (363) soon raised doubts, indicating that L-dopa may relieve dystonic posture, but can increase dynamic dystonia. Haloperidol may improve the latter side effects. The literature has remained controversial on the use of L-dopa, apomorphine, haloperidol, or amantadine in the torsion dystonias or spasmodic torticollis (365–368) but there is no doubt that there is a small subgroup of patients who respond dramatically. In our own series of 14 cases, this response has occurred and been maintained 4 times. It is of interest that all 4 such cases were of the autosomal dominant type. Perhaps this is related to the above-mentioned findings of Wooten and collaborators (364).

(c) *Athetosis.* A number of extrapyramidal symptoms can result from brain damage in utero or at birth. These have been described in detail in a recent review by Spiegel & Baird (369). Since athetoid cerebral palsy is largely due to damage of the basal ganglia (370), it was almost inevitable that L-dopa would be used in this disorder. Rosenthal and co-workers (332) claimed favorable results, but this has not been the experience of others (8, 365, 369). In our own practice, Diazepam still remains the drug of choice, albeit of very moderate efficacy.

CONCLUSION

The introduction of L-dopa into the therapy of Parkinson's disease has permitted the clinico-biochemical delineation of the principal symptoms, and particularly of the differentiation between akinesia and rigidity. The side effects produced by L-dopa, such as the abnormal involuntary movements, have again focussed the attention of researchers upon the metabolism of cerebral amines in disorders of the basal ganglia. These observations have been the impetus for new experimental therapeutic approaches in Huntington's chorea, torsion dystonia, and other extrapyramidal disorders. The present review can only be considered an introductory chapter into the fascinating pharmacology of these diseases, but it should be sufficient to indicate that these chronic neurological disorders *can* be treated. Accepting this very conclusion is in itself the revolution of the last few years in neurology.

ACKNOWLEDGMENTS

Original studies from the author's laboratory were supported in part through grants from the Medical Research Council of Canada, the Department of National Health and Welfare, Canada, the United Parkinson Foundation, the Committee to Combat Huntington's Disease (Los Angeles Chapter), and the W. Garfield Weston Foundation.

Literature Cited

1. Jung, R., Hassler, R. 1960. *Handbook of Physiology,* Sect. I–Neurophysiology, ed. J. Field, H. W. Magoun, V. E. Hall, 2:837–927. Washington DC: Am. Physiol. Soc.
2. Barbeau, A. 1971. *Nervous System, Birth Defects, Orig. Art. Ser.* 7:156–66. Washington DC: Nat. Found.
3. Martin, J. P. 1967. *The Basal Ganglia and Posture,* pp. 1–152. London: Pitman Med. Publ.
4. Pinder, R. M. 1972. *Progr. Med. Ther.* 9:191–274
5. Winkelman, A. C., Di Palma, J. R. 1971. *Seminars in Drug Treatment* 1: 10–62
6. Brogden, R. N., Speight, T. M., Avery, G. S. 1971. *Drugs* 2:262–400
7. Rinne, U. K. 1972. *Acta Neurol. Scand.* 48, Suppl. 51:49–103
8. Barbeau, A. 1969. *Can. Med. Assoc. J.* 101:791–800
9. Wanger, S. L. 1972. *Med. Clin. N. Am.* 56:693–709
10. McMasters, R. E. 1971. *Mod. Treat.* 8:245–57
11. Yahr, M. D. 1972. *Med. Clin. N.Am.* 56:1377–92
12. Barbeau, A. 1970. *NY State J. Med.* 19:2437–43
13. Yahr, M. D., Duvoisin, R. C. 1972. *New Engl. J. Med.* 287:20–24
14. Korczyn, A. D. 1972. *Neuropharmacology* 11:601–07
15. Andén N. E., Roos, B. E., Werdinius, B. 1964. *Life Sci.* 3:149–58
16. Christensen, E., Moller, J. E., Faurbye, A. 1970. *Acta Neurol. Scand.* 46:14–23
17. Crane, G. E., Paulson, G. W. 1967. *Int. J. Neuropsychiat.* 3:286–91
18. Fog, R. L., Randrup, A., Pakkenberg, H. 1968. *Psychopharmacologia* 12: 428–32
19. Gey, K. F., Pletscher, A. 1961. *J. Pharmacol. Exp. Ther.* 133:18–24
20. Munkvad, I., Pakkenberg, H., Randrup, A. 1968. *Brain Behav. Evol.* 1: 89–100
21. Uhrbrand, L., Faurbye, A. 1960. *Psychopharmacologia* 1:408–18
22. Florio, V., Longo, V. G. 1971. *Neuropharmacology* 10:45–54
23. Janssen, P. A. J., 1967. *Int. J. Neuropsychiat.* 3, Suppl. I:10–18
24. Gessa, R., Tagliamonte, A., Gessa, G. L. 1972. *Lancet* 2:981–82
25. York, D. H. 1972. *Brain Res.* 37: 91–99
26. Hunter, R., Earl, C. J., Thronicroft, S. 1964. *Proc. Roy. Soc. Med.* 57:758–62

27. Hunter, R., Blackwood, W., Smith, M. C., Cummings, J. N. 1968. *J. Neurol. Sci.* 7:263–73
28. Paulson, G. W. 1969. *Geriatrics* 23: 105–10
29. Crane, G. E. 1968. *Am. J. Psychiat.* 124, Suppl.:40–48
30. Faurbye, A. 1970. *Compr. Psychiat.* 11: 205–24
31. Turek, I., Kurland, A. A., Hanlon, T. E., Bohm, M. 1972. *Brit. J. Psychiat.* 121:605–12
32. Klawans, H. L., McKendall, R. R. 1971. *J. Neurol. Sci.* 14:189–92
33. Rubovits, R., Klawans, H. L. 1972. *Arch. Gen. Psychiat.* 27:502–07
34. Calne, D. B. 1971. *Brit. Med. J.* 3: 683–97
35. Barbeau, A. 1960. *Neurology* 10: 442–51
36. Barbeau, A. 1961. *Arch. Neurol.* 4:97–102
37. Barbeau, A. 1962. *Can. Med. Assoc. J.* 87:802–07
38. Barbeau, A. 1968. *Proc. Aust. Assoc. Neurol.* 5:95–100
39. Barbeau, A. 1972. *Rev. Neurol.* 127 (2):253–64
40. Ehringer, H., Hornykiewicz, O. 1960. *Klin. Wochenschr.* 38:1236–39
41. Hornykiewicz, O. 1966. *Pharm. Rev.* 18:925–64
42. Hornykiewicz, O. 1971. *Biogenic Amines and Physiological Membranes In Drug Therapy,* ed. J. H. Biel, L. G. Abood, 5:Pt. B, 173–258. NY: Decker
43. Barbeau, A., Murphy, G. F., Sourkes, T. L. 1961. *Science* 133:1706–07
44. Jéquier, E., Dufresne, J. J. 1971. *Neurology* 21:15–21
45. Papeschi, R., Molina-Negro, P., Sourkes, T. L., Hardy, J., Bertrand, C. 1970. *Neurology* 20:991–1001
46. Lloyd, K. G., Hornykiewicz, O. 1970. *Science* 170:1212–13
47. Barbeau, A. 1961. *Excerpta Med. Int. Congr. Ser.* 38:152–53
48. Birkmayer, W., Hornykiewicz, O. 1961. *Wien. Klin. Wochenschr.* 73:787–88
49. Cotzias, G. C., Van Woert, M. H., Schiffer, L. 1967. *New Engl. J. Med.* 276:374–79
50. Cotzias, G. C., Papavasiliou, P. S., Gellene, R. 1969. *New Engl. J. Med.* 280: 337–45
51. Schwab, R. S., Zieper, I. 1965. *Psychiatria et Neurologia* 150:345–57
52. Joubert, M., Barbeau, A. 1969. *Progress in Neuro-Genetics,* ed. A. Barbeau, J. R. Brunette, 366–76. Amsterdam: Excerpta Medica
53. Barbeau, A. 1972. *Parkinson's Disease (Rigidity, Akinesia, Behavior),* ed. J. Siegfried, 1:152–74. Bern: Hans Huber
54. Barbeau, A. 1973. *Biology of Brain Dysfunction,* Vol. 2, ed. G. E. Gaull. NY: Plenum
55. Barbizet, J. 1971. *La Presse Méd.* 79: 2033–37
56. Brumlik, J., Boshes, B. 1966. *Neurology* 16:337–44
57. Klawans, H., Ilahi, M.M., Shenker, D. 1970. *Acta Neurol. Scand.* 46:409–41
58. Barbeau, A. 1972. *Monogr. Human Genet.* 6:114–36
59. Barbeau, A. 1971. *Monoamines, Noyaux Gris Centraux et Maladie de Parkinson,* ed. J. de Ajuriaguera, 385–402. Paris: Masson
60. Ng, L.K.Y., Chase, T. N., Colburn, R. W., Kopin, I. J. 1972. *Neurology* 22: 688–96
61. Sandler, M., Ruthven, C. R. J. 1969. *Progr. Med. Chem.* 6:200–65
62. Sandler, M. 1972. *Handb. Exp. Pharmacol.* 33:845–99
63. Cotzias, G. C. 1969. *JAMA* 210: 1255–62
64. Yahr, M. D., Duvoisin, R. C., Schear, M. J., Barrett, R. E., Hoehn, M. M. 1969. *Arch. Neurol.* 21:343–54
65. Calne, D. B. 1970. *Parkinsonism: Physiology, Pharmacology and Treatment,* 1–136. London: Arnold
66. Calne, D. B., Spiers, A. S. D., Stern, G. M., Laurence, D. R., Armitage, P. 1969. *Lancet* 2:973–76
67. McDowell, F. H., et al 1970. *Ann. Int. Med.* 72:29–35
68. Barbeau, A., McDowell, F. H. 1970. *L-DOPA and Parkinsonism,* 1–433. Davis: Philadelphia
69. Barbeau, A. 1970. *Ariz. Med.* 27:1–4
70. Cotzias, G. C. 1971. *JAMA* 218: 1903–08
71. Schwartz, A., et al 1972. *Can. Med. Assoc. J.* 107:973–76
72. Yahr, M. D., 1972. *Res. Publ. Assoc. Nerv. Ment. Dis.* 50:973–76
73. Hornykiewicz, O. 1973. *Fed. Proc.* 32: 182–90
74. Klawans, H. L. 1968. *Dis. Nerv. Syst.* 29:805–16
75. Bertler, A., Rosengren, E. 1959. *Acta Physiol. Scand.* 47:350–61
76. Sano, I. et al 1959. *Biochim. Biophys. Acta* 32:586–89
77. Carlsson, A. 1959. *Pharmacol. Rev.* 11:490–93

78. Barolin, G. S., Bernheimer, H. Hornykiewicz, O. 1964. *Schweiz. Arch. Neurol Neurochir. Psychiat.* 94:241–48

79. Hornykiewicz, O. 1966. *Biochemistry and Pharmacology of the Basal Ganglia*, ed. E. Costa, L. J. Côté, M. D. Yahr, 171–81. Raven: New York

80. Carlsson, A., Rosengren, E., Bertler, A., Nilsson, J. 1957. *Psychotropic Drugs*, ed. S. Garattini, N. V. Uitgeners, 363–72. Elsevier: Amsterdam

81. Hornykiewicz, O. 1963. *Wien. Klin. Wochenschr.* 75:309–12

82. Bernheimer, H., Birkmayer, W. Hornykiewicz, O. 1963. *Klin. Wochenschr.* 41:465–69

83. Andén, N. E. et al 1964. *Life Sci.* 3:523–30

84. Andén, N. E. et al 1966. *Acta Physiol. Scand.* 67:313–26

85. Andén, N. E., Dahlström, A., Fuxe, K. Larsson, K. 1966. *Acta Pharmacol.* 24:263–74

86. Heller, A., Moore, R. Y. 1965. *J. Pharmacol. Exp. Ther.* 150:1–9

87. Poirier, L. J., Sourkes, T. L. 1965. *Brain* 88:181–92

88. Goldstein, M. et al 1969. *J. Neurochem.* 16:645–48

89. Poirier, L. J. et al 1969. *Brain Res.* 14:147–55

90. McGeer, P. L., McGeer, E. G., Wada, J. A. 1971. *Neurology* 21:1000–07

91. Metzel, E., Weinmann, D., Riechert, T. 1969. *Third Symp. Parkinson's Dis.* ed. F. J. Gillingham, I. M. Donaldson, 47–50. Livingstone: Edinburgh

92. Barbeau, A., Trombitas, S. See Ref. 52, pp. 352–56

93. Goodall, McC., Alton, H. 1969. *J. Clin. Invest.* 48:2300–09

94. Barbeau, A. 1970. *Can. Med. Assoc. J.* 103:824–32

95. Barbeau, A. 1968. *Agressologie* 9:195–200

96. Barbeau, A. See Ref. 91, pp. 66–73

97. Barbeau, A., Jasmin, G. 1961. *Rev. Can. Biol.* 20:837–38

98. Barbeau, A. et al 1972. *Experientia* 28:289–91

99. Hornykiewicz, O. See Ref. 53, pp. 127–49

100. Sourkes, T. L. 1970. *Biochem. Med.* 3:321–25

101. Goodall, McC., Alton, H. 1972. *Biochem. Pharmacol.* 21:2401–08

102. Abrams, W. B., Coutinho, C. B., Leon,

A. S., Spiegel, H. E. 1971. *JAMA* 218:1912–14

103. Peaston, M. J. T., Bianchine, J. R. 1970. *Brit. Med. J.* 1:400–03

104. Hare, T. A., Vanna, S., Beasley, B., Chambers, R., Vogel, W. H. 1971. *J. Lab. Clin. Med.* 77:319–25

105. Calne, D. B., Karoum, F., Ruthven, C. R. J., Sandler, M. 1969. *Brit. J. Pharmacol.* 37:47–61

106. Jéquier, E., Dufresne, J.-J. 1972. *Neurology* 22:12–21

107. Yamada, K., Minnich, J., Donaldson, J., Barbeau, A. 1973. *J. Neurol. Sci.* 18:311–15

108. Routh, J. I., Bannow, R. E., Fincham, R. W., Stoll, J. L. 1971. *Clin. Chem.* 17:867–71

109. Sandler, M. 1970. *L-DOPA and Parkinsonism*, ed. A. Barbeau, F. H. McDowell, 72–75. Philadelphia: Davis

110. Tyce, G. M., Muenter, M. D., Owen, C. A. 1970. *Mayo Clin. Proc.* 45:438–43

111. Ibid 45:645–56

112. McGeer, P. L., Boulding, J. E., Gibson, W. C., Foulkes, R. G. 1961. *JAMA* 177:665–70

113. Duvoisin, R. C. 1967. *Arch. Neurol.* 17:124–36

114. Steg, G. 1964. *Acta Physiol. Scand.* 61, Suppl. 225:1–100

115. Arvidsson, J., Roos, B.-E., Steg, G. 1966. *Acta Physiol. Scand.* 67:398–404

116. Barbeau, A. 1973. *Huntington's Chorea, 1872–1972*, ed. A. Barbeau, T. N. Chase, G. W. Paulson, 473–524. New York: Raven

117. Langrall, H. M., Joseph, C. 1972. *Neurology* 22(2):3–16

118. McDowell, F. H., Markham, C. H., Lee, J. E., Treciokas, L. J., Ansel, R. D. 1971. *Recent Advances in Parkinson's Disease* ed. F. H. McDowell, C. H. Markham, 175–201. Philadelphia: Davis

119. Barbeau, A., Mars, H., Gillo-Joffroy, L. See Ref. 118, 203–37

120. Barbeau, A. 1972. *Union Med. Can.* 101:849–52

121. Constantinidis, J., Bartholini, G., Tissot, R., Pletscher, A. 1968. *Experientia* 24:130–31

122. Constantinidis, J., Bartholini, G., Gleisbühler, R., Tissot, R. 1970. *Experientia* 26:381–83

123. De la Torre, J. C. 1971. *J. Neurol. Sci.* 12:77–93

124. Bartholini, G., Burkard, W. P.,

Pletscher, A., Bates, H. M. 1967. *Nature* 215:852–53
125. Bartholini, G., Pletscher, A. 1968. *J. Pharmacol. Exp. Ther.* 161:14–20
126. Bartholini, G., Pletscher, A. 1969. *J. Pharm. Pharmacol.* 21:323–24
127. Bartholini, G., Blum, J. E., Pletscher, A. 1969. *J. Pharm. Pharmacol.* 21:297–301
128. Bartholini, G., Constantinidis, J., Tissot, R., Pletscher, A. 1971. *Biochem. Pharmacol.* 20:1243–47
129. Pletscher, A., Bartholini, G. 1971. *Clin. Pharmacol. Ther.* 12:344–52
130. Lotti, V. J., Porter, C. C 1970. *J. Pharmacol. Exp. Ther.* 172:406–15
131. Birkmayer, W., Mentasti, M. 1967. *Archiv. Psych. Nervenkrank* 210:29–35
132. Birkmayer, W. 1971. *Wien. Klin. Wochenschr.* 83:221–27
133. Siegfried, J. 1970. *Rev. Neurol.* 4:243–48
134. Rinne, U. K., Sonninen, V., Siirtola, T. 1972. *Z. Neurol.* 202:1–20
135. Barbeau, A., Gillo-Joffroy, L., Mars, H. 1971. *Clin. Pharmacol. Ther.* 12:353–59
136. Barbeau, A., Mars, H., Botez, M. I., Joubert, M. 1972. *Can. Med. Assoc. J.* 106:1169–74
137. Barbeau, A. 1973. *Advances in Neurology,* ed. M. D. Yahr, 2:173–98. New York: Raven
138. Calne, D. B. et al 1971. *Brit. Med. J.* 1:729–32
139. Rao, S. K., Vakil, S. D., Calne, D. B., Hilson, A. 1972. *Postgrad. Med. J.* 48:653–56
140. Papavasiliou, P. S. et al 1972. *New Engl. J. Med.* 286:8–14
141. Chase, T. N., Watanabe, A. M. 1972. *Neurology* 22:384–92
142. Fermaglich, J., O'Doherty, D. S. 1971. *Neurology* 21:408
143. Sweet, R. D., Lee, J. E., McDowell, F. H. 1972. *Clin. Pharmacol. Ther.* 13:23–27
144. Fermaglich, J., Chase, T. N. 1973. *Lancet* 1:1261–62
145. Goldberg, L. I. 1972. *Pharmacol. Rev.* 24:1–23
146. Goldberg, L. I., Whitsett, T. L. 1971. *JAMA* 218:1921–23
147. Duvoisin, R. C., Yahr, M. D., Côté, L. 1969. *Trans. Am. Neurol. Assoc.* 94:81–84
148. Jameson, H. D. 1970. *JAMA* 211:1700
149. Leon, A.-S., Spiegel, H. E., Thomas, G., Abrams, W. B. 1971. *JAMA* 218:1924–27

150. Yahr, M. D., Duvoisin, R. C., Côté, L., Cohen, G. 1972. *Role of Vitamin B₆ in Neurobiology, Advances in Biochemical Psychopharmacology,* ed. M. S. Ebadi, E. Costa, 4:185–194. New York: Raven
151. Golden, R. L., Mortati, F. S., Schroeter, G. A. 1970. *JAMA* 213:628
152. Cotzias, G. C., Papavasiliou, P. S. 1971. *JAMA* 215:1504–05
153. Yahr, M. D. 1971. *JAMA* 216:2141
154. Yahr, M. D. 1973. *The Treatment of Parkinsonism: The Role of Dopa Decarboxylase Inhibitors,* ed. M. D. Yahr, 1–303. New York: Raven
155. Cuche, J. L., Kuchel, O., Barbeau, A., Boucher, R., Genest, J. 1972. *Clin. Sci.* 43:481–91
156. Tolosa, E. S., Martin, W. E., Cohen, H. P. 1973. *Lancet* 1:942
157. Anonymous. 1973. *Lancet* 1:979–80
158. Hornykiewicz, O. 1972. *Handb. Neurochem.* 7:465–501
159. Asso, D. 1969. *Brit. J. Psych.* 115:555–56
160. Ball, B. 1882. *Encéphale* 2:22–32
161. Riklan, M., Levita, E. 1969. *Subcortical Correlates of Human Behavior: A Psychological Study of Thalamic and Basal Ganglia Surgery.* Baltimore: Williams & Wilkins
162. Warburton, J. W. 1967. *Brit. J. Med. Psychol.* 40:169–71
163. Riklan, M., Weiner, H., Diller, L. 1959. *J. Nerv. Ment. Dis.* 129:263–72
164. Schwab, R. S., England, A. C., Peterson, E. 1959. *Neurology* 9:65–72
165. Botez, M. I., Barbeau, A. 1973. See Ref. 99, Vol. 2
166. Hoehn, M. M., Yahr, M. D. 1967. *Neurology* 17:427–35
167. Arbit, J., Boshes, B., Blonsky, R. See Ref. 68, pp. 329–36
168. Cole, J. O. See Ref. 68, pp. 343–47
169. Marsh, G. G., Markham, C. H., Ansel, R. 1971. *J. Neurol. Neurosurg. Psychiat.* 34:209–18
170. Guthrie, T. C., Dunbar, H. S., Weider, A. 1970. *Trans. Am. Assoc.* 95:250–52
171. Boshes, B., Arbit, J. 1970. *Trans. Am. Neurol. Assoc.* 95:59–63
172. Beardsley, J. V., Puletti, F. 1971. *Arch. Neurol.* 25:145–50
173. Meier, M. J., Baker, A. B., Martin, W. E. 1970. *Trans. Am. Neurol. Assoc.* 95:64–68
174. Loranger, A. W., Goodell, H., Lee, J. E., McDowell, F. H. 1972. *Arch. Gen. Psychiat.* 26:163–68
175. Klaiber, R., Siegfried, J., Ziegler, W. H., Perret, E. 1971. *Eur. J. Clin. Pharmacol.* 3:172–75

176. Riklan, M. 1972. *Neurology* 22(2): 43–55
177. Garron, D. C., Klawans, H. L., Narin, F. 1972. *J. Nerv. Ment. Dis.* 154: 445–52
178. Celesia, G. G., Barr, A. N. 1970. *Arch. Neurol.* 23:193–200
179. Keenan, R. E. 1970. *Neurology* 20: 46–59
180. Goodwin, F. K. 1971. *JAMA* 218: 1915–20
181. Bunney, W. E. 1970. *Am. J. Psychiat.* 127:361–62
182. Malitz, S. 1972. *L-DOPA and Behavior,* ed. S. Malitz, 1–144. New York: Raven
183. Riklan, M. 1973. *L-DOPA and Parkinsonism: A Psychological Assessment,* 1–402. Springfield: Thomas
184. Barbeau, A. See Ref. 182, pp. 9–33
185. Schildkraut, J. J. 1965. *Am. J. Psychiat.* 122:509–22
186. Snyder, S. H., Taylor, K. M., Coyle, J. T., Meyerhoff, J. L. 1970. *Am. J. Psychiat.* 127:199–207
187. Barbeau, A. 1971. *Lancet* 1:995
188. Barbeau, A. 1972. *Neurology* 22(2): 22–24
189. Markham, C. H. 1972. *Neurology* 22(2):17–21
190. Barbeau, A. 1974. *Proceedings of Princeton Symposium,* ed. F. H. McDowell, A. Barbeau. New York: Raven. In press
191. Boudin, G., Pépin, B., Guillard, A., Fabiani, J. M., Haguenau, M. 1972. *Les Médiateurs Chimiques,* ed. P. Girard, R. Couteaux, 79–97. Paris: Masson
192. Calne, D. B., 1974. *Proceedings of Princeton Symposium,* ed. F. H. McDowell, A. Barbeau. New York: Raven. In press
193. Anonymous. 1973. *Brit. Med. J.* 1:373
194. Blaschko, H., Chrusciel, T. L. 1960. *J. Physiol.* 151:272–75
195. Barbeau, A., Sourkes, T. L., Murphy, G. F. 1962. *Monoamines et Système nerveux Central,* ed. J. de Ajuriaguerra, 247–62. Paris: Masson
196. Andén, N.-E., Butcher, S. G., Engel, J. 1970. *J. Pharm. Pharmacol.* 22:548–50
197. Ungerstedt, U. et al 1973. *Eur. J. Pharmacol.* 21:230–37
198. Cotzias, G. C., Papavasiliou, P. S., Mena, I. 1973. *JAMA* 223:83
199. Roth, R. H., Giarman, N. J. 1970. *Biochem. Pharmacol.* 19:1087–90
200. Laborit, H., Kind, A., De Leon Regil, C. 1961. *Presse Méd.* 69:1216–18
201. Camba, R., Rudas, N., Boero, G. C., Caboni, F., Gessa, G. L. 1965. *Rev. Sarda Criminol.* 1:435–45

202. Gessa, G. L. et al 1966. *Life Sci.* 5: 1921–25
203. Gessa, G. L. et al 1967. *Boll. Soc. Ital. Biol. Sper.* 53:1–13
204. Gessa, G. L., Caabai, F., Vargiu, L., Spano. P. F. 1968. *J. Neurochem.* 15: 377–81
205. Spano, P. H., Tagliamonte, A., Tagliamonte, P., Gessa, G. L. 1971. *J. Neurochem.* 18:1831–36
206. Boncinelli, A. et al 1971. *Riv. Farmacol. Terap.* 2:29–32
207. Papavasiliou, P. S., Cotzias, G. C., Mena, I., Bell, M. 1973. *JAMA* 224: 130
208. Bartholini, G., Kuruma, I., Pletscher, A. 1970. *Brit. J. Pharmacol.* 40:462–66
209. Bartholini, G., Kuruma, I., Pletscher, A. 1971. *Nature* 230:533–35
210. Gauthier, G. et al 1971. *Presse Méd.* 79:91–98
211. De Ajuriaguerra, J. et al 1971. *Presse Méd.* 79:1396–99
212. Chase, T. N. 1972. *Neurology* 22:417
213. Muenter, M. D., Sharpless, N. S., Tyce, G. M. 1972. *Neurology* 22:416–17
214. Goldstein, M., Nakajima, K. 1967. *J. Pharmacol. Exp. Ther.* 157:96–99
215. Braham, J. 1970. *Brit. Med. J.* 3:540–41
216. Hidaka, H. 1971. *Nature* 231:54–55
217. Mena, I., Court, J., Cotzias, G. C. 1971. *JAMA* 218:1829
218. Barbeau, A., Duchastel, Y. 1962. *Can. Psych. Assoc. J.* 7:S-91-S-95
219. Hunter, K. R., Stern, G. M., Laurence, D. R., Armitage, P. 1970. *Lancet* 2:566
220. Kuchel, O. et al 1970. See Ref. 68, pp. 293–305
221. Ericsson, A. L. 1971. *J. Neurol. Sci.* 14:193
222. Schwab, R. S., England, A. C., Poskanzer, D. C., Young, R. R. 1969. *JAMA* 208:1168–70
223. Schwab, R. S., England, A. C. 1969. *Trans. Am. Neurol. Assoc.* 94:85–87
224. Parkes, J. D., Zilkha, K. J., Calver, D. M., Knill-Jones, R. P. 1970. *Lancet* 1: 259–62
225. Voller, G. W. 1970. *Deut. Med. Wochenschr.* 95:934–37
226. Fieschi, C. et al 1970. *Lancet* 1:945–46
227. Shealy, C. N., Weeth, J. B., Mercier, D. 1970. *JAMA* 212:1522–23
228. Hunter, K. R., Stern, G. M., Laurence, D. R., Armitage, P. 1970. *Lancet* 1: 1127–29
229. Parkes, J. D., Zilkha, K. J., Marsden, P., Baxter, R. C. H. 1970. *Lancet* 1: 1130–33
230. Funfgeld, E. W. 1970. *Deut. Med. Wochenschr.* 95:1834–36

231. Gilligan, B. S., Veale, J., Wodak, J. 1971. *Med. J. Aust.* 25:634
232. Pearce, J., Rao, N. S. 1970. *Lancet* 2: 1091–92
233. Barbeau, A., Mars, H., Botez, M. I., Joubert, M. 1971. *Can. Med. Assoc. J.* 105:42–47
234. Mann, D. C., Pearce, L. A., Waterbury, L. D. 1971. *Neurology* 21:958–62
235. Schwab, R. S., Poskanzer, D. C., England, A. C., Young, R. R. 1972. *JAMA* 222:792–95
236. Castaigne, P., Laplane, D., Dordain, G. 1972. *La Nouv. Presse Méd.* 1:533–36
237. Godwin-Austin, R. B., Frears, C. C., Bergmann, S., Parkes, J. D., Knill-Jones, R. P. 1970. *Lancet* 2:383–85
238. Scotti, G. 1970. *Lancet* 1:1394–95
239. Sigwald, J., Raymondeau, C. 1971. *La Nouv. Presse Méd.* 1:1237–39
240. Rinne, U. K., Sonninen, V., Siirtola, T. 1972. *Eur. Neurol.* 7:228–40
241. Grelak, R. P., Clark, R., Stump, J. M., Vernier, V. G. 1970. *Science* 169:203–4
242. Scatton, B., Cheramy, A., Besson, M. J., Glowinski, J. 1970. *Eur. J. Pharmacol.* 13:131–33
243. Strömberg, U., Svensson, T. H., Waldeck, B. J. 1970. *J. Pharm. Pharmacol.* 22:959–62
244. Von Voigtlander, P. F., Moore, K. E. 1971. *Science* 174:408–10
245. Fletcher, E. A., Redfern, P. H. 1970. *J. Pharm. Pharmacol.* 22:957–58
246. Rinne, U. K., Sonninen, V., Hyyppä, M. 1972. *Experientia* 28:57–58
247. Herblin, W. F. 1972. *Biochem. Pharmacol.* 21:1993–95
248. Baldessarini, R. J., Lipinski, J. F., Chace, K. V. 1972. *Biochem. Pharmacol.* 21:77–87
249. Symchowicz, S., Korduba, C. A., Veals, J. 1973. *Eur. J. Pharmacol.* 21:155–60
250. Solatunturi, E., Paasonen, M. K., Kivalo, E. 1971. *Scand. J. Clin. Lab. Invest.* 27, Suppl. 116:77
251. Maj, J., Sowinska, H., Baran, L. 1972. *Psychopharmacologia* 24:296–307
252. Jones, D. G., Turnbull, M. J., Lenman, J. A. R., Robertson, M. A. H. 1972. *J. Neurol. Sci.* 17:245–53
253. Narotzky, R., Griffith, D., Stahl, S., Bondareff, W., Zeller, E. A. 1973. *Exp. Neurol.* 38:218–30
254. Brumlik, J., Yap, C. B. 1970. *Normal Tremor: A Comparative Study,* 1–93. Springfield: Thomas
255. Van Buskirk, C., Wolbarsht, M. L., Stecher, K. 1966. *Neurology* 16:217–20
256. Marshall, J., Walsh, E. G. 1956. *J. Neurol. Neurosurg. Psychiat.* 19:260–67

257. Dana, C. L. 1887. *Am. J. Med.* 94:386
258. Critchley, M. 1949. *Brain* 72:113–39
259. Davis, C. H., Kunkle, E. C. 1951. *Arch. Int. Med.* 87:808–16
260. Larsson, T., Sjögren, T. 1960. *Acta Psychiat. Neurol. Scand.* 36, Suppl. 144: 1–176
261. Marshall, J. 1962. *J. Neurol. Neurosurg. Psychiat.* 25:122–26
262. Gybels, J. 1963. *The Neural Mechanism of Parkinsonian Tremor,* 1–161. Brussels:Presses Acad. Eur.
263. Cordeau, J. P. 1961. *Rev. Can. Biol.* 20:147–57
264. Bertrand, G., Jasper, H. H. 1965. *Confin. Neurol.* 26:205–8
265. Lamarre, Y., Cordeau, J. P. 1964. *J. Physiol.* 56:589–91
266. Poirier, L. J. et al 1969. *Rev. Neurol.* 120:15–22
267. Olivier, A., Parent, A., Simard, H., Poirier, L. J. 1970. *Brain Res.* 18: 273–82
268. Ambani, L. M., Van Woert, M. H. 1972. *Brit. J. Pharmacol.* 46:344–47
269. Rix, A., Fisher, R. G. 1972. *S. Med. J.* 65:1385–89
270. Wilson, J. W., Kunkle, E. C. 1953. *Trans. Am. Neurol. Assoc.* 78:282–84
271. Constas, C. 1962. *J. Neurol. Neurosurg. Psychiat.* 25:116–21
272. Marsden, C. D., Foley, T. H., Owen, D. A., McAllister, R. G. 1967. *Clin. Sci.* 33:53–65
273. Herring, A. B. 1964. *Lancet* 2:892
274. Owen, D. A., Marsden, C. D. 1965. *Lancet* 2:1252–62
275. Strang, R. R. 1965. *J. Neurol. Neurosurg. Psychiat.* 28:404–06
276. Vas, C. J. 1966. *Lancet* 1:182–83
277. Thompson, M. K. 1972. *Lancet* 2:388
278. Abramsky, O., Carmon, A., Lavy, S. 1971. *J. Neurol. Sci.* 14:491–94
279. Winkler, G. F., Young, R. R. 1971. *Trans. Am. Neurol. Assoc.* 96:66–68
280. Pakkenberg, H. 1972. *Lancet* 1:633
281. Gilligan, B. 1972. *Lancet* 2:980
282. Murray, T. J. 1972. *Can. Med. Assoc. J.* 107:984–86
283. Barbeau, A. 1973. *Union Méd. Can.* 102:899–902
284. Ernst, A. M. 1967. *Psychopharmacologia* 10:316–23
285. Ungerstedt, U., Butcher, L. L., Butcher, S. G., Andén, N. E., Fuxe, K. 1969. *Brain Res.* 14:461–70
286. Schwab, R. S., Amador, L. V., Lettvin, J. Y. 1951. *Trans. Am. Neurol. Assoc.* 76:251–53

287. Cotzias, G. C., Papavasiliou, P. S., Fehling, C., Kaufman, B., Mena, I. 1970. *New Engl. J. Med.* 232:31–33
288. Düby, S. E., Dahl, L. K., Cotzias, G. C. 1971. *Trans. Assoc. Am. Phys.* 84: 289–96
289. Düby, S. E., Cotzias, G. C., Steck, A. 1971. *Fed. Proc.* 30(2):216
290. Düby, S. E., Cotzias, G. C., Papavasiliou, P. S., Lawrence, W. H. 1972. *Arch. Neurol.* 27:474–80
291. Braham, J., Sarova-Pinhas, I., Goldhammer, Y. 1970. *Brit. Med. J.* 3:768
292. Castaigne, P., Laplane, D., Dordain, G. 1971. *Res. Comm. Chem. Pathol. Pharmacol.* 2:154–58
293. Corrodi, H., Fuxe, K., Ungerstedt, U. 1971. *J. Pharm. Pharmacol.* 23:989–91
294. Goldstein, M., Battista, A. F., Ohmoto, T., Anagnoste, B., Fuxe, K. 1973. *Science* 179:816–17
295. Van Woert, M. H., Bowers, M. B. 1970. *Experientia* 26:161–62
296. Sourkes, T. L., Poirier, L. J. 1966. *Can. Med. Assoc. J.* 94:53–60
297. Bernheimer, H., Birkmayer, W., Hornykiewicz, O. 1961. *Klin. Wochenschr.* 39:1056–60
298. Everett, G. M., Borcherding, J. W. 1970. *Science* 168:849–50
299. Rodríguez, R. 1972. *Life Sci.* 11(1): 535–44
300. Van Woert, M. H., Ambani, L. M., Levine, R. J. 1972. *Dis. Nerv. Syst.* 33: 777–80
301. Strang, R. R. 1965. *Brit. Med. J.* 2: 33–38
302. Laitinen, L. 1969. *Acta Neurol. Scand.* 45:109–20
303. Chase, T. N. 1970. *Lancet* 2:1029
304. Chase, T. N., Ng, L. K. Y., Watanabe, A. M. 1972. *Neurology* 22:479–84
305. Hall, C. D., Weiss, E. A., Morris, C. E., Prange, A. J. 1972. *Neurology* 22: 231–37
306. Granit, R. 1970. *The Basis of Motor Control.* London: Academic
307. Steg, G. See Ref. 19, pp. 26–31
308. Greenblatt, D. J., Shader, R. I. 1973. *New Engl. J. Med.* 288:1215–19
309. Coyle, J. T., Snyder, S. H. 1969. *Science* 166:899–901
310. Hitomi, M. et al 1972. *Drug Res.* 22: 953–61
311. Hitomi, M., Watanabe, N., Kumadaki, N., Kumada, S. 1972. *Drug Res.* 22: 961–66
312. Ohashi, T., Akita, H., Tamura, T., Noda, K., Honda, F. 1972. *Drug Res.* 22:966–72

313. Farnebo, L. O., Fuxe, K., Hamberger, B., Ljungdahl, A. 1970. *J. Pharm. Pharmacol.* 22:733–37
314. Fuxe, K., Goldstein, M., Ljungdahl, A. 1970. *Life Sci.* 9(1):811–24
315. Molina-Negro, P., Illingworth, R. A. 1971. *Union Méd. Can.* 100:1947–51
316. Ibid. 1973. *Union Méd. Can.* 102: 303–08
317. Kastin, A. J., Ross, G. T. 1964. *Endocrinology* 75:187–91
318. Kastin, A. J. et al 1969. *Endocrinology* 84:20–24
319. Kastin, A. J., Schally, A. V., Viosca, S. 1971. *Proc. Soc. Exp. Biol. Med.* 137: 1437
320. Kastin, A. J. 1967. *New Engl. J. Med.* 276:1041
321. Plotnikoff, N. P. et al 1971. *Life Sci.* 10:1279–81
322. Plotnikoff, N. P. et al 1972. *Proc. Soc. Exp. Biol. Med.* 140:811–12
323. Kastin, A. J., Barbeau, A. 1972. *Can. Med. Assoc. J.* 107:1979–81
324. Carman, J. S. 1973. *Lancet* 1:1247
325. O'Reilly, S., Strickland, G. T., Weber, P. M., Beckner, W. M., Shipley, L. 1971. *Arch. Neurol.* 24:385–90
326. O'Reilly, S., Pollycove, M., Tono, M., Herradora, L. 1971. *Arch. Neurol.* 24: 481–88
327. O'Reilly, S., Weber, P. M., Oswald, M., Shipley, L. 1971. *Arch. Neurol.* 25: 28–32
328. Goldstein, N. P., Tauxe, W. N., McCall, J. T., Randall, R. V., Gross, J. B. 1971. *Arch. Neurol.* 24:391–400
329. Barbeau, A., Friesen, H. 1970. *Lancet* 1:1180
330. Morgan, J. P., Preziosi, T. J., Bianchine, J. R. 1970. *Lancet* 2:659
331. Klawans, H. L. 1971. *Confin. Neurol.* 33:133–45
332. Rosenthal, R. K., McDowell, F. H., Cooper, W. 1972. *Neurology* 22:1–11
333. Klawans, H. L. 1970. *Eur. Neurol.* 4: 148–63
334. Klawans, H. L., Paulson, G. W., Barbeau, A. 1970. *Lancet* 2:1185–86
335. Klawans, H. L., Paulson, G. W., Ringel, S. P., Barbeau, A. 1972. *New Engl. J. Med.* 286:1332–34
336. Fog, R., Pakkenberg, H. 1970. *Acta Neurol. Scand.* 46:249–51
337. Barbeau, A., Chase, T. N., Paulson, G. W. See Ref. 116, pp. 1–826
338. Klawans, H. L., Shenker, D. M. 1972. *J. Neurol. Transmis.* 33:73–81
339. Lee, D. K., Markham, C. H., Clark, W. G. 1968. *Life Sci.* 7:707–12

340. Barbeau, A. 1969. *Lancet* 2:1066
341. Klawans, H. L., Rubovits, R., Ringel, S. P., Weiner, W. J. 1972. *Arch. Neurol.* 26:282–84
342. Chase, T. N., Watanabe, A. M., Brodie, H. K. H., Donnelly, E. F. 1972. *Arch. Neurol.* 26:282–84
343. Anonymous. 1972. *Lancet* 2:573–75
344. Dalén, P. 1973. *Lancet* 1:107–08
345. Mattsson, B. 1973. *Lancet* 1:718
346. Manyam, N. V. B., Bravo-Fernandez, E. 1973. *Lancet* 1:1010
347. Dalén, P., Steg, G. 1973. *Lancet* 1: 936–37
348. Chalmers, A., McGeer, E. G., Wickson, V., McGeer, P. L. 1970. *Comp. Gen. Pharm.* 1:385–90
349. Fahn, S., Côté, L. J. 1968. *J. Neurochem.* 15:209–13
350. Barbeau, A. 1972. *Union Méd. Can.* 101:1377–79
351. Feltz, P. 1971. *Can. J. Physiol. Pharmacol.* 49:1113–15
352. Perry, T. L., Hansen, S., Kloster, M. 1973. *New Engl. J. Med.* 288:337–42
353. Bird, E. D., Mackay, A. V. P., Rayner, C. N., Iversen, L. L. 1973. *Lancet* 1: 1090–92
354. Chapel, J. L., Brown, N., Jenkins, R. L. 1964. *Am. J. Psychiat.* 121:608–10

355. Shapiro, A. K., Shapiro, E. 1968. *Brit. J. Psychiat.* 114:345–50
356. Yvonneau, M. 1972. *Rev. Neurol.* 126: 65–70
357. Eldridge, R. 1970. *Neurology* 20(2): 1–78
358. Barbeau, A. 1970. *Neurology* 20(2):96–102
359. Chase, T. N. 1970. *Neurology* 20(2): 122–30
360. Coleman, M. P., Barnet, A. 1969. *Proc. Am. Neurol. Assoc.* 94:91
361. Coleman, M. P. 1970. *Neurology* 20 (2): 114–21
362. Mandell, S. 1970. *Neurology* 20(2): 103–06
363. Barrett, R. E., Yahr, M. D., Duvoisin, R. C. 1970. *Neurology* 20 (2):107–13
364. Wooten, G. F., Eldridge, R., Axelrod, J., Stern, R. S. 1973. *New Engl. J. Med.* 288:284–87
365. Parkes, J. D., Knill-Jones, R. P., Clements, P. J. 1971. *Postgrad. Med. J.* 47: 116–19
366. Rajput, A. H. 1973. *Lancet* 1:432
367. Braham, J., Sarova-Pinhas, I. 1973. *Lancet* 1:432–33
368. Shaw, K. M., Hunter, K. R., Stern, G. M. 1973. *Lancet* 1:1399
369. Spiegel, E. A., Baird, H. W. 1968. *Handb. Clin. Neurol.* 6:440–75
370. Towbin, A. 1960. *The Pathology of Cerebral Palsy.* Springfield: Thomas

PHARMACOLOGICAL RESEARCH IN INDIA

❖6584

P. C. Dandiya and J. S. Bapna

Department of Pharmacology, S.M.S. Medical College, Jaipur, India

INTRODUCTION

An exhaustive review entitled "Highlights of Pharmacology Research in India" was written by Mukerji and associates in the 1963 issue of *Annual Review of Pharmacology* (1). Subsequently "Trends in Pharmacology Research in India" by Dandiya & Bapna (2) and "CNS Active Drugs from Plants Indigenous to India," by Dandiya & Chopra (3) have been published. A comprehensive review on *Ayurvedic Medicine—Past and Present* has been recently written by Sharma (4). In the present article an attempt has been made to summarize the research work done in India during the past decade, including research on the active materials isolated from plants indigenous to India, which has received considerable attention during the last twelve years.

Pharmacology research in India has been traditionally sponsored by the medical colleges. Several factors have provided impetus to the trend. The growth and expansion of medical education was very rapid generally after 1950 and particularly during the 1960s. New institutions were fortunate in having on their staffs a number of Indian pharmacologists trained abroad under the auspices of various international agencies, some trained under eminent pharmacologists in western countries. Besides, pharmacological research, like research in other medical sciences, was promoted and supported with substantial financial assistance by the Indian Council of Medical Research (ICMR). In 1962 an independent committee was constituted by the ICMR to encourage research on indigenous drugs. A year later ICMR appointed a separate expert group to evaluate research proposals on pharmacology, and thus separated the responsibility that had hitherto been undertaken by the combined committee for physiology and pharmacology. The research projects on indigenous drugs have now been assigned to the Central Council of Research on Indian Medicine and Homoeopathy. For some years this Council has been running composite research units of indigenous drugs comprising subunits of chemistry, pharmacology, pharmacognosy, and clinical trials, the last being housed mostly in the hospitals of indigenous systems of medicine.

115

The Central Drug Research Institute (CDRI) at Lucknow, functioning under the control of the Council of Scientific and Industrial Research, has been another promoter of drug research in India. Significant work has been done in the last few years in this Institute. Private enterprise in pharmacology research is yet in its infancy in India, the solitary exception being CIBA research center. Lately, the Hoechst Pharmaceuticals have also made a beginning in this direction. These developments have contributed to the advancement of pharmacological research in the country from 1960 onwards. The rate of growth and the quality of work could have been higher but for the following reasons: (a) the opening of too many new medical colleges in the 1960s led to the migration of the professional talent from the few institutions then existing to a large number of teaching colleges. Some of the departments left with skeleton manpower that could barely manage the teaching load were unable to indulge in the luxury of research; (b) due to stress of expansion of medical education, government funds were directed more and more towards undergraduate teaching while grants for purchasing equipment for postgraduate training and advanced research gradually shrank. The paucity of foreign exchange was another limiting factor in the procurement of sophisticated equipment; (c) a good number of pharmacologists who had received training abroad returned to the western countries where superior research facilities were available. This was particularly so in the case of nonmedical pharmacologists who were not easily accepted on the faculties of medical colleges in India. Further, the progress of biochemistry in India was slow and this adversely influenced the growth of pharmacological research; (d) the facilities for clinical research were not available to the pharmacologists of this country, the sole exception being the pharmacology department of the Seth G.S. Medical College in Bombay, where a clinical research unit has existed under the leadership of Dr. U. K. Sheth for quite a few years.

CENTRAL NERVOUS SYSTEM

Natural Substances

The sanskrit word "Gandha" means smell and since time immemorial sarpa-gandha (snake smelling) i.e. *Rauwolfia serpentina;* ugra-gandha (strong smelling) i.e. *Acorus calamus;* and ashwa-gandha (horse smelling) i.e. *Withania somnifera,* were the main herbs employed for mental ailments in India. The isolation of reserpine from *Rauwolfia serpentina,* which possessed marked CNS depressant and antihypertensive actions, led to the investigation of the other two herbs.

The active principles from the roots and rhizomes of *A. calamus* were isolated and identified as α-asarone (asarone) and β-asarone i.e. *trans-* and *cis-*2,4,5-trimethoxy-1-propenylbenzene respectively (5). Asarone was found to have a marked CNS depressant effect in mice, rats, and monkeys. It decreased spontaneous locomotor activity in mice (6) and rats (7) and produced a calming effect in monkeys which lasted for 24 hr (8). The onset of action of asarone was quicker than reserpine and it counteracted the stimulant effect of *d*-amphetamine, LSD, methylphenidate, and mescaline but only partially antagonized the effect of imipramine in rats and mice (8). It also offered complete protection to aggregated mice treated with toxic doses of *d*-amphetamine, where it was found to be more effective than chlorpromazine (9). It prolonged the hypnosis induced by pentobarbital, hexobarbital, and ethanol, an effect which could not be prevented by LSD or iproniazid (10). It caused hypothermia in mice (10) and counteracted LSD-induced hyperpyrexia (8). It prevented pentylenetetrazol-induced convulsions and electroshock seizures, but facilitated picrotoxin-induced convulsions in rats (10, 11). It potentiated the effect of reserpine on electroconvulsions (12), blocked conditioned avoidance response of trained rats, and potentiated the effect of reserpine on this response. It also antagonized fighting behavior due to foot shock and increased the number of shocks accepted by experimental animals in conflict neurosis (13).

The work done on its mechanism of action revealed that unlike reserpine it did not deplete the brain contents of 5-HT (12) or norepinephrine (NE) (6). It caused sedation in mice treated with iproiazid similar to that of chlorpromazine (6, 8). Because the chemical structure of asarone resembled a part of the reserpine molecule, an attempt was made to find out if both these agents acted on a common receptor site. α-Methyltyrosine pretreatment, which lowered brain NE by about 65%, enhanced the sedative action of both asarone and reserpine (14, 15). However, unlike tetrabenazine, asarone did not block the sedative action of reserpine, suggesting a different site of action (6).

Asarone elicited a mild hypotensive effect in anesthetized dogs and exhibited a varying degree of antiacetylcholine, antihistamine, and antiserotonin activity on isolated muscle preparations (9, 16). It prevented the depletion of adrenal ascorbic acid in rats subjected to cold stress.

In search for more useful and less toxic asarone analogs a number of trimethoxybenzene derivatives: i.e. phenylalkyl derivatives (17, 18), benzamides (17, 19–25), phenylesters, anilides, tetrazoles (22, 26), piperazines (27), azlactones (26, 28, 29), styrenes and cinnamic acids (17, 30, 31), and hydantoins and 2-thiohydantoins (32, 33) were synthesized by Dandiya and co-workers and interesting structure activity relationships were established (34).

The work done on ashwagandha (*W. Somnifera*) revealed that its total alkaloid fraction, ashwagandholine and two saponins becoside A and B, possessed mild CNS depressant activity (35, 36).

Besides these, a few other CNS active principles were obtained from plants. A glycoside saponin principle "hersaponin" isolated from *Herpestis monniera,* which is used in the Ayurvedic system of medicine in insanity, epilepsy, and hysteria, has been shown to produce a sedative effect in rats and guinea pigs. It potentiated hexobarbitone induced sleep in mice, caused hypothermia (37), and was reported to deplete brain NE and 5-HT content in rats (38). Bhide (39) has reported the presence of a tranquilizing principle in the husk of millet from *Paspalum scrobiculatum.* A sesquiterpene Jatamansone, syn. velaranone, having a weak tranquilizing, hypotensive (40, 41), and antihyperkinetic activity (42), has been isolated from *Nardostachys jatamansi.*

Stereotyped Behavior

A successful attempt has been made to analyze the influence of hallucinogens (LSD, mescaline), CNS stimulants (amphetamine, methylphenidate, caffeine), and antidepressants (imipramine, iproniazid, pargyline) on the open field performance in rats (43, 44). Two distinct behavioral actions, namely the horizontal activity (ambulation) and vertical activity (rearing), were observed when rats were subjected to the open field test. The horizontal activity, a function of increasing doses of hallucinogens like LSD and mescaline, was considered as simple stereotypy, while the vertical activity was taken as complex stereotypy, which was found to be a characteristic behavioral pattern of amphetamine and methylphenidate (44–47). The antidepressants, however, failed to modify the behavioral actions in rats in the open field test. Lately, with the aid of enzyme inhibitors and precursors the possible role of brain biogenic amines in the stereotyped behavior was analyzed (48) and it was found that complex stereotypy was mediated by brain dopaminergic mechamism while the simple stereotypy was a function of brain NE (49).

Sethy et al (50) suggested the use of "amphetamine stereotypy" as a test for CNS stimulant or depressant drugs. It was also shown that small doses of CNS depressants could enhance amphetamine activity when given in combination (51).

Monoamines and CNS Drugs

The role of catecholamines (CA) and 5-HT in the action of psychotropic drugs was studied by Dandiya and associates employing specific enzyme inhibitors that are known to block their synthesis at the rate-limiting step. It was found that α-methyltyrosine, which lowered brain CA, remarkably enhanced the sedative actions of reserpine, chlorpromazine (14, 52), and asarone (6) and antagonized the excitatory actions of mescaline, amphetamine, morphine, and cocaine (53). It was further reported that α-methyltyrosine protected aggregated mice from the toxicity of amphetamine (15), suggesting that CA play an important role in the actions of the above-mentioned drugs. The excitation caused by reserpine in pargyline-treated rats was also suggested to be more closely related to CA than 5-HT (54, 55). These workers have also reported the beneficial influence of a number of monoamine oxidase inhibitors and some other antidepressants on the efficacy of diphenylhydramine in preventing drug-induced parkinson-like signs in rats and mice (56, 57).

Influence of Drugs in Stress

Dandiya et al (58) have investigated the antistress actions of some tranquilizers. Physiological stress caused a varying degree of biochemical alterations in the animals. A fall in adrenal ascorbic acid content, serum cholesterol, and serum sodium levels was reported after subjecting the animals to cold stress (58, 59). Heat stress lowered brain glutathione and acetylcholine contents but increased 5-HT and NE levels (59, 60). Both chlorpromazine and reserpine offered protection to these heat stress-induced changes. Mescaline and LSD produced a lowering of brain glutathione levels and aggravated the heat stress-induced reduction in glutathione level (59). Sharma and associates showed that both reserpine and chlorpromazine prevented the rise in stress-induced cardiac and plasma CA and acetylcholine contents

(61, 62). α-Methyltyrosine was able to prevent the fall in myocardial glycogen and blood glucose in rats (63). Pohujani and co-workers have reported the protective influence of a number of barbiturates, glucocorticoids, and chlorpromazine against the effects of centrifugal stress on rat adrenals (64–66).

Analgesics and Muscle Relaxants

Sheth and his colleagues investigated the mechanism of morphine- and meperidine-induced analgesia. The ED_{50} of meperidine significantly increased in mice pretreated with reserpine or p-chlorophenylalanine (PCPA) when tested by tail clip and electroshock method (67, 68). Similarly the ED_{50} of tremorine also increased in mice treated with reserpine, PCPA, or diethyldithiocarbamate when tested for analgesic activity (69). It was suggested that morphine released dopamine in the CNS which in turn excited the central dopaminergic receptors (70).

Sinha et al (71, 72) demonstrated the muscle relaxing property of tricyclic antidepressants and some β-adrenergic blocking agents. On intravenous administration, imipramine, desmethylimipramine, and amitriptyline showed neuromuscular blocking properties, and amitriptyline was found to be the most potent. The nature of blockade appeared to be competitive. Bhargava et al (73) studied the muscle relaxant properties of methaqualone and its derivatives and found that dimethaqualone was more potent than methaqualone and mephenesin as a muscle relaxant.

Emesis

Bhargava & Dixit (74) suggested the presence of histaminergic receptors in the chemoreceptor trigger zone, which were possibly responsible for the mechanism of emesis. They suggested that reserpine may be acting directly on the CT-zone and not by depleting the CA (75). Gupta et al (76) have ruled out the possibility of cholinergic mediation in the central integration of emesis and showed that antidepressants blocked reserpine- and apomorphine-induced emesis (77).

The alcoholic extract of the root of *Cyperus rotundus* has been found to protect dogs against apomorphine-induced emesis (78).

Sleep

Haranath and co-workers (79, 80) studied the role of cholinergic mechanism in sleep and REM sleep, using cholinergic agonists and antagonists. By perfusing the cerebral ventricles of anesthetized and unanesthetized dogs with cholinergic agents, these workers demonstrated that the release of acetylcholine diminished before and at the time of sleep but increased during REM sleep (81–83). They further showed that quaternary ammonium compounds, like curare, gallamine, and atropine, and NE passed into cerebrospinal fluid when given intravenously (84–86).

CARDIOVASCULAR SYSTEM

Antiarrhythmics

Antiarrhythmic activity of a number of drugs: i.e. some phenothiazines (87–89), ajmaline and its esters (90), phencarbamide (91), BP-400, cyproheptadine, chlorphenoxamine (92), glucagon (93), propranolol (94), INPEA (95), MJ-1999 (96) pronethalol (97), and H66/29 was reported. It was found that β-adrenergic receptor blocking drugs were most effective in blocking experimental cardiac arrhythmias (95, 96, 98). However, Madan et al (98) suggested that this activity was independent of β-receptor antagonism.

Studies on the role of various neurochemical substances like acetylcholine (99–101), CA (102), and 5-HT (103) in the genesis of cardiac arrhythmias indicated that acetylcholine may be involved (100, 104). Madan & Gupta (99) found that acetylcholine and atropine acted synergistically rather than antagonistically on the myocardium. Bhargava et al (102) reported that CA may be responsible in the centrogenic cardiac arrhythmias induced by aconitine, which could be blocked by prior reserpinization, bilateral adrenelactomy, thoracic splanchnic nerve section, or β-receptor blocking drugs. Aconitine also increased the 5-HT content of the heart, which returned to control value when normal rhythm was restored by quinidine (103).

Cardiotonics

Arora et al (105) found that peruvoside, a cardiac glycoside obtained from *Thevetia neriifolia,* produced positive inotropic and chronotropic effects on cat heart. Its toxicity, potency, and clinical efficacy were similar to ouabain. Singh & Rastogi (106, 107) isolated asclepin, a cardenolide from *Asclepias curassavica,* and determined its chemical structure. Its action was similar to digoxin but lasted longer. The extract obtained from *Nerium indicum* was also reported to possess cardiotonic activity (108, 109).

Hypertension

The effects of neurochemical substances like choline (110), histamine (111), 5-HT (112), and CA (113) on the central vasomotor loci have been studied. It was shown that cerebroventricular (ICV) administration of choline caused initial pressor followed by depressor response. These responses were explained on the basis of the peripheral and central release of CA by choline (110). 5-HT produced a depressor response in dogs, which was prevented by pretreatment with dibenzylene or morphine, suggesting the pressence of undifferentiated receptors for 5-HT which could be blocked by M or D types of blockers (112). Phenylephrine or NE caused bradycardia, whereas isoprenaline caused tachycardia, which could be blocked by α- and β-receptor blocking agents respectively (113). The injection of propranolol into the lateral ventricles elicited a biphasic response, i.e. an initial short-lived pressor phase with tachycardia followed by a prolonged depressor effect and bradycardia (114). The role of CA in renal hypertension was studied using 6-hydroxydopamine and it was suggested that the functional sympathetic nervous system was important in the development of renal hypertension in rats (115, 116). Gulati and co-workers studied the mechanism of antihypertensive action of guanethidine and supported the hypothesis of a cholinergic link in sympathetic transmission (117, 118).

Dhar and co-workers isolated a number of alkaloids from *Croton sparsiflorus morong* and reported that N-methylcrotsparine produced a moderate hypotension in anesthetized dogs. A derivative of this alkaloid, N-methylapocrotsparine, produced a marked hypotension due to its central and peripheral actions (119, 120).

MISCELLANEOUS

Chemotherapy

Berberine-containing plants like *Berberis aristata* have been used in the Indian system of medicine for a long time as a stomachic, bitter tonic, and in the treatment of leprosy, snake bite, and jaundice (121). Dutta & Panse (122) found that the effect of berberine in experimental cholera was comparable to chloramphenicol (123). The alkaloid was also reported to possess antibacterial activity against a wide variety of microorganisms such as fungi, *Vibrio cholerae*, and *Entamoeba histolytica* (124–130). It also protected rabbits from cholerogenic toxins (131). Desai et al (132) have studied the cytotoxic actions of *Abrus precatorius* and reported that the seed extract produced chromosomal aberrations in ciliates (133–135).

Among the antifilarial agents synthesized, 3-ethyl-8-methyl-1,3,8-triazabicyclo(4,4,0)decan-2-one was found to be more effective than diethylcarbamazine in cotton rats (136). Rao & Narasimharao (137) isolated champamycin B from *Streptomyces champavatii*, which protected mice from sublethal doses of *Candida albicans*.

Anti-inflammatory Drugs

Studies on determining the association of histamine, 5-HT (138, 139), and CA (140, 141) with the inflammatory process revealed that only histamine or 5-HT may be involved in it at the exudative and reparative stages of the response (138). Reserpine, which depleted 5-HT, antagonized the inflammatory process (139). Studies carried out on the anti-inflammatory activity of a large number of substances obtained from natural products have shown that triterpenoids, saponins, flavonoids, β-glycyrrhetinic acid, β-amyrin, and turmeric (142–148) possessed moderate antiinflammatory action. Among the flavonoids, taxifolin, isolated from *Madhuca butyracea*, possessed potent anti-inflammatory activity (149).

Antidiabetic Activity

In India a number of herbs have been used in the indigenous system of medicine for the treatment of diabetes mellitus. In the 1960s an extensive effort was made by the Indian pharmacologists to determine their efficacy and the pharmacological basis of their use. It was reported that *Ficus bengalensis* Linn contained three flavonoid compounds, each possessing a hypoglycemic action in fasting rabbits (150–152). The extracts of several other plants such as *Gymnema sylvestre* (153), *Vinca rosea, Cassia auriculata, Eugenia jambolana* (154), and *Momordica charantia* (155) were shown to possess similar properties. The fact that these investigators have practically given up further investigation of these materials indicates the low degree of blood sugar lowering property possessed by them.

Antifertility Agents

Anand and co-workers synthesized a number of furans (156), benzofurans (156–158), arylophenones (159–163), coumarins, chromans, and chromenes (164) and reported antiimplantation activity in many of these. The most effective compound was 3, 4-*trans*-2, 2-dimethyl-3-phenyl-1, 4-(*p*-β-pyrrolidinoethoxyphenyl)-7-methoxychroman (164). A single oral dose administered postcoitum completely prevented conception in mice, rats, dogs, and monkeys (165).

Sympathomimetics

The sympathomimetic action of acetylcholine on nictitating membrane of dog (117) and rat ileum (166) was demonstrated by Gulati and co-workers. This action was blocked by adrenergic neurone blocking agents and regenerated by indirectly acting sympathomimetics (167, 168), tetrodotoxin, and NE (118). These workers also reported the α-adrenergic blocking activity of β-blockers (169) and the excitatory action of tyramine on human umbilical cord (170).

In conclusion, one could state categorically that pharmacology has been developing steadily in India during the last twelve years, and a larger number of pharmacologists than before are tending to specialize in specific fields. More intensive work is being carried out on the CNS than in other fields. Behavioral studies, too, have found their place in Indian pharmacology.

The cost of modern drugs, in terms of the earning capacity of the masses of India, remains high and is rising every year. Intensive efforts made to discover new and potent drugs from a plethora of plant drugs, employed empirically in the Indigenous system of medicines, have so far been unrewarding. This makes the situation desperate. The average man in India is not interested in the discovery of a new drug in a western country, because it will be beyond his means. For example, he is not looking forward to a miracle cure of cancer. Today, he is challenging the Indian pharmacologist to bring out effective drugs that are inexpensive, so that his suffering is alleviated at low cost. The need is so urgent that it will be logical to expect that in the next few years Indian pharmacologists in collaboration with chemists, biochemists, and physicians will take up the search for less expensive, readily available agents having antifertility, antiamoebic, and broad spectrum anthelmintic properties with low side effects, and which could be manufactured from raw materials available indigenously. Whether they will respond to these challenges and train themselves to solve these national problems is a matter of conjecture.

ACKNOWLEDGMENTS

The authors are thankful to Mr. S. K. Kulkarni and Mr. N. K. Gurbani for their valuable support in the preparation of the manuscript.

Literature Cited

1. Mukerji, B., De, N. N., Kohli, J. D. 1962. *Ann. Rev. Pharmacol.* 2:17–30
2. Dandiya, P. C., Bapna, J. S. 1968. *East. Pharm.* 11:29–35
3. Dandiya, P. C., Chopra, Y. M. 1970. *Indian J. Pharm.* 2:67–90
4. Sharma, S. 1971. *Progr. Drug. Res.* 15: 11–67
5. Baxter, R. M., Dandiya, P. C., Kandel, S. I., Okany, A., Walker, G. C. 1960. *Nature* 185:466–67
6. Menon, M. K., Dandiya, P. C. 1967. *J. Pharm. Pharmacol.* 19:170–75
7. Sharma, J. D., Dandiya. P. C. 1962. *Arch. Int. Pharmacodyn.* 137:218–30
8. Dandiya, P. C., Menon, M. K. 1964. *J. Pharmacol. Exp. Ther.* 145:42–46
9. Dandiya, P. C., Menon, M. K. 1965. *Life Sci.* 4:1635–41
10. Dandiya, P. C., Sharma, J. D. 1962. *Indian J. Med. Res.* 50:46–60
11. Sharma, J. D., Dandiya, P. C., Baxter, R. M., Kandel, S. I. 1961. *Nature* 192: 1299–1300
12. Dandiya, P. C., Menon, M. K. 1963. *Brit. J. Pharmacol.* 20:436–42
13. Chak, I. M., Sharma, J. N. 1965. *Indian J. Exp. Biol.* 3:252–54
14. Menon, M. K., Dandiya, P. C., Bapna, J. S. 1967. *J. Pharmacol. Exp. Ther.* 156:63–69
15. Menon, M. K., Dandiya, P. C. 1967. *J. Pharm. Pharmacol.* 19:596–602
16. Das, P. K., Malhotra, C. L., Dhalla, N. S. 1962. *Arch. Int. Pharmacodyn.* 135: 167–77
17. Dandiya, P. C., Sharma, P. K., Menon, M. K. 1962. *Indian J. Med. Res.* 50: 750–60
18. Sheth, N. A., Dadkar, N. K., Sheth, U. K., Deliwala, C. V., Petigara, R. B. 1969. *Indian J. Pharmacol.* 1:33–49
19. Menon, M. K., Dandiya, P. C. 1963. *Indian J. Med. Res.* 51:1037–47
20. Sogani, S. K., Dandiya, P. C. 1965. *J. Med. Chem.* 8:139–40
21. Sogani, S. K., Menon, M. K., Dandiya, P. C. 1965. *Indian J. Pharm.* 27:173–76
22. Sharma, P. K., Dandiya, P. C., Bose, B. C., Vijayvargiya, R. 1965. *Indian J. Med. Res.* 53:1191–95
23. Hemnani, K. L., Menon, M. K., Dandiya, P. C. 1966. *Indian J. Pharm.* 28: 292–96
24. Dandiya, P. C., Hemnani, K. L., Sharma, H. L. 1966. *Indian J. Physiol. Pharmacol.* 10:153–61
25. Chaturvedi, A. K., Chaudhari, A., Parmar, S. S. 1972. *J. Pharm. Sci.* 61:1157

26. Dandiya, P. C., Menon, M. K., Hemnani, K. L., Chandra, S. 1966. *Proc. Recent Advan. Pharm. Sci.*, Chandigarh 62–72
27. Petigara, R. B., Deliwala, C. V., Mandrekar, S. S., Dadkar, N. K., Sheth, U. K. 1969. *J. Med. Chem.* 12:865–70
28. Sharma, P. K., Menon, M. K., Dandiya, P. C. 1964. *J. Pharm. Sci.* 53: 1055–58
29. Chandra, S., Dandiya, P. C. 1970. *Indian J. Hosp. Pharm.* 7:151–55
30. Chandra, S., Sharma, P. K., Varma, R. R., Dandiya, P. C. 1969. *Indian J. Pharm.* 31:91–94
31. Chandra, S., Dandiya, P. C., Mital, R. L., Bapna, J. S. 1969. *Indian J. Hosp. Pharm.* 6:238–44
32. Chandra, S., Dandiya, P. C. 1969. *Can. J. Chem.* 47:3704–5
33. Mishra, A. K. 1971. *Preparation and pharmacological screening of some newer hydantoin and 2-thiohydantoin derivatives.* PhD thesis. Univ. Rajasthan, Jaipur, India
34. Dandiya, P. C. 1970. *Indian J. Physiol. Pharmacol.* 14:87–94
35. Malhotra, C. L., Mehta, V. L., Prasad, K., Das, P. K. 1965. *Indian J. Physiol. Pharmacol.* 9:8–15
36. Kulshrestha, D. K., Rastogi, R. P. 1972. *Proc. VIII Int. Symp. Chem. Natural Prod.* 190
37. Malhotra, C. L., Das, P. K., Dhalla, N. S. 1960. *Arch. Int. Pharmacodyn.* 129: 290–302
38. Malhotra, C. L., Prasad, K., Dhalla, N. S., Das, P. K. 1961. *J. Pharm. Pharmacol.* 13:447–49
39. Bhide, N. K. 1962. *Brit. J. Pharmacol.* 18:7–18
40. Arora, R. B. 1965. *Indian Council Med. Res. Suppl. Rep.* 51
41. Arora, C. K., Arora, R. B., Sheth, U. K., Shah, M. J. 1967. *Indian J. Med. Sci.* 21:455–60
42. Arora, R. B., Chatterji, A. K., Gupta, R. D., Arora, C. K., Tondon, P. N. 1966. *CSIR Symp. CNS Drugs,* 118
43. Dandiya, P. C., Gupta, B. D., Gupta, M. L., Patni, S. K. 1969. *Psychopharmacologia* 15:333–40
44. Dandiya, P. C., Gupta, B. D., Gupta, M. L. 1970. *Indian J. Med. Res.* 58: 487–94
45. Dandiya, P. C., Gupta, B. D., Gupta, M. L. 1970. *Pharmakopsychiat. Neuro Psychopharmakologie* 3:349–54

46. Gupta, B. D., Dandiya, P. C., Gupta, M. L., Gabba, A. K. 1971. *Eur. J. Pharmacol.* 13:341–46
47. Gupta, B. D., Dandiya, P. C., Gupta, M. L. 1971. *Jap. J. Pharmacol.* 21: 293–98
48. Kulkarni, S. K., Dandiya, P. C. 1972. *Psychopharmacologia* 27:367–72
49. Dandiya, P. C., Patni, S. K. 1973. *Indian J. Med. Res.* 61:891–95
50. Sethy, V. H., Naik, S. R., Sheth, U. K. 1967. *Indian J. Med. Sci.* 21:109–11
51. Sethy, V. H., Naik, P. Y., Sheth, U. K. 1970. *Psychopharmacologia* 18:19–25
52. Bapna, J. S., Dandiya, P. C. 1970. *Psychopharmacologia* 17:361–66
53. Menon, M. K., Dandiya, P. C., Bapna, J. S. 1967. *Psychopharmacologia* 10: 437–44
54. Chopra, Y. M., Dandiya, P. C. 1969. *Arch. Int. Pharmacodyn.* 181:47–56
55. Bapna, J. S., Dandiya, P. C. 1972. *Pharmakopsychiat. Neuro Psychopharmakol.* 5:241–48
56. Dandiya, P. C., Bhargava, L. P. 1968. *Arch. Int. Pharmacodyn.* 176:157–67
57. Patni, S. K., Dandiya, P. C. 1972. *Jap. J. Pharmacol.* 22:301–8
58. Dandiya, P. C., Varma, R. R., Sogani, R. K., Khuteta, K. P. 1967. *J. Pharm. Sci.* 56:300–1
59. Varma, R. R., Khuteta, K. P., Dandiya, P. C. 1968. *Psychopharmacologia* 12: 170–75
60. Menon, M. K., Dandiya, P. C. 1969. *Eur. J. Pharmacol.* 8:285–91
61. Sharma, V. N., Godhwani, J. L. 1970. *Indian J. Med. Res.* 58:1063–72
62. Godhwani, J. L., Sharma, V. N. 1970. *Indian J. Med. Res.* 58:1728–35
63. Prabhu, S., Sharma, V. N., Singh, V. 1972. *Brit. J. Pharmacol.* 44:814–16
64. Pohujani, S. M., Chittal, S. M., Raut, V. S., Sheth, U. K. 1969. *Indian J. Med. Res.* 57:1081–86
65. *Ibid.* 57:1087–90
66. *Ibid.* 57:1091–94
67. Sethy, V. H., Pradhan, R. J., Mandrekar, S. S., Sheth, U. K. 1970. *Indian J. Med. Res.* 58:1453–58
68. Sethy, V. H., Pradhan, R. J., Mandrekar, S. S., Sheth, U. K. 1970. *Psychopharmacologia* 17:320–26
69. Sethy, V. H., Naik, S. R., Sheth, U. K. 1971. *Psychopharmacologia* 19:73–80
70. Dhasmana, K. M., Dixit, K. S., Jaju, B. P., Gupta, M. L. 1972. *Psychopharmacologia* 24:380–83
71. Sinha, J. N., Dixit, K. S., Srimal, R. C., Chandra, O., Bhargava, K. P. 1966. *Arch. Int. Pharmacodyn.* 162:79–83
72. Sinha, J. N., Jaju, B. P., Srimal, R. C. 1966. *Jap. J. Pharmacol.* 16:250–56
73. Bhargava, K. P., Rastogi, S. K., Sinha, J. N. 1972. *Brit. J. Pharmacol.* 44: 805–6
74. Bhargava, K. P., Dixit, K. S. 1968. *Brit. J. Pharmacol.* 34:508–13
75. Bhargava, K. P., Dixit, K. S., Gupta, G. P. 1967. *Brit. J. Pharmacol.* 29:37–41
76. Gupta, G. P., Dhawan, K. N., Sinha, J. N. 1968. *Jap. J. Pharmacol.* 18:266–67
77. Gupta, G. P., Saxena, R. C., Chandra, O., Dhawan, K. N. 1969. *Psychopharmacologia* 15:255–59
78. Singh, N., Kulshrestha, V. K., Gupta, M. B., Bhargava, K. P. 1970. *Indian J. Med. Res.* 58:103–9
79. Haranath, P. S. R. K., Sunanda-Bai, K., Venkatakrishna-Bhatt, H. 1967. *Brit. J. Pharmacol.* 29:42–54
80. Haranath, P. S. R. K., Indiranarayan, G. 1971. *Indian J. Physiol. Pharmacol.* 15:59–60
81. Haranath, P. S. R. K., Venkatakrishna-Bhatt, H. 1972. *Indian J. Med. Res.* 60:1682–88
82. Haranath, P. S. R. K., Venkatakrishna-Bhatt, H. 1971. *Indian J. Physiol. Pharmacol.* 15:58–59
83. Haranath, P. S. R. K., Shyamalakumari, S., Devasankaraiah, G. 1971. *Indian J. Physiol. Pharmacol.* 15:59
84. Draskoci, M., Feldberg, W., Haranath, P. S. R. K. 1960. *J. Physiol. London* 150:34–49
85. Haranath, P. S. R. K., Premalatha, K., Sunanda-Bai, K. 1966. *Brit. J. Pharmacol.* 27:10–16
86. Haranath, P. S. R. K., Devasankaraiah, G., Krishnamurty, A. 1971. *Indian J. Pharmacol.* 3:41
87. Singh, K. P., Sharma, V. N. 1969. *Arch. Int. Pharmacodyn.* 177:168–78
88. Singh, K. P. 1968. *Arch. Int. Pharmacodyn.* 172:475–86
89. Singh, K. P. 1969. *Indian J. Physiol. Pharmacol.* 13:223–32
90. Arora, R. B., Bagchi, N., Sharma, J. N. 1967. *Indian J. Med. Res.* 55:389–95
91. Madan, B. R., Madan, V., Pendse, V. K., Gupta, R. S. 1970. *Arch. Int. Pharmacodyn.* 185:53–65
92. Sharma, V. N., Vyas, D. S., Madan, B. R. 1968. *Indian J. Med. Res.* 56:871–78
93. Madan, B. R. 1971. *Brit. J. Pharmacol.* 43:279–86
94. Madan, B. R., Jain, B. K., Gupta, R. S. 1971. *Arch. Int. Pharmacodyn.* 194: 78–82
95. Singh, N. et al 1970. *Jap. J. Pharmacol.* 20:467–72

96. Sharma, P. L. 1967. *Indian J. Med. Res.* 55:1357–65
97. Manekar, M. S., Rajapurkar, M. V. 1967. *Arch. Int. Pharmacodyn.* 168: 109–15
98. Madan, B. R., Mishra, S. N., Khanna, N. K. 1969. *Arch. Int. Pharmacodyn.* 182:121–29
99. Madan, B. R., Gupta, R. S. 1969. *Arch. Int. Pharmacodyn.* 178:43–52
100. Madan, B. R., Khanna, N. K., Soni, R. K. 1970. *J. Pharm. Pharmacol.* 22:621
101. Dutta, S. N., Sanyal, R. K., Tripathi, O. N. 1969. *Brit. J. Pharmacol.* 36:380–85
102. Bhargava, K. P., Kohli, R. P., Sinha, J. N., Tayal, G. 1969. *Brit. J. Pharmacol.* 36:240–52
103. Madan, B. R., Khanna, N. K., Godhwani, J. L., Pendse, V. K. 1969. *Indian J. Physiol. Pharmacol.* 13:233–37
104. Khanna, N. K. 1972. *Eur. J. Pharmacol.* 17:309–11
105. Arora, R. B., Sharma, J. N., Bhatia, M. L. 1967. *Indian J. Exp. Biol.* 5:31–36
106. Singh, B., Rastogi, R. P. 1969. *Indian J. Chem.* 7:1105–10
107. Singh, B., Rastogi, R. P. 1972. *Phytochemistry* 11:757–62
108. Kohli, R. P., Singh, N., Kulshrestha, V. K., Srivastava, R. K. 1969. *J. Res. Indian Med.* 4:54–57
109. Singh, N., Kulshrestha, V. K., Kohli, R. P. 1970. *J. Res. Indian Med.* 5:32–37
110. Srimal, R. C., Jaju, B. P., Sinha, J. N., Dixit, K. S., Bhargava, K. P. 1969. *Eur. J. Pharmacol.* 5:239–44
111. Sinha, J. N., Gupta, M. L., Bhargava, K. P. 1969. *Eur. J. Pharmacol.* 5: 235–38
112. Dhawan, K. N., Dhawan, B. N., Gupta, G. P. 1967. *Jap. J. Pharmacol.* 17: 435–38
113. Bhargava, K. P., Mishra, N., Tangri, K. K. 1972. *Brit. J. Pharmacol.* 45:596–602
114. Srivastava, R. K., Kulshrestha, V. K., Singh, N., Bhargava, K. P. 1973. *Eur. J. Pharmacol.* 21:222–29
115. Grewal, R. S., Kaul, C. L. 1971. *Brit. J. Pharmacol.* 42:497–504
116. Gupta, P. P., Srimal, R. C., Dhawan, B. N. 1972. *Eur. J. Pharmacol.* 20:215–23
117. Arya, P. C., Gulati, O. D. 1968. *Brit. J. Pharmacol.* 33:413–25
118. Gulati, O. D., Jaykar, S. 1971. Brit. J. Pharmacol. 42:352–63
119. Bhakuni, D. S., Dhar, M. M. 1968. *Experientia* 24:10–11
120. Bhakuni, D. S., Sheo, S., Dhar, M. M. 1970. *Phytochemistry* 9:2573–80
121. Chopra, R. N., Dikshit, B. B., Chowhan, J. S. 1932. *Indian Med. Gaz.* 67: 194–97
122. Dutta, N. K., Panse, M. V. 1962. *Indian J. Med. Res.* 50:732–36
123. Lahiri, S. C., Dutta, N. K. 1967. *J. Indian Med. Assoc.* 48:1–11
124. Subbaiah, T. V., Amin, A. H. 1967. *Nature* 215:527–28
125. Amin, A. H., Subbaiah, T. V., Abbasi, K. M. 1969. *Can. J. Microbiol.* 15: 1067–76
126. Dutta, N. K., Iyer, S. N. 1968. *J. Indian Med. Assoc.* 50:349–52
127. Modak, S., Modak, M. J., Venkataraman, A. 1970. *Indain J. Med. Res.* 58: 1510–22
128. Sharada, D. C. 1970. *J. Indian Med. Assoc.* 54:22–24
129. Sabir, M., Bhide, N. K. 1971. *Indian J. Physiol. Pharmacol.* 15:111–32
130. Kulkarni, S. K., Dandiya, P. C., Varandani, N. L. 1972. *Jap. J. Pharmacol.* 22:11–16
131. Dutta, N. K., Marker, P. H., Rao, N. R. 1972. *Brit. J. Pharmacol.* 44:153–59
132. Desai, V. B., Sirsi, M., Shankarappa, M., Kasturibai, A. R. 1971. *Indian J. Exp. Biol.* 9:369–71
133. Desai, V. B., Sirsi, M., Shankarappa, M., Kasturibai, A. R. 1966. *Indian J. Exp. Biol.* 4:164–66
134. Desai, V. B., Sirsi, M. 1966. *Indian J. Pharm.* 28:164–65
135. Reddy, V. V. Subba, Sirsi, M. 1969. *Cancer Res.* 29:1447–51
136. Saxena, R., Iyer, R. N., N. Anand, Chatterjee, R. K., Sen, A. B. 1970. *J. Pharm. Pharmacol.* 22:306–7
137. Rao, N., Narasimharao, P. L. 1967. *Indian J. Exp. Biol.* 5:39–43
138. Bhatt, K. G. S., Sanyal, R. K. 1963. *J. Pharm. Pharmacol.* 15:78–79
139. Ibid. 1964. 16:385–93
140. Bhalla, T. N., Sinha, J. N., Tangri, K. K., Bhargava, K. P. 1970. *Eur. J. Pharmacol.* 13:90–96
141. Ibid. 1972. 20:366–68
142. Tangri, K. K., Seth, P. K., Parmar, S. S., Bhargava, K. P. 1965. *Biochem. Pharmacol.* 14:1277–81
143. Tangri, K. K., Bhalla, T. N., Gupta, M. B., Seth, P. K., Bhargava, K. P. 1969. *Aspects Aller. Appl. Immunol.* 2: 151–60
144. Bhargava, K. P., Gupta, M. B., Gupta, G. P., Mitra, C. R. 1970. *Indian J. Med. Res.* 58:724–30
145. Gupta, M. B., Bhalla, T. N., Gupta, G. P., Mitra, C. R., Bhargava, K. P. 1969. *Eur. J. Pharmacol.* 6:67–70

146. Gupta, M. B., Gupta, G. P., Tangri, K. K., Bhargava, K. P. 1969. *Biochem. Pharmacol.* 18:531–32
147. Gupta, M. B., Bhalla, T. N., Tangri, K. K., Bhargava, K. P. 1971. *Biochem. Pharmacol.* 20:401–5
148. Arora, R. B., Basu, N., Kapoor, V., Jain, A. P. 1971. *Indian J. Med. Res.* 59:1289–95
149. Gupta, M. B., Bhalla, T. N., Gupta, G. P., Mitra, C. R., Bhargava, K. P. 1971. *Jap. J. Pharmacol.* 21:377–82
150. Brahmachari, H. D., Augusti, K. T. 1962. *J. Pharm. Pharmacol.* 14:617
151. Brahmachari, H. D., Aususti, K. T. 1964. *Indian J. Physiol. Pharmacol.* 8: 60–64
152. Gupta, S. S. 1966. *Indian J. Med. Res.* 54:354
153. Gupta, S. S., Variyar, M. C. 1964. *Indian J. Med. Res.* 52:200–7
154. Shrotri, D. S., Kelkar, M., Deshmukh, V. K., Aiman, R. 1963. *Indian J. Med. Res.* 51:464–67
155. Chatterjee, K. P. 1963. *Indian J. Physiol. Pharmacol.* 7:240–44
156. Grover, P. K., Chawla, H. P. S., Anand, N., Kamboj, V. P., Kar, A. B. 1965. *J. Med. Chem.* 8:720–21
157. Rastogi, S. N., Anand, N., Prasad, C. R. 1972. *J. Med. Chem.* 15:286–91
158. Chawla, H. P. S., Grover, P. K., Anand, N., Kamboj, V. P., Kar, A. B. 1970. *J. Med. Chem.* 13:54–59
159. Iyer, R. N., Gopalachari, R. 1966. *Indian J. Chem.* 4:520–23
160. Iyer, R. N., Gopalachari, R., Kamboj, V. P., Kar, A. B. 1967. *Indian J. Exp. Biol.* 5:169–70
161. Iyer, R. N., Gopalachari, R. 1969. *Indian J. Pharm.* 31:49–54
162. Gopalachari, R., Iyer, R. N., Kamboj, V. P., Kar, A. B. 1970. *Contraception* 2:199
163. Gopalachari, R., Iyer, R. N. Kamboj, V. P., Kar, A. B. 1971. *Indian J. Exp. Biol.* 9:104–5
164. Ray, S., Grover, P. K., Anand, N. 1970. *Indian J. Chem.* 8:961–63
165. Kamboj, V. P., Kar, A. B., Ray, S., Grover, P. K., Anand, N. 1971. *Indian J. Exp. Biol.* 9:103–4
166. Gokhale, S. D., Gulati, O. D., Panchal, D. I. 1967. *Brit. J. Pharmacol.* 30:35–45
167. Gokhale, S. D., Gulati, O. D., Udwadia, B. P. 1966. *Arch. Int. Pharmacodyn.* 160:321–29
168. Gulati, O. D., Dave, B. T., Gokhale, S. D., Shah, K. M. 1966. *J. Clin. Pharmacol. Ther.* 7:510–14
169. Gulati, O. D., Gokhale, S. D., Parikh, H. M., Udwadia, B. P., Krishnamurthy, V. S. R. 1969. *J. Pharmacol. Exp. Ther.* 166:35–43
170. Gulati, O. D., Kelkar, V. V. 1971. *Brit. J. Pharmacol.* 42:155–58

TOXICOLOGY OF FOOD COLORS[1]

❖6585

Jack L. Radomski

University of Miami, Miami, Florida

[1]Key to Chemical Names of Colors Referred to:
FD&C Blue No. 1 (Brilliant Blue FCF); disodium salt of 4-{[4-(N-ethyl-p-sulfobenzylamino)-phenyl]-(2-sulfoniumphenyl)-methylene{-[1-(N-ethyl-N-p-sulfobenzyl)-Δ²,⁵-cyclohexadienimine]: FD&C Blue No. 2 (Indigotine); disodium salt of 5,5'-indigotindisulfonic acid: FD&C Green No. 1 (Guinea Green B); monosodium salt of 4-[4-(N-ethyl-p-sulfobenzyl-amino)-diphenylmethylene]-[1-(N-ethyl-N-p-sulfoniumbenzyl)-Δ²,⁵-cyclohexadienimine]: FD&C Green No. 2 (Bright Green FS); disodium salt of 4-{[4-(N-ethyl-p-sulfobenzylamino)-phenyl] (4-sulfoniumphenyl)-methylene{-[1-(N-ethyl-N-p-sulfobenzyl)-Δ²,⁵-cyclohexadi-enimine]: FD&C Green No. 3 (Fast Green FCF); disodium salt of 4-{[4-(N-ethyl-p-sulfobenzyl-amino)-phenyl]-(4-hydroxy-2-sulfoniumphenyl)-methylene{-[1-(N-ethyl-N-p-sulfobenzyl)-Δ²,⁵-cyclohexadienimine]: FD&C Yellow No. 3 (Yellow AB); 1-Phenylazo-2-naphthylamine: FD&C Yellow No. 4 (Yellow OB); 1-o-Tolylazo-2-naphthylamine: FD&C Yellow No. 5 (Tartrazine); trisodium salt of 3-carboxy-5-hydroxy-1-p-sulfophenyl-4-p-sulfophenylazo-pyrazole: FD&C Yellow No. 6 (Sunset Yellow FCF); disodium salt of 1-p-sulfophenylazo-2-naphthol-6-sulfonic acid: FD&C Orange No. 1 (Orange 1); monosodium salt of 4-p-sulfo-phenylazo-1-naphthol: FD&C Orange No. 2 (Orange FS); 1-o-Toylazo-2-naphthol: FD&C Red No. 1 (Ponceau 3R); disodium salt of 1-pseudocumylazo-2-naphthol-3,6-disulfonic acid: FD&C Red No. 2 (Amaranth); trisodium salt of 1-(4-sulfo-1-naphthylazo)-2-naphthol-3,6-disulfonic acid: FD&C Red No. 3 (Erythrosine); disodium salt of 9-o-carboxyphenyl-6-hydroxy-2,4,5,7-tetraiodo-3-isoxanthone: FD&C Red No. 4 (Ponceau SX); disodium salt of 2-(5-sulfo-2,4-xylylazo)-1-naphthol-4-sulfonic acid: FD&C Red No. 32 (Oil Red XO); 1-Xylylazo-2-naphthol: FD&C Violet No. 1; monosodium salt of 4-{[4-(N-ethyl-p-sulfobenzylamino)-phenyl]-[4-(N-ethyl-p-sulfoniumbenzylamino)-phenyl]-methylene{-(N,N-dimethyl-Δ²,⁵-cyclohexadienimine): Citrus Red No. 2; 2,5-dimeth-oxyphenyl-azo-2-naphthol: Ponceau MX; disodium salt of 1-(2,4-xylylazo)-2-naphthol-3,6-disulfonic acid: Ponceau 4R; trisodium salt of 1-(4-sulfo-1-naphthylazo)-2-naphthol-6,8-disulfonic acid: D&C Red No. 9; barium salt of 1-(4-chloro-o-sulfo-5-tolylazo)-2-naphthol: D&C Red No. 10; monosodium salt of 2-(2-hydroxy-1-naphthylazo)-1-naphthalene-sulfonic acid.

127

INTRODUCTION

When beginning a discussion of food colors it is customary to point out that man has been artificially coloring his food since ancient times and that color is an important characteristic of food, usually the first to be perceived. On the other hand, it appears that the use of artificial food coloring is largely the economic matter of rendering foods more attractive to the consumer.

Not much attention was paid to the safety of coloring materials for food until the early 1950s when two instances of toxicity to humans took place. The first of these was an occurrence of diarrhea in children produced by a black and orange colored Halloween taffy. Investigations at the US Food and Drug Administration of the cathartic effect of the components of this candy traced the active ingredient to FD&C Orange No. 1, an azo food color. It was soon found that this color had approximately the same cathartic potency as phenolphthalein. A similar consumer complaint was subsequently received by FDA concerning popcorn that had been colored by FD&C Red No. 32. This food coloring was also found to be a cathartic. It was then observed that FD&C Yellow No. 4 (the latter two colors at that time being used extensively in coloring butter and margarine) was also cathartic (1). As a result of these occurences, a flurry of interest in the possible harmful effects of food colors occurred, and a considerable amount of chronic toxicity testing was initiated, largely at the toxicology laboratories of FDA.

Because these colors find their way into a vast number of food products ingested by virtually everyone in the country, there is no certain way of knowing whether or not lifetime ingestion of food colors is adversely affecting the population. Outside of the above-named incidents, there is no direct evidence that the use of food coloring materials has been injurious. Use of animal testing procedures for chronic toxicity determinations allows the identification of the most potentially harmful colors.

For little apparent good reason, the specific food colors in use vary widely from country to country. Because of space considerations, this review is limited to food colors used in the United States. The reader is referred to two reviews covering food colors used in the United Kingdom (2, 3). The Food and Agriculture Association of WHO has thoroughly reviewed the toxicology and chemical composition of the food colors used around the world in hopes of achieving standardization of this chaotic situation. The results of their deliberations and their recommendations are available (4–6).

TRIPHENLYMETHANE COLORS

The triphenylmethane colors include FD&C Blue No. 1 (Brilliant Blue FCF), FD&C Green No. 1 (Guinea Green B), FD&C Green No. 2 (Bright Green FS), FD&C Green No. 3 (Fast Green FCF), and FD&C Violet No. 1. All of these colors contain sulfonic acid groups and are therefore highly water soluble. They are also all poorly absorbed from the gastrointestinal tract, undoubtedly due to their low pKs. When these colors were given orally to rats, more than 90% of the administered dose was recovered in the feces with the exception of FD&C Green No. 2. With this color, only 68% was found in the feces, due apparently to decomposition in the GI tract. When administered to dogs, small amounts (1–3% of the dose) were found to be excreted in the bile, with the exception of FD&C Violet No. 1 where no excretion was observed (7). Thus it is apparent that these colors, because of their strongly acidic nature, are very poorly absorbed after oral administration and are largely excreted unchanged in the feces.

The triphenylmethane colors have an additional characteristic in common. It was first reported in 1937 that FD&C Green No. 2 induced sarcomas at the site of injection when a dose of 3 ml of a 2% solution was injected subcutaneously (8). The observation was later confirmed (9) and extended to the other triphenylmethane colors. In an experiment lasting 99 weeks, 76% or more of the rats developed sarcomas at the site of injection when 1 ml of a 2 or 3% solution of FD&C Blue No. 1, FD&C Green No. 2, and FD&C Green No. 3 was injected subcutaneously. FD&C Green No. 1 apparently had a much lower tendency to produce this effect, for only one tumor was observed in 18 rats tested (10). A considerable controversy over the significance of this observation exists. In a study of the mechanism of the effect, it was concluded that the production of sarcomas in rats by this technique is a reflection of the physical properties of the colors, primarily a lowering of surface tension, and not a true test for chemical carcinogenesis (11–13).

Triphenylmethane colors, for instance, gentian violet, have long been used in topical applications for controlling bacterial and fungal infections of the skin (14). Tests involving repeated application of high concentrations indicate that these substances generally are primary irritants (15).

Much more relevant to the matter of the possible harmful effects of these food colors are chronic feeding experiments. FD&C Blue No. 1 was fed to rats at concentrations up to 5% in the diet for 2 years. No effect was observed even at this high level (16). The three FD&C green colors were fed to rats, dogs, and mice for two years at concentrations up to 5% in the diet. Considering the massive amounts fed, few toxic effects were observed. The only possibly meaningful pathologic effect was an increase in hepatic tumor incidence in rats fed 5% FD&C Green No. 1. FD&C Green No. 2 produced some growth inhibition at the 2 and 5% feeding levels. FD&C Green No. 3 survived this intensive testing procedure showing no tumorigenic or toxic effects (17). It would appear that the triphenylmethane colors have a low degree of toxicity to experimental animals when fed orally. These experiments did not confirm an earlier observation of the induction of malignant lymphomas in rats fed 4% of FD&C Greens No. 1 and 3 (18).

FD&C Blue No. 2 (Indigotine) is a related sulfonated water-soluble color that does not have the triphenylmethane structure. It appears to have similar properties, producing fibrosarcomas at the site of repeated subcutaneous injection in rats. Chronic toxicity studies conducted in rats and dogs over a two year period and in pigs for 90 days indicate this substance is substantially innocuous even at the highest feeding level (5%) (16, 19).

SULFONATED NAPHTHALENE AZO COLORS

This is a group of water-soluble mono-, di-, and trisulfonated colors containing a naphthalene ring and an azo linkage to either a second naphthalene or benzene ring. It is comprised of FD&C Orange No. 1 (Orange 1), FD&C Yellow No. 6 (Sunset Yellow FCF), FD&C Red No. 1 (Ponceau 3R), FD&C Red No. 2 (Amaranth), and FD&C Red No. 4 (Ponceau SX). At the time of the investigation into the consumer complaint concerning FD&C Orange No. 1, it was observed that this color was readily split at the azo linkage by reductive fission by the bacterial flora of the gut of humans and animals (20). This phenomenon was subsequently observed to be a general one with this group of colors (21–24). This property suggests that effects observed with these colors may be due to their reduction products (25–27).

FD&C Orange No. 1 has a significant cathartic effect at 100–200 mg in dogs and beginning at 80 mg in man (28). Mice fed 15–20 mg of FD&C Orange No. 1 per week for 58 weeks did not develop a significantly increased incidence of tumors (29). In rats fed this color for 2 years at levels of 0.5, 1.0, and 2.0% of the diet, considerable toxicity was observed. At the higher feeding levels, increased mortality occurred along with splenic enlargement, leucocytosis, anemia, diarrhea, and growth suppression. Even at the 0.5% level congested kidneys, chronic nephritis, and splenic enlargement with increased pigmentation was observed. Dogs fed 0.2% in the diet survived 5 years without showing any ill effects. Higher concentrations, however, produced decreased survival though no specific pathologic effects were found (30, 31).

Of the three red colors in this group, FD&C Red No. 2 has been regarded as the least toxic. Several long-term feeding studies have been conducted on rats at concentrations of up to 5% in the diet in which no pathological effects or increase in tumors was observed (18, 32, 33). Recently, however, it was reported that this color produced liver damage including vacuolization and fatty degeneration accompanied by a rise in serum albumen and β-globulin when fed to rats for 18 months at 0.12% in the diet (34). Dogs fed 2% of the color in the diet for 7 years showed no evidence of any pathologic effect (35). Feeding studies in mice showed no tumorigenic effect (29). An embryotoxic effect was observed with FD&C Red No. 2 in female rats although no teratogenicity was found (36, 37). Studies published in the Russian literature indicated that FD&C Red No. 2 may be carcinogenic by oral administration. When this color was fed at 4% (reduced to 2.5%) in the diet for 25 months, peritoneal sarcomas were found in 11 of 18 rats (38). Of 48 animals fed FD&C Red No. 2 at 2% of the diet, 13 developed malignant tumors in another experiment lasting 33 months (39). Since carcinogenic effects were not revealed in comprehensive rat, mice, and dog experiments conducted in this country, it is possible that the effects reported above are due to an impurity (40). Colors are frequently mixtures of compounds and the composition of the same color may vary in different countries.

The other two red water-soluble azo colors, FD&C Red No. 1 and FD&C Red No. 4, appear to have somewhat greater toxicity. Although no toxic or tumorigenic effects were observed in rats and mice fed levels as high as 5% of FD&C Red No. 4 in the diet for 2 years, this color produced pathological changes in dogs when fed at a 1% level in the diet for 7 years. There was atrophy of the adrenal zona glomerulosa and chronic follicular cystitis with hematomatous projections into the urinary bladder and small hemosiderotic foci in the liver (41). It must be remembered when considering the significance of these changes that these dogs consumed huge amounts of the color.

An isomer of FD&C Red No. 4, Ponceau MX, appears to be more toxic. Pathologic effects in rats including liver cell adenomas, tubular degeneration of the kidneys, and glomerular changes were observed at all feeding levels down to 1.2% (42–44).

The most toxic of these red colors appears to be FD&C Red No. 1. At feeding concentrations to rats of 0.5–5%, this color produced increased mortality, growth inhibition, and most significantly, malignant liver tumors (45, 46). This color also produced mortality and liver pathology in dogs (45). It would appear that the toxicity and carcinogenicity of this color may be related to its metabolic products, in particular mesidine and pseudocumidine, the trimethyl aniline derivatives produced by reductive fission of the azo linkage. Tests conducted on 2,4-, 2,5-, and 2,6-xylidine in rats and dogs indicate that these substances are hepatotoxic (25, 47–50).

Perhaps the least toxic of these water soluble colors has been found to be FD&C Yellow No. 6. This color has been extensively tested for carcinogenicity and chronic toxicity in mice, rats, and dogs. No pathologic or toxicologic effects were noted even at 2–5% of the diet. The dog studies were conducted for a total of 7 years (51, 52). FD&C Yellow No. 6 has also been tested in pigs for 98 days at levels up to 100 mg/day. No toxicological abnormalities were observed (53).

One is tempted to generalize concerning the relationship of the structure to toxicity of this series of compounds. The less toxic members of this series, FD&C Yellow No. 6, FD&C Red No. 2, and FD&C Red No. 4 (slightly more toxic) are sulfonated on both aromatic rings adjacent to the azo group. They would therefore yield only sulfonated fission products which are certain to be poorly absorbed. With the more toxic FD&C Red No. 1 and FD&C Orange No. 1, sulfonic acid groups are limited to one of the aromatic rings. The other nucleus which would be released upon reductive fission would therefore be unsulfonated and probably absorbed. This suggestion is supported by the low toxicity of Ponceau 4R (not used in this country) (54–56) and the greater toxicity of D&C Red No. 10 (57) and D&C Red No. 9 (58).

FD&C Yellow No. 5 (Tartrazine) is a water soluble azo color with similar biological properties but differing somewhat in structure due to the presence of a heterocyclic ring adjacent to the azo group. This color is quite nontoxic and has been extensively tested in mice, rats, and dogs in feeding concentrations up to 5% for periods up to 2 years. No toxic or pathologic effects or increased incidence of tumors were observed (18, 32, 33, 59, 60).

OIL-SOLUBLE AZO COLORS

The oil-soluble azo colors as a group are the most toxic. These include FD&C Orange No. 2 (Orange FS), FD&C Red No. 32 (Oil Red XO), Citrus Red No. 2,

FD&C Yellow No. 3 (Yellow AB), and FD&C Yellow No. 4 (Yellow OB). These colors all contain a naphthalene residue on one side and a benzene residue on the other side of the azo linkage, and are completely unsulfonated. Somewhat surprisingly, the oil-soluble azo colors are also reduced by the intestinal flora of rats, rabbits, and dogs although at a slower rate than the water-soluble ones (61, 62).

After the incident with popcorn colored with FD&C Red No. 32, this color was found to exhibit a cathartic action in dogs and rats (61). Chronic toxicity experiments with FD&C Red No. 32 revealed this compound to be highly toxic. Pathological changes including liver damage, increased mortality, decreased growth rate, and right side heart pathology were observed at the lowest feeding level of 0.1% over a 2 year period in rats. Similar effects were observed with dogs (63). A less extensive study with the closely related FD&C Orange No. 2 showed similar toxicity (63).

Because of the desirability of having an oil-soluble red or orange color for the purpose of coloring the skin of oranges, the dye industry developed a replacement for FD&C Red No. 32 named Citrus Red No. 2. This color has the same chemical structure as FD&C Red No. 32 except that the methyl groups on the benzene ring are replaced by methoxy groups. Chronic toxicity tests in dogs, mice, and rats, however, have not indicated that this color is significantly less toxic than FD&C Red No. 32 (64). Hyperplasia with thickening of the bladder wall and the production of a papillary carcinoma in one mouse were noted in an experiment in which rats and mice were fed diets containing 0.05 and 0.25% Citrus Red No. 2 for 24 months. Unfortunately, bladder stones were present in most of the animals and it was not possible to determine if these stones were responsible for the tumor and/or hyperplasia produced. However, the lesions in rats and mice were likened to those observed with the proven bladder carcinogen, 4-ethylsulfonylnaphthalene-1-sulfonamide (65). Perhaps undue significance was attached to this observation because of the identification of the O-glucuronide and the ethereal sulfate conjugates of 1-amino-2-naphthol in the urine of rats, rabbits, and dogs given Citrus Red No. 2 (66). Ortho-hydroxy amines were considered for years to be the active carcinogenic metabolite of the bladder cancer-producing aromatic amines. However, more recent results have indicated that the active carcinogenic metabolites are the N-hydroxy metabolites rather than ortho-hydroxy metabolites (67–69). There is no evidence of the production of N-hydroxy metabolites of Citrus Red No. 2 or any other azo color. It would seem, therefore, that the significance of this observation must stand on its own. In one experiment in which mice were given subcutaneous injections of the color, the female mice showed an increased incidence of malignant tumors, including adenocarcinomas of the lung and lymphosarcomas (70).

FD&C Yellows No. 3 and 4 (Yellows AB and OB) were formerly used in the United States for coloring oleomargarine. These colors are derived by coupling either aniline or orthotoluidine with 2-naphthylamine. This in itself would seem to be adequate justification for eliminating these dyes as food colors. In addition, it has been reported that azo colors of this type in dilute acid solution may undergo a reversal of the coupling reaction (71). This could result in the liberation of 2-naphthylamine in the acid milieu of the stomach. While no evidence of the metabolism of FD&C Yellow No. 4 to 2-naphthylamine in animals' stomachs has been obtained, evidence of the formation of an imidazole resulting from the reaction of the azo color with naturally occurring aldehydes was obtained (72). FD&C Yellows No. 3 and 4 were tested for chronic toxicity in rats and dogs and found to be hepatotoxic (73). Right side cardiac atrophy and hypertrophy were observed in a 2 year feeding experiment with rats. Only at 0.05% in the diet did the rats survive without pathologic effects. In a 1 year feeding experiment, dogs suffered weight loss and toxicity at concentrations in the diet down to 0.05% (74, 75). A related color, 1-phenylazo-2-naphthol, formerly used in margarine in England, has also been found to be highly toxic and possibly a carcinogen. Kirby & Peacock found it to induce hepatomas after injection in stock mice (76), and carcinogenic changes in the bladder epithelium were observed in rabbits fed this color (77).

MISCELLANEOUS COLORS

FD&C Red No. 3 (Erythrosine) is a food color of rather unusual composition containing 4 iodine atoms. Not being an azo color, it does not undergo reductive fission in the intestine. It is one of the more nontoxic of the food colors. It has been extensively tested in rats, dogs, mice and gerbils. Dogs fed levels up to 2% in the diet for 2 years showed no toxic effects (78). In several experiments in mice, tumorigenicity tests both by feeding and by injection revealed no evidence of tumor production (59, 78). A series of feeding experiments in rats with levels up to 5% for 2 years revealed no significant pathologic changes (10, 18, 78–80). Gerbils fed levels up to 4% for 2 years were also without significant toxicologic effects (78). A slight but statistically significant mutagenic effect on *Escherichia coli* was observed at high concentrations of the color, however (81, 82). Apparently very little of the color is absorbed; a majority is excreted unchanged in the feces, which is perhaps an explanation for the lack of toxicity of the compound. This property, however, has caused some difficulty. A case was reported of a young boy passing red stools who was unfortunately subjected to extensive hospital diagnostic procedures before it was concluded that the source of the red was erythrosine used to color the cereal he was fond of (83). Another unusual property of erythrosine is its ability to produce elevated protein-bound iodine measurements (84, 85). At first this was thought to be due to an effect on thyroid function. However, careful study has demonstrated that it is merely a matter of interference of circulating erythrosine with the conventional analytical determination for protein-bound iodine (86, 87). There is evidence that ingestion of erythrosine-containing foods can contribute to dietary iodine intake (88).

FD&C Red No. 3, FD&C Yellow No. 6, and FD&C Blue No. 2 were tested for Heinz body formation in cats without finding significant effects (79).

It should be pointed out that people may become allergic to food colors. Production of asthma from FD&C Yellow No. 5 has been reported (89). Positive allergic reactions have been obtained with others (89–92). This fact should be kept in mind in the investigation of food allergies in patients.

NATURAL FOOD COLORS

Despite the reassuring connotation of the word "natural" there is little logic to the previous categoric assumption of the safety of these substances. Highly toxic and even lethal compounds abound in nature. The principal natural food colors permitted in the United States about which toxicological information is available are the following: the carotenoids, annatto extracts, chlorophyll, riboflavin, turmeric, and carbon black.

The carotenoids are widely present in both plants and animals and frequently have Vitamin A activity. Since the withdrawal of FD&C Yellows No. 3 and 4 as food colors, carotenoids have been widely used as fat-soluble colors (butter and oleomargarine). β-carotene, the most important natural precursor of Vitamin A, is now produced synthetically. Ingestion of large amounts by man and experimental animals, while it may produce hypercarotenemia (yellowing of the skin), surprisingly does not produce hypervitaminosis A (93). High dietary levels are not absorbed (94). A four-generation rat study at 1000 ppm of β-carotene in the diet for 110 weeks produced no adverse effects (95). β-apo-8'-carotenal and β-apo-8'-carotenoic acid, methyl or ethyl ester, have very similar biological properties to β-carotene (96, 97). Canthaxanthine is a closely related carotenoid that does not have provitamin A activity. It has been fed to rats for 2 years at levels up to 5% in the diet, and to dogs at 400 mg/kg daily for 15 weeks without producing toxic effects (98).

The annatto colors are obtained from the seeds of a tropical tree (*Bixa orellana* L.). The principal color present is the carotenoid bixin. Annatto extracts have been fed to mice and rats for their life span at levels up to 0.5% in the diet as well as injected subcutaneously. No toxicity or carcinogenicity was observed (99, 100). Chlorophyll and its copper complex are considered to be innocuous largely on the basis of their total failure to be absorbed after ingestion and their prolonged human usage. The copper complex has been fed to rats for their life span at dietary levels up to 3% without toxic effects (101). The vitamin riboflavin is used as a food color. Only short-term toxicity tests in dogs and rats have been carried out, but in view of the extensive experience with this substance and its role as an essential nutrient it has been judged to be harmless (102). Turmeric has been tested in 2 dogs for 1 year at 1% in the diet and for 420 days in rats at 0.5% in the diet without producing significant toxicity (103).

Many other substances such as dehydrated beets, caramel, grape skin extract, corn endosperm oil, paprika, and carbon black are used for coloring foods. With the exception of carbon black, no toxicity data have been reported; they have been assumed to be safe on the basis of long prior usage. With carbon black, the question has existed whether 3,4-benzpyrene and other polynuclear hydrocarbons were produced during the production of carbon black by combustion. Evidence indicates that carbon black produced by the low temperature impingement process is free of such substances and therefore safe. Carbon black is not absorbed after oral administration (104).

SUMMARY OF THE PRESENT STATUS OF FOOD COLORS

In the United States, at the present time the triphenylmethane colors FD&C Blue No. 1, FD&C Blue No. 2, and FD&C Green No. 3 are permitted to be used in foods on the basis of their almost complete excretion in the feces and their low chronic toxicity. The production of local sarcomas by repeated injection of large doses is not considered relevant to the use of these colors in foods. FD&C Violet No. 1, formerly a permitted color, was delisted. The water-soluble sulfonated azo colors FD&C Yellow No. 5, FD&C Yellow No. 6, and FD&C Red No. 2 are permitted food colors, as is FD&C Red No. 3. In view of its toxicity, FD&C Red No. 4 is permitted only for coloring maraschino cherries. The oil-soluble azo dyes are judged to be too toxic for use in foods except for Citrus Red No. 2, which is permitted only for coloring the skin of oranges.

The World Health Organization has reviewed the toxicology of food colors rather intensively and concurred with the judgments of the US Food and Drug Administration except for the limited special uses of FD&C Red No. 4 and Citrus Red No. 2.

Literature Cited

1. Vos, B. J., Radomski, J. L., Fuyat, Henry N. 1953. *Fed. Proc.* 12:376
2. Food Standards Committee. 1964. *Report on the Review of the Colouring Matter in Food Regulations, 1957.* London: HMSO. 23 pp.
3. Golberg, L. 1967. *J. Soc. Cosmet. Chem.* 18:421–32
4. Food and Agriculture Organization of the United Nations World Health Organization. 1966. *Specifications for Identity and Purity and Toxicological Evaluation of Food Colours, Geneva, 8–17 Dec. 1964,* Rep. Ser. No. 38B. 212 pp.
5. Food and Agriculture Organization of the United Nations World Health organization. 1969. *Toxicological Evaluation of Some Food Colours, Emulsifiers, Stabilizers, Anti-caking Agents and Certain Other Substances,* Rep. Ser. No. 46A. 161 pp.
6. Food and Agriculture Organization of the United Nations World Health Organization. 1970. *Specifications for the Identity and Purity of Some Food Colours, Emulsifiers, Stabilizers, Anti-caking Agents and Certain Other Substances,* Rep. Ser. No. 46B. 138 pp.
7. Hess, S. M., Fitzhugh, O. G. 1955. *J. Pharmacol. Exp. Ther.* 114:38–42
8. Schiller, W. 1937. *Am. J. Cancer* 31:486–90
9. Harris, P. N. 1947. *Cancer Res.* 7:35–36
10. Nelson, A. A., Hagan, E. C. 1953. *Fed. Proc.* 12:397–98
11. Gangolli, S. D., Grasso, P., Golberg, L. 1967. *Food Cosmet. Toxicol.* 5:601–21
12. Grasso, P., Gangolli, S. D., Golberg, L., Hooson, J. 1971. *Food Cosmet. Toxicol.* 9:463–78
13. Gangolli, S. D., Grasso, P., Golberg, L., Hooson, J. 1972. *Food Cosmet. Toxicol.* 10:449–62
14. Rosenkranz, H. S., Carr, H. S. 1971. *Brit. Med. J.,* 3:702–3
15. Björnberg, A., Mobacken, H. 1972. *Acta Dermato-Venereol.* 52:55–60
16. Hansen, W. H., Fitzhugh, O. G., Nelson, A. A., Davis, K. J. 1966. *Toxicol. Appl. Pharmacol.* 8:29–36
17. Hansen, W. H., Long, E. L, Davis, K. J., Nelson, A. A., Fitzhugh, O. G. 1966. *Food Cosmet. Toxicol.* 4:389–410
18. Willheim, R., Ivy, A. C. 1953. *Gastroenterology* 23:1–19
19. Gaunt, I. F., Kiss, I. S., Grasso, P., Gangolli, S. D. 1969. *Food Cosmet. Toxicol.* 7:17–24
20. Radomski, J. L. Unpublished
21. Ryan, A. J., Wright, S. E. 1961. *J. Pharm. Pharmacol.* 13:492–95
22. Radomski, J. L., Mellinger, T. J. 1962. *J. Pharmacol. Exp. Ther.* 136:259–66
23. Roxon, J. J., Ryan, A. J., Wright, S. E. 1967. *Food Cosmet. Toxicol.* 5: 367–69
24. Ryan, A. J., Roxon, J. J., Sivayavirojana, A. 1968. *Nature* 219: 854–55

25. Lindstrom, H. V., Hansen, W. H., Nelson, A. A., Fitzhugh, O. G. 1963. *J. Pharmacol. Exp. Ther.* 142:257–64
26. Lindstrom, H. V., Wallace, W. C., Hansen, W. H., Nelson, A. A., Fitzhugh, O. G. 1963. *Fed. Proc.* 22:188
27. Bowie, W. C., Arnault, L. T., Brouwer E. A., Lindstrom, H. V. 1965. *Fed. Proc.* 24:392
28. Radomski, J. L., Deichmann, W. B. 1956. *J. Pharmacol. Exp. Ther.* 118:322–27
29. Cook, J. W., Hewett, C. L., Kennaway, E. L., Kennaway, N. M. 1940. *Am. J. Cancer* 40:62–77
30. Bourke, A. R., Nelson, A. A., Fitzhugh, O. G. 1956. *Fed. Proc.* 15:404
31. FAO/WHO. 1966. See Ref. 4, pp. 67–70
32. Farbstoff Kommission. 1957. *Deutsche Forschungsgemeinschaft,* Bad Godesberg, Fed. Rep. Ger. Mitteilung 6
33. Mannell, W. A., Grice, H. C., Lu, F. C., Allmark, M. G. 1958. *J. Pharm. Pharmacol.* 10:625–34
34. Gales, V., Preda, N., Popa, L., Sendrea, D., Simu, G. 1972. *Eur. J. Toxicol.* 5:167–73
35. FAO/WHO. 1966. See Ref. 4, p. 25
36. Shtenberg, A. I., Gavrilenko, E. V. 1970. *Vop. Pitan.* 29:66–73
37. Collins, T. F. X., McLaughlin, J., Gray, G. C. 1972. *Food Cosmet. Toxicol.* 10:619–24
38. Bajguseva, M. M. 1968. *Vop. Pitan.* 27:46–50
39. Andrianova, M. M. 1970. *Vop. Pitan.* 29:61–65
40. *Food Cosmet. Toxicol.* 1969. 7:679
41. Davis, K. J., Nelson, A. A., Zwickey, R. E., Hansen, W. H., Fitzhugh, O. G. 1966. *Toxicol. Appl. Pharmacol.* 8:306–17
42. Ikeda, Y., Horiuchi, S., Furuya, T., Omori, Y. 1966. *Food Cosmet. Toxicol.* 4:485–92
43. Hall, D. E., Lee, F. S., Fairweather, F. A. 1966. *Food Cosmet. Toxicol.* 4:375–82
44. Grasso, P., Lansdown, A. B. G., Kiss, I. S., Gaunt, I. F., Gangolli, S. D. 1969. *Food Cosmet. Toxicol.* 7:425–42
45. Hansen, W. H., Davis, K. J., Fitzhugh, O. G., Nelson, A. A. 1963. *Toxicol. Appl. Pharmacol.* 5:105–18
46. Mannell, W. A. 1964. *Food Cosmet. Toxicol.* 2:169–74
47. Lindstrom, H. V., Hansen, W. H. 1962. *Fed. Proc.* 21:450
48. Barrett, J. F., Pitt, P. A., Ryan, A. J., Wright, S. E. 1965. *Biochem. Pharmacol.* 14:873–79
49. Lindstrom, H. V., Bowie, W. C., Wallace, W. C., Nelson, A. A., Fitzhugh, O. G. 1969. *J. Pharmacol. Exp. Ther.* 167:223–34
50. Magnusson, G., Bodin, N. O., Hansson, E. 1971. *Acta Pathol. Microbiol. Scand.* 79A:639–48
51. FAO/WHO. 1966. See Ref. 4, pp. 85–86
52. Gaunt, I. F., Farmer, M., Grasso, P., Gangolli, S. D. 1967. *Food Cosmet. Toxicol.* 5:747–54
53. Gaunt, I. F., Kiss, I. S., Grasso, P., Gangolli, S. D. 1969. *Food Cosmet. Toxicol.* 7:9–16
54. Allmark, M. G., Mannell, W. A., Grice, H. C. 1957. *J. Pharm. Pharmacol.* 9:622–28
55. Gaunt, I. F., Farmer, M., Grasso, P., Gangolli, S. D. 1967. *Food Cosmet. Toxicol.* 5:187–194
56. Gaunt, I. F., Grasso, P., Creasey, M., Gangolli, S. D. 1969. *Food Cosmet. Toxicol.* 7:443–49
57. Davis, K. J., Fitzhugh, O. G. 1963. *Toxicol. Appl. Pharmacol.* 5:728–34
58. Davis, K. J., Fitzhugh, O. G. 1962. *Toxicol. Appl. Pharmacol.* 4:200–05
59. Waterman, N., Lignac, G. O. E. 1958. *Acta Physiol. Pharmacol. Neerl.* 7:35–55
60. Davis, K. J., Fitzhugh, O. G., Nelson, A. A. 1964. *Toxicol. Appl. Pharmacol.* 6:621–26
61. Radomski, J. L. 1961. *J. Pharmacol. Exp. Ther.* 134:100–9
62. Childs, J. J., Nakajima, C., Clayson, D. B. 1967. *Biochem. Pharmacol.* 16:1555–61
63. Fitzhugh, O. G., Nelson, A. A., Bourke, A. R. 1956. *Fed. Proc.* 15:422
64. FAO/WHO. 1969. See Ref. 5, pp. 30–32
65. Dacre, J. C. 1965. *Proc. Univ. Otago Med. Sch.* 43:31–33
66. Radomski, J. L. 1962. *J. Pharmacol. Exp. Ther.* 136:378–85
67. Radomski, J. L., Brill, E. 1970. *Science* 167:992–93
68. Radomski, J. L., Brill, E. 1971. *Arch. Toxikol.* 28:159–75
69. Radomski, J. L., Conzelman, G. M. Jr., Rey, A. A., Brill, E. 1973. *J. Nat. Cancer Inst.* 50:989–95
70. Sharratt, M., Frazer, A. C., Paranjoti, I. S. 1966. *Food Cosmet. Toxicol.* 4:493–502

71. Harrow, L. S., Jones, J. H. 1954. *J. Assoc. Off. Agr. Chem.* 37:1012–20
72. Radomski, J. L., Harrow, L. S. 1966. *Ind. Med. Surg.* 35:882–88
73. Allmark, M. G., Grice, H. C., Lu, F. C. 1955. *J. Pharm. Pharmacol.* 7:591–603
74. Hansen, W. H., Fitzhugh, O. G., Nelson, A. A. 1958. *Fed. Proc.* 17:375
75. Hansen, W. H., Nelson, A. A., Fitzhugh, O. G. 1963. *Toxicol. Appl. Pharmacol.* 5:16–35
76. Kirby, A. H. M., Peacock, P. R., 1949. *Glasgow Med. J.* 30:364–72
77. Bonser, G. M. 1962. *Acta Unio Int. Contra Cancrum* 18:538–44
78. FAO/WHO. 1969, See Ref. 5, p. 35
79. Oettel, H., Frohberg, H., Nothdurft, H., Wilhelm, G. 1965. *Arch. Toxikol.* 21: 9–29
80. Umeda, M. 1956. *Gann* 47:51–77
81. Lück, H., Rickerl, E., 1969 *Z. Lebensm.-Unters.-Forsch.* 122:157–63
82. Lück, H., Wallnöefer, P., Bach, H. 1963. *Pathol. Microbiol. Basel* 26:206–24
83. Payne, J. V. 1972. *Pediatrics* 49:293–94
84. Bowie, W. C., Wallace, W. C., Lindstrom, H. V. 1966. *Fed. Proc.* 25:556
85. Hung, W. 1966. *Pediatrics* 37:677–80
86. Andersen, C. J., Keiding, N. R., Nielsen, A. B. 1964. *Scand. J. Clin. Lab. Invest.* 16:249
87. *Food Cosmet. Toxicol.* 1967. 5:109
88. Vought, R. L., Brown, F. A., Wolff, J.

1972. *J. Clin. Endrocrinol. Metab.* 34:747–52
89. Chafee, F. H., Settipane, G. A. 1967. *J. Allergy* 40:65–72
90. Klevansky, H., Kingsley, H. J. 1964. *S. Afr. Med. J.* 38:216
91. Mitchell, J. C. 1971. *Arch. Dermatol.* 104:329–30
92. Lockey, S. D. 1972. *Ann. Allergy* 30:638–41
93. Greenberg, R., Cornbleet, T., Jeffay, A. I. 1959. *J. Invest. Dermatol.* 32:599–604
94. FAO/WHO. 1966. See Ref. 4, pp. 38–42
95. Bagdon, R. E., Zbinden, G., Studer, A. 1960. *Toxicol. Appl. Pharmacol.* 2:225–36
96. FAO/WHO. 1966. See Ref. 4, pp. 43–45
97. FAO/WHO. 1966. See Ref. 4, pp. 34–37
98. FAO/WHO. 1966. See Ref. 4, pp. 31–33
99. van Esch, G. J., van Genderen, H., Vink, H. H. 1959. *Z. Lebensm.-Unters.-Forsch.* 111:93–108
100. Engelbreth-Holm, J., Iversen, S. 1955. *Acta Pathol. Microbiol. Scand.* 37:483–91
101. Harrisson, J. W. E., Levin, S. E., Trabin, B. 1954. *J. Am. Pharm. Assoc. Sci. Ed.* 43:722–37
102. FAO/WHO. 1969. See Ref. 5, pp. 20–21
103. FAO/WHO. 1969. See Ref. 5, p. 23
104. Radomski, J. L. 1968. unpublished report to the American Toilet Goods Association

TOXICITY OF CHLORINATED BIPHENYLS

❖6586

Lawrence Fishbein
National Center for Toxicological Research, Jefferson, Arkansas

Despite the fact that polychlorinated biphenyls (PCBs) have been available commercially for 40 years, it is only within the last 5 years that they have been recognized to be of environmental and potential toxicologic concern.

PCBs are produced by a comparatively small number of manufacturers in the USA, France, Germany, and Japan and marketed under a number of commerical trade names, e.g. Aroclor, Clophen, Phenoclor, and Kaneclor.

The series of Aroclors (Monsanto) are marketed under various numbers and consist of mixtures of chlorinated biphenyls and terphenyls. The first two digits represent the molecular type: 12-chlorinated biphenyls; 25 and 44-blends of chlorinated biphenyls and chlorinated terphenyls (75% biphenyl and 60% biphenyl, respectively); 54-chlorinated terphenyls. The last two digits give the weight percent of chlorine, e.g. Aroclor 1242 is a chlorinated biphenyl containing 42% chlorine.

The PCBs have been employed in a broad spectrum of applications because of their chemical stability, low volatility, high dielectric content, nonflammability, and general compatability with chlorinated hydrocarbons. The major areas of utility include: heat exchanger and dielectric fluids, hydraulic and lubricating fluids, plasticizers for plastics and coatings, ingredients of caulking compounds, printing inks, paints, adhesives, and carbonless duplicating paper, flame retardants, and extender for pesticides.

The rates and routes of transport of the PCBs in the environment (1), and their accumulation in ecosystem (2–16), have been cited. Salient features of the chemical (3, 4, 7, 11, 14–17), analytical (3–18), biological (3, 7, 9, 14–20, 28, 30–38), aspects of the PCBs as well as their occurrence in human diets (2–4, 14, 15, 39–42), and tissue (14–16, 33–38, 43–47), have all been reported.

The major objective of this review is to highlight the status of the toxicologic, carcinogenic, teratogenic, and mutagenic aspects of the PCBs that are of greatest relevance to man.

Compared to the chlorinated hydrocarbon pesticides, definitive aspects of acute, subacute, and chronic toxicity still remain rather poorly known. The toxicological characterization of PCBs is confounded by the fact that the commercial products are mixtures of isomers, and significant traces of chlorinated dibenzofurans and naphthalenes have been found in several preparations (e.g. Clophen A-60 and Phenoclor Dp-6) (48).

ANIMAL TOXICITY

Early studies of acute oral, dermal, and vapor pressure of the PCBs have involved in many cases mixtures or compounds of undefined specifications and hence have been rather difficult to interpret unambiguously.

a. Acute and Subacute Toxicity

Table 1 summarizes measurements of the oral and dermal toxicity of seven Aroclor mixtures to rats and rabbits respectively, and indicates that the PCBs are of a low order of toxicity when administered as a single dose. These results suggest that while the oral toxicity to rats decreases with increasing chlorination, there is no apparent trend of toxicity with chlorination in the data for rabbits. Miller (49), studied the toxicity of a PCB mixture equivalent to Aroclor 1242 and indicated that the guinea pig was the most sensitive of the three species, followed by the rabbit and the rat in that order.

Table 1 Toxicity of Aroclors*

	Aroclors										
	1221	1232	1242	1248	1260	1262	1268	4465	5442	5460	2565
Oral LD_{50} mg/Kg (rats)	3980^a	4470^a	8650^a	$11,000^a$	$10,000^b$	$11,300^b$	$10,900^b$	$16,000^b$	$10,600^b$	$19,200^c$	6,310
Skin MLD mg/Kg (rabbits)	$>2000^a$	$>1260^a$	$>794^a$	$>794^a$	$>1260^b$	$>1260^b$		$>2000^b$	$>1260^b$	$>7940^c$	$>2000^a$
	$<3169^a$	$<2000^a$	$<1269^a$	$<1269^a$	$<2000^b$	$<3160^b$	$<2500^c$	$<3160^b$	$<2000^b$		<3160

*FDA Status Report on the Chemistry and Toxicology of Polychlorinated Biphenyls (PCB) or Aroclors as of June 1, 1970 (Ref. 30).
[a]Undiluted.
[b]Administered as 50% solution in corn oil.
[c]Administered as 33.3% solution in corn oil.

Analogously with the chlorinated hydrocarbon pesticides the most important effects are long-range sublethal effects. Aroclor 1254 at 1000 ppm in the diet was fatal to ¾ male rats in 43 days and it was reported by Tucker & Crabtree (50) that a total intake of 500–2000 mg/kg was the lethal level under these conditions. The single-dose oral LD_{50} for Aroclor 1260 and 1254 in rats is considerably higher (Table 1), hence the lethal effect appears to be of a highly cumulative nature.

Rehfeld et al (51) studied the subacute toxicity of Aroclor 1248 in 10-day-old chickens. The mortality after 25 days feeding at 50, 40, 30, and 10 ppm in the diet was 16/30, 4/20, 1/30, and 0/10 respectively. Only 2–4 out of 10 chicks survived on diets containing 100 and 150 ppm. Kohanawa et al (52) found Kannachlor-400

(~48% chlorination) to be fatal to 10/10 chicks within 8 days at a concentration of 300 ppm, while at 100 ppm there were no mortalities in 20 days. It is important to note that different batches or sources of PCBs of similar degrees of chlorination appear to vary as to potency, as reported by Vos & Koeman (53) in their studies in chickens with special reference to porphyria, edema formation, liver necrosis, and tissue residues. Aroclor 1260 caused only 15% mortality in chicks after 8 weeks, with an average time of death of approximately 3 weeks. The greater toxicity of the latter preparation was attributed to the presence of trace amounts of chlorinated dibenzofurans (probably tetrachloro- and pentachlorodibenzofuran) (48).

Table 2 depicts pathologic changes induced by PCB, and illustrates some interesting differences between mammals and birds. For example, the most striking findings in mammals are alterations to the liver, whereas fluid in the pericardial sac, kidney damage, and reduced spleen are found in birds. PCB-induced death in rats, rabbits, and guinea pigs is accompanied by liver lesions, including fatty infiltration, centrolobular atrophy necrosis (49, 52), and in the case of rats, by hyaline degeneration. Except for chloracne-like lesions occurring at the point of skin injection or intradermal injection, other organs in these species are not prominently affected. In birds, the most consistently observed lesions are hydropericardium and ascites as seen in the chicken (52–55), Japanese Quail (52), and bob whites (56). Other lesions in birds experimentally poisoned with PCBs include kidney damage (52–54), liver damage (52, 54), enteritis and intestinal hemorrhages (54), subcutaneous edema (52, 55), and dermatitis (53).

Nishizumi (57) studied the effects on mouse and monkey liver of chlorinated biphenyls [48% chlorine, equivalent to three to four atoms of chlorine per molecule, with a trace (0.01% of naphthalenes]. Groups of 30 female mice were given a dosage level of 0.2 ml rice bran oil containing 1600 ppm or 0.5% PCB in olive oil by stomach tube each day for 4–26 weeks resulting in marked liver enlargement. (Light microscopy revealed only slight liver changes but electron microscopy disclosed marked alterations in the liver cells.) A similar study with 8 monkeys (5 cynomolgus and 3 squirrel) given chlorinated biphenyls in dosage levels of 1.4–1.6 mg/day in their diet for 40–48 days showed both liver cell enlargement and fatty degeneration. The major abnormality reported for the administration of chlorinated biphenyls to mice and monkeys was an increase in the smooth endoplasmic reticulum in the liver cells.

The administration of high doses of Aroclor 1242 to rats by oral intubation produced diarrhea, chromodacryorrhea, loss of body weight, unusual stance and gait; lack of response to pain stimuli and central nervous system depression apparently contributed to each fatality. Histopathological changes appeared only in the liver and kidneys as foci of sudanophilic vacuolation (58).

Rats given 100 mg Aroclor 1242/kg every other day for 3 weeks showed similar histopathological changes but no overt signs of toxicity (58). A single 100 mg/kg ip injection increased rat liver weight, total hepatic cytochrome P450, and cytochrome b_5 levels. The hepatic microsomal enzyme activity remained elevated 10

Table 2 Pathologic changes induced by PCBs

Treatment	Animal	Liver	Kidney	Pericardium & Peritoneum	Other Observable Changes	References
Single oral dose of 69 mg (42% Cl)	Guinea Pig Rat Rabbit	Small droplets through lobules, slight to moderate central atrophy, focal necrosis noted in a few animals.	Essentially normal	No noteworthy changes	Adrenals, spleen & pancreas showed no noteworthy changes.	Miller (99)
300 mg daily for 6 days (65% Cl)	Rat	Cells swollen, hyaline granules present. Most died within few days.				Bennett et al (106)
50 mg daily for up to 6 months (65% Cl)	Rat	Enlarged (33% weight increase), large number of hyaline globules in cytoplasm. Several died during experiment.				Bennett et al (106)
25, 50 & 100 ppm in diet for 15 days (21-68% Cl Aroclors)	Rat	Increase in weight, effect increasing with increasing chlorine content. Aroclor 1232-10%, 1252-12%, 1254-14%, 1268-24% at 50 ppm				Street et al (25)
100 ppm in diet 200 ppm in diet 400 ppm in diet 800 ppm in diet (Aroclor 1242)	Chicken	No effect No effect Enlarged & Mottled Damaged	Damaged	Slight Hydropericardium Hydropericardium Hydropericardium Hydroperitoneum Enlarged		McCune et al (55)
200 & 400 ppm in diet for 3 weeks (42%)	Chicken	No changes noted	Paleness at 200 ppm, extensive hemorrhage, and enlargement at 400 ppm.	Increased fluid in pericardial sac at the higher concentration.	Paleness of pancreas, enlargment of adrenal and small spleen at low concentrations. At higher concentrations pale cream-colored pancreas, adrenals hemorrhagic.	Flick et al (54)
Various doses (54% Cl, Aroclor)	Bengalese Finch	No weight changes	Weight was 32.4% of brain weight for controls and 53.5% for those dying from PCB poisoning.	Slight weight increase, a few showed liquid in pericardial sac.		Presst et al (108)
400 ppm in diet for 60 days (60% Cl[a])	Chicken	Centrolobular necrosis (compd. 1 & 2). Liver weight increased from 2.76 g/100 g to 4.31 g/100 g (compd. 3). Fatty degeneration.	Tubular dilation, (compd. 1 & 2). Rare with compd. 3.	Hydropericardium common with compds. 1 & 2. Rare with compd. 3.	Increased porphyria, spleen small with reduction of red pulp and atrophy of white pulp (compd. 1 & 2). Spleen decreased from 0.14 g/100 g to 0.136 g/100 g (compd. 3).	Vos & Koeman (5

[a]Phenoclor DP 6 (compd. 1), Clophen A60 (compd. 2), and Aroclor 1260 (compd. 3) were used. Differential effects noted under compd. numbers. All chickens died on compd. 1 and 2 within 60 days; only 15% mortality on compd. 3.

days after a single dose of Aroclor 1242, suggesting that PCBs may be important in altering biological responses of mammals subjected to environmental chemical stress.

Koller & Zinkl (59) compared the clinical and anatomical pathological effects produced by administering Aroclors 1221, 1242, and 1254 orally to rabbits once a week for 14 weeks. The livers in the 1254- and 1242-treated rabbits were significantly enlarged compared to the 1221-treated and control animals. The earliest change was megalohepatocytosis, followed by subcapsular midzonal necrosis. Fibrous connective tissue replaced the necrotic part of the lobules in the more severely affected livers. The rough endoplasmic reticulum in the livers of the 1254-treated rabbits appeared to have been destroyed, and there was also atrophy of the uteri in the 1254 treated rabbits.

Dermal toxicity studies in rabbits of technical PCB samples that contain an average of 60% chlorine (Phenoclor DP6, Clophen A60, and Aroclor 1260) as well as fractions containing tetra and pentachlorodibenzofuran have been recently described by Vos & Beems (60). PCB-induced skin lesions were hyperplasia and hyperkeratosis of the epidermal and follicular epithelium following application of 118 mg of the three PCBs (5 times per week for 38 days) in the back skin of adult female New Zealand rabbits. Histopathology of the liver included centrolobular degeneration, centrolobular liver cell atrophy, focal necrosis, and cytoplasmic hyalin degeneration. PCB-induced kidney lesions were hydropic degeneration of the convoluted tubules and tubular dilation with the presence of casts. Definitive hyperplasia and hyperkeratosis of the follicular epithelium of the ear skin were seen after the topical application of fractions of Phenoclor and Clophen (eluted from chromatographic columns with 25% diethyl ether in hexane), while the fraction from Aroclor caused a minimal hyperplasia and hyperkeratosis of the follicular epithelium. Other effects elicited by the dermal application of the PCBs included thymus atrophy and lymphopenia as well as elevated excretion of fecal coproporphyria and protoporphyria.

From the response of the back skin and the liver of the rabbit to the three PCB mixtures, and from the response of the ear to the 25% diethyl ether-hexane fractions it was concluded that there were definite quantitative differences in toxicity, at least between the samples used in the above study (60) and prior studies (48). The extent to which these samples are representative of the normal commercial output has not been established and emphasizes the difficulty in the evaluation of toxicity data of PCBs in which the samples may differ in the amount and nature of toxic impurities.

Vos & Beems (60) also raised the possibility that since PCB is a porphyrogenic chemical, the skin lesions in man due to PCB may be caused by a combination of chloracne and acquired porphyria cutanea tarda.

Vos & Notenboom-Ram (61) compared the toxicity of Aroclor 1260 with a single isomer 2,4,5,2',4',5'-hexachlorobiphenyl in New Zealand rabbits. Dermal applications of a total 120 mg Aroclor 1260 (5 times/wk for 28 days) resulted in early macroscopic skin lesions. The lesions in a 2,4,5,2',4',5'-hexachlorobiphenyl group of rabbits treated similarly appeared later and were less severe. Hyperplasia and hyperkeratosis of the follicular and epidermal epithelium were more severe in the Aroclor group. Enhanced liver weights were found in both test groups. Liver injury, as judged by light microscopic lesions and elevated serum transaminase levels, was somewhat more severe in the hexachlorobiphenyl group. Light microscopic findings included subcapsular necrosis, zonal necrosis, hydroscopic degeneration as well as peripheral and perinuclear shift of cell organelles, and focal cytoplasmic hyalin degeneration.

In electron microscopy the shift was due to a proliferation of smooth surfaced membranes of the endoplasmic reticulum (SER) resulting in a displacement of rough surfaced membranes (RER).

From the observed acnelike lesions, both from the PCB mixture and 2,4,5,2',4', 5'-hexachlorobiphenyl, and assuming that the hexachlorobiphenyl is free from contamination with chlorinated dibenzofuran, we can conclude that this particular compound of the mixture PCB has a slight acnegenic action of itself. The major acnegenic action of crude PCB mixtures comes from chlorinated dibenzofurans and hepatic prophyria comes only from PCB itself.

It is important also to stress the toxic nature of the polychlorodibenzofurans. For example, tri- and tetrachlorodibenzofuran in a single oral dose of 0.5–1.0 mg/kg caused severe and often lethal liver necrosis in rabbits (62). The related compound 2,3,7,8-tetrachlorodibenzo-p-dioxin caused a lethal liver necrosis in the rabbit after a single oral dose of 0.05 mg/kg, and when applied to the ear again in a dose 10 times lower than that found to be effective in the case of chlorinated dibenzofuran, resulted in chloracne. Vos & co-workers (48) calculated a maximum dose/egg of 0.2 μg pentachlorodibenzofuran (obtained from Clophen A60), that caused 100% embryonic mortality when injected into the air cell of chicken eggs. The analogous effect was obtained with 0.05 μg hexachlorodibenzo-p-dioxin (63). The relationship between the toxic nature of PCB and the chick edema factor 1,2,3,7,8,9-hexachlorodibenzo-p-dioxin has been described by Flick and co-workers (54).

b. Chronic Toxicity

The effects of low-level feeding (1,10, and 100 ppm) of Aroclors 1242, 1254, and 1260 to rats and dogs have been reported by Keplinger et al (64, 65). The only effect noted in dogs after 12 months of feeding was with Aroclor 1260 in a reduced rate of weight gain, increased liver weights, and elevated serum alkaline phosphatase in males at 100 ppm, and a reduced rate of weight gain in females at both 10 and 100 ppm. The effects seen in rats after 15 months of feeding were elevated liver and kidney weights (noted only with Aroclor 1260). However, the feeding of all three Aroclors led to an increase of liver weights and liver-weight-to-body-weight ratios at 24 months. Fatty degeneration, focal hyperplasia, and focal hypertrophy were also observed in some of the livers (64).

Kimbrough et al (66, 67) described morphological changes in livers of male and female Sherman strain rats fed 20, 100, 500, and 1000 ppm of Aroclors 1260 and 1254 in their diet for 8 months. Light microscopic changes consisted of hypertrophy of the liver cells, inclusions in the cytoplasm, brown pigment in Kupffer cells, lipid accumulation and, at the higher dietary levels, adenofibrosis. Ultrastructural changes of the livers of exposed animals consisted of an increase in smooth endoplasmic reticulum and a typical mitochondria. Lipid vacuoles were occasionally surrounded by concentric membranes. The epithelial component of adenofibrosis consisted of goblet cells and cells that resembled the epithelium that lines the bile ducts. In general, the effect of Aroclor 1254 on the liver was more pronounced than that of Aroclor 1260.

Adenofibrosis was found in: (a) 1/10 males and 6/10 females at the dosage level of 100 parts per million Aroclor 1254 in the diet for about 8 months; (b) in 1/10 female rats at 100 parts per million Aroclor 1260 in the diet for about 8 months; and (c) in several male rats at 1000 parts per million Aroclor 1260 in the diet for 8 months (none at 500 parts per million).

The findings of Kimbrough et al in the above studies (66, 67), suggesting that the mammalian toxicity decreases as the level of chlorination increases, are in agreement with the conclusions of Lichtenstein et al (68) and Vos (26).

c. Reproductive Effects

A definite effect on reproduction in rats was produced by feeding 100 ppm of Aroclor 1254 (67). The first breeding was performed after 76 days on the treated diets and resulted in fewer offspring. The offspring at weaning were smaller and the survival was decreased compared to control animals. An increase in the liver weight in the F_{2a} generation of the weanlings at a dietary level of 20 ppm Aroclor 1254 was also found. A dosage of Aroclor 1260 equivalent to 100 mg/kg/day during the 7th and 15th days of pregnancy reduced the survival and number of young.

In another reproduction study in rats reported by FDA (29), Aroclors 1242, 1254, and 1260 were administered at levels of 1, 10, and 100 ppm in the diet. While Aroclor 1242 had no effect on the first generation, mating indices were low in the second generation at 100 ppm. The number of pups delivered and the number surviving to weaning were reduced in both the second and third litters with Aroclor 1254. Aroclor 1260 at a level of 100 ppm increased the number of stillborn animals. No effect was observed at levels of 1 and 10 ppm.

Keplinger et al (64) reported low mating indices and decreased survival of pups for animals receiving Aroclor 1242 at 100 ppm, and decreased survival of pups receiving Aroclor 1254 at 100 ppm. No reproductive effects were found with Aroclor 1260 at 1, 10, or 100 ppm, or with Aroclor 1242 or 1254 at 1 or 10 ppm (65). These studies suggest that in mammals reproductive effects decrease with increasing chlorination.

Keplinger et al (65), also reported that chickens fed 10 or 100 ppm of Aroclor 1242 or 100 ppm of 1254 exhibited loss of body weight, decreased thickness of egg shells, and poor hatchability of eggs. However, at 1, 10, and 100 ppm of Aroclor there were no adverse effects. While decreased hatchability was observed at 8 ppm of Aroclor 1242, there were no observed effects at 6, 4, or 2 ppm (64).

Studies reported by FDA (29) indicated that decreased egg production by chickens occurred at 100 ppm with Aroclors 1242 and 1254, but not with Aroclor 1260. Levels of 10 and 100 ppm of Aroclor 1242, and 100 ppm of Aroclor 1254 resulted in decreased eggshell thickness, which was not observed with Aroclor 1260 even at

100 ppm. The hatchability of eggs was lowered at 10 and 100 ppm of Aroclor 1242 but not at 100 ppm of Aroclor 1254 or Aroclor 1260.

Scott et al (69) found decreased egg production at dietary levels of 10 and 20 ppm of Aroclor 1254 (10–13% reduction after 8 weeks). Hatchability of eggs was reduced at 10 and 20 ppm (up to 50% and 2.4%, respectively, after 8 weeks).

With a PCB level in the eggs of 2.2 ppm, hatchability of 3 and 4.5 ppm in eggs, the hatchability was reduced to about 56% of normal and almost to zero, respectively.

d. Carcinogenic, Teratogenic, and Mutagenic Effects

Kimbrough (67) observed bladder cancers in two rats fed 100 ppm of Aroclor 1260 over an 8-month period. Nagasaki et al (70) reported the hepatocarcinogenicity of Kaneclor-500 in male dd mice fed 500 ppm of PCB. The hepatomas appeared similar to those induced by δ-isomer of benzene hexachloride (71, 72), whereas Kaneclor-400 and Kaneclor-300 had no carcinogenicity activity in the liver of mice.

Kimura & Baba (72) described neoplastic changes in the rat liver induced by Kaneclor-400. The PCB administered to rats in the diet at 38.5–462 ppm induced a benign neoplastic change in the liver, which appeared exclusively in the female. All the rats that ultimately ingested $>$ 700 mg of Kaneclor-400 showed hypertrophy of the liver, while pinhead to pear-sized round and pale brown flecks or modules were scattered on the surface and on the cut surface of the liver of all female rats ingesting $>$ 1200 mg, but on none of the male rat livers. Fatty degeneration and multiple adenomatous nodules in the liver, lung abscesses, pneumonia, spleenatrophy, and intracranial abscesses were found frequently in experimental animals of both sexes, and depilation was observed in females ingesting $>$ 600 mg of Kaneclor-400.

Allen & Norback (73) reported the induction of hyperplasia and dysplasia of the gastric mucosa in subhuman primates (male rhesus monkeys ranging in age from 1.5–2 years and having an average weight of 2.9 kg) fed a diet containing 300 ppm of Aroclor 1248 or 5000 ppm of polychlorinated triphenyl (Aroclor 5460) (PCT) for 3 months. During the course of the experiment, the animals were given access to 400 g of the experimental diet daily. Within 1 month, all of the PCB fed animals and within 6 weeks, all of the PCT fed animals (6) had hair loss from the head, neck, and back. A progressive, generalized, subcutaneous edema, particularly of the face, was manifested as swollen eyelids and lips.

The concentration of PCB within the experimental diet was less than an order of magnitude greater than that occurring in random food samples sold in the United States and less than levels that have occurred in food products as a result of industrial accidents. The increased cellularity, abnormal dyplastic growth pattern, and invasion of the adjacent tissue region indicate compromised gastric function and were believed by the authors to be *suggestive* of an eventual neoplastic transformation. However, the carcinogenic potential could not be evaluated from a short-term study.

McLaughlin et al (74) reported that Aroclor 1242 gave no hatch at a level of 25 mg when injected into chicken yolk sac. At a level of 10 mg/egg embryos were found with back deformities, edema, and growth retardation. Carlson & Duby (75) found that injection of Aroclor 1242 into chicken eggs on day 0 of incubation severely limited hatchability at levels above 2.5 ppm. The 1254 and 1260 isomers were less effective in this respect, requiring 10 ppm or more. Embryonic mortality occurred during the period of organ formation, suggesting an effect on inductive mechanisms (several malformations in chicks that developed until day 21). The effects induced by the day 0 injection of the 1242 isomer were permanent, as growth rates were severely depressed during the 2 week period following hatching.

Aroclor 1254 was found to be fetotoxic to the rabbit at amounts of 12.5 mg/kg and above as evidenced by abortions, maternal deaths, and stillborns (76). The fetotoxic effect did not appear to be dose related nor was it influenced by the period of administration. The rat did not appear to be as sensitive a species, as doses up to 100 mg/kg did not cause fetal deaths or malformations. Dead fetuses from treated animals showed no consistent skeletal abnormalties. Oral administration of 12.5–50 mg/kg/day did induce abortions and was fetopathic to rabbits when treated for the first 28 days of gestation. In a preliminary study (76) the oral administration of 50/mg/kg of Acroclor 1254 to 6 pregnant rabbits 5 days a week during their gestation period also caused abortions and fetal deaths.

Peakall et al (77) reported that embryos from the second generation of Ring doves *(Streptopelia risoria)* fed 10 ppm Aroclor 1254 exhibited a high frequency of chromosomal aberrations and a high incidence of embryonic death.

No chromosomal aberrations were observed in human lymphocyte cultures exposed to Aroclor 1254 at 100 ppm (78), and Keplinger et al (64), employing a dominant lethal assay, reported no evidence of mutagenic effects of Aroclors.

Green et al (79) described the cytogenetic effects of Aroclor 1242 on rat bone marrow and spermatogonial cells. Aroclor 1242 was given to albino Osborne-Mendel rats as an acute dosage (PO) at 5000, 2500, and 1250 mg/kg or as a subacute regimen at 500 mg/kg and as a solution in corn oil at the other levels.

The results from the bone marrow study showed no significant increases in chromosomal abnormalities or inhibition of cellular division. The study of spermatogonial cells showed significant increase in abnormalties but statistically significant decreases in the number of dividing spermatogonial cells ($P < 0.05$). This effect was noted at 500 X 5 and 5000 X 1 dosages. It was concluded that Aroclor 1242 does not produce chromosomal abnormalities in rat bone marrow or spermatogonia but does cause, at relatively high dosages, a decrease in the number of dividing spermatogonial cells.

e. *Immunosuppressive Effects*

An interaction of PCBs with duck hepatitis virus was found by Friend & Trainer (80). Ten-day-old ducklings fed Aroclor 1254 at 25, 50, and 100 ppm of PCBs for 10 days suffered no apparent clinical intoxication but when challenged with duck hepatitis virus 5 days later suffered higher mortality than ducklings not exposed to PCB but challenged with the virus.

The effect of PCB (Clophen A-60 and Aroclor 1260) feeding at levels of 0, 10, 50, and 250 ppm on the humoral and cell-mediated immune response was described by Vos & Van Driel-Grootenhuis (81). A suppression to the humoral immunity was found at the 50 ppm level in guinea pigs, after stimulation with one dose of tetanus toxoid (alum-adsorbed). The number of tetanus antitoxin-producing cells in the stimulated popliteal lymph nodes was reduced. Stress was not considered responsible for the reduced immunological responses. A high mortality occurred at the 250 ppm level. Cachexia and depletion of the lymphoid system and liver damage were the most important findings in these animals.

The immunosuppressive activity of Aroclor 1260 (10 and 50 ppm over 8 weeks) on the humoral immune response in female albino guinea pigs was studied by Vos & Deroij (82), using tetanus toxoid as a function test of the immunological system in half the animals. Cellulose acetate electrophoresis was used to determine the seven proteins, including the γ-globulin level. The number of γ-globulin containing cells in the popliteal lymph nodes was determined semiquantatively with the direct fluorescent antibody technique. (Both techniques were sensitive parameters for the immunosuppressive action of PCB in the tetanus toxoid stimulated animals.)

Vos & Beems (60) found a reduced number of white blood cells, atrophy of the cortex of the thymus, and a reduction in the number of germinal centers in the spleen and lymph nodes after dermal application of high doses of PCBs in rabbits. This suggests the possibility of an immunosuppressive action.

Feeding guinea pigs 10 ppm Aroclor 1260 for 8 weeks (26) resulted in a decreased number of antibody-forming cells in the popliteal lymph nodes, after stimulation of the humoral lymphoid system with tetanus toxoid. Vos (26) suggested that this suppression may explain the higher sensitivity of PCB-fed ducklings for duck hepatitis virus (80).

Small spleens were noted in chickens fed PCBs, showing atrophy of the lymphoid system (52, 53).

f. Human Effects

In 1968, an outbreak of poisoning that involved at least 1000 people occurred in Northern and Western Japan where rice bran oil was contaminated with Kaneclor-400. This PCB contains 48% chlorine and has as its main components 2,4,3',4'-, 2,5,3',4'-, 2,3,5,4'- and 3,4,3',4'-tetrachlorobiphenyl, and 2,3,5,3',4'-pentachlorobiphenyl (83). The disease was named "Kanemi Yusho" (34, 84). The contamination occurred because PCBs used as heat exchangers in the manufacturing process leaked into the oil through pin holes in the pipes. Umeda claimed (33) that there are an estimated 15,000 victims of Kanemi Yusho although only 1081 persons have been officially diagnosed as such.

Exposure levels to the oil were calculated to approximate 15,000 mg/day. The lowest reported figures allow an estimate of a minimal positive effect level at 3 mg PCB per day over several months. However, the average doses associated with significant disease in the "Yusho" incident were much higher and were in the range of 30 mg/day (15, 28). The latency period between ingestion of the oil and the onset of clinical signs and symptoms was estimated at 5–6 months (3).

The clinical aspects associated with Yusho included: chloracne, blindness, systemic gastrointestinal symptoms with jaundice, edema, and abdominal pain. Chloracne is very persistent, with some patients showing evidence of it after 3 years. Table

Table 3 Subjective symptoms complained of by Yusho patients[a, b]

Symptom	Male (%)	Female (%)
Dark brown pigmentation of nails	83.1	75.0
Distinction of hair follicles	64.0	56.0
Increased sweating at palms	50.6	55.0
Acnelike skin eruptions	87.6	82.0
Red plaques on limbs	20.2	16.0
Itching	42.7	52.0
Pigmentation of skin	75.3	72.0
Swelling of limbs	20.2	41.0
Stiffened sole and palm	24.7	29.0
Pigmented mucous membrane	56.2	47.0
Increased eye discharge	88.8	83.0
Hyperaemia of conjunctiva	70.8	71.0
Transient visual disturbance	56.2	55.0
Jaundice	11.2	11.0
Swelling of upper eyelids	71.9	74.0
Feeling of weakness	58.4	52.0
Numbness in limbs	32.6	39.0
Fever	16.9	19.0
Hearing difficulties	18.0	19.0
Spasm of limbs	7.9	8.0
Headache	30.3	39.0
Vomiting	23.6	28.0
Diarrhea	19.1	17.0

[a]Eighty-nine male and 100 female patients diagnosed before October 31, 1968 were examined.

[b]From a report of "Yusho, A Poisoning Caused by Rice Oil Contaminated with Chlorobiphenyls" (Ref. 84).

3 lists the subjective symptoms of 89 male and 100 female Yusho patients. The severity of the disease varied with age, being greatest from adolescence through 40 years (85). The disorder generally cleared when exposure to the offending agent was discontinued.

Newborn infants of poisoned mothers had skin discoloration due to the presence of PCB via placental passage. (The dark skin discoloration regressed after a period of 2–5 months). Gingival hyperplasia with pigmentation was seen in several cases. Decreased birth weights were also noted, but no evidence could be obtained in regard to the possible retardation in physical and mental activities of the babies (86). The skin of stillborn infants showed hyperkeratosis and atrophy of the epidermis, and cystic dilation of the hair follicles. Residues of PCB have been found in fetal tissue (87, 88).

Examination of autopsy tissues of two Yusho fatalities revealed the presence of chlorobiphenyls in all of the examined organs, especially mesenterial fatty tissues, skin, and bone marrow (87, 89). PCBs were found with longer retention times (probably pentachlor- and higher chlorinated biphenyls) in autopsy tissues, and it was assumed that their presence might have been responsible for the observed long duration of the intoxication symptoms.

Additional detailed clinical and experimental studies have been made regarding the clinical features of Yusho and concerning toxicological effects on laboratory animals (34–37). Among the miscellaneous observations of biochemical and physiological abnormalities in Yusho patients are: increased urinary 17-ketosteroid excretion, respiratory distress with secondary infection of the upper respiratory tract, a hematological picture suggestive of acute or chronic inflammation, and elevated blood-serum triglycerides.

Chloracnegen effects were reported as early as 1936, following industrial exposure to the PCBs (32, 90–96). Approximately 10 cases of fatal intoxication involving persons who handled or were exposed to chlorinated biphenyls or naphthalenes in their occupations have been described (94, 96). In all cases histological examination revealed liver fatty degeneration necrosis and cirrhosis.

In contrast to the reports of industrial PCB poisoning, the outstanding difference in Yusho disease is the frequent occurrence of hyperpigmentation of the skin, as seen in 72% of women and 75% of men, which may be due to the differences in route of intake. The Yusho cases resulted from oral intake while industrial cases resulted from dermal exposure. Liver damage (in contrast to occupational poisoning) was not marked in the Yusho cases.

Two surveys of human adipose tissue in the USA (44, 45) gave broadly similar results with means of the order 1.0 ppm PCB. Biros et al (43), however, have reported 200 and 600 ppm of PCB in samples of human adipose tissue, and Price (44) reported that one autopsy case contained 115–240 ppm in fat.

Mean levels of PCB in human blood plasma were reported by Finklea et al (38) to be in the order of 2.0 ppb. In this study, rural Negroes had much lower levels in blood plasma (0.35 ppb) than the overall. Rural whites had slightly higher levels (near 3.2 ppb). Interestingly, this pattern was opposite to that of Σ DDT, in which rural Negroes had by far the highest levels (38).

Risebrough & Brodine (47) reported the mean PCB level in human milk from two cities in California to be about 60 ppb. Mean levels in human milk in Sweden and Germany were 16 ppb and 100 ppb respectively (41, 46). It has been calculated that, based on a daily milk intake of 150g/kg, breast-fed infants in California ingest some $9/\mu g/kg/day$ of PCBs. The toxicological consequences of body burdens of PCBs are difficult to assess at this time.

g. Miscellaneous Toxicological and Biological Effects

Aroclor 1254 was found to potentiate the toxicity of carbon tetrachloride in a manner similar to that reported for DDT (28). The studies of Grant et al (97) suggest that the liver is the main site of Aroclor 1254 metabolism, because rats with carbon tetrachloride damaged livers were unable to metabolize this mixture of chlorinated biphenyls as rapidly as rats with normal livers. Aroclor 1254 significantly increased the size of the liver and also the percentage of lipid in the liver. The same study revealed that the components of Aroclor 1254 with the shorter GLC retention times, presumably with the lowest chlorine content (98), were metabolized to a greater degree than those with the longer retention times. This effect is in agreement with the studies of Phenochlor DP6 fed to Japanese quail (99).

Street and co-workers (25) studied the effects of diets of 50 ppm to 100 ppm of 10 Aroclors ranging in chlorine content, and 21%–68% fed to rats for 15 days. Their effect on sleeping time induced by hexobarbital, in vitro rates of aniline hydroxylation, and demethyation of p-nitroanisole, and the rate of excretion were all found to be increased with increasing chlorine content. Aroclor 1221 (50 ppm) reduced hexobarbital sleeping time by 11%, whereas for Aroclor 1248 and 1268 the figures were 35% and 48%, respectively. Liver weights also increased with increasing chlorine content of the Aroclors. The storage of dieldrin was decreased in relationship to the chlorine content. For example, with Aroclors containing 60% chlorine or more, the storage in adipose tissue was reduced to the levels found in untreated control animals. The induction of PCBs of hepatic microsomal hydroxylating enzymes has been demonstrated in the American kestrel (Peakall & Lincer 7) and pigeons (Risebrough et al 5).

Villeneuve et al (101) studied the effects of PCB administration on microsomal enzyme activity in pregnant rabbits. The nil-effect level of Aroclor 1254 for enzyme induction in the pregnant rabbit is between 1.0 and 10 mg/kg body weight when administered for 28 days during gestation. Aroclor 1221 induced no enzyme activity in the does, fetus, or placenta, so its nil-effect level must be considered higher than that for Aroclor 1254. Placental transfer was shown to occur for both Aroclor 1254 and 1221 but causes no changes in the biochemical physiological parameters measured, e.g. total amount of Vitamin A stored per liver, protein levels, aniline hydroxylase enzyme activity, serum cholesterol, no effect in reproductive processes. The drug-metabolizing enzymes aniline hydroxylase and aminopyrine-n-demethylase were both induced by 10 mg/kg Aroclor 1254.

Litterst & Van Loon (100) studied enzyme induction by equimolar dietary amounts of DDT, phenobarbital, and Aroclor 1254 after 30 days of treatment. At 150 μ mole/kg of food, the PCB was far more effective than phenobarbital, and at least as effective as DDT. At 15 μ mole, phenobarbital, DDT, and Aroclor 1254 produced substrate-specific increases in enzymatic activity.

Ito and co-workers (102) found that the administration of PCBs to rabbits increases the total lipid, triglyceride, and cholesterol content of liver and decreases the total liver phospholipid content. (The concentration of serum triglycerides was abnormally increased.)

Lincer & Peakall (24) demonstrated an inductive effect on estradiol metabolism from the administration of Aroclor 1254 and Aroclor 1262 to American kestrels. Aroclors 1221, 1232, 1242, and 1248 also have an estrogenic effect on the rat uterus, which was not shown with Aroclors of higher chlorination (22). The estrogenic activity was evaluated using the 18-hr glycogen response to the immature rat after a single subcutaneous injection.

Platonow & Funnell (23) reported an antiandrogenic-like effect in cockerels when Aroclor 1254 was incorporated in the diet at 250 ppm for as little as 6 weeks. Vos (26) suggested that both increased steroid metabolism as cited by Rehfeld et al (51) and the estrogenic activity could be responsible for the depression of secondary sexual characteristics such as decreased development of comb and wattles noted in cockerels (23).

Örberg et al (21) described the prolongation of estrus cycle in NMRI-strain mice given single ip administrations of DDT (40 mg/kg) and Clophen A-60 (20 mg/kg). The prolongation appeared to decrease with time, the lengths returning to normal after 3 cycles. The effects observed probably indicated that the chlorinated hydrocarbons affected the catabolism of steroid hormones. No changes were found in the frequences of cornified cells after the ingestions. A prolonged estrus cycle implies less frequent periods of sexual receptivity in the female and hence could cause a decline in the reproductive capacity of the animals.

Ogawa (103) demonstrated neuropathy in rats following administration of PCB (0.3–0.5 ml/kg/day) for 14 or 21 days as evidenced by marked or moderately impaired motor function, decreased motor conduction velocity, and loss of large nerve fibers.

Norback & Allen (104, 105) reported that ingestion of PCBs by rats for 1–5 weeks resulted in liver hypertrophy, with proliferation of the smooth surfaced membranes of the endoplasmic reticulum (SER) and formulation of large concentric membrane arrays within the cytoplasm of the hepatic cells. These concentric membrane arrays were suggested by Vos (26) as probably representing the hyalin bodies described by Bennett et al (106) and Miller (49) and could have an enzymatic function similar to that associated with the SER (104, 105).

Yap et al (107) reported that PCBs inhibit the activity of fish ATPases in vitro. Both Mg^{2+}ATPase and NA^{+}-K^{+}-ATPase were inhibited in brain, kidney, and liver at concentrations as low as 0.03 ppm. An analogous effect for DDT has been cited in the above study.

h. Summary and Conclusions

Despite the increasing number of mammalian toxicological investigations, aspects of *definitive* acute, subacute, and chronic toxicity of the polychlorinated biphenyls still remain poorly known as regards man. The chemical and physical properties, e.g. the stability, complexity, and heterogeneity of the commercial formulations per se, the difficulty of separation and analysis as well as the non- or ill-defined nature of the material actually used or reported in many studies, conspire in making the evaluation of toxicity and biological data difficult.

A number of the more salient biological and toxicological aspects of the PCBs are summarized in Table 4. It is possible to distinguish two actions of the PCBs on mammals, e.g. liver damage and skin lesions. Liver damage has been predominantly manifest in mice, rats, guinea pigs, rabbits, and monkeys in feeding and to a lesser extent in inhalation studies. Liver damage and transplacental transmission as shown in abnormal pigmentation and miscarriages have also been observed in the Yusho poisonings in Japan. Skin lesions have been observed in rabbits in dermal toxicity studies. In addition, chloracnegenic and porphyrogenic as well as edema effects in many species have been caused by commerical PCB preparations. The liver damage and skin lesions are believed to be caused primarily by chlorinated dibenzofuran contaminants and to a minor extent by PCB itself. These contaminants are also responsible for the edema formation observed in fowl, while the PCBs are suggested to the causative agent for the hepatic prophyria.

In contrast to the acute toxicity, aspects of subacute and chronic toxicity appear to be of far greater concern. In rats the acute LD_{50} is of the order of 5–10 g/kg. Chronic intake of relatively small doses of PCBs, however, has been demonstrated to have adverse effects in man and other vertebrates. For example, in man it has been estimated that as little as 10 mg/kg over 50 days causes chloracne. It has also been shown that toxic effects during continuous exposure at low levels may only appear after extremely prolonged intake, e.g. certain reproductive effects of Aroclors 1242 and 1254 in rats were not manifest until after 15 months of prolonged intake.

Although deaths from exposure, either acute or chronic, have not been clearly documented for man, aspects of the toxicity as described above coupled with increasing reports of the ubiquity of the presence of PCBs in humans (analogous to DDT and DDE) suggest further study is essential to elaborate more definitely the potential toxicity of this environmental pollutant. In this regard further toxicologi-

Table 4 Some toxicological and biological effects of the PCBs

1. Acute oral LD_{50} in mammals varies from approximately 2–10 g/kg. (Apparent increase in mammalian toxicity with decrease in chlorine content.)
2. Induction of hyperplasia and dysplasia of gastric mucosa in subhuman primates.
3. Enlargement of the liver and vacuolar or fatty degeneration of liver cells in rats, guinea pigs, and monkeys.
4. Hepatocarcinogenicity in mice and bladder carcinogenicity in rats.
5. Production of hydropericardial edema in chickens and Japanese quail.
6. Teratogenic effect in chick embryo.
7. Fetotoxicity in rabbit.
8. Adverse reproductive effects in rats at levels of ca 100 ppm in diet.
9. Adverse reproductive effects in mink.
10. Enhanced chromosomal aberrations and embyonic death in ring doves.
11. Effects on hatchability in chickens, Japanese quail.
12. Skin, liver, and kidney lesions in rabbits following dermal exposure.
13. Immunosuppressive effects in rabbits.
14. Chemical porphyrogenic effects in many species.
15. Chloracnegenic and hepatotoxic effects in man.
16. Hyperglyceridemic effects in man.
17. Human miscarriages, stillbirths, and transplacental transmission in abnormal pigmentation from "rice-oil disease" (Yusho).
18. Hepatoxic, chloracnegenic, and porphyrogenic effects of chlorinated dibenzofuran contaminants in several species.
19. Potentiating of toxicity (e.g. carbon tetrachloride) in rats.
20. Chloracnegenic effects of chlorinated naphthalene contaminants in man.
21. Generally, enzyme induction increases with increase in chlorination of PCBs.
22. Induction of hepatic hydroxylating microsomal enzymes and increased estrogenic activity in the rat.
23. Inductive effect on estradiol metabolism and anti-androgenic effects in kestrels.
24. Prolongation of estrus cycle in mice.
25. Inhibition of ATPases in vitro.

cal and biological studies involving key individual characterized PCB isomers, trace contaminant chlorinated dibenzofuran and naphthalenes, definitive pharmacokinetic elaborations (perhaps in primates), and more definitive mutagenic and teratologic studies should all help in this most needed assessment.

Literature Cited

1. Nisbet, I. C. T., Sarofim, A. F. 1972. *Environ. Health Perspect.* 1:21–38
2. Risebrough, R. W., Delappe, B. 1972. *Environ. Health Perspect.* 1:39–44
3. Nelson, N. 1972. Polychlorinated Biphenyls—Environmental Impact. *Environ. Res.* 5:253–362
4. Jensen, S. 1973. *Ambio* 1:123–31
5. Risebrough, R. W. et al 1968. *Nature* 220:1078–1102
6. Gustafson, C. G. 1970. *Environ. Sci. Technol.* 4:814–19
7. Peakall, D. B., Lincer, J. L. 1970. *Bioscience* 20:958–64
8. Hammond, A. L. 1972. *Science* 175:155–60
9. Savage, E. P., Tessari, I. 1971. *J. Environ. Health* 35:30–34
10. Veith, G. C., Lee, G. F. 1970. *Water Resour.* 4:265–71
11. Reynolds, L. M. 1971. *Residue Rev.* 34:27–81
12. Holden, A. V. 1970. *Nature* 228:1220–24
13. Zitko, V. 1971. *Bull. Environ. Contam. Toxicol.* 6:464–70
14. Zitko, V., Choi, P. M. K. 1971. PCB and other industrial halogenated hydrocarbons in the environment. *Fisheries Res. Board of Canada Tech. Rept.* No. 272:2–54
15. Polychlorinated Biphenyls and the Environment. 1972. Interdepartmental Task Force on PCBs. *Nat. Tech. Info. Serv.* Springfield, Va. 1–181
16. Fishbein, L. 1972. *J. Chromatogr.* 68: 345–426
17. Cook, J. W. 1972. *Environ. Health Perspect.* 1:3–13
18. Sissons, D., Welti, D. J. 1971. *J. Chromatogr.* 60:15–32
19. Bitman, J., Cecil, H. C., Harris, S. J. 1972. *Environ. Sci. Perspect.* 1:145–49
20. Norback, D. H., Allen, J. R. 1972. *Environ. Sci. Perspect.* 1:137–49
21. Örberg, J., Johansson, N., Kihlstrom, J. E., Lundberg, C. 1972. *Ambio* 1: 148–49
22. Botman, J., Cecil, H. C. 1970. *J. Agr. Food Chem.* 18:1108–14
23. Platonow, N. S., Funnell, H. S. 1971. *Vet. Rec.* 89:109–10

24. Lincer, J. L., Peakall, D. B. 1970. *Nature* 228:783–84
25. Street, J. C. et al 1969. *Comparative effects of PCBs and organochlorine pesticides in induction of hepatic microsomal enzymes.* Presented at Am. Chem. Soc. Meet., New York, Sept. 8–12
26. Vos, J. G. 1972. *Environ. Health Perspect.* 1:105–17
27. Stalling, D., Mayer, F. C. 1972. *Environ. Health Perspect.* 1:159–69
28. Kolbye, A. C. Jr. 1971. *Current status of toxicological effects of PCBs.* FDA, Wash. DC Sept. 1 & 29
29. Burke, J., Fitzhugh, O. G. 1970. Suppl. 1, *Status Rept. of Chemistry & Toxicology of PCBs.* FDA, Wash. DC Dec. 1
30. Cook, J. W. 1970. *Status Report on the Chemistry and Toxicology of PCBs.* FDA, Wash. DC, June 1
31. Schwartz, L. 1936. *U. S. Publ. Health Bull.* Pt. 2:229
32. Meigs, J. W., Albom, J. J., Castin, B. L. 1954. *J. Am. Med. Assoc.* 154:1417–18
33. Umeda, G. 1972. *Ambio* 1:132–44
34. Kuratsune, M. et at 1972. *Environ. Health Perspect.* 1:119–28
35. Kuratsune, M. 1972. *Environ. Health Perspect.* 1:129–36
36. Reports of the Study Group for "Yusho" (Chlorobiphenyls Poisoning). 1969. *Fukuoka Acta Med.* 60:403–533
37. The Second Report of the Study for "Yusho" (Chlorobiphenyls Poisoning). 1971. *Fukuoka Acta Med.* 62:1–176
38. Finklea, J. F. et al 1971. *Polychlorinated Biphenyl Residues in Human Plasma.* Presented at 99th Am. Publ. Health Assoc. Meet., Minneapolis, Minn. Oct. 11–15
39. Kolbye, A. C. 1972. *Environ. Health Perspect.* 1:85-88
40. Westöö, G., Norén, K. 1970. *Vår Föda* 22:93–146
41. Westöö, G., Norén, K., Andersson, M. 1970. *Vår Föda* 22:10–42
42. Isono, N. 1971. *Critical News* 1:1–2
43. Biros, F. J., Walker, A. C., Medberry, A. 1970. *Bull. Environ. Contam. Toxicol.* 5:317–23

44. Price, H. A. 1972. *Environ. Health Perspect.* 1:73–78
45. Yobs, A. R. 1972. *Environ. Health Perspect.* 1:79–82
46. Acker, L., Schulte, E. 1970. *Naturwissenschaften* 57:497–500
47. Risebrough, R., Brodine, V. 1970. *Environment* 12:16–27
48. Vos, J. G. et al 1970. *Food Cosmet. Toxicol.* 8:625–33
49. Miller, J. W. 1944. *U. S. Publ. Health Rept.* 59:1085–93
50. Tucker, R. K., Crabtree, D. G. 1970. *Handbook of Toxicity of Pesticides to Wildlife,* U. S. Dept. of Interior, Bureau of Sport Fisheries & Wildlife, Publ. 84, Wash. DC
51. Rehfeld, B. M., Bradley, R. L. Jr., Sunde, M. L. 1971. *Poultry Sci.* 50: 1090–96
52. Kohanawa, M., Shoya, S., Ogura, Y. et al 1969. *Nat. Inst. Anim. Health Quart.* 9:213–19
53. Vos, J. G., Koeman, J. H. 1970. *Toxicol. Appl. Pharmacol.* 17:656–68
54. Flick, D. F., O'Dell, A. G., Childs, V. A. 1965. *Poultry Sci.* 44:1460–65
55. McCune, E. L., Savage, J. E., O'Dell, B. L. 1962. *Poultry Sci.* 41:295–99
56. Heath, R. G., Spann, J. W., Kreitzer, J. F. 1970. *Effects of Polychlorinated Biphenyls on Birds.* Presented at XV Congr. Ent. Ornithol. Den Haag, Sept. 3–7
57. Nishizumi, M. 1970. *Arch. Environ. Health* 21:620–26
58. Bruckner, J. V., Knanna, K. L., Cornish, H. H. 1973. *Toxicol. Appl. Pharmocol.* 24:434–38
59. Koller, L. D., Zinkl, J. G. 1973. *Am. J. Pathol.* 70:363–73
60. Vos, J. G., Beems, R. B. 1971. *Toxicol. Appl. Pharmacol.* 19:617–33
61. Vos, J. G., Notenboom-Ram, E. 1972. *Toxicol. Appl. Pharmacol.* 23:563–78
62. Bauer, H., Schulz, K. H., Spiegelberg, U. 1961. *Arch. Gewerbepathol. Gewerbehyg.* 18:538–42
63. Higginbotham, G. R. et al 1968. *Nature* 220:702–5
64. Keplinger, M. L. et al 1972. *Toxicological Studies with Polychlorinated Biphenyls.* PCB Conf. Quail Roost. Conf. Center, Rougemont, NC, Dec. 1971
65. Keplinger, M. L., Fancher, 'O. E., Calandra, J. C. 1971. *Toxicol. Appl. Pharmacol.* 19:402–3
66. Kimbrough, R. D., Linder, R. E., Gaines, T. B. 1972. *Arch. Environ. Health.* 25:354–64
67. Kimbrough, R. D. 1971. Interagency Meet. PCBs, Dept. HEW, Wash. DC, Aug. 5
68. Lichtenstein, E. P., Schulz, K. R., Fuhremann, T. W. 1969. *J. Econ. Entomol.* 62:761–65
69. Scott, M. L. et al 1971. *Results of experiments on the effects of PCBs on laying hen performance.* Proc. 1971 Cornell Nutrition Conf. Feed Mfrs. 56–64
70. Nagasaki, H. et al 1972. *Gann* 63: 805
71. Nagasaki, H. 1971. *Gann* 62:431–32
72. Kimura, N. T., Baba, T. 1973. *Gann* 64:105–8
73. Allen, J. R., Norback, D. H. 1972. *Science* 179:498–99
74. McLaughlin, J., Marliac, J. P., Verrett, M. J., Mutchler, M. K. Fitzhugh, O. G. 1963. *Toxicol. Appl. Pharmacol.* 5: 760–61
75. Carlson, R. W., Duby, R. T. 1973. *Bull. Environ. Contam. Toxicol.* 9:261–66
76. Villeneuve, D. C., Grant, D. L., Khera, K. 1971. *Environ. Physiol.* 1:67–71
77. Peakall, D. B., Lincer, J. L., Bloom, S. E. 1972. *Environ. Health Perspect.* 1: 103–4
78. Hoopingarner, R., Samuel, A., Krause, D. 1972. *Environ. Health Perspect.* 1: 155–58
79. Green, S., Palmer, K. A., Oswald, E. J. 1973. Abstr. 12th Ann. Meet. Soc. Toxicol., New York, March 18–22
80. Friend, M., Trainer, D. O. 1970. *Science* 170:1314–16
81. Vos, J. G., Van Driel-Grootenhuis, L. 1972. *Sci. Total Environ.* 1:289–302
82. Vos, J. G., Deroij, T. 1972. *Toxicol. Appl. Pharmacol.* 21:549–55
83. Saeki, S., Tsutsui, A., Oguri, K., Yoshimura, H., Hamana, M. 1971. *Fukuoka Acta Med.* 62:20–23
84. Kuratsune, M. et al 1969. *Fukuoka Acta Med.* 60:513–32
85. Goti, M., Higuchi, K. 1969. *Fukuoka Acta Med.* 60:409–31
86. Yamaguchi, A., Yoshimura, T., Kuratsune, M. 1971. *Fukuoka Acta Med.* 62: 117–21
87. Kojima, T., Fukumoto, H., Makisumi, J. 1969. *Jap. J. Legal Med.* 23:415–17
88. Inagami, K., Koga, T., Tomita, Y. 1969. *Shokuhin Eisei Gaku Zasshi* 10: 312–15
89. Kikuchi, M. O., Mikagi, Y., Hashimoto, M., Kojima, T. 1971. *Fukuoka Acta Med.* 62:89–93

90. Schwartz, L. 1936. *Am. J. Publ. Health* 26:58–61
91. Schwartz, L. 1943. *J. Am. Med. Soc.* 122:158–62
92. Schwartz, L. Barlow, F. A. 1942. *U. S. Public Health Repts.* 57:1747–50
93. Jones, J. W., Alden, H. S. 1936. *Arch. Dermatol. Syphilol.* 33:1022–26
94. Flinn, F. B., Jarvik, D. E. 1936. *Proc. Soc. Exp. Biol. Med.* 35:118–22
95. Greenburg, L., Mayers, M. R., Smith, A. R. 1939. *J. Indian Hyg. Toxicol.* 21:29–33
96. Drinker, C. K., Warren, M. F., Bennett, G. A. 1937. *J. Indian Hyg. Toxicol.* 19:283–87
97. Grant, T. L., Phillips, W. E. J., Villeneuve, D. C. 1971. *Bull. Environ. Contam. Toxicol.* 6:102–08
98. Bagley, G. E., Reichel, W. L., Cromartie, E. 1970. *J. Assoc. Offic. Anal. Chem.* 53:251–55
99. Koeman, J. H., Ten Noever de Brauw, M. L., De Vos, R. H. 1969. *Nature* 221:1126–30
100. Litterst, C. L., Van Loon, E. J. 1972. *Proc. Soc. Environ. Biol. Med.* 141:765–68
101. Villeneuve, D. C. et al 1971. *Bull. Environ. Contam. Toxicol.* 6:120–26
102. Ito, Y., Uzawa, H., Notumi, A. 1971. *Fukuoka Acta Med.* 62:48–54
103. Ogawa, M. 1971. *Fukuoka-Igaku-Zasshi* 62:74–77
104. Norback, D. H., Allen, J. R. 1970. *Fed. Proc.* 29:816–18
105. Norback, D. H., Allen, J. R. 1972. *Environ. Health Perspect.* 1:137–43
106. Bennett, G. A., Drinker, C. K., Warren, M. F. 1938. *J. Indian Hyg. Toxicol.* 20:97–100
107. Yap, H. H., Desaiah, D., Cutkomp, L. K. 1971. *Nature* 223:61–63
108. Presst, I., Jefferies, D. J., Moore, N. W. 1970. *Environ. Pollut.* 1:3–25

CHEMOTHERAPY OF CANCER   ❖6587

Stephen K. Carter and Milan Slavik
Division of Cancer Treatment, National Cancer Institute, Bethesda, Maryland

INTRODUCTION

Cancer is one of the oldest diseases afflicting mankind, and the efforts at treatment have been recorded as long ago as the use of arsenic pastes in ancient Egypt. Today, cancer is second only to cardiovascular disease as the major cause of death in the United States. Each year an estimated 650,000 new cases are diagnosed and over one million known patients continue treatment. The major difficulties in mounting a rapid scientific assault on cancer are that it encompasses more than 100 clinically distinct diseases and is inextricably linked to fundamental life processes that still are not completely understood.

THERAPEUTIC APPROACHES

Several modes of therapy, including surgery, radiotherapy, and chemotherapy, are effective against cancer and have been developed to a point of practical use as either single or combined modalities. In many instances, cure can be achieved through removal or destruction of localized cancer, before it has spread to distant areas, by surgery and/or radiotherapy. Surgery is sometimes more successful when both the tumor and involved regional lymph nodes are excised. Radiotherapy is used to destroy localized tumors that are not accessible to surgery.

Unfortunately, although they may eradicate the primary disease, the local modalities often fail as a result of the spread of disease to other parts of the body. In such instances, the demonstrated capacity of chemotherapy for controlling disseminated disease offers the greatest hope for reducing mortality in a number of different cancers (1).

Like the other therapeutic measures, chemotherapy can be curative or palliative to varying degrees depending on the individual tumor (Table 1). "Cure" means that the treated cancer patient has a "normal" life expectancy, i.e. the same as that of a matched cohort in the general population.

Cures, or at least possible cures, by antitumor drugs alone have been achieved in such diseases as choriocarcinoma, Burkitt's lymphoma, acute lymphocytic leukemia, testicular cancer, and Hodgkin's disease. Chemotherapy combined with

157

Table 1 Chemotherapeutic potential in cancer

Effect of Chemotherapy	Cancer Type		
	Hematologic Malignancies	Adult Solid Tumors	Pediatric Solid Tumor
With optimal treatment, some patients survive free of disease for long periods	Acute lymphocytic leukemia Advanced (stage III & usually IV) Hodgkin's disease Burkitt's tumor	Trophoblastic carcinoma (choriocarcinoma) Testicular tumors	Wilms' Tumor[a] Ewing's sarcoma [a] Embryonal rhabdomyosarcoma[a] Retinoblastoma[a]
Significant number of patients achieve objective regression with survival gain	Non-Hodgkin's malignant lymphoma Multiple myeloma Acute granulocytic leukemia Chronic lymphocytic leukemia	Adenocarcinoma of the breast Adenocarcinoma of the ovary	Neuroblastoma[a]
Transient disease regression in some patients, but survival gain not established	Blast crisis of chronic granulocytic leukemia	Bronchogenic carcinoma GI adenocarcinoma Prostatic, bladder and thyroid carcinomas Soft tissue sarcoma Squamous cell carcinoma of the head and cervix Malignant melanoma	Osteogenic sarcoma

[a]Optimal use of chemotherapy requires combination with radiotherapy and/or surgery.

surgery and/or radiotherapy promises cure in many patients with childhood solid tumors such as Wilms' tumor, embryonal rhabdomyosarcoma, and Ewing's sarcoma. In other tumors, chemotherapeutic agents produce a significant degree of tumor cell kill that is reflected in a high rate of objective tumor regression and enhanced survival, although cure cannot be shown at present. These tumors include adenocarcinomas of the breast and ovary, non-Hodgkin's lymphoma, multiple myeloma, chronic leukemias, and acute granulocytic leukemia. In many of the other diseases, chemotherapy can achieve objective regression and palliative benefits in one fifth to one third of the treated patients.

Table 2 charts the drugs commonly used in the chemotherapy of the major types of cancer in the United States. The commercially available drugs considered useful in cancer therapy are listed in Table 3, together with their dosages and routes of administration, toxic effects, antitumor activity, and mechanisms of action. Table 4 details the experimental drugs that have shown definite antitumor effectiveness. All of the experimental drugs are usually available from the National Cancer Institute under the Food and Drug Administration regulations governing use of investigational drugs.

RECENT PROGRESS IN CHEMOTHERAPY

Since 1954, the National Cancer Institute has led a national effort to achieve chemical control of cancer. This systematic effort was undertaken by the government simply because its cost could not be met solely by private industry, the academic community, and independent clinical and laboratory institutions. The chemotherapy program area of the NCI encompasses every phase of drug research and development, from the acquisition of potential anticancer agents through the completion of clinical trials and introduction of active drugs into medical practice.

Each year a large number of compounds are tested for possible antitumor activity. Most of these candidate agents are obtained from random sources, but an increasing number of rationally designed synthetic compounds are being examined as a direct consequence of recent advances in molecular biology. In 1972, the NCI evaluated 30,800 new compounds, including about 16,000 synthetic chemicals and 14,800 natural products derived from fermentation processes or plant and animal sources. During this period, tests in various animal tumors and in vitro cell systems increased 79% over those performed in 1971.

The qualitative and quantitative effects of experimental drugs in animal model systems are studied to establish effective dose levels and schedules of administration that will be applicable in the clinical situation. Similarly, investigations of drug toxicology are conducted to estimate safe dose levels for man and predict the toxic effects that may be encountered during clinical trials.

Over the years a large number of antitumor agents have been placed in clinical trial through the drug research and development program of the National Cancer Institute. The following have been among the most interesting drugs under investigation in recent years:

Adriamycin

This anthracycline antibiotic was isolated from a culture of *Streptomyces peucetius* var. *caesius* and, structurally, is a hydroxylated analog of daunorubicin (58, 59). Its mechanism of action is postulated as binding to DNA by intercalation between base pairs (60, 61) and inhibition of DNA and RNA synthesis (62, 63).

The experimental antitumor activity of adriamycin is superior to daunorubicin in L1210 leukemia (64) and P388 leukemia in mice (65), as well as in other systems such as Ehrlich ascites tumor and Sarcoma 180 in mice (66). Pharmacokinetic studies in mice and rats show that adriamycin is rapidly cleared from plasma; concentrated in the liver, spleen, kidney, heart, and lung; and excreted slowly in the urine and bile (67, 68). Alopecia, total depression of hematopoiesis, thrombocytopenia, blood coagulation changes, and hyperazotemia are the major organ toxicities in dogs and rabbits (69).

In man, adriamycin is rapidly cleared from plasma and slowly excreted in the urine and bile, being predominantly metabolized in the liver (70, 71). Data from over 2000 patients analyzed in the Cancer Therapy Evaluation Program of the NCI Division of Cancer Treatment (52) demonstrate significant objective response rates in a wide range of solid tumors, particularly adenocarcinoma of the breast (35%), malignant sarcomas (25%), and bronchogenic carcinoma (22%), as well as in malignant lymphomas (37%) and acute leukemias (25%).

Alopecia, myelosuppression, stomatitis, and nausea and vomiting are the most frequent toxic effects observed in man, but the most serious side effect is cardiac toxicity. This may be fatal if the total administered dose of the drug exceeds 550 mg/m² (72).

Table 2 Drugs commonly used for treatment of major types of cancer

Cancer Type	Primary Approach	Secondary Approach	Other Drugs with Reported Activity
HEMATOLOGIC MALIGNANCIES			
Acute lymphocytic leukemia	Induction: Vincristine sulfate + Prednisone Maintenance: Mercaptopurine Methotrexate with periodic use of "induction" regimen	Daunorubicin[a] Asparaginase[a] Cyclophosphamide Cytarabine hydrochloride	Thioguanine Carmustine[a]
Acute granulocytic leukemia	Cytarabine hydrochloride + Thioguanine	Daunorubicin[a]	Mercaptopurine Methotrexate Prednisone Cyclophosphamide Asparaginase[a]
Chronic granulocytic leukemia	Busulfan	Dibromannitol[a] Hydroxyurea	Mercaptopurine Melphalan
Chronic lymphocytic leukemia	Chlorambucil Cyclophosphamide	Prednisone	Cytarabine
Multiple myeloma	Melphalan or Cyclophosphamide + Prednisone	Carmustine[a]	Chlorambucil
Hodgkin's disease (Stage III & IV)	"MOPP" Combination: Mechlorethamine (nitrogen mustard) Oncovin (generic, vincristine sulfate) Procarbazine hydrochloride Prednisone	Vinblastine sulfate Lomustine[a] Bleomycin[a]	Adriamycin[a] Dacarbazine[a] Methotrexate Cyclophosphamide Chlorambucil Thiotepa Carmustine[a]
Non-Hodgkin's lymphoma	"COP" Combination: Cyclophosphamide Oncovin (generic, vincristine sulfate) Prednisone	Adriamycin[a] Bleomycin[a]	Carmustine[a] Procarbazine hydrochloride Methotrexate Vinblastine sulfate Chlorambucil Mechlorethamine
Burkitt's tumor	Cyclophosphamide	Carmustine[a]	
Mycosis fungoides	Methotrexate		
Malignant insulinoma	Streptozotocin[a]		
Renal cell	Medroxyprogesterone	Vinblastine sulfate (poor) Lomustine[a]	Hydroxyurea (poor)
Malignant melanoma	Dacarbazine[a]	Carmustine[a] Vincristine sulfate	Cyclophosphamide Dactinomycin Chlorambucil Melphalan Hydroxyurea Thiotepa
Miscellaneous sarcomas	Adriamycin + Dacarbazine[a] Dactinomycin	Cyclophosphamide Vincristine sulfate	Methotrexate
Primary brain neoplasms	Carmustine[a] Lomustine[a] Dexamethasone (to control edema)	Vincristine sulfate Methotrexate	
PEDIATRIC SOLID TUMORS			
Wilms' tumor	Dactinomycin Vincristine sulfate (with radiation and/or surgery)	Adriamycin[a]	
Ewing's sarcoma	Cyclophosphamide Dactinomycin Vincristine sulfate (with radiation and/or surgery)	Adriamycin[a]	
Embryonal rhabdomyosarcoma	Cyclophosphamide Dactinomycin Vincristine sulfate (with radiation and/or surgery)	Adriamycin[a]	Thiotepa Methotrexate
Neuroblastoma	Cyclophosphamide Vincristine sulfate	Adriamycin[a]	Vinblastine sulfate Daunorubicin Prednisone
Retinoblastoma	Triethylenemelamine (+ radiation)		
Gestational trophoblastic neoplasms (choriocarcinoma)	Methotrexate Dactinomycin Vinblastine sulfate		

Table 2 (continued)

Cancer Type	Primary Approach	Secondary Approach	Other Drugs with Reported Activity
SOLID TUMORS			
Breast cancer	Diethylstilbestrol	Adriamycin[a]	Lomustine[a]
	Testosterone	Medroxyprogesterone	Vinblastine sulfate
	Combination utilizing some or all of the following:		Thiotepa
	Fluorouracil		Ethinyl estradiol
	Methotrexate		Fluoxymesterone
	Vincristine sulfate		Melphalan
	Prednisone		
	Cyclophosphamide		
Ovarian cancer	Melphalan or Cyclophosphamide	Fluorouracil	Vinblastine sulfate
		Hexamethylmelamine[a]	Dactinomycin
			Methotrexate
			Thiotepa
Bronchogenic carcinoma	Mechlorethamine (nitrogen mustard)	Lomustine[a]	Procarbazine hydrochloride
	or Cyclophosphamide	Hexamethylmelamine[a]	Bleomycin+ Vincristine sulfate
	Methotrexate		Thiotepa
			Adriamycin[a]
GI adenocarcinoma (large bowel, pancreas, stomach)	Fluorouracil	Carmustine[a]	Mitomycin C[a]
		Lomustine[a]	
		Cyclophosphamide	
Prostate	Diethylstilbestrol		Ethinyl estradiol
Squamous cell head and neck	Methotrexate	Fluorouracil	
		Bleomycin[a]	
Squamous cell of cervix	Methotrexate	Fluorouracil	
	Cyclophosphamide	Bleomycin[a]	
		Vincristine sulfate	
Endometrial carcinoma	Hydroxyprogesterone		
	Medroxyprogesterone		
Adrenal cortical carcinoma	Mitotane		
Testicular seminoma	Melphalan		
Testicular carcinoma	Vinblastine sulfate		
	Dactinomycin		
	Mithramycin		
	Bleomycin[a]		

[a]Available for investigational use only.

Different dose schedules have been used but, based on pharmacokinetic studies in man, a single dose of 60–75 mg/m² iv repeated every 3 weeks is recommended.

5-Azacytidine

This antitumor agent was isolated from a fermentation of *Streptoverticillium ladakanus* (73, 74) and independently synthesized by Piskala & Sorm (75). The mechanism of action has been elucidated in a number of studies (67–84). 5-Azacytidine is an analog of cytidine and is rapidly phosphorylated and incorporated in both RNA and DNA. By disrupting the processes of translation of nucleic acid sequences into protein, the synthesis of protein is inhibited. Moreover, it affects de novo pyrimidine synthesis by inhibiting orotidylic acid decarboxylase (85).

The drug has exhibited experimental antitumor activity against L1210 leukemia (86), lymphoid leukemia in AK mice (87), and Ehrlich ascites tumor in mice (88). Pharmacokinetic studies in mice show that 5-azacytidine is rapidly cleared from

Table 3 Commercially available cancer chemotherapeutic drugs

Drug	Usual Dosage	Toxicity		Major Indications	Mechanism of Action
		Acute	Delayed		
ALKYLATING AGENTS					
Mechlorethamine (nitrogen mustard; HN$_2$ Mustargen)	0.4 mg/kg, iv in single or divided dose	Nausea and vomiting	Moderate depression of peripheral blood count	Hodgkin's disease and other lymphomas, bronchogenic carcinoma	The alkylating agents act by transfer of alkyl groups to biologically important cell constituents such as an amino, carboxyl, sulfhydryl, or phosphate group, whose function is then impaired. Alkylation of the N^7 of guanine in DNA is one of the crucial reactions and leads to (a) alteration of guanine so that it forms an abnormal base pair with thymine (miscoding); (b) cleavage of the imidazole ring of guanine (destroying it); (c) linking of guanine pairs, producing cross-linked DNA strands which cannot replicate; & (d) depurination of DNA, causing actual breakage of the DNA strands (2–8).
Thiotepa (triethylenethiophosphoramide)	0.2 mg/kg, iv x 5 day	None	Bone marrow depression	Hodgkin's disease, bronchogenic & breast carcinomas	
Chlorambucil (Leukeran)	Start 0.1–0.2 mg/kg/ day PO, adjust for maintenance	None	Bone marrow depression (anemia, leukopenia & thrombocytopenia) can be severe with excessive dosage	Chronic lymphocytic leukemia Hodgkin's disease, non-Hodgkin's lymphoma, trophoblastic neoplasms	
Cyclophosphamide (Cytoxan)	40 mg/kg iv in single or in 2–8 daily doses or 2–4 mg/kg/day PO for 10 day, adjust for maintenance	Nausea and vomiting	Bone marrow depression; alopecia; cystitis	Hodgkin's disease and other lymphomas, multiple myeloma, lymphocytic leukemia, many solid cancers	
Triethylenemelamine (TEM)	2.5–5 mg PO, 2 times weekly for 4 weeks initially	Nausea and vomiting	Bone marrow depression; alopecia; cystitis	Retinoblastoma	
Melphalan (1-phenylalanine mustard; Alkeran)	0.25 mg/kg/day x 4 PO; 2–4 mg/day as maintenance or 0.1–0.15 mg/kg/day for 2–3 weeks	None	Bone marrow depression	Multiple myeloma, malignant melanoma, ovarian carcinoma, testicular seminoma	
Busulfan (Myleran)	2–8 mg/day for 2–3 wks PO: stop for recovery; then maintenance	None	Bone marrow depression	Chronic granulocytic leukemia	
ANTIMETABOLITES					
Methotrexate (amethopterin; MTX)	2.5–5.0 mg/day PO; 0.4 mg/kg rapid iv daily 4–5 day (not over 25 mg) or 0.4 mg/kg rapid iv twice wk	Occasional diarrhea, hepatic necrosis	Oral and gastrointestinal ulceration; bone marrow depression (anemia, leukopenia, thrombocytopenia); cirrhosis	Acute lymphocytic leukemia, choriocarcinoma carcinoma of cervix and head and neck area, mycosis fungoides, solid cancers	Competitively inhibits dihydrofolate reductase, thus restricting the availability of tetrahydrofolic acid (THF) to cells. THF is critically important to metabolic transfer of one-carbon units in a variety of biochemical reactions.

Table 3 (continued)

Drug	Usual Dosage	Toxicity		Major Indications	Mechanism of Action
		Acute	Delayed		
Mercaptopurine (6-MP; Purinethol)	2.5 mg/kg/day PO	Occasional nausea vomiting, usually well tolerated	Bone marrow depression occasional hepatic damage	Acute lymphocytic and granulocytic leukemia chronic granulocytic leukemia	Converted intracellularly to its corresponding ribonucleotide (6-thioinosinic acid), which may have several effects: (a) suppression of de novo purine biosynthesis via "pseudo-feedback inhibition" of the formation of ribosylamine 5-phosphate from glutamine & PRPP (5-phosphoribosyl-1-pyrophosphate); (b) inhibition of formation of adenylic and guanylic acid from inosinic acid; (c) inhibition of interconversion reactions among intermediate compounds in purine metabolism (12–16)
Thioguanine (6-TG)	2 mg/kg/day PO	Occasional nausea and vomiting usually well tolerated	Bone marrow depression	Acute leukemia	Is metabolized, along pathways similar to those of 6-MP to the nucleotide structurally corresponding to guanine and partially inhibits purine metabolizing enzymes. Its growth-inhibiting action seems to be substitution for guanine in nucleic acid synthesis, producing functionally altered polynucleotides.
Fluorouracil (5-FU; FU)	12.5 mg/kg/day iv x 3–5 day or 15 mg/kg/wk x 6	Nausea	Oral and gastrointestinal ulceration; stomatitis and diarrhea; bone marrow depression	Breast, large bowel, and ovarian cancer	Thymidylic acid is the deoxyribonucleotide of thymine (5-methyluracil), the pyrimidine base unique to DNA. Methylation of 2-deoxyuridine-5'-phosphate to yield this nucleic acid is ultimately catalyzed by thymidylate synthetase. 5-FU, when

The topmost mechanism text (above Mercaptopurine row):

These include biosynthesis of thymidylic acid from deoxyuridine 5'-monophosphate (thymidylic acid is the nucleotide specific to DNA), and the biosynthesis of inosinic acid, the precursor of adenine and guanine nucleotides in de novo purine biosynthesis (9–11)

Table 3 (continued)

Drug	Usual Dosage	Toxicity		Major Indications	Mechanism of Action
		Acute	Delayed		
					converted in vivo to the deoxynucleotide, has an affinity for the thymidylate synthetase system but is not itself incorporated into DNA. Thus, the primary cytotoxic action of the drug is to block thymidylate (and thereby DNA) synthesis. In addition, 5-FU is incorporated as the nucleotide into RNA, probably thereby depressing RNA synthesis directly by blocking incorporation of uracil and orotic acid into RNA (17–20).
Cytarabine hydrochloride (arabinosyl cytosine; Cytosar)	2–3 mg/kg/day iv until response or toxicity or 1–3 mg/kg iv over 24 hr for up to 10 day	Nausea and vomiting	Bone marrow depression; megaloblastosis	Acute leukemia	Originally proposed that inhibition is produced by phosphorylated derivative of ara C blocking conversion of cytidine diphosphate to deoxycytidine diphosphate. Later shown that tumor cell reductase is poorly inhibited by the di- or triphosphate (ara-CTP) of ara C. Most generally accepted is that ara-CTP inhibits DNA polymerase by competitive inhibition of deoxycytidine triphosphate rather than inhibiting polymerase synthesis (20–22).
NATURAL PRODUCTS (PLANT ALKALOIDS AND ANTIBIOTICS)					
Vinblastine sulfate (Velban)	0.1–0.2 mg/kg/wk iv or q 2 wks	Nausea and vomiting, local irritant	Alopecia; stomatitis; bone marrow depression; loss of reflexes	Hodgkin's disease and other lymphomas, solid cancers	Reversible mitotic arrest by binding drug to a cytoplasmic precursor of the spindle, probably during S-phase, and inhibition of RNA synthesis by effects on DNA-dependent RNA polymerase system. Vinca alkaloids also cause rearrangement of binding sites in protein of microtubular units in the mitotic spindle, permitting polymerization of protein to protofibrils (23–25).
Vincristine sulfate (Oncovin)	0.01–0.03 mg/kg/wk iv	Local irritant	Areflexia; peripheral neuritis; paralytic ileus; mild bone marrow depression	Acute lymphocytic leukemia, Hodgkin's disease and other lymphomas, solid cancers	

Table 3 (continued)

Drug	Usual Dosage	Toxicity Acute	Toxicity Delayed	Major Indications	Mechanism of Action
Dactinomycin (actinomycin D; Cosmegen)	0.015–0.05 mg/kg/wk (1–2.5 mg) 3–5 wk iv; wait for marrow recovery (3–4 wk), then repeat course	Nausea and vomiting; local irritant	Stomatitis; oral ulcers; diarrhea; alopecia; mental depression; bone marrow depression	Testicular carcinoma, Wilms' tumor, rhabdomyosarcoma, Ewings and osteogenic sarcoma, and other solid cancers	Dactinomycin forms a stable complex with DNA, producing inhibition of DNA-dependent RNA synthesis (26–29).
Mithramycin (Mithracin)	0.025–0.050 mg/kg q 2 day for up to 8 doses, iv	Nausea and vomiting; hepatotoxicity	Bone marrow depression (thrombocytopenia); hypocalcemia	Testicular carcinoma, trophoblastic neoplasms	Like dactinomycin, it inhibits DNA-dependent RNA synthesis without affecting DNA synthesis per se. It is thought to stabilize secondary structure of DNA by forming bridges between complementary strands of the helix (30).
OTHER SYNTHETIC AGENTS					
Procarbazine hydrochloride (Methyl hydrazine; ibenzmethyzin; Matulane)	Start 1–2 mg/kg/d PO; increase over 1 wk to 3 mg/kg; maintain for 3 wk then reduce to 2 mg/kg/day until toxicity	Nausea and vomiting	Bone marrow depression; CNS depression	Hodgkin's disease, non-Hodgkin's lymphoma, bronchogenic carcinoma	Uncertain. Exerts inhibitory effects on synthesis of protein, RNA, and DNA in cells in vitro. Its oxidative breakdown products degrade DNA in vivo. These derivatives may, in vivo, liberate formaldehyde, azomethine, N = hydroxymethyl derivatives, and hydrogen peroxide, which could produce the inhibitory effects. N-methylation of procarbazine occurs in vivo and a selective effect of the compound on methylation of transfer RNA could contribute to carcinostatic activity (31–35).
Hydroxyurea (Hydrea)	80 mg/kg PO single dose q 3 day or 20–30 mg/kg/day PO	Mild nausea and vomiting	Bone marrow depression	Chronic granulocytic leukemia	Directly inhibits DNA synthesis, primarily by inhibiting ribonucleoside diphosphate reductase. The effect is specific for the S-phase of the cell cycle (36–41).
Mitotane (ortho para' DDD; o, p' DDD; Lysodren)	6–15 mg/kg/day PO	Nausea and vomiting	Dermatitis, diarrhea; mental depression	Adrenal cortical carcinoma	Destruction of adrenal glands (42).
HORMONES					
Prednisone	10–100 mg/day PO	None	Hyperadrenocorticism	Acute and chronic lymphocytic leukemia, Hodgkin's disease, non-Hodgkin's lymphoma,	The precise mechanism of hormones is unknown. Steroids must bind to cytoplasmic receptor proteins of tumor cells to exert

Table 3 (continued)

Drug	Usual Dosage	Toxicity		Major Indications	Mechanism of Action
		Acute	Delayed		
Diethylstilbestrol (DES)	1, 5 or 14 mg/day PO (1 mg in prostate)	None	Fluid retention; hypercalcemia; feminization; uterine bleeding; if during pregnancy, may cause vaginal carcinoma in offspring	breast carcinoma, multiple myeloma	antitumor effects. Loss of specific steroid-binding protein can be correlated with resistance to anticancer effects of certain steroids in breast cancer and lymphomas. Adrenocortical hormones injure specific cell types through unknown means. They interfere with lymphoid proliferation, cause dissolution of lymphocytes and regression of lymphatic tissue, and inhibit growth in certain mesenchymal tissues. The anti-inflammatory activity of adrenal steroids may be similar to their therapeutic action in certain tumors (43–47).
				Breast and prostate carcinoma	
Ethinyl estradiol (Estinyl)	3 mg/day PO	None	Fluid retention; hypercalcemia; feminization; uterine bleeding	Breast and prostate carcinoma	
Testosterone enanthate (Testosterone heptanoate)	600–1200 mg/wk, im	None	Fluid retention; masculinization	Breast carcinoma	
Testolactone (Teslac)	100 mg 3 × wk, im	None	Fluid retention, masculinization	Breast carcinoma	
Testosterone propionate (Oreton)	50–100 mg, im 3 × wk	None	Fluid retention; masculinization	Breast carcinoma	
Fluoxymesterone (Halotestin)	10–20 mg/day PO	None	Fluid retention; masculinization; cholestatic jaundice	Breast carcinoma	
Dromostanolone propionate	100 mg 3 × wk, im	None	Fluid retention; masculinization; hypercalcemia	Breast carcinoma	
Hydroxyprogesterone caproate (delalutin)	1 g im twice/wk	None	None	Endometrial carcinoma	
Medroxyprogesterone acetate (Provera)	100–200 mg/day PO; 200–600 mg twice/wk	None	None	Endometrial carcinoma, renal cell, breast cancer	

Table 4 Investigational drugs[a]

| Drug | Usual Dosage | Toxicity | | Major Indications |
		Acute	Delayed	
Carmustine (bischloroethyl nitrosourea; BCNU) (48)	100 mg/m^2/day × 2 iv; not to be repeated for 6 wk	Nausea and vomiting; hepatotoxicity	Leukopenia and thrombocytopenia	Primary and secondary CNS neoplasms, Hodgkin's disease, multiple myeloma, malignant melanoma, GI adenocarcinoma, Burkitt's tumor, non-Hodgkin's lymphoma
Lomustine (cyclohexyl chloroethyl nitrosourea; CCNU) (48)	130 mg/m^2, PO, single dose repeated at 6 wk intervals	Nausea and vomiting; hepatotoxicity	Leukopenia and thrombocytopenia	Hodgkin's disease, primary and secondary CNS neoplasms, GI adenocarcinoma, bronchogenic carcinoma, renal cell
Hexamethylmelamine (49)	12 mg/kg/day × 21, PO	Nausea and vomiting	Bone marrow depression	Bronchogenic and ovarian carcinoma
Daunorubicin (daunomycin; Rubidomycin; Cerubidine) (50)	30–60 mg/m^2/day × 3 iv or 30–60 mg/m^2/wk, iv	Nausea, fever, red urine (not hematuria)	Bone marrow depression; cardiotoxicity; alopecia	Acute lymphocytic and granulocytic leukemia
Adriamycin (51, 52)	60–90 mg/m^2 iv, single dose or over 3 day; repeated q 3 wk	Nausea, red urine (not hematuria)	Bone marrow depression; cardiotoxicity; alopecia; stomatitis	Soft tissue, osteogenic & miscellaneous sarcomas, Hodgkin's disease, non-Hodgkin's lymphoma, bronchogenic & breast carcinoma
Bleomycin (53)	10–15 mg/m^2/wk or twice weekly, iv or im to total dose 300–400 mg	Nausea, vomiting, and fever; very toxic	Edema of hands; pulmonary fibrosis; stomatitis; alopecia	Hodgkin's disease, non-Hodgkin's lymphoma
Dacarbazine (DTIC; DIC) (54)	3.5 mg/kg/day iv × 10 repeated 28 day	Nausea and vomiting ("flu-like" syndrome")	Bone marrow depression (rare)	Malignant melanoma, Hodgkin's disease
Streptozotocin (55)	1 g/m^2/wk iv × 4 continued if response is observed	Nausea and vomiting	Renal damage	Malignant insulinoma, carcinoid
Asparaginase (Elspar) (56, 57)	200 IU/kg/day iv × 28 day	Nausea, fever, and possible anaphylactic reaction	Hepatotoxicity; pancreatitis; CNS depression	Acute lymphocytic leukemia

[a]Experimental drug; not yet approved by the FDA and may be available only from the Investigational Drug Branch, Cancer Therapy Evaluation Program, National Cancer Institute. Dosage is tentative.

plasma, concentrates in lymphatic tissues, and is rapidly excreted in the urine as both unchanged drug and metabolites (89, 90). The pharmacokinetics in man indicate a plasma half-life of 3.5 hr after iv administration, with 85% of the radioactivity being excreted within 48 hr (91).

Phase I clinical studies established the maximum tolerated doses as 533 mg/m² iv single weekly dose, 160–200 mg/m² daily X 5 repeated every 3 weeks (92), and 1.6 mg/kg (60 mg/m²) iv daily for 10 days (93). The principal toxic effects are severe nausea and vomiting, which are apparently dose related, and marrow suppression.

Although antitumor activity against solid tumors was originally reported (93), it does not appear to be confirmed in Phase II clinical trials (94). However, promising results are reported in the treatment of acute myeloblastic leukemia (95, 96) confirming the original reports from Czechoslovakia (97).

Bleòmycin

This agent is actually a mixture of sulfur-containing glycopeptide antibiotics isolated from a strain of *Streptomyces verticillus* (98). In the presence of sulfhydryl compounds, bleomycin binds to DNA and causes single strand scission (99, 100) which appears to be responsible for the inhibition of thymidine incorporation into DNA (101).

The drug has demonstrated antitumor activity against a number of experimental animal tumors including Ehrlich ascites carcinoma in mice, virus-induced tumors (102), and methyl cholanthrene-induced dermoid carcinoma transplanted intramuscularly in mice (103). While bleomycin is fairly active against a spectrum of experimental mouse tumors, including Lewis lung carcinoma, it has only minimal activity against L1210 and P388 leukemias. The drug accumulates in high concentration in skin and tumor tissue of experimental animals, as detected by measurements 30 min after iv administration (104). Similar findings of drug accumulation in skin and tumor tissue are reported in man, with urinary excretions of about 40% of the iv-administered drug in 24 hr (104).

The clinical data available to the Cancer Therapy Evaluation Program for 1174 patients treated with bleomycin reveals significant response rates in squamous cell carcinomas at various anatomical sites, malignant lymphomas, and testicular carcinoma (53). Drug toxicities include cutaneous reaction, stomatitis, alopecia, pyrexia, nausea and vomiting, and potentially fatal pulmonary fibrosis. However, the drug is remarkable in its lack of bone marrow toxicity even at very high doses. The most commonly used dose schedule appears to be 15 mg/m² iv twice weekly.

cis-Platinum (II) Diamminedichloride

This antineoplastic agent is one of a group of platinum compounds first noted to have antibiotic effect by Rosenberg and his colleagues, and since found to exhibit antitumor activity in animals (105–108). Structurally, it is a complex formed by a central atom of platinum surrounded by two chlorine or ammonia moeities in *cis*-position (107).

Although this compound inhibits incorporation of labeled precursors of DNA, RNA, and protein in mammalian cells in vitro (109), experiments in mice bearing Ehrlich ascites tumor cells indicate a selective inhibition of DNA synthesis (110). Interference with DNA synthesis is apparently caused by cross-linking of complementary strands of DNA (111).

The drug exhibits antitumor activity against a number of experimental systems, including B16 melanoma in mice, Walker 256 carcinosarcoma in rats (112), sarcoma 180 in mice (108), and DMBA-induced mammary tumors in rats (113). The selection of the drug for clinical studies stems from its significant activity in the L1210 system over a variety of ip dosage schedules. The drug has no activity by the oral route (Venditti, unpublished data of NCI).

cis-Platinum exhibits synergism in experimental tumors when combined with a variety of anticancer compounds including alkylating agents (114), pyrimidine and purine antimetabolites (115), ICRF 159 (116), and vinca alkaloids (115).

Pharmacokinetic observations in man show that platinum is rapidly removed from the circulation and widely distributed in the tissues. Less than 10% of the platinum remains in the plasma at 1 hr (117). The initial half-life ranges between 41 and 49 min, while the secondary one is between 58.5 and 73 hr (118). About 90% of the plasma radioactivity is protein bound; 19.2–33.9% and 25–43.6% of the administered drug is excreted by urine within 24 and 96 hr respectively (118).

Platinum has been used in Phase I clinical studies on various dose schedules: single iv dose repeated every 3 weeks (118, 119); daily iv dose X 5 days, repeated every 3 weeks (119, 120); and, daily doses by iv push until toxicity (121). The reported toxic effects include predictable and reversible myelosuppression, reversible renal insufficiency, high frequency ototoxicity detectable by audiometry, and GI intolerance. Phase II studies in major signal tumors are now in progress using either a high intermittent dose (50 mg/m2/day iv, repeated every 3 weeks) or 15–20 mg/m2/day iv X 5. Although some activity against malignant lymphomas and solid tumors was reported in the Phase I studies, it is too early to draw definite conclusions on antitumor activity in man.

Chromomycin A_3

This anticancer antibiotic of Japanese origin was isolated from a culture of *Streptomyces griseus* No. 7 (122) and is commercially available in Japan as "Toyomycin." Chromomycin A_3 is an aureolic acid analog consisting of an aglycone moiety (chromomycinone) and five attached pentoses (123–125). Studies of the mechanism of action show that Chromomycin A_3, in the presence of Mg^{2+}, inhibits DNA-dependent RNA polymerase (126–128). The interaction of the drug with DNA requires the presence of a guanine base (126, 127, 129). Inhibition of DNA polymerase has been demonstrated by Hartman et al (130).

The drug was selected for clinical trial on the basis of its activity against P388 leukemia in mice, where it shows superiority to both mithramycin and olivomycin. Cytostatic activity is also reported in a number of experimental animal tumors including Yoshida's sarcoma, Sarcoma 180, Ehrlich ascites, and others (131–133). Little activity has been reported against L1210 leukemia in mice.

Preclinical pharmacokinetic studies show that the drug is rapidly excreted in bile and urine, and almost totally cleared from the plasma in 3 hr after iv administration (134). Chromomycin A_3 has been used as a single agent in more than 500 Japanese and South African patients with a wide variety of neoplastic diseases (135, 136). Objective responses are reported in malignant lymphomas (137–141) and in solid tumors including bronchogenic carcinoma, GI adenocarcinomas, carcinomas of the female genital tract, malignant gliomas, and soft tissue sarcomas (139, 140, 142). The drug has also been used in combination with radiotherapy (140, 143) and with alkylating agents, where a synergistic effect is noted (144, 145).

Toxicity reported in Japanese and South African studies is surprisingly low, consisting of nausea and vomiting after daily doses of 1 mg or higher (139, 140), moderate leucopenia (137, 139, 140), and local reaction at the injection site with necrosis after extravasal administration. Recent Phase I studies in the United States reveal that renal toxicity is dose limiting when a daily iv dose for 5 days is escalated above 0.9 mg/m². Hypocalcemia, which has not been detected in previous studies, is also reported. Other dose schedules are now being explored and Phase II studies using lower doses are being proposed to avoid the dose-limiting side effects.

1,2-Di(3,5-dioxopiperazine-1-yl)propane

This compound, known as ICRF 159, was developed by the Imperial Cancer Research Fund facilities in London, England (146). Although the exact mechanism of action has not been fully elucidated, the cytotoxic effect occurs during late prophase and early metaphase (G_2-M) and involves inhibition of DNA synthesis (147, 148).

ICRF 159 was selected for clinical trials on the basis of antitumor activity in L1210 leukemia and in the Lewis lung system. The drug exhibits definite schedule dependency in L1210, where it is most active on an intermittent schedule and less active when administered daily. The most exciting data have been observed in the Lewis lung tumor which, when implanted in the flank of a mouse, metastasizes spontaneously to the lungs. Salsbury et al (149) examined this property of the tumor in a series of experiments comparing the ability of ICRF 159 and cyclophosphamide to prevent the metastases. ICRF 159 completely inhibited metastases formation at doses having little influence on the rate of growth of the primary tumor implant. Inhibition was produced by the effect of ICRF 159 on the development of blood vessels in the invading margins of the primary tumor. Cyclophosphamide did not prevent metastatic spread when used on schedules similar to ICRF 159 but did decrease the number and size of the metastases. All the untreated control mice developed metastases.

Initial clinical trials in Great Britain have been performed on a schedule of daily oral doses of 20–30 mg/kg/day in divided doses administered until the occurrence of hematologic toxicity (150–153). Leukopenia and thrombopenia occur within a few days of treatment initiation and are dose related (5 g total dose is the current British restriction). Dramatic decreases in the number of circulating blast cells are described in leukemia patients, and no cross-resistance to their antileukemic drugs has been noted.

Two studies with ICRF 150 have been completed in the United States (154, 155). Based on the pharmacokinetic study in man, the recommended dose for Phase II clinical studies is 3000 mg/m² po given once weekly. Phase II studies in the major signal tumors are in progress.

5(3,3-Dimethyl-1-triazeno)-imidazole-4-carboxamide (DTIC)

This drug is one of the new synthetic anticancer agents developed by the Division of Cancer Treatment of the National Cancer Institute (156–158). The postulated mechanisms of action include alkylating activity (159), inhibition of DNA synthesis, de novo purine synthesis, and SH interaction (160).

Experimental antitumor activity was originally reported against L1210 leukemia in mice (157) and is also seen in sarcoma 180, adenocarcinoma 755, and Ehrlich ascites carcinoma in mice (161). The drug does not appear to be schedule dependent (162) or cell cycle stage specific (163). Pharmacokinetic studies in man show a short plasma half-life and rapid urinary excretion by a renal tubular secretory mechanism. About 46% of the administered drug is excreted in 6 hr, 21% as DTIC, and 20% as AIC (5-amino-4-imidazole carboxamide), which is the final metabolite of the DTIC metabolic pathway (164–167).

Clinically, the drug is usually given in daily schedules, either 70–160 mg/m²/day × 10 repeated every 28 days or 250 mg/m²/d × 5 repeated every 21 days (54). However, high intermittent doses of 1050–1250 mg/m² repeated every 4–5 weeks have been reported (168). DTIC toxicities in man include bone marrow depression, nausea and vomiting, and a flu-like syndrome. Although the drug has been tested against various solid tumors, its most significant activity in man is in malignant melanoma. Data reported to the Cancer Therapy Evaluation Program reveal objective responses in 166 of 758 melanoma patients for a response rate of 22%, which is remarkable in its consistency throughout various clinical trials. The drug has been studied in combination with other active drugs in malignant melanoma and sarcomas.

1,3-bis(2-Chloroethyl)-1-nitrosourea (BCNU)

BCNU was the first of an exciting new group of compounds, the nitrosoureas, developed and clinically tested in studies sponsored by the Division of Cancer Treatment, NCI. It was synthesized, during the rational search for active congeners of 1-methyl-1-nitrosourea, as the twenty-third analog evaluated against L1210 leukemia in mice (169). Studies on the mechanism of action have shown alkylating activity by formation of a diazohydroxide and/or 2-chlorethylamine (170), selective interference with the utilization of histidine in 1-carbon metabolism through inhibition of formininotransferase (171), increased NADase activity and decreased concentration of tumor NAD⁺ (172), and decreased DNA nucleotidyltransferase activity (173).

BCNU has antitumor activity against L1210 mouse leukemia (174), where it shows no schedule dependency for maximum activity and is equally effective as a single dose every other day for 8 doses, once every fourth day for 4 doses, or every

3 hr X 8 each fourth day for 4 courses. It is also active against intracranially implanted L1210 as well as leukemia L1798 and Dunning leukemia (175, 176).

BCNU has a wide range of effectiveness in a spectrum of other experimental tumors such as Wagner osteogenic sarcoma, Sarcoma 180, Ehrlich ascites carcinoma, Krebs II ascites carcinoma, and Taper ascites hepatoma in mice as well as Flexner-Jobling carcinoma, Jensen sarcoma, Yoshida sarcoma, Sugiura-Brown fibrosarcoma, and Iglesia's ovarian and adrenal tumors in rats (177). Moreover, it is also active against B16 melanoma, adenocarcinoma E0771, Ridgeway osteogenic sarcoma, and Sarcoma T241 (178).

Pharmacokinetic studies in experimental animals and man indicate that BCNU is rapidly metabolized; intact drug is not detected in body fluids shortly after administration. Studies with ^{14}C-labeled drug show prolonged levels of isotope in tissues of monkeys and man, probably representing radioactive fragments of the parent compound. DeVita et al (179) suggest that the breakdown products of the drug may be associated with its delayed toxicity. The radioactive compound is rapidly excreted by mice, suggesting biliary excretion and enterohepatic circulation, but the pattern of excretion is slower in both man and monkeys.

BCNU has received extensive clinical trial in a variety of tumors, and the compiled data of the Cancer Therapy Evaluation Program reveal high response rates in advanced Hodgkin's disease (75/149 = 50%), brain tumors (34/78 = 42%), multiple myeloma (12/31 = 39%), malignant melanoma (17/108 = 16%), and large bowel cancer (17/123 = 13%). In most cases, BCNU has been given at 200–300 mg/m^2 administered intravenously over 2–3 days. The current recommended dose regimen is 100 mg/m^2/day X 2 iv with courses repeated every 6 weeks.

Organ toxicities in man include delayed leukopenia and thrombocytopenia, nausea and vomiting, and hepatotoxicity. The few cases of pulmonary toxicity that have been reported to the Cancer Therapy Evaluation Program suggest that the effect may be drug related.

1-(2-Chloroethyl)-3-cyclohexyl-1-nitrosourea (CCNU)

This agent was the first analog of BCNU selected for clinical studies because of its superior experimental activity in leukemia L1210 and great lipid solubility (48).

Unlike BCNU, CCNU has an asymmetrical structure which enables identification of its breakdown products (cyclohexylamine, cyclohexylisocyanate, and N,N'-dicyclohexylurea). Studies in L1210 ascites leukemia show that only CCNU or cyclohexylisocyanate prolong the S-phase to twice the normal period, while the other products are inactive (180). CCNU inhibition of DNA nucleotidyltransferase activity is about the same as that produced by BCNU (181). Recent studies on the binding of the breakdown products of ^{14}C-labeled CCNU reveal that radioactivity from cyclohexyl-labeled CCNU is extensively bound to proteins and not to the nucleic acids, while radioactivity from the ethyl-labeled CCNU is nucleic acid bound with only a fraction bound to proteins (182). These data suggest that CCNU interacts with proteins through cyclohexylcarbamoylation (183) and with nucleic acids by alkylation.

The antitumor activity of CCNU is superior to BCNU in L1210 leukemia, and it is also significantly active against Walker 256 carcinosarcoma in rats and B16 melanoma (48).

Pharmacokinetic studies in rodents show that 75% of the ^{14}C cyclohexyl- or ethyl-labeled CCNU is excreted in the urine in 24 hr after oral or ip administration, while about 10–20% of carbonyl- or ethyl-labeled CCNU is expired as $^{14}CO_2$ (184). CCNU is rapidly metabolized in dogs and monkeys and excreted predominantly in the urine (184). Pharmacokinetic studies with C^{14}-labeled drug in man show rapid metabolism, prolonged plasma half-life of radiolabeled compounds ranging from 16–48 hr, and urinary excretion of 50% of administered dose within 24 hr and 75% within 4 days with no parent drug detectable in the urine (185).

Clinically, clear superiority of CCNU over BCNU has been demonstrated in a controlled study of Hodgkin's disease (186) and activity is reported against malignant gliomas (187), gastrointestinal cancer (188), carcinoma of the breast, hypernephroma, bladder cancer, malignant melanoma, and squamous cell carcinomas in various anatomical sites. The toxic effects of CCNU include nausea, vomiting, and delayed leukopenia and thrombocytopenia (189). The recommended dose is 130 mg/m² (po), repeated every 6 weeks.

1-(2-Chloroethyl)-3-(4-methyl-cyclohexyl)-1-nitrosourea (Methyl CCNU)

This is a methylated analog of CCNU selected for clinical trial because of its superiority to both BCNU and CCNU in the advanced Lewis lung tumor in mice (48). The drug also has antitumor activity against L1210 leukemia by both the iv and oral routes.

Pharmacokinetic studies in man after single oral doses of either cyclohexyl- or chloroethyl-labeled methyl-CCNU show rapid absorption of both moieties of the parent compound, with significant plasma levels of radioactivity as early as 10 min after administration (190). The average peak plasma levels of radioactivity occur at 3 hr for the cyclohexyl moiety and at 6 hr for the chloroethyl moiety. These peak levels correspond to plasma concentrations of between 2 and 4 μg/ml of drug equivalence. The disappearance of radioactivity from plasma for the chloroethyl moiety is single phased with a half-life of 36 hr, while the cyclohexyl moiety disappears biphasically with an early exponential phase having a half-life of 24 hr, followed by a slower phase with a half-life of 72 hr. No parent drug is detectable in any plasma sample.

Phase II clinical trials of methyl-CCNU are proceeding in a number of institutions and cooperative groups. The data accumulated by the Cancer Therapy Evaluation Program for more than 300 patients indicate methyl-CCNU activity against adenocarcinoma of the colon, malignant gliomas, malignant melanoma, malignant lymphomas, and squamous cell carcinomas at different anatomical sites. However, the numbers are still small and more data are needed to confirm these findings.

The toxic effects of methyl-CCNU include nausea and vomiting at doses of 170 mg/m² or higher, and delayed bone marrow toxicity that is dose limiting (191). The recommended dose is 200 mg/m² po every 6 weeks with individual adjustment.

NEW DIRECTIONS IN CHEMOTHERAPY

Recently, the chemotherapy program area has been expanded and integrated into the Division of Cancer Treatment in the NCI under the new emphasis of the National Cancer Plan. The immediate objectives of the DCT program are to increase the number of patients responding to cancer therapy and prolong the length of the disease-free period of remission. The ultimate goal is the cure or control of cancer.

The increased scope of the DCT program includes not only the drug development and clinical testing aspects of the former chemotherapy program but also the improvement of therapy by combined modality approaches. These efforts will proceed largely on disease-oriented lines, with the major emphasis on effective treatment for the solid tumors that are the major cause of cancer deaths in the United States.

The major thrust in combined modality treatment will seek an integration of chemotherapy with surgery and/or radiotherapy, and perhaps with immunotherapy. This is a logical approach in view of the fact that chemotherapy is the only modality of unquestioned effectiveness against tumor cells found anywhere in the body. As pointed out earlier, chemotherapy, either alone or with other modalities, can cure some patients with at least eight different kinds of cancer.

The philosophic base of the combined modality approach is the recognition that surgery and radiotherapy have reached a plateau in their ability to cure solid tumors. These localized modalities kill tumor cells only where they are applied, and it is not technically feasible to increase the scope of their application for tumors in which they are effective. They fail to cure many patients, even when they remove all the tumor visible to the naked eye or diagnostic X-ray film. The reason for this failure is felt to be the presence of disseminated disease foci at the time of surgical excision of the primary tumor, which many times includes the surrounding tissue and part of the regional lymph nodes.

Chemotherapy, when used optimally, has the potential to eradicate these metastatic foci. The drug regimens that have shown the highest degree of activity in advanced disease will be the prime candidates for use in the combined modality approach. The degree of cell kill necessary to shrink a bulky solid tumor mass by greater than 50% is quite large. If this degree of cell kill could be directed against the relatively small tumor burden remaining after surgical excision, perhaps eradication of the last neoplastic cell can be achieved.

The major successes of chemotherapy have been in the hematologic malignancies, especially acute lymphocytic leukemia and advanced Hodgkin's disease. These triumphs of cure and long disease-free survival have not been translated to the common solid tumors, which are the major cause of cancer mortality in this country. Many reasons have been put forth for this disparity of results, among them the differing kinetics of the tumors and the relative accessibility of the tumor cells to significant drug concentrations. One additional factor, which is often neglected, involves the point on the treatment strategy for a given disease at which chemotherapy is introduced.

As a general rule, the major potential for cure in any tumor lies in the initial therapeutic approach. In leukemia, a disseminated disease, chemotherapy is the treatment of choice at all stages of the disease (Figure 1). The optimum drug regimens are used in early disease, while new drugs or regimens are tried in later stages and the successful ones are integrated into the initial therapeutic approach. On the other hand, surgery and/or radiotherapy are the primary approaches in solid tumors without disseminated disease. Chemotherapy is relegated, almost exclusively, to secondary or tertiary treatment after the local modalities fail and the disease is advanced and disseminated. The secondary or tertiary treatment is rarely curative in any tumor, including hematological malignancies. It is understandable, therefore, that the chemotherapy presently used in solid tumors is not curative, although tumor regression, palliative benefit, and some survival increases are achieved. Any comparison of the results of chemotherapy in solid tumors and hematological malignancies should take into consideration the differences in the therapeutic approaches.

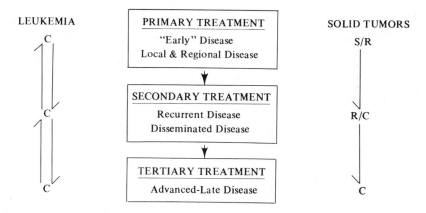

Figure 1 Comparison of therapeutic modalities in leukemia and solid tumors. C = chemotherapy; R = radiotherapy; S = surgery.

The proposed therapeutic strategy for increasing cure rates in solid tumors involves the integration of chemotherapy into combined modality approaches for primary treatment (Figure 2). In this scheme, new drugs or drug combinations would be tested in advanced disease and those showing positive results would be studied in the primary therapy of disseminated disease. An optimum regimen developed in this manner would then be integrated into combined modality treatment in local and regional disease.

Figure 3 outlines this type of approach to a therapeutic attack against breast cancer. The solid arrows show the standard flow of therapy, beginning with mastectomy and moving through hormonal manipulation and eventually to chemotherapy. The broken arrows indicate the concerted efforts of the NCI Division of Cancer

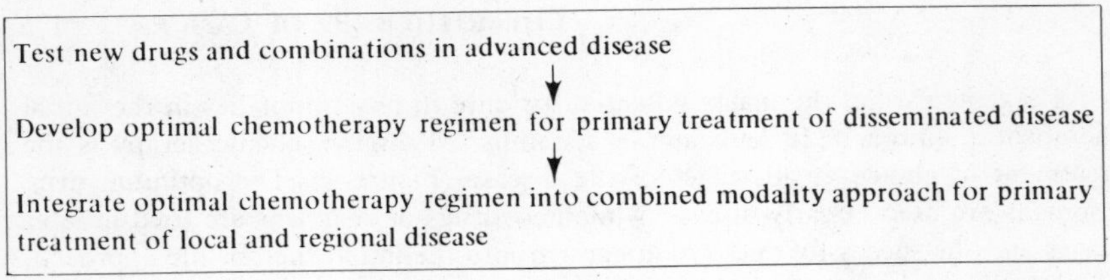

Test new drugs and combinations in advanced disease

↓

Develop optimal chemotherapy regimen for primary treatment of disseminated disease

↓

Integrate optimal chemotherapy regimen into combined modality approach for primary treatment of local and regional disease

Figure 2 Proposed strategy for developing combined modality therapy for solid tumors.

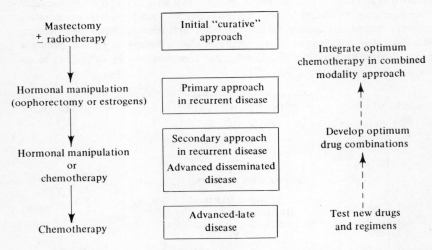

Figure 3 Proposed integration of chemotherapy into the treatment of breast cancer.

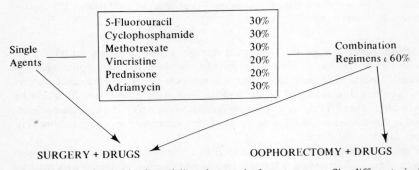

Figure 4 Plan of combined modality therapy in breast cancer. Six different single agents produce 20–30% objective response and combinations of these can yield an approximate 60% response rate.

Treatment and the Breast Cancer Task Force aimed at the use of chemotherapy in the earlier stages of treatment. A specific plan of combined modality therapy in breast cancer is shown in Figure 4.

Of all the major solid tumors, breast cancer is one of the most responsive to chemotherapy. Various agents have the ability to produce a significant number of objective regressions, as shown in the Cancer Therapy Evaluation Program summary of pooled results for single agents given in Table 5. In general, five drugs have been most active: 5-FU, Cytoxan, methotrexate, vincristine, and prednisone (which alone has an overall response rate of $\sim$ 20%).

Table 5 Summary of single agents active against advanced breast cancer

Drug	No. Evaluable Patients	No. Objective Responses	Response (%)
Alkylating agents			
Cyclophosphamide	165	52	31.5
Nitrogen mustard	92	32	35
Phenylalanine mustard	86	20	23
Chlorambucil	54	11	20.4
Thio-TEPA	162	48	30
Antimetabolites			
5-fluorouracil	1052	310	29
Methotrexate	259	87	33.6
6-Mercaptopurine	45	6	13
Arabinosyl cytosine	64	6	9
Vinca Alkaloids			
Vincristine	164	32	19.5
Vinblastine	95	19	20
Antibiotics			
Actinomycin D	44	5	11
Mithramycin	32	5	16
Mitomycin	60	23	38
Miscellaneous agents			
Hydroxyurea	21	4	20
BCNU	40	15	37

The basic tools, therefore, for a combined approach have existed for a long time. Greenspan (192), at Mt. Sinai Hospital in New York, first reported that a combination of methotrexate and thio-TEPA gave a 60% response rate (25 of 40 patients). In 1966 he reported (193) that multiple drug therapy consisting of thio-TEPA, methotrexate, cyclophosphamide, 5-FU, and testosterone produced regressions in 59 of 73 patients (81%).

At the American Association for Cancer Research Meeting in 1969, Dr. Richard Cooper of the Buffalo Medical Group presented a study combining five drugs as follows: 5-fluorouracil: 12 mg/kg/day × 4, then 500 mg/wk iv; methotrexate: 25–50 gm/wk iv; vincristine: 35 μg/kg/wk iv; cyclophosphamide: 2.5 mg/kg/day po; and prednisone: 0.75 mg/kg/day po (194). He reported responses in 90% (54 of 60) of patients treated. This initial report stimulated wide-ranging studies of combination regimens, and data now are available on 323 patients treated with intensive combination chemotherapy. Objective responses have been reported in 244, or more than 75%. Even if the results of Cooper are excluded, the overall response is still 56% and indicates a significant potential for cell kill in a large percentage of patients with advanced breast cancer. Responses to various therapeutic modalities available are compared in Table 6.

Table 6 Comparison of therapeutic modalities in breast cancer

Modality	Response (%)
Oophorectomy	40–50
Hormonal ablative surgery	30–40
Androgens	20
Estrogens	35
Single agent chemotherapy	30
Combination chemotherapy	56–75

Clearly, chemotherapy should be involved in the therapeutic approach at an earlier stage of disease and treatment, perhaps in combination with other therapeutic modalities so as to attempt to use the large cell kill potential when, theoretically at least, the amount of residual disease is smaller. It is hoped this will lead to an increased incidence of disease-free survival.

CONCLUSION

Chemotherapy is still a relatively new modality of cancer therapy, dating back only to 1946 with the initial clinical trials of nitrogen mustard. A wide range of active agents with a broad variety of applications has since developed. As a result, a Subspeciality Board of Medical Oncology has been approved by the American Board of Internal Medicine. The curative potential of chemotherapy alone, or combined with surgery and/or radiotherapy, has been established in at least eight tumors which, unfortunately, account for only a little over 10% of cancers. In five other tumors, chemotherapy is associated with enhanced survival, and it is thought that combined modality approaches offer an immediate chance of even greater survival gains and possible cure. This is especially true for adenocarcinoma of the breast and ovary, two of the major cancers causing death in women.

Palliation for advanced solid tumors is a major role of chemotherapy today, and its value to patients should not be downgraded. It is often forgotten that most of internal medicine practice is palliation of disease after the excitement of making the differential diagnosis. Still, the ultimate future of chemotherapy for solid tumors does not lie in palliation alone but in combination with surgery and radiotherapy in the treatment of primary disease. The localized modalities of surgery and radiation therapy fail in many cases, not because they do not eradicate the primary disease but because microscopic metastatic foci exist outside the treated area. It is hoped that in palliative treatment for advanced disease, regimens of cytotoxic potential will be uncovered which, when used in the primary therapeutic approach as an adjuvant to surgical therapy or radiotherapy, will destroy metastatic foci and increase the number of patients who survive free of disease indefinitely.

Literature Cited

1. Carter, S. K. 1972. *Yearb. Cancer 1972*, ed. R. L. Clark, R. W. Cumley, 475–98. Chicago: Yearb. Med. Publ. 515 pp.
2. Schmidt, L. H., Fradkin, R., Sullivan, R., Flowers, A. 1965. *Cancer Chemother. Rep. Suppl. 2:1–1528*
3. Lawley, P., Brookes, P. 1967. *J. Mol. Biol.* 25:143–60
4. Karnofsky, D. A. 1958. *Ann. NY Acad. Sci.* 66:657–1266
5. Fairley, K. F., Simister, J. M. 1965. *Cyclophosphamide* Baltimore: Williams & Wilkins
6. Van Duuren, B. L. 1969. *Ann. NY Acad. Sci.* 163:589–1029
7. Wheeler, G. P. 1962. *Cancer Res.* 22: 651–88
8. Livingston, R. B., Carter, S. K. 1970. *Single Agents in Cancer Chemotherapy.* New York:Plenum. 405 pp.
9. Bertino, J. R. 1963. *Cancer Res.* 23: 1286–1306
10. Werkheiser, W. C. 1963. *Cancer Res.* 23:1277–85
11. Bertino, J. R., Huennekens, F. M. 1971. *Ann. NY Acad. Sci.* 186:1–519
12. Burchenal, J., Ellison, R. 1961. *Clin. Pharmacol. Ther.* 2:523–41
13. Calabresi, P., Welch, A. 1962. *Ann. Rev. Med.* 13:147–202
14. Elion, G., Callahan, S., Rundles, R. W., Hitchings, G. H. 1963. *Cancer Res.* 23: 1207–17
15. Brockman, R. 1963. *Cancer Res.* 23: 1191–1201
16. Hitchings, G. H., Rhoads, C. P. 1954. *Ann. NY Acad. Sci.* 60:183–508
17. Heidelberger, C. et al 1957. *Nature* 179:663
18. Bosch, L., Harbers, E., Heidelberger, C. 1958. *Cancer Res.* 18:335–43
19. Harbers, E., Chaudhuri, N., Heidelberger, C. 1959. *J. Biol. Chem.* 234: 1255–62
20. Chu, M., Fischer, G. 1962. *Biochem. Pharmacol.* 11:423–30
21. Moore, E., Cohen, S. 1967. *J. Biol. Chem.* 242:2116–18
22. Furth, J., Cohen, S. 1968. *Cancer Res.* 28:2061–67
23. Creasey, W. 1968. *Fed. Proc.* 27:760
24. Madoc-Jones, H., Mauro, F. 1968. *J. Cell. Physiol.* 72:185
25. Bensch, K., Malawista, S. 1969. *J. Cell. Biol.* 40:95–107
26. Young, C. W. 1969. *Am. J. Clin. Path.* 52:130–37
27. Ro, T., Narayan, K., Busch, H. 1966. *Cancer Res.* 26:780–85
28. Schwartz, H., Sodergren, J., Ambaye, R. 1968. *Cancer Res.* 28:192–97
29. Kessel, D., Wodinsky, I. 1968. *Biochem. Pharmacol.* 17:161–64
30. Kersten, W., Kersten, H., Szybalski, W. 1966. *Biochemistry* 5:236–44
31. Hope-Stone, H. 1965. In *Natulan (Ibenzmethyzin)*, ed. A. Jelliffe, J. Marks, 15–19. New York: Wright
32. Sartorelli, A., Tsunamura, S. 1966. *Mol. Pharmacol.* 2:275
33. Berneis, K., Kofler, M., Bollag, W., Kaiser, A., Langemann, A. 1963. *Experientia* 19:132–33
34. Kreis, W., Yen, W. 1965. *Experientia* 21:284
35. Kreis, W. 1970. *Cancer Res.* 30:82–89
36. Young, C., Hodas, S. 1964. *Science* 146:1172
37. Turner, M., Abrams, R., Lieberman, I. 1966. *J. Biol. Chem.* 241:5777–80
38. Elford, H. 1968. *Biochem. Biophys. Res. Commun.* 33:129
39. Krakoff, I., Brown, N., Reichard, P. 1968. *Cancer Res.* 28:1559–65
40. Schabel, F. 1968. In *The Proliferation and Spread of Neoplastic Cells*, 379–408. Baltimore: Williams & Wilkins

41. Brockman, R. W., Shaddix, S., Laster, W. R. 1970. *Cancer Res.* 30:2358–68
42. Hutter, A. M., Kahoe, D. E. 1966. *Am. J. Med.* 41:572–81
43. American Cancer Society. 1965. *Cancer* 18:1517–1666
44. Baxter, J. D., Harris, A. W., Tomkins, G. M., Cohn, M. 1971. *Science* 171: 189–91
45. Krakoff, I. 1967. In *Cancer Chemotherapy,* ed. I. Brodsky, 77–83. New York: Grune & Stratton
46. Pincus, G., Vollmer, E., Eds. 1960. *Biological Activities of Steriods in Relation to Cancer.* New York: Academic
47. Tait, J. F., Burstein, S. 1964. *The Hormones* 5:441–557
48. Carter, S. K., Schabel, F. M., Broder, L. E., Johnston, T. P. 1972. *Advan. Cancer Res.* 16:273–332
49. Blum, R. H., Livingston, R. B., Carter, S. K. 1973. *Eur. J. Cancer* 9:195–202
50. Bernard, J., Paul, R., Boiron, M., Jacquillat, C., Moral, R., Eds. 1969. *Recent Results in Cancer Research. Rubidomycin—A New Agent Against Cancer.* New York: Springer. 178 pp.
51. Carter, S. K., DiMarco, A., Ghione, M., Krakoff, I. H., Mathe G. 1972. *Int. Symp. Adriamycin.* New York: Springer. 251 pp.
52. Blum, R. H., Carter, S. K. 1973. *Ann. Intern. Med.* Submitted for publication
53. Blum, R. H., Carter, S. K., Agre, K. 1973. *Cancer* 31:903–14
54. Friedman, M. A., Carter, S. K. 1972. *Eur. J. Cancer* 8:85–92
55. Broder, L. E., Carter, S. K. 1973. *Ann. Intern. Med.* 79:108–18
56. Tallal, L. et al 1970. *Cancer* 25:732–34
57. Whitecar, J. P., Bodey, G., Harris, J., Freireich, E. J. 1970. *N. Engl. J. Med.* 282:732–34
58. Arcamone, F. et al 1969. *Biotechnol. Bioeng.* 11:1101–10
59. Arcamone, F. et al See Ref. 51, pp. 9–22
60. Calendi, E. et al 1965. *Biochim. Biophys. Acta* 103:25–49
61. Lambertenghi-Deliliers, G. See Ref. 51, pp. 26–34
62. Silvestrini, R., Gambarucci, D., Dasdia, T. 1970. *Tumori* 56:137–48
63. Wang, J., Chervinsky, D. S., Rosen, J. 1971. *Proc. Am. Assoc. Cancer Res.* 12:77
64. Goldin, A. 1972. See Ref. 51, pp. 64–74
65. Sandberg, J. S., Howsden, F. L., DiMarco, A., Goldin, A. 1970. *Cancer Chemother. Rep.,* Pt. 1, 54:1–7
66. DiMarco, A., Gaetani, M., Scarpinato, B. 1969. *Cancer Chemother. Rep.* 53: 33–37
67. Yesair, D. W. et al 1972. *Cancer Res.* 32:1177–83
68. Arena, E. 1971. *Arzeim. Forsch.* 81: 1258–63
69. Bertazzoli, C., Chieli, T., Ferni, G., Ricevuti, G., Solcia, E. 1972. *Toxicol. Appl. Pharmacol.* 21:287–301
70. Benjamin, R. S. 1972. *Int. Congr. Hematol., XIV, Sao Paulo, Brazil,* Abstr. No. 508
71. Bachur, N. et al 1973. *Proc. Am. Assoc. Cancer Res.* 14:56
72. Gottlieb, J. A. et al 1973. *Proc. Am. Assoc. Cancer Res.* 14:88
73. Hanka, L. J., Evans, J. S., Mason, D. J., Dietz, A. 1966. *Antimicrob. Ag. Chemother.* 619–24
74. Bergy, M. E., Herr, R. R. 1967. *Antimicrob. Ag. Chemother.* 625–30
75. Piskala, A., Sorm, F. 1964. *Collect. Czech. Chem. Commun.* 29:2060–76
76. Jurovcik, M., Raska, K. Jr., Sormova, Z., Sorm, F. 1965. *Collect. Czech. Chem. Commun.* 30:3370–76
77. Jurovcik, M., Raska, K. Jr., Sormova, Z., Sorm, F. 1965. *Collect. Czech. Chem. Commun.* 30:3215–17
78. Cihak, A., Tykva, R., Sorm, F. 1966. *Collect. Czech. Chem. Commun.* 31: 3015–19
79. Raska, K. Jr. et al 1966. *Collect. Czech. Chem. Commun.* 31:2809–15
80. Cihak, A., Vesely, J., Sorm, F. 1967. *Collect. Czech. Chem. Commun.* 32: 3427–36
81. Doskocil, J., Paces, V., Sorm, F. 1967. *Biochim. Biophys. Acta* 145:771–79
82. Doskocil, J., Paces, V., Sorm, F. 1967. *Biochim. Biophys. Acta* 145:780–91
83. Paces, V., Doskocil, J., Sorm, F. 1968. *FEBS Lett.* 1:55–58
84. Paces, V., Dosckocil, J., Sorm, F. 1968. *Biochim. Biophys. Acta* 161:352–60
85. Vesely, J., Cihak, A., Sorm, F. 1968. *Biochem. Pharmacol.* 17:519
86. Venditti, J. M. 1971. *Cancer Chemother. Rep.,* Pt. 3, 2:35–59
87. Sorm, F., Vesely, J. 1964. *Neoplasma* 11:123–30
88. Sorm, F., Piskala, A., Cihak, A., Vesely, J. 1964. *Experientia* 20:202–3
89. Raska, K. et al 1965. *Collect. Czech. Chem. Commun.* 30:3001–6
90. Sorm, F. et al 1966. *Rev. Roum. Biochim.* 3:139–47
91. Troetel, W. M., Weiss, A. J., Stambaugh, J. E., Laucius, J. F., Manthei, R. W. 1972. *Cancer Chemother. Rep.* 56: 405–11

92. Karon, M., Sieger, L., Finkelstein, J., Nesbit, M. 1972. *Abstr. Am. Soc. Clin. Oncol.* No. 33
93. Weiss, A. J., Stambaugh, J. E., Mastrangelo, M. J., Laucius, J. F., Bellet, R. E. 1972. *Cancer Chemother. Rep.* 56: 413–19
94. Moertel, C. G., Schutt, A. J., Reitemeier, R. J., Hahn, R. G. 1972. *Cancer Chemother Rep.* 56:649–52
95. Karon, M., Sieger, L., Leimbrock, S., Nesbit, M., Finkelstein, J. 1973. *Proc. Amer. Assoc. Cancer Res.* 14:94
96. McCredie, K. B. et al 1973. *Cancer Chemother. Rep.* 57:319–23
97. Hrodek, O., Vesely, J. 1971. *Neoplasma* 18:493–503
98. Umezawa, H., Maeda, K., Takeuchi, T., Okami, Y. 1966. *J. Antibiot. A* 19: 200–9
99. Sûzuki, H., Nagai, K., Yamaki, H., Tanaka, N., Umezawa, H. 1968. *J. Antibiot. A* 21:379–86
100. Suzuki, H., Nagai, K., Yamaki, H., Tanaka, N., Umezawa, H. 1969. *J. Antibiot. A* 22:446–48
101. Kunimoto, T., Hori, M., Umezawa, H. 1967. *J. Antibiot. A* 20:277–81
102. Ishizuka, M., Takayama, H., Takeuchi, T., Umezawa, H. 1967. *J. Antibiot. A* 20:15–24
103. Jorgensen, S. J. 1970. *Eur. J. Cancer* 6:93–97
104. Fujita, M., Kimura, K. 1970. *Progr. Antimicrob. Anticancer Chemother.* 2:309–14
105. Rosenberg, B., VanCamp, L., Krigas, T. 1965. *Nature* 205:698–99
106. Rosenberg, B., VanCamp, L., Grimley, E. B., Thomson, A. J. 1967. *J. Biol. Chem.* 242:1347–52
107. Rosenberg, B., VanCamp, L., Trosko, J. E., Mansour, V. H. 1969. *Nature* 222: 385–86
108. Rosenberg, B., VanCamp, L. 1970. *Cancer Res.* 30:1799–1802
109. Harder, H. C., Rosenberg, B. 1970. *Int. J. Cancer* 6:207–16
110. Howle, J. A., Gale, G. R. 1970. *Biochem. Pharmacol.* 19:2757–62
111. Roberts, J., Pascoe, J. 1972. *Nature* 235:282–84
112. Kociba, R. J., Sleight, S. D., Rosenberg, B. 1970. *Cancer Chemother. Rep.* 54: 325–28
113. Welsch, C. W. 1971. *Proc. Am. Assoc. Cancer Res.* 12:25
114. Sirica, A., Venditti, J. M., Kline, I. 1971. *Proc. Am. Assoc. Cancer Res.* 12:4
115. Speer, R. J. 1971. *Wadley Med. Bull.* 1:103–9

116. Woodman, R. J., Venditti, J. M., Schepartz, S. A., Kline, I. 1971. *Proc. Am. Assoc. Cancer Res.* 12:24
117. Hill, J. M. et al 1971. *Abstr. Int. Congr. of Chemother., VII, Prague*
118. DeConti, R. C., Lange, R. C., Harder, H. C., Creasey, W. A. 1972. *Proc. Am. Assoc. Cancer Res.* 13:96
119. Rossof, A. H., Slayton, R. E., Perlia, C. P. 1972. *Abstr. Am. Soc. Clin. Oncol.* No. 55
120. Talley, R. W., O'Bryan, R. M., Brownlee, R. W., Gastesi, R. A. 1972. *Proc. Am. Assoc. Cancer Res.* 13:81
121. Lippman, A., Helson, C., Helson, L., Kaufman, R., Krakoff, I. H. 1972. *Proc. Am. Assoc. Cancer Res.* 13:40
122. Tatsuoka, S. et al 1958. *Gann Suppl.* 49:23
123. Miyamoto, M. et al 1964. *Tetrahedron Lett.* 34:2367–70
124. Miyamoto, M., Kawamatsu, Y., Kawashima, K., Shinohara, M., Nakanishi, K. 1966. *Tetrahedron Lett.* 6:545–52
125. Miyamoto, M. et al 1967. *Tetrahedron Lett.* 23:421–37
126. Behr, W., Honikel, K., Hartmann, G. 1969. *Eur. J. Biochem.* 9:82–92
127. Kaziro, Y., Kamiyama, M. 1965. *Biochem. Biophys. Res. Commun.* 19: 433–37
128. Kaziro, Y., Kamiyama, M. 1967. *J. Biochem. Tokyo* 62:424–29
129. Ward, D., Reich, E., Goldberg, I. 1965. *Science* 149:1259–63
130. Hartmann, G., Goller, H., Koschel, K., Kersten, W., Kersten, H. 1964. *Biochem. Z.* 341:126–28
131. Kaziwara, K., Watanabe, J., Komeda, T., Usui, T. 1960. *Ann. Rep. Takeda Res. Lab.* 19:68–96
132. Kaziwara, K., Watanabe, J., Komeda, T., Usui, T. 1961. *Cancer Chemother. Rep.* 13:99–106
133. Sato, K., Okamura, N., Utagawa, K., Ito, Y., Watanabe, M. 1960. *Sci. Rep. Res. Inst. Tohoku Univ. Med.* 9:224– 32
134. Aramaki, Y. et al 1960. *Ann. Rep. Takeda Res. Lab.* 19:109–30
135. Slavik, M., Carter, S. K. 1972. *Clinical Brochure on Chromomycin A₃* Bethesda, Md: Nat. Cancer Inst.
136. Slavik, M., Carter, S. K. 1974. *Advan. Pharmacol. Chemother.* 12: In press
137. Kuru, M. 1961. *Cancer Chemother. Rep.* 13:91–97
138. Ishigami, S. et al 1963. *Jikken Chiryo* 371:67
139. Falkson, G., Falkson, H., Sandison, A. 1964. *Med. Proc. S. Africa* 10:264– 68

140. Falkson, G., Sandison, A., Falkson, H., Fichardt, T. 1966. *S. Afr. J. Radiol.* 4: 38–39
141. Takatsu, T., Taguchi, N. 1965. *Gan no Rinsho* 11:333–34
142. Saito, T., Ohira, S. 1964. *Shindan To Chiryo* 52:35–46 (Abstract in 1964. *Cancer Chemother. Abstr.* 4:518)
143. Ishigami, S., Kurahori, T., Morii, K., Yamaguchi, S., Watanabe, Y. 1964. *Nippon Naika Gakkai Zasshi* 53:668–69 (Abstract in 1965. *Cancer Chemother. Abstr.* 6:582)
144. Saito, T. 1966. *Gan no Rinsho* 12:225–232 (Abstract in 1966. *Cancer Chemother. Abstr.* 7:739)
145. Suzuki, Y. 1966. *Nippon Jibiinkoka Gakkai Kaiho* 69, Suppl. 2:11–19 (Abstract in 1966. *Cancer Chemother. Abstr.* 7:505)
146. Creighton, A. M., Hellmann, K., Whitecross, S. 1969. *Nature* 222: 384–85
147. Creighton, A. M., Birnie, G. D. 1970. *Int. J. Cancer.* 5:47–54
148. Sharpe, H. B. A., Field, E. O., Hellmann, K. 1970. *Nature* 226:524–26
149. Salsbury, A. J., Burrage, K., Hellmann, K. 1970. *Brit. Med. J.* 4:344–45
150. Hellmann, K., Newton, K. A., Whitmore, D. N., Hanham, I. W. F., Bond, J. V. 1969. *Brit. Med. J.* 1:822–24
151. Hellmann, K. 1970. In *Advances in the Treatment of Acute (Blastic) Leukemias,* 52–53. New York: Springer
152. Mathe, G. et al. See Ref. 151, pp. 54–55
153. Hellmann, K., Burrage, K. 1970. *Int. Cancer Congr. Abstr.* 10:682
154. Bellet, R. E., Mastrangelo, M. J., Dixon, L. M., Yarbro, J. W. 1973. *Cancer Chemother. Rep.* 57:185–89
155. Creaven, P. J., Taylor, S. G. 1973. *Proc. Am. Assoc. Cancer Res.* 14:20
156. Shealy, Y. F., Struck, R. F., Holum, L. B., Montgomery, J. A. 1961. *J. Org. Chem.* 26:2396
157. Shealy, Y. F., Montgomery, J. A., Laster, W. R. Jr. 1962. *Biochem. Pharmacol.* 11:674–76
158. Shealy, Y. F., Krauth, C. A. 1966. *J. Med. Chem.* 9:34
159. Skibba, J. L., Johnson, R. O., Bryan, G. T. 1970. *Proc. Am. Assoc. Cancer Res.* 11:73
160. Saunders, P. P., Schultz, G. A. 1970. *Biochem. Pharmacol.* 19:911–19
161. Hano, K. et al 1965. *Gann* 56:417
162. Hoffman, G. et al 1968. *Cancer Chemother. Rep.* 52:715
163. Wilkoff, L. J., Dulmadge, E. A., Dixon, G. J. 1968. *Cancer Chemother. Rep.* 52:725
164. Housholder, G. E., Loo, T. L. 1969. *Life Sci.* 8:533
165. Skibba, J. L., Ramirez, G., Beal, D. D., Bryan, G. T. 1969. *Cancer Res.* 20: 1944–51
166. Skibba, J. L., Ramirez, G., Beal, D. D., Bryan, G. T. 1970. *Int. Cancer Congr. Abstr.* 10:498
167. Skibba, J. L., Beal, D. D., Ramirez, G., Bryan, G. T. 1970. *Cancer Res.* 30: 147–50
168. Cowan, D., Bergsagel, D. 1971. *Cancer Chemother. Rep.* 55:175–81
169. Johnston, T. P., McCaleb, G. S., Montgomery, J. A. 1963. *J. Med. Chem.* 6: 669–81
170. Wheeler, G. P., Chumley, S. 1967. *J. Med. Chem.* 10:259–61
171. D'Angelo, J. M., Groth, D. P., Vogler, W. R. 1970. *Int. Cancer Congr. Abstr.* 10:408–9
172. Green, S., Bodansky, O. 1967. *Proc. Am. Assoc. Cancer Res.* 8:23
173. Wheeler, G. P., Bowdon, B. J. 1968. *Cancer Res.* 28:52–59
174. Schabel, F. M. 1970. In *Proceedings of Chemotherapy Conference on Chemotherapy of Solid Tumors: An Appraisal of 5-FU and BCNU,* ed. S. K. Carter, 159–80. Bethesda, Md.: Nat. Cancer Inst.
175. Schabel, F. M. et al 1963. *Cancer Res.* 23:725
176. Wodinsky, I., Kensler, C. J. 1967. In *Abstracts of Papers, Proc. Int. Cancer Congr., 9th,* 380 New York: Springer
177. Sugiura, K. 1967. *Cancer Res.* 27: 179
178. Tarnowski, G. S., Schmid, F. A., Cappuccino, J. G., Stock, C. C. 1968. *Cancer Chemother. Rep.,* Pt 2, 1:403–534
179. DeVita, V. T., Denham, C., Davidson, J. D., Oliverio, V. T. 1967. *Clin. Pharmacol. Ther.* 8:566–77
180. Bray, D., Oliverio, V., Adamson, R., DeVita, V. 1970. *Proc. Am. Assoc. Cancer Res.* 11:12
181. Wheeler, G. P., Bowdon, B. J. 1968. *Cancer Res.* 28:52
182. Cheng, C. J., Fujimura, S., Grunberger, D., Weinstein, B. 1972. *Cancer Res.* 32:22–27
183. Schmall, B., Cheng, C. J., Fujimura, S., Grunberger, D., Weinstein, B. 1972. *Proc. Am. Assoc. Cancer Res.* 13:65
184. Oliverio, V. T., Vietzke, W. M., Williams, M. K., Adamson, R. H. 1968. *Proc. Am. Assoc. Cancer Res.* 9:56
185. Oliverio, V. T., Walker, M. D., Hayes, S. L., DeVita, V. T. 1970. *Proc. Am. Assoc. Cancer Res.* 11:61

186. Selawry, O. S., Hansen, H. H. 1972. *Proc. Am. Assoc. Cancer Res.* 13:46
187. Walker, M. D., Rosenblum, M. L., Smith, K. A., Reynolds, A. F. 1971. *Proc. Am. Assoc. Cancer Res.* 12:51
188. Moertel, C. G., Schutt, A. J., Reitemeier, R. J., Hahn, R. G. 1972. *Cancer Res.* 32:1278
189. Hansen, H. H., Selawry, O. S., Muggia, F. M., Walker, M. D. 1971. *Cancer Res.* 31:223–27

190. Sponzo, R. W., DeVita, V. T., Oliverio, V. T. 1973. *Cancer* 31:1154–59
191. Young, R. C. et al 1973. *Cancer* 31: 1164–69
192. Greenspan, E. M., Fieber, M. M., Geeson, L., Edelman, S. 1963. *J. Mt. Sinai Hosp.* 30:246–67
193. Greenspan, E. M. 1966. *J. Mt. Sinai Hosp.* 33:1–27
194. Cooper, R. G. 1969. *Proc. Am. Assoc. Cancer Res.* 10:15

CARCINOGENICITY AS RELATED TO AGE[1]

❖6588

R. Schoental
Department of Pathology, Royal Veterinary College, Royal College Street, London, England

INTRODUCTION

Cancer is considered a disease of old age. The highest mortality from cancer occurs indeed after the age of 50, but the tumors are likely to have been initiated long before any symptoms of the disease become apparent, possibly in childhood or even in utero.

The majority of tumors that occur in late life may be caused by multiple carcinogenic agents; they represent great difficulties when attempting to trace the aetiological factors involved. The difficulties are becoming ever more formidable with the increasing complexities of modern life.

Though not numerous, tumors occur in the newborn, in early childhood, and even in the fetus (1–3). Childhood tumors have been reported to be one of the main causes of mortality among the young, and their frequency appears to be increasing in the last years (4). The tracing of the aetiology of tumors that occur in the fetus or in early childhood has better chances of success. Though the causative agents need not be the same as those operating in later life, the recognition and possible elimination of even a single agent would be of practical value. The combination of the remaining carcinogenic factors would obviously be less effective, and the appearance of the tumors accordingly delayed, hopefully, beyond the lifespan of the individual.

Evidence from animal experiments brought to light the fact that in order to induce tumors, exposure to carcinogenic agents does not need to be continuous; single or a few doses may be sufficient; these may give no warning in the form of a recogniz-

[1]The following abreviations are used in this review: PAH = polycyclic aromatic hydrocarbons; MCHA = 3-methylcholanthrene; 7,12-DMBA = 7,12-dimethylbenz[a]anthracene; OC = oral contraceptives; Enovid = 17α-ethynyl-19-hydroxyestren-3-one; DES = 3,4-di-(4-hydroxyphenyl)-hex-3-ene = diethylstilbestrol; AAT = N-2-fluorenylacetamide; Zearalenone =[6(10-hydroxy-6-oxo-*trans*-1-undecenyl)]-β-resorcinic acid lactone; MNU = N-methyl-N-nitrosourea; ENU = N-ethyl-N-nitrosourea; DEN = N-nitrosodiethylamine; DDT = 1,1,1-trichloro-2,2-di-(4-chlorophenyl)-ethane.

185

able illness for a long time. The latent period before tumors appear is to some extent related to the dose: the lower the dosage, the longer will usually be the latent period. Cancer seen in old age might have been initiated early in life.

Age is conventionally calculated from the time of birth, though the individual's existence starts at conception. However, biologically, the consignment of cells, which in time develop into the future ova, exist in the female's ovary since its organogenesis in her mother's uterus (5).

The existence of a mammalian organism can be roughly subdivided into the following stages:

1. The quiescent presence of the germ cell in the ovary
2. Maturation of the germ cell into an ovum in the mother's ovary
3. Maturation of the male germ cells into spermatozoa in the father's gonads
4. Fertilization of the ovum by the spermatozoon
5. Implantation of the fertilized ovum and embryogenesis
6. Organogenesis and the development of the fetus
7. Parturition
8. Infancy (suckling, or milk diet)
9. Childhood (with adoption of mixed diet)
10. Adolescence (hormonal influence due to maturing gonads)
11. Adulthood
12. Senescence

Assuming certain genetic susceptibility, exposure at appropriate stages to carcinogenic agents, viral, physical, or chemical, could have lethal, cytotoxic, mutagenic, or teratogenic effects, or could initiate the chain of events that result in cancer.

This paper considers the induction of tumors by chemical carcinogens in relation to age. Viral agents have been reviewed by Gross, 1970 (6); radiation carcinogenesis by Stewart, 1971 (7).

In the introduction to his classical paper "Occurrence and significance of congenital malignant neoplasms," Wells (1940) stated (1):

> In glaring contrast (to the long time usually needed for tumors to develop as a result of experimental or industrial exposure to carcinogenic agents) is the fact that certain types of malignant growth are seen almost exclusively in the very young and that sometimes a malignant growth may develop in the fetus, even producing widespread metastases, before the brief span of intra-uterine existence has been accomplished. Surely these tumors must differ in some fundamental way from the ordinary sorts of cancer, which require so long a period for development, and this difference may throw some light on the mystery of malignancy.

During the two scores of years since this was written, new carcinogens came to light, "natural" and synthetic ones, which can induce in rodents tumors similar to those seen in man (8–11); and also in the fetus, when given to pregnant females during the second half of pregnancy (12). Treatment of pregnant females during the early stages of gestation, leads to death of the embryo, its absorption, or abortion, or malformations, but rarely to tumors (4). However, even in the transplacentally treated offspring, tumors appear late in their life. Animal models, which would result in tumors during the intrauterine existence, have still to be devised. Whether such early tumors may be the result of exposure to carcinogenic agents of the ovum or of the spermatozoa before they leave the parental gonads, requires detailed investigation. In experiments in which female mice were treated with PAH (MCHA or 7,12-DMBA) and were allowed to breed, degeneration of the ovarian follicles, reduced fertility, or sterility followed (13). Ovarian and mammary tumors developed in the treated females; their incidence varied depending on the strain of the mice used (13). However, as regards the offspring, no detailed examinations have been made.

In such experiments, any progeny should be carefully examined microscopically. Many malformations and incipient neoplasms may remain unrecognized on naked eye examination when dealing with an aborted or stillborn fetus (14).

TRANSPLACENTAL CARCINOGENESIS

Estrogens

Transplacental carcinogenesis has been the subject of a symposium sponsored by the WHO and by the International Agency for Research on Cancer in 1971, the proceedings of which have been published (12). The interest in the transplacental effects of chemicals has been stimulated by the tragic epidemic-like occurrence of malformations in Germany among babies of mothers that were given the sedative-hypnotic drug, thalidomide, during pregnancy (15, 16). More recently, a chance finding of seven cases of vaginal cancer in one hospital among young women 14–22 years of age attracted attention, because of the rarity of this type of neoplasia in the young. The tumors have been traced to be the result of treatment of the patients' mothers with large doses of diethylstilbestrol (up to 125 mg/day) or steroidal estrogens for threatened abortion (17). Since then, a number of additional cases of vaginal abnormalities and tumors in young women came to light, which are of similar iatrogenic origin (18). As yet, no reports are available whether the treatments had carcinogenic sequalae in the treated women or in their male offspring. As the latent period for the clinical appearance of the vaginal tumors in the very susceptible young was 14–22 years, a longer time interval would be expected to elapse before tumors could become apparent in the mothers. The consequences of high estronization of the male fetus require specific investigation. Masculinization of the female offspring as a result of treatment of their mothers during pregnancy with progestins or estrogens has been reported (19).

Medications involving relatively high doses of estrogens are given sporadically to women to suppress lactation (5–15 mg/day), for the treatment of mammary carcinoma (10–20 mg/day), as postcoital contraceptives (25 mg twice/day, for 5 days) (20) etc. Epidemiological investigations now in progress should pay attention to the long term effects of hormonal imbalance, not only in the treated women, but also to those that arise in their progeny, male or female, who may be conceived at any time subsequent to treatment.

The effects of smaller dosage are likely to take longer to become clinically recognizable. The continuous use of oral contraceptives (OC), which contain small doses of estrogens in conjunction with progestogens, would be expected to have cumulative effects, which have yet to be adequately investigated. An increased risk, tenfold of thromboembolic (21) and twofold of gall bladder diseases has been reported among the users of OC as compared with nonusers (22). Serious malformations occurred among the offspring of women who have taken OC as "pregnancy tests" or without realizing that pregnancy already existed (23).

Recently, jaundice among breast-fed infants has been correlated with the use of OC by their mothers, long before these babies were conceived (24).

In mice fetal malformations have been produced experimentally by the administration of daily doses of OC corresponding to 1–3 times the doses that prevent pregnancy in this species (25).

Since the first demonstration by Lacassagne in 1932 (26) that folliculin (oestrone) can induce mammary tumors in male mice, estrogens have been known to be carcinogenic. They are able to induce tumors in several target organs (breast, uterus, vagina, anterior pituitary, ovary, etc), in susceptible animals under appropriate conditions (27, 28). The younger the animals, the more susceptible they are to the action of estrogens (and other hormones). Newborn animals are particularly sensitive. A single dose of DES induced multiple cysts of the epididymis in male mice and tumors of the vagina, uterus, and myoblastoma in female mice (29); similar results were obtained with the OC Enovid (30). Continuous administration of large doses of Enovid in diet, induced uterine tumors in all the treated mice (30). In spite of the small scale of these experiments, the results are highly significant.

The foundations of chemical carcinogenesis have been the result of careful observations made on small numbers of patients or animals by experienced and interested scientists who could recognize the significance of the tumors found, even though these were few in numbers. It would be of interest to know whether the present tendency to use very large numbers of animals (mega-mouse experiments have been suggested) and in consequence to have to rely on observations made by unskilled technical staff and on statistical evaluation by computers, will lead to an improvement as regards the reliability of the results and the discovery of new (unprogrammed) facts.

Besides affecting target organs, estrogens have been found to induce renal tumors in male hamsters (*Cricetus auratus*) (31); whether they play some role in diseases of the kidneys in other species remains to be investigated. Sex hormones can greatly modify the response to carcinogenic agents. They are responsible for the differences in the incidence and/or in the localization of tumors observed in response to the same treatment, depending on age, sex, and pregnancy. Most hepatocarcinogens are usually more effective in males than in females, and castration or treatment with the respective sex hormones appropriately modify the response. This has been found to be so in the case of N-2-fluorenylacetamide (AAF) and its congeners (32–34), azo-dyes (35), N-4-(4'-fluorobiphenyl)acetamide (36), pyrrolizidine alkaloids (10), cycasin (11), and aflatoxins (8). However, the cirrhogenic action of carbon tetrachloride (37) and the carcinogenic response of the liver to diethylnitrosamine have been reported to be more accentuated in the females (38). Estrogens have a modifying effect on the carcinogenic action of polycyclic aromatic hydrocarbons (MCHA and 7,12-DMBA) on mouse gonads (13); they also enhance the induction of tumors of the mammary gland in Sprague-Dawley rats (39); when ovariectomized the rats have a very low incidence of mammary tumors, but develop renal tumors (40).

The modifying effects of sex hormones is no doubt related to their multifarious actions: on food consumption, metabolism, induction of enzymes (41); on development and growth, etc. The normal liver is usually able to metabolize, conjugate, and inactivate estrogenic agents, but in certain pathological conditions, it might be unable to cope with an excessive intake; the circulating estrogens can then affect the gonads and other organs.

An interesting observation has been recently reported from Australia: C3H A^{vy} mice, which have a high incidence of mammary and hepatic tumors in the Laboratories of the National Cancer Institute (NIH) in USA, have been found to develop fewer tumors when imported to Australia; the incidence declined strikingly in the subsequent generations bred in Australia. However, when the mice were given the American diet, the incidence of their mammary tumors increased and was restored to the American level when their bedding was replaced by shavings of red cedar (*Juniperus virginiana*), which is used at NIH (42). The authors suspect that the red cedar shavings contain carcinogens. This is indeed likely, in view of the carcinogenic activity of 3,4,5-trimethoxycinnamaldehyde, a derivative of certain α,β-unsaturated aldehydes, which are normal constituents of wood lignins (43, 44). Other specific carcinogenic compounds may also be present in red-cedar wood. However, the enhancing effect of the American diet on the induction of mammary cancer may be related to its content of estrogens (see below). This remarkable instance of modification of the incidence of "spontaneous" tumors, believed to be genetically determined, by environmental factors, appears of great importance and warrants closer examination.

Synthetic estrogens, mainly DES, have been used as additives to livestock diets in order to accelerate their growth and fattening-up and to obtain a better food conversion. The Food and Drug Administration of the USA has prohibited the addition of DES to animal fodder or the implantation of its pellets into the ears of livestock (45); however, estrogenic material, "Ralgro," has been developed to replace DES. This preparation has similar estrogenic activity, but is of different structure (46); it consists of two stereoisomers, the hydroxylic reduction products of zearalenone, a secondary metabolic product of *Fusarium graminearum (Gibberella zeae)* and certain related fungi, which often contaminate cereals and other foodstuffs. The estrogenic activity of zearalenone has been discovered during investigation of a pathological condition in pigs, known as "vulvo-vaginitis," which has been traced to contamination of the pig's diet with Fusaria (46).

Plants used as food also contain substances that have estrogenic activity. In Figure 1 are given the chemical structures of representative compounds of several types of known estrogenic agents. The physiological female sex hormones are steroidal compounds, Figure 1 (*I*); estrone has been found also in plant materials, e.g. date palm kernels (47). Genistein (Figure 1 *III*), the 5,7,4'-trihydroxyisoflavone, is present in red clover, *Trifolium subterraneum,* (Leguminosae) and in related plant species. Though its estrogenic activity is only 10^{-5} of that shown by DES or estradiol, it has been found to be responsible for sterility in sheep that grazed on subterranean clover in Australia due to the high content of this constituent (48). A number of related isoflavonoids present in plants are also estrogenic (49). Coumestrol (Figure 1 *IV*) and its congeners are coumarin derivatives, which have a higher estrogenic activity than the isoflavonoids, and are present in soya beans and other plants used as food (50). There are still others (51).

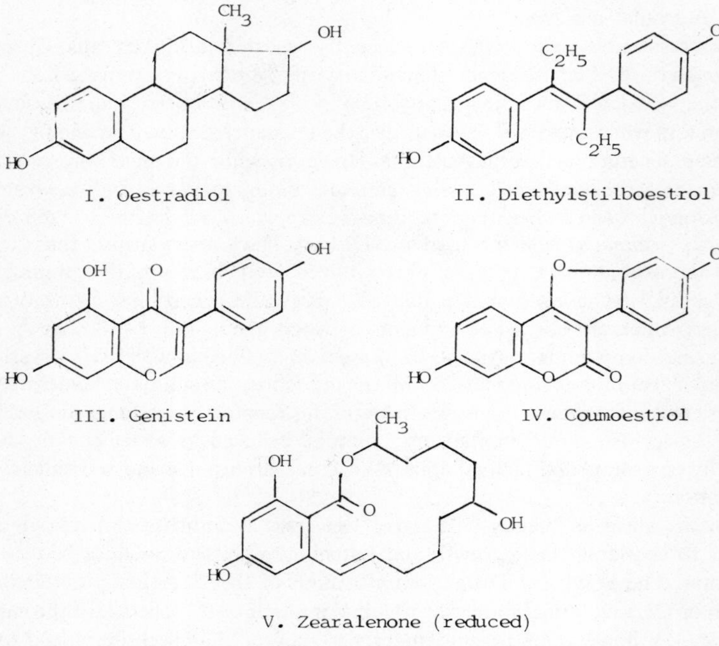

I. Oestradiol

II. Diethylstilboestrol

III. Genistein

IV. Coumoestrol

V. Zearalenone (reduced)

Figure 1 Structures of compounds that have estrogenic activity.

Though the various estrogenic compounds differ in their chemical structures, they show marked similarity as regards the positions of the hydroxyl groups, which are essential for the estrogenic action. Indeed, of the two stereoisomeric reduction products of zearalenone, which differ in the configuration of the hydroxyl at C-6 (Figure 1 *V*), one is much more active than the other (46).

The various plant and fungal estrogenic compounds have yet to be tested for carcinogenic action. However, their effects on the target organs are likely to be similar to those found with DES and with the steroidal estrogens. The activity of both the steroidal and the synthetic estrogens depends on the presence of hydroxyl-groups at the extremities of their molecules (estrone has only about 1/10th of the activity of estradiol, to which it is metabolically reduced in the animal body). The hydroxyls are involved in the binding with specific receptor proteins present in the cytosol of cells in the target organs. The resulting complexes are then carried into the nucleus where they become tightly bound to acceptor proteins. This process can be detected in vivo and in vitro; it is susceptible to inhibition by thiol reagents (52).

In the environment of animals and man, the load of estrogenic agents has been steadily increasing. Some of the consequences, which may include changes in sexual and social behavior, are not easy to evaluate in animal experiments. Attempts should be made to restrict the present liberal uses of estrogenic substances to the unavoidable minimum.

The high incidence of mammary (53) and/or uterine tumors in women all over the world is a sufficient indication that man is a species susceptible to the action of estrogenic agents.

Chemical Carcinogens

Most of the chemical carcinogens, especially in their activated form, have cytotoxic, mutagenic, teratogenic, as well as carcinogenic action; there is, however, no direct parallelism among these activities.

Cytotoxic effects are the least specific and can be caused by a variety of compounds acting at appropriate concentration. The relation between mutagenesis and carcinogenesis (54, 55) will not be fully understood, until the active forms of indirectly acting carcinogens become known.

Teratogenic action (56) causing morphological and/or functional abnormalities in the fetus implies that the carcinogen when given to pregnant females at an appropriate stage of gestation can cross the placenta or exert its effect indirectly, e.g. by interference with blood supply etc. Severe malformations are usually not compatible with survival beyond the intrauterine existence; these can be detected by removing the fetus from the uterus a few days after treatment, before it is lost due to resorption or abortion. A number of carcinogens show teratogenic effects under such conditions, including certain polycyclic aromatic hydrocarbons, azo-dyes, 2AAF, antitumor agents, estrogens (57), pyrrolizidine alkaloids (58), cycasin (59), various nitroso- and related compounds (60). The effects depend on many factors, including genetic susceptibility, the species and strain of the test animal, also on the stage of development of the fetus at the time of administration of the compound. Thus, aflatoxin B_1 induced malformations in hamsters and in C3H mice when treated at the most sensitive period between the days 8–12 of gestation, but induced only growth retardation in rats (60).

The concentration of the acting substance appears to be critical for teratogenic effects; repeated small doses are not additive, in contradistinction to carcinogenic responses, which are the result of summation or potentiations of even very small individual doses. Many teratogens are not carcinogenic (56); the evidence for thalidomide is equivocal (61).

Neoplastic transformation is a very rare cellular event, which affects only a few among the billions of cells that come in contact with a carcinogen introduced into the animal body. Evidently, a cell has to be in a very specific receptive stage for the "fateful" interaction to take place.

In the majority of studies on the induction of tumors by chemical agents weanling or young adult rodents were used, and the treatments were either continuous or repeated over long periods (62). More recently, newborn animals given such treatments proved to be more susceptible than adults to the action of many carcinogens. These include polycyclic aromatic hydrocarbons, aromatic amines, azo-compounds, urethane and certain nitroso and other compounds (compare 63–65), pyrrolizidine alkaloids (66) cycasin (59), aflatoxins (8), N-4-(4'-fluorobiphenyl)acetamide (36) and others. The reviews by Toth in 1968 (63) and by Della Porta & Terracini in 1969 (64) illustrate the difficulties involved in trying to evaluate the many variables (number of doses and their size, frequency and route of administration, solvents used, etc) inherent in such experiments. Comparisons *sensu stricto* of susceptibility to carcinogens at various ages became possible with the recognition that certain compounds are able to induce tumors with a *single* dose. The first indication of this has been obtained in experiments with a pyrrolizidine alkaloid, lasiocarpine (67), soon confirmed in the case of dimethylnitrosamine (68), nitroso-N-methylurethane (69), and retrorsine (70). However, the incidence of tumors in these cases was rather low; among the rats surviving for more than 1 year after a single dose of retrorsine, the incidence of hepatomas did not exceed 20% (70).

Using pure strains of rats, inbred for 50–100 generations (71) and having more than 70 nitroso and related compounds (mostly synthesized by Preussmann), Druckrey and his co-workers were able to extend greatly the studies of single dose carcinogenesis (72, 73).

The finding that a single dose of MNU will induce tumors in a variety of organs including the brain (72) had particularly significant consequences. MNU is more effective when given to newborn animals than to weanlings (74); when given intravenously it will induce in the rat preferentially tumors of the nervous system (75). When given intravenously to pregnant rats during the second week of gestation, the fetuses develop malformations (76, 77), while the treated mothers may develop tumors of the gonads (78). Methylnitrosourea probably does not require enzymic activation and though very unstable at alkaline pH, it evidently retains its activity for the short time required to be carried in the blood stream throughout the animal body.

The higher homologue, ENU, which is more stable, proved more effective and convenient for comparative studies of its transplacental and postnatal action (79–83) and has been used extensively by many workers (84–89). The examples given in Table 1 illustrate the effects in rats of single doses of MNU and ENU in relation to the age at the time of treatment, the size of the dose, and the route of administration. When a single dose of MNU was given orally, mainly gastrointestinal and kidney neoplasias developed (90), but intravenously it induced also neurogenic tumors (72).

When the carcinogenic efficacies of MNU and ENU were directly compared by giving one equimolecular dose of each (0.14 mM/kg body weight) to rats of the same strain at the end of pregnancy, the incidence of neurogenic tumors in the offspring was 39.7% (with MNU) and 97.4% (with ENU) respectively (86). This may be due to the instability and higher toxicity of MNU. Its toxicity (possibly

Table 1 Tumors and/or malformations induced in rats with a single dose of carcinogen in relation to the age at the time of treatment

Compound	Strain	Age in days	Dose mg/kg body wt	Route[a]	Tumors present in				Malform.	Refs
					Nervous System	Stomach	Kidney	Others		
N-methyl-N-nitrosourea $O=N-N\diagdown{}^{CH_3}_{CONH_2}$	BD	(-13)→(-8)	10, 20	iv					++	76
	White	(-14)→(-10)	10	ip					++	77
	White	(-1)	20, 40	iv	+				++	4
	BD	>60	70-100	iv	+	++	+	++		72
	White	>60	90	ig	+	++	+	+		90
N-ethyl-N-nitrosourea $O=N-N\diagdown{}^{C_2H_5}_{CONH_2}$	BD IX	(-8)	40, 80	iv	+++				++	79
		(-8)	5-80	iv	+++					79-81, 83
		(-11)→(-1)	60	iv	+++					80
		(-1)	5-60	iv	+++					81
		1	5-80	sc	+++		+	+		81
		10	10-80	sc, o	+++	+		+		81
		30	20-80	iv	+++		+	++		81
		>60	60-200	iv	++	+	+	++		81
	10 various BD strains	(-8)	50	iv	+++			+		82
	Long Evans	(-6)	10	iv	+++					84
	Sprague Dawley	(-3)	50	iv	+++		+			85

[a] iv = intravenous; ig = intragastic; sc = subcutaneous; o = oral.

related to the alkylating action) prevents the use of doses high enough to give an "effective" concentration of the carcinogenic entity in the fetus after passage through a fully developed placenta. The barrier characteristics of the placenta are likely to vary with the progress of pregnancy; compounds may pass more freely before the placenta is fully developed and at the end of gestation when it is undergoing degeneration (96).

With alkylnitrosobiurets (91, 92) the results are similar to those obtained with alkylnitrosoureas, but higher dose levels were required. After a single dose, given to adult rats, intragastrically, stomach tumors preferentially developed and also tumors of the kidneys and other organs. However, when N-ethyl-N-nitrosobiuret was given to pregnant rats, exclusively neurogenic tumors were found in the offspring. The effective dose was about one fifth of that required for the adult rat (92).

Examples in Table 2 illustrate the differences in the response to azoxy compounds (59, 93–95). The younger the animals, the smaller is the dose that is required to induce neoplasias. The respective hydrazo and azo compounds are readily oxidized in the body to azoxyderivatives and accordingly give similar results (94).

ENU proved to be a very suitable carcinogen for the transplacental induction of almost exclusively neurogenic tumors in the rat (80). A dose that corresponds to 2% of the LD_{50} for the adult rat will induce neurogenic tumors in the majority of the offspring, when given on the 15th day of gestation (the –8 day of age) or later.

The neoplasias thus induced often represent tumors of considerable size in the hemispheres, in the cerebellum, the spinal cord, the cranial or peripheral nerves; they include oligodendrogliomas, astrocytomas, mixed gliomas, ependymomas, neurinomas (97). Similar neurogenic tumors were obtained by a number of workers in different laboratories who gave ENU to other strains of rats at various times during the third week of pregnancy (84–87). However, the incidence of the tumors can vary, depending on the strain of the rats (82).

Hamsters develop also neurogenic tumors when given ENU during the second half of pregnancy (4, 80), but mice similarly treated respond with lung and lymphoid tumors (88); mice of the strains A and C3Hf that are liable to "spontaneous" hepatomas also develop liver neoplasias. It thus appears that as a result of transplacental action of ENU, the neoplasias in the offspring develop mainly in organs that respond with tumors when the animals are treated postnatally. Mice of many strains appear to be resistant to neurogenic tumors, but a few mice (about 10%) of the strains IF and DBA developed neurogenic tumors including medulloblastomas, when given as newborns a single, subcutaneous dose of ENU (10–120 mg/kg of body weight) (89). No such tumors were found in similarly treated mice of the strains A or C57BL (89).

Similar species and strain differences have been observed in transplacental and/or postnatal studies of various carcinogens: cycasin, or its aglycone, methylazoxymethanol (11, 95, 98), urethane (99–104), pyrrolizidine alkaloids (105, 106), and others. The striking differences in response to carcinogens of different animal species, different strains, and even among animals of the same strain when kept under varied conditions are usually referred to genetic, immunological, or viral factors, however, the exact mechanism that determines susceptibility or resistance has not been ex-

Table 2 Tumors and/or malformations induced in rodents with a single (or a few) doses of carcinogen in relation to the age at the time of treatment

Compound	Species (strain)	Age in days	Dose mg/kg body wt	Route[a]	Tumors present in				Malform.	Refs.
					Kidney	Intestine	Nervous System	Others		
Azoxymethane.	Rats (BD)	(-13)→(-8)	30	iv	-	-	-	-	-	93
$CH_3 - N = N - CH_3$ ↓O		(-13)→(-8)	30	sc	-	-	-	-	-	
		(-1)	30	sc	+		+			
		1	4	sc	+	+	+			
		3	6	sc	++	+	+			
		10	12	sc	+	+	+			
		30	20	sc	+	++	+			
		>60	40	sc	++	++				
Methylazoxymethanol	rats Fischer	(-8)→(-7)	20	iv	++	++	+		+	59, 95
$CH_3 - N = N - CH_2OH$ ↓O		60	20	iv	++	++		+		
	golden hamster	(-13)	20	iv					+++	
Azoxyethane	rats BD1X	(-13)	50	iv					++	94
$H_5C_2 - N = N - C_2H_5$ ↓O		(-8)	150	iv			+++			
		(-1)	150	iv			+++			
		>60	210	iv			+			

[a] iv = intravenous; sc = subcutaneous.

plained. This is one of the most important problems for investigation; understanding of the factors responsible for resistance to tumor induction may give a lead to cancer prevention.

The transplacental studies have demonstrated the greater sensitivity to carcinogens of the fetus in relation to that of its adult mother. In some instances, the presence of the carcinogen given to the pregnant female has been detected in the fetus (103, 107–109). Using labeled 3-methylcholanthrene the quantities detected in the mouse fetus represented 0.26% of the dose given to the mother. It would appear that 2 ng/mg of fetal lung tissue is sufficient to induce lung tumors in later life (109). The carcinogens appear to persist longer in the fetus than in the adult (103).

Transplacental studies are very suitable for such investigation. When direct comparison is made of the response of the fetus and the adult to the same dose of carcinogen, experimental errors are eliminated that might arise due to leakage or to licking of the material by the mother, when newborns are injected; moreover, the carcinogen can undergo activation in the mother's tissues, regardless of the metabolic competence of the fetus. The problem of the passage of carcinogens through the placenta at various stages of pregnancy remains to be investigated.

Evidence for the in vivo Formation of Nitroso Carcinogens from Precursors

In view of the very small dose of ENU required for the transplacental induction of malformations and tumors of the nervous system in rats (5 mg/kg body weight), pregnant females were used in experiments intended to detect whether ENU can be formed in the animal body from ethylurea and nitrite in sufficient concentrations to induce such effects. Positive results have been reported for both teratogenic action (110, 111) and for the induction of neurogenic tumors in the offspring (112, 113).

It is of great interest that administration of ascorbic acid prior to the nitrite prevented the development in the fetus of hydrocephalic lesions (111) in direct confirmation of the observation of Mirvish et al (114) that in the animal stomach, ascorbic acid reacts with nitrite and therefore prevents the nitrosylation of the alkylamino compounds to carcinogens.

CARCINOGENS IN MILK

The great susceptibility at the perinatal period to many carcinogens indicates the need for paying particular attention to the possibility that carcinogens ingested by lactating females may be excreted in the milk and present a hazard to the suckling young. Surprisingly, in spite of the milk's vital importance as the main foodstuff of the very young few experimental data are available on this problem.

"Natural" carcinogens are of particular interest in this connection. Poisoning of livestock, cows, sheep, and chicken by plants containing the hepatocarcinogenic (Senecio) pyrrolizidine alkaloids (PA) has been known for many years (115). When given to lactating rats, the suckling young developed acute and chronic liver and other lesions; the treated mother rats did not show ill effects, and their lactation remained unimpaired (116).

The form in which the PA are excreted in the milk is not yet known. More extensive studies would be needed, in order to establish whether and under which conditions the suckling young could survive long enough and develop tumors. The carcinogenic toxin of the bracken fern, *Pteridium aquilinum* has been reported to pass into the milk when fed to cows (117).

The fungal carcinogens, aflatoxin B_1 and G_1 are excreted in the milk in traces together with their equally toxic metabolites, aflatoxin M_1 and GM_1 (8), when given to several species of animals, including rats and cows, during lactation. Similarly, when the carcinogenic cycasin and its aglycone, methylazoxymethanol, were given to nursing rats, these compounds could be detected in the milk and in the tissues of the suckling young, and also some related metabolic products, whose structure has not yet been identified (107). The suckling young of cows, pigs, or rats fed cycas meal during lactation developed liver and other lesions that were more pronounced than those induced in the treated mothers (118).

Urethane, given to lactating mice, induces lung adenomas and lymphoid leukemias in the suckling young (102).

Mice nursed by mothers treated with methylcholanthrene also develop increased incidence of lung and lymphoid tumors (119); the presence of the hydrocarbon in the milk has been detected (109, 120).

As for the carcinogenic nitrosocompounds, hamsters nursed by mothers given daily small doses of DEN during lactation developed tumors of the upper respiratory tract, including the lung, trachea, and nose; similar tumors were present also in the nursing mothers (121). Rats nursed by mothers given a few large doses of DEN intragastrically during lactation developed aesthesioneuroepithelioma of the nasal ethmo-turbinals, which spread into the brain; some had also liver tumors; among their mothers, liver and kidney tumors were found. (122). The ready induction of various tumors by the milk of rodents treated with DEN raises the problem whether the nitrosamine is excreted into the milk in sufficient concentration to account for the results or whether the milk contains also some carcinogenic metabolites of DEN, perhaps related to the hydroxyethyl-N-nitroso-N-ethylamine and the respective carboxylic oxidation products that have been identified in the rat's urine (123).

The work on transplacental carcinogenesis made it clear that pregnant women have to be protected from exposure to carcinogens. Similar protection is needed for women who nurse their babies. An appropriate surveillance of dried milk and other infant foods is also obviously needed.

In this connection the problem of formation of nitroso compounds in the stomach from nitrite and alkylamides, mentioned previously, is relevant. A variety of non-neurogenic tumors has been induced by the administration to adult animals of nitrite in conjunction with various alkylamido and related compounds (124–126). These results raise the possibility that in human life, similar formation of nitroso carcinogens may occasionally occur, e.g. when certain medicines are taken and food is consumed that contains nitrite as preservative (126).

Epidemiological investigation disclosed an association between drugs administered during pregnancy and congenital abnormalities of the fetus (127). This problem is at present receiving much attention. The discovery of the protective action of ascorbic acid (111, 114, 125) suggests a simple solution; starting meals with citrus fruit might be adopted with advantage.

ETIOLOGY OF CHILDHOOD TUMORS

The problem of the etiology of childhood tumors is of much greater significance than their incidence (2–3% of all cancer cases) may appear to suggest. Neoplasias of childhood are likely to have originated pre- or during the intrauterine existence (128). The etiological factors of childhood tumors may be easier to trace than those of adults; yet the same agents may be responsible for tumors that appear later in life, if they acted at lower dosage levels or at different stages of the individual's development.

Neoplasias are only one of the manifestations of the action of carcinogenic agents. Some of these can cause also cytotoxic, mutagenic, and teratogenic effects and may be responsible for some of the congenital malformations and other abnormalities, often considered of genetic or viral etiology (128). Experimental evidence has already been obtained that the offspring of rats given cycasin during pregnancy may develop tumors or malformations of the brain and of the retina (95) or may exhibit "intellectual deficit" demonstrable in specific tests (129).

Multigeneration studies have been reported. Their aim was to explore the possible effects of continuous exposure to traces of carcinogenic contaminants that may be present in human environment or as a result of the use of insecticides [DDT (130, 131)], of methylthiouracil (77), or of diets contaminated with aflatoxins (132), PAH (133, 134) etc.

Other investigations have begun to appear that deal with the consequences in offspring (and in subsequent generations of their progeny) of the administration of carcinogens during pregnancy or before mating (135). The tentative results so far obtained require to be extended by varying the experimental conditions and by paying attention to the causes of death of the fetuses and newborns that may occur in the F2 and F3 generations.

MECHANISM OF THE INDUCTION OF TUMORS

As this review shows, substances of a variety of chemical structures can induce tumors in young animals with a *single* dose. The localization of the tumors in particular organs and the cell type from which the tumors originate appear to depend on the concentration of the active entity that reaches the tissue and on the presence at the critical time of cells in a "receptive" stage.

The mechanism of action of many carcinogens has been interpreted by alkylations, involving nucleophilic substitution of nitrogen, carbon, or oxygen in nucleic acids, or in proteins (136–138). In the course of the last few years, however, it became evident that alkylations, especially of the bases of nucleic acids (which attracted most attention) did not correlate with the development of tumors (137, 139), or with the results of mutagenic studies (140, 141).

Reactions that are relevant for the induction of tumors and probably also for the mutagenic action are likely to involve both the nucleic acids and the proteinaceous constituents of chromatin (142).

Studies of the metabolism of various carcinogens in the animal body have shown that the parent compounds undergo mainly oxidation before their stepwise further degradation. Among the oxidation products that appear to represent the activated carcinogenic entities are epoxides, e.g. those formed at the K zone of polycyclic aromatic hydrocarbons (143); at the double bond $\Delta^{1,2}$ of the pyrrolizidine moiety of Senecio alkaloids (144); at the terminal double bond of the dihydrodifurano moiety of aflatoxins (144); at the α,β-double bond of unsaturated aldehydes (43) (Figure 2).

In the case of dialkylnitrosamines, ω- or β-oxidation products of one of the alkyls have been identified as urinary metabolites (123, 145). The hydroxymethyl derivatives probably form the respective aldehydes before their oxidation to the respective carboxylic acids. Metabolites with an aldehyde or keto function have been suggested to be the activated carcinogenic forms of dialkylnitrosamines, methylazoxymethanol, and related compounds (142).

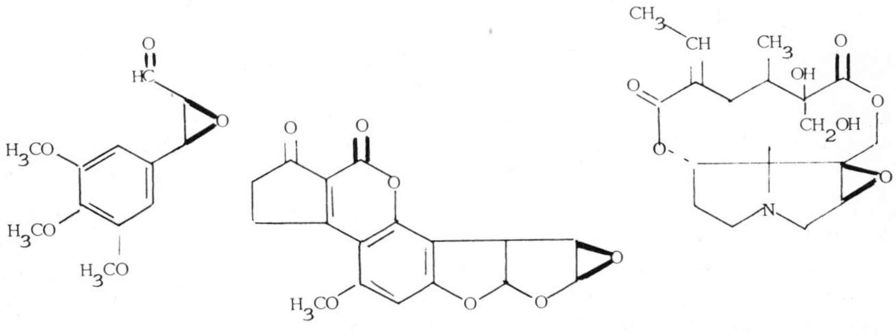

Figure 2 Suggested structures for epoxides of 3,4,5-trimethoxycinnamaldehyde (*left*), aflatoxin B$_1$ (*middle*), and retrorsine (*right*).

It is not unlikely that at a particular stage of the cell's existence, chromatin assumes a configuration in which a free amino group of a nucleic acid base may be present in close vicinity to two thiols of peptide chains. Such a configuration would allow the aldehydic carbonyl to condense with the amino group to form a Schiff-base type of bond, while the thiols could reduce the nitroso group and form a covalent bond. As a result, a firm bridge (possibly in the form of a six- or seven-membered ring) would bind the protein to the nucleic acid. Such binding may be irreversible and have long lasting, fateful consequences, as is the case of carcinogens which can induce tumors with even a single dose.

The particular sensitivity of the young and their actively developing tissues to the action of carcinogens may be related to their higher content of cells in the receptive state. In addition, the paucity of certain enzyme systems at the perinatal age will slow down the formation and also the degradation of the activated form of the carcinogens. The net balance results in the higher probability that both interactants will meet in the appropriate state.

However, the interplay of other factors, genetic, viral, and immunological will determine whether and which of the cells affected by a carcinogen will die and which ones will survive, start dividing, and form the center of a new growing tissue with neoplastic characteristics.

The idea that a specific organotropism is an inherent characteristic of a carcinogen is no more tenable. It is clear from the reviewed results that a carcinogen can induce tumors in almost any organ or tissue that contains cells in appropriate receptive state at the time when it is reached by the activated carcinogenic entity in appropriate concentration.

The answers to the fundamental questions—where and how is the activated carcinogenic entity formed, and when formed, how long can it survive the passage in the blood stream and through the inter- and intracellular membranes so as to reach the recipient site in adequate concentration, and what are the essential characteristics of the activated entity—all seem to need reconsideration.

The various alkylating forms, so far proposed (136, 137) may not be relevant for the carcinogenic process. An alternative hypothesis has been suggested (149).

More than one step is likely to be involved in the activation of the parent molecules. Are these steps accomplished at the same or at different sites of the cell or possibly in different organs?

The liver may not be an over-important organ in dealing with the activation of carcinogens. Drug metabolizing enzyme systems have been reported in other organs, e.g. the lung (146).

Though we may not yet be able to give satisfactory explanations to all these questions, the demonstration that many organs are particularly sensitive to carcinogens during the perinatal period indicates that metabolic studies on the molecular level in the newborn may give better chances for the identification of the reactions relevant for the induction of tumors.

SUMMARY

The reviewed evidence derived from animal experiments performed in the last few years by many workers shows the following:

A single dose of carcinogen, which may not cause immediate ill effects, can induce tumors after a prolonged latent period.

The susceptibility of the fetus or of the newborn to carcinogens is much greater than that of weanlings or adults.

The type and the localization of the tumors induced depends not only on the characteristics of the carcinogen, its route of entry, and the size of the dose, but to a large extent on the biological age of the recipient and on the developmental and functional state of the organs at the time of treatment.

Exposure of females to carcinogens during the early stages of pregnancy has usually cytotoxic effects, which cause resorption or abortion of the embryo; during the second trimester of pregnancy malformations may be produced, while tumors develop in the offspring when the carcinogen acts during the second half of gestation. The tumors induced in rodents transplacentally become apparent only many months later.

Hormones, especially estrogens, can induce neoplasias in their target organs; they may have, in addition, modifying effects on the action of other carcinogens.

The possibility is discussed that exposure of pregnant or lactating females to an increased load of compounds with estrogenic and other hormonal activities may present teratogenic or carcinogenic hazards to both sexes of the offspring.

Formation of carcinogenic nitroso-compounds in the stomach from noncarcinogenic constituents possibly present in food and medicines may represent an additional teratogenic and carcinogenic hazard.

In order to reproduce in animals a situation in which tumors would appear in the fetus or in the newborn (as in clinical experience), preconception exposure of the parents' gonads to carcinogens might be required, possibly in addition to intrauterine exposure of the embryo to noncytotoxic concentrations of carcinogenic agents.

Epidemiological studies in the USA disclosed an increased incidence of childhood tumors and leukemias in the offspring of parents who were exposed to irradiation long before conception, especially when the offspring was additionally irradiated prenatally or postnatally (for references see 147). Such a situation may have its counterpart also in the case of the "radiomimetic" chemical carcinogens.

ACKNOWLEDGMENTS

I wish to thank Mrs. N. P. Brewster for her excellent and devoted secretarial help.

Note added in proof: The recent finding of the very rare benign hepatomas in seven young women, 25–39 years old, possibly associated with the use of oral contraceptives for up to 12 years (148), adds to the misgivings expressed in this review as regards the use of OC.

Literature Cited

1. Wells, H. G. 1940. *Arch. Pathol.* 30: 535–601
2. Willis, R. A. 1962. *The Pathology of Tumours of Children.* Edinburgh: Oliver and Boyd
3. Morison, J. E. 1970. *Foetal and neonatal pathology.* London: Butterworth. 3rd ed.
4. Napalkov, N. P. 1973. In *Transplacental Carcinogenesis,* ed. L. Tomatis, U. Mohr, W. Davis. IARC Publ. No. 4, 1–13
5. Zuckerman, S., Mandl, A. M., Eckstein, P., Eds. 1968. *The Ovary.* London: Academic
6. Gross, L. 1970. *Oncogenic Viruses.* Oxford: Pergamon. 2nd ed.
7. Stewart, A. 1971. *Advan. Cancer Res.* 14:359–90
8. Detroy, R. W., Littlehoj, E. B., Ciegler, A. 1971. In *Fungal Toxins,* ed. A. Ciegler, S. Kadis, S. J. Ajl, 6:4–178, London: Academic
9. Magee, P. N., Barnes, J. M. 1967. *Advan. Cancer Res.* 10:163–246
10. Schoental, R. 1968. *Cancer Res.* 28: 2237–46
11. Lacqueur, G. L., Spatz, M. 1968. *Cancer Res.* 28:2262–67
12. Tomatis, L., Mohr, U., Davis, W., Eds. 1973. *Transplacental Carcinogenesis.* IARC Publ. No. 4
13. Orr, J. W. See Ref. 5, 2:533–65
14. Stewart, A. M. 1973. *Brit. J. Cancer* 27:465–72
15. Lenz, W. 1962. *Am. J. Dis. Child.* 112: 99–106
16. Karnofsky, D. A. 1965. *Ann. Rev. Pharmacol.* 5:447–72
17. Herbst, A. L., Ulfelder, H., Poskanzer, D. C. 1971. *N. Engl. J. Med.* 284: 878–81

18. Herbst, A. L., Kurman, R. J., Scully, R. E., Poskanzer, D. C. 1972. *N. Engl. J. Med.* 287:1259–63
19. Wilkins, L. P. 1960. *J. Am. Med. Assoc.* 172:1028–32
20. Kuchera, L. K. 1971. *J. Am. Med. Assoc.* 218:562–63
21. Doll, R. 1971. *Brit. Med. Bull.* 27: 25–31
22. Report from the Boston Collaborative Drug Surveillance Programme. 1973. *Lancet* i:1399–1404
23. Nora, J. J., Nora, A. H. 1973. *Teratology* 7:Abstr. 24
24. Wong, Y. K., Wood, B. S. B. 1971. *Brit. Med. J.* iv:403–4
25. Andrea, F. P., Christensen, H. D., Williams, T. L., Thompson, M. G., Wall, M. E. 1973. *Teratology* 7:A11 (Abstr., Proc. Meet. Teratol. Soc., 13th)
26. Lacassagne, A. 1932. *C. R. Acad. Sci. Paris* 195:630–32
27. Gardner, W. U. 1959. *Ann. NY Acad. Sci.* 75:543–64
28. Mühlbock, O. 1972. *J. Nat. Cancer Inst.* 48:1213–16
29. Dunn, T. B., Green, A. W. 1963. *J. Nat. Cancer Inst.* 31:425–55
30. Dunn, T. B. 1969. *J. Nat. Cancer Inst.* 43:671–92
31. Kirkman, H. 1972. *Progr. Exp. Tumor Res. Basel* 16:201–40
32. Sidransky, H., Wagner, B. P., Morris, H. P. 1961. *J. Nat. Cancer Inst.* 26: 151–87
33. Firminger, H. I., Reuber, M. D. 1961. *J. Nat. Cancer Inst.* 27:559–95
34. Morris, H. P., Firminger, H. I. 1956. *J. Nat. Cancer Inst.* 16:927–49
35. Runsfeld, H. W. Jr., Miller, W. L. Jr., Baumann, C. A. 1951. *Cancer Res.* 11: 814–19
36. Stromberg, K., Reuber, M. D. 1970. *J. Nat. Cancer Inst.* 44:1047–54
37. Reuber, M. D., Glover, E. L. 1967. *J. Nat. Cancer Inst.* 38:891–99
38. Reuber, M. D., Lee, C. W. 1968. *J. Nat. Cancer Inst.* 41:1133–40
39. Huggins, C., Briziarelli, G., Sutton, H. 1959. *J. Exp. Med.* 109:25–42
40. Jasmin, G., Riopelle, J. L. 1970. *Cancer Res.* 30:321–26
41. Gillette, J. R. 1971. *Ann. NY Acad. Sci.* 179:43–66
42. Sabine, J. R., Horton, B. J., Wicks, M. B. 1973. *J. Nat. Cancer Inst.* 50: 1237–42
43. Schoental, R., Gibbard, S. 1972. *Brit. J. Cancer* 26:504–06
44. Schoental, R. 1973. *Lab. Anim.* 7: 47–49
45. Editorial. 1973. *Nature* 243:6
46. Mirocha, C. J., Christensen, C. M., Nelson, G. H. See Ref. 8, 7:107–38
47. Butenandt, A., Jacobi, H. 1933. *Hoppe-Seyler's Z. Physiol. Chem.* 218:104–2
48. Bradbury, R. B., White, D. E. 1954. *Vitam. Horm. New York* 12:207–33
49. Liener, J. E. 1969. In *Toxic constituents of plant foodstuffs*, ed. J. E. Liener, 409–48. London: Academic
50. Bickoff, E. M. et al 1957. *Science* 126: 969–70
51. Bickoff, E. M., Livingston, A. L., Hendrickson, A. P., Booth, A. N. 1962. *J. Agr. Food Chem* 10:410–12
52. Jensen, E. V., DeSombre, E. R. 1972. *Ann. Rev. Biochem.* 41:203–30
53. Campbell, H. 1972. *Proc. Roy. Soc. Med.* 65:641–45
54. Malling, H. V., de Serres, F. J. 1969. *Ann. NY Acad. Sci.* 163:788–800
55. Röhrborn, G. See Ref. 12, pp. 168–74
56. Clegg, D. J. 1971. *Ann. Rev. Pharmacol.* 11:409–24
57. Di Paolo, J. A., Kotin, P. 1966. *Arch. Pathol.* 81:3–23
58. Green, C. R., Christie, G. S. 1961. *Brit. J. Exp. Pathol.* 42:369–78
59. Spatz, M. 1969. *Ann. NY Acad. Sci.* 163:848–59
60. Di Paolo, J. A. 1969. *Ann. NY Acad. Sci.* 163:801–12
61. Roe, F. J. C., Walters, M. A., Mitchley, B. C. V. 1967. *Brit. J. Cancer* 21:331–33
62. Hartwell, J. L. 1941. *US Publ. Health Serv. Publ.* No. 149; Shubik, P., Hartwell, J. L. 1957. Suppl. 1; 1969. Suppl. 2, ed. J. A. Peters
63. Toth, B. 1968. *Cancer Res.* 28:727–38
64. Della Porta, G., Terracini, B. 1969. *Progr. Exp. Tumor Res.* 11:334–63
65. Roe, F. J. C., Walters, M. A. 1968. *Food Cosmet. Toxicol.* 6:581–82
66. Schoental, R. 1970. *Nature,* 227:401–2
67. Schoental, R., Magee, P. N. 1957. *J. Pathol. Bacteriol.* 74:305–19
68. Magee, P. N., Barnes, J. M. 1959. *Acta Unio Int. Contra. Cancrum* 15:187–90
69. Schoental, R. 1960. *Nature* 188:420–21
70. Schoental, R., Bensted, J. P. M. 1963. *Brit. J. Cancer* 17:242–51
71. Druckrey, H. 1971. *Arzneim. Forsch.* 21:1274–78
72. Druckrey, H., Steinhoff, D., Preussmann, R., Ivankovic, S. 1964. *Z. Krebsforsch.* 66:1–10
73. Druckrey, H., Preussmann, R., Ivankovic, S., Schmähl, D. 1967. *Z. Krebsforsch.* 69:103–201

74. Terracini, B., Testa, M. C. 1970. *Brit. J. Cancer* 24:588–98
75. Jänisch, W., Schreiber, D., Stengel, R., Steffen, V. 1967. *Exp. Pathol.* 1:243–255
76. Kreybig, T. von 1965. *Z. Krebsforsch.* 67:46–50
77. Napalkov, N. P., Alexandrov, V. A. 1968. *Z. Krebsforsch.* 71:32–50
78. Alexandrov, V. A. 1969. *Nature* 222:1064–65
79. Druckrey, H., Ivankovic, S., Preussmann, R. 1966. *Nature London* 210:1378–79
80. Ivankovic, S., Druckrey, H. 1968. *Z. Krebsforsch.* 71:320–60
81. Druckrey, H., Schagen, B., Ivankovic, S. 1970. *Z. Krebsforsch.* 74:141–61
82. Druckrey, H., Landschütz, Ch., Ivankovic, S. 1970. *Z. Krebsforsch.* 73:371–86
83. Druckrey, H., Preussmann, R., Ivankovic, S. 1969. *Ann. NY Acad. Sci.* 163:676–95
84. Grossi-Paoletti, E., Paoletti, P., Schiffer, D., Fabiani, A. 1970. *J. Neurol. Sci.* 11:573–81
85. Koestner, A., Swenberg, J. A., Wechsler, W. 1971. *Am. J. Pathol.* 63:37–56
86. Jänisch, W., Schreiber, D., Warzok, R., Schneider, J. 1972. *Arch. Geschwulstforsch.* 39:99–106
87. Jones, E. L., Searle, C. E., Smith, W. T. 1973. *J. Pathol.* 109:123–39
88. Rice, J. M. 1969. *Ann. NY Acad. Sci.* 163:813–26
89. Searle, C. E., Jones E. L. 1973. *Nature* 240:559–60
90. Leaver, D. D., Swann, P. F., Magee, P. N. 1969. *Brit. J. Cancer* 23:177–87
91. Druckrey, H., Landschütz, C., Preussmann, R., Ivankovic, S. 1971. *Z. Krebsforsch.* 75:229–39
92. Druckrey, H., Landschütz, C. 1971. *Z. Krebsforsch.* 76:45–58
93. Druckrey, H., Lange, A. 1972. *Fed. Proc.* 31:1482–84
94. Druckrey, H. et al 1968. *Experientia* 24:561–62
95. Laqueur, G. L., Spatz, M. See Ref 12, pp. 59–64
96. Ginsburg, J. 1971. *Ann. Rev. Pharmacol.* 11:387–408
97. Wechsler, W. et al 1969. *Ann. NY Acad. Sci.* 159:360–408
98. Hirono, I. 1972. *Fed. Proc.* 31:1493–97
99. Mirvish, S. S. 1968. *Advan. Cancer Res.* 11:1–42
100. Matsuyama, M., Suzuki, H., Naka-mura, T. 1969. *Brit. J. Cancer,* 23:167–71
101. Kommineni, V. R., Greenblatt, M., Mihailovich, N., Vesselinovitch, S. D. 1970. *Cancer Res.* 30:2552–55
102. Nomura, T. 1973. *Cancer Res.* 33:1677–83
103. Nomura, T., Takebe, H. Okamoto, E. 1973. *Gann* 64:29–40
104. Goldfeder, A. 1972. *Cancer Res.* 32:2771–77
105. Schoental, R., Cavanagh, J. B. 1972. *J. Nat. Cancer Inst.* 49:665–71
106. Schoental, R. Unpublished results
107. Spatz, M., Laqueur, G. L. 1968. *Proc. Soc. Exp. Biol. Med.* 127:281
108. Tomatis, L. et al 1971. *J. Nat. Cancer Inst.* 47:645–51
109. Takahashi, G., Yasuhira, K. 1973. *Cancer Res.* 33:23–38
110. Alexandrov, V. A., Jänisch, W. 1971. *Experientia* 27:538–39
111. Ivankovic, S., Preussmann, R., Schmähl, D., Zeller, J. 1973. *Z. Krebsforsch.* 79:145–47
112. Ivankovic, S., Preussmann, R. 1970. *Naturwissenschaften,* 57:460
113. Osske, G., Warzok, R., Schneider, J. 1972. *Arch. Geschwulstforsch.* 40:244
114. Mirvish, S., Wallcave, L., Eagen, M., Shubik, P. 1972. *Science* 177:65–68
115. McLean, E. K. 1970. *Pharmacol. Rev.* 22:429–83
116. Schoental, R. 1959. *J. Pathol. Bacteriol.* 77:485–95
117. Evans, I. A., Jones, R. S., Mainwaring-Burton, R. 1972. *Nature* 237:107–8
118. Mickelsen, O., Campbell, E., Yang, M., Mugera, G., Whitehair, C. K. 1964. *Fed. Proc.* 23:1363–65
119. Shay, H., Gruenstein, M., Weinberger, M. 1952. *Cancer Res.* 12:29
120. Shay, H., Friedmann, B., Gruenstein, M. 1950. *Cancer Res.,* 10:797–800
121. Mohr, U., Althoff, J., Emminger, A., Bresch, K., Spielhoff, R. 1972. *Z. Krebsforsch.* 78:73–77
122. Schoental, R. Unpublished results
123. Blattmann, L., Preussmann, R. 1973. *Z. Krebsforsch.* 79:3–5
124. Sander, J. 1971. *Arzneim. Forsch.* 21:1707–13, 2034–39; 1970. 20:418–19
125. Greenblatt, H. M., Mirvish, S. S. 1973. *J. Nat. Cancer Inst.* 50:119–24
126. Lijinsky, W., Taylor, H. W., Snyder, C., Nettesheim, P. 1973. *Nature* 244:176–78
127. Nelson, M. M., Forfar, J. O. 1971. *Brit. Med. J.* i:523–27
128. Miller, R. W. See Ref. 12, pp. 175–80

129. Haddad, R. K., Rabe, A., Laqueur, G. L., Spatz, M., Valsamis, M. P. 1969. *Science* 163:88
130. Shabad, L. M., Kolesnichenko, T. S., Nikonova, T. V. 1973. *Int. J. Cancer* 11:688–93
131. Terracini, B., Testa, M. C., Cabral, J. R., Day, N. 1973. *Int. J. Cancer* 11: 747–64
132. Alfin-Slater, R. B., Aftergood, L., Hernandez, H. J., Stern, E., Melnick, D. 1969. *Am. Oil Chemists' Soc.* 46:493, quoted in Ref 8
133. Tomatis, L. 1965. *Proc. Soc. Exp. Biol. Med.* 119:743–47
134. Tomatis, L., Goodall, C. M. 1969. *Int. J. Cancer* 4:219–25
135. Tanaka, T. See Ref. 12, pp. 100–11
136. Druckrey, H. See Ref. 12, pp. 45–58
137. Magee, P. N. See Ref. 12, pp. 143–48
138. Culvenor, C. C. J., Downing, D. T., Edgar, J. A., Jago, M. V. 1969. *Ann. NY Acad. Sci.* 163:837–47
139. Schoental, R. 1967. *Biochem. J.* 102:5C
140. Rosenkranz, H. S., Rosenkranz, S., Schmidt, R. M. 1969. *Biochim. Biophys. Acta* 195:262–65
141. Singer, B., Fraenkel-Conrat, H. 1969. *Biochemistry* 8:3266–69
142. Schoental, R. 1973. *Brit. J. Cancer.* In press
143. Grover, P. L. et al 1971. *Proc. Nat. Acad. Sci. USA* 68:1098–1101
144. Schoental, R. 1970. *Nature* 227:401–2
145. Okada, M., Suzuki, E. 1972. *Gann* 63: 391–92
146. Fouts, J. R., Devereux, T. R. 1972. *J. Pharmacol. Exp. Ther.* 183:458–68
147. Miller, R. W. 1972. *J. Nat. Cancer Inst.* 49:1221–27 and references therein
148. Baum, J. K., Bookstein, J. J., Joltz, F., Klein, E. W. 1973. *Lancet* ii:926–29
149. Schoental, R. 1974. In press

FACTORS DETERMINING THE TERATOGENICITY OF DRUGS

❖6589

James G. Wilson

Children's Hospital Research Foundation and Departments of Pediatrics and Anatomy, University of Cincinnati, Cincinnati, Ohio

Because knowledge of this subject has expanded tremendously in the past several years, it is no longer possible to do more than outline it in a review of this length. The main objective, therefore, is to enumerate the aspects of the subject that are now recognized as important determinants; however, certain areas where concepts are currently undergoing change are reviewed in detail. The considerations presently known to be involved in determining whether a drug will be teratogenic are listed in Table 1. Before discussing these individually it should be emphasized that the term teratogenicity is used here in the broad sense of developmental toxicity, encompassing all deviations in developmental processes originating between fertilization and postnatal maturity, including death, malformation, growth retardation, and functional deficiency.

Table 1 Factors determining teratogenicity of drugs

1. Type of drug (chemical and pharmacological properties)
2. Level and duration of dosage
3. Maternal modulation of dosage
4. Access to the conceptus
5. Developmental stage at time of dosage
6. Disposition within the conceptus
7. Susceptibility of species and individual

TYPES OF DRUGS

The types of drugs shown to be teratogenic in laboratory mammals number in the hundreds and cannot be listed, although some impression of their variety is given

205

in Table 2. In most of the experimental situations in which such compounds have been shown to be embryotoxic, the doses used were much larger than those recommended for human therapeutic use or, in the case of environmental chemicals, than likely exposure levels to human populations. More extensive but by no means exhaustive lists have been compiled elsewhere (1–5). The multitude of substances thus implicated suggests that all chemical agents are teratogenic. In fact, most investigators in the field accept as a working hypothesis the principle that all chemicals are capable of producing some embryotoxic effect under the right conditions of dosage, developmental stage, and species selection (6, 7). It may be difficult to demonstrate embryotoxicity, however, when high maternal toxicity intercedes.

Table 2 Types of drugs and environmental chemicals shown to be teratogenic[a] in one or more species of mammals[b]

Salicylates (e.g. aspirin, oil of wintergreen)

Certain alkaloids (e.g. caffeine, nicotine, colchicine)

Tranquilizers (e.g. meprobamate, chlorpromazine, reserpine)

Antihistamines (e.g. buclizine, meclizine, cyclizine)

Antibiotics (e.g. chloramphenicol, streptonigrin, penicillin)

Hypoglycemics (e.g. carbutamide, tolbutamide, hypoglycins)

Corticoids (e.g. triamcinolone, cortisone)

Alkylating agents (e.g. busulfan, chlorambucil, cyclophosphamide, TEM)

Antimalarials (e.g. chloroquine, quinacrine, pyrimethamine)

Anesthetics (e.g. halothane, urethan, nitrous oxide, pentobarbital)

Antimetabolities (e.g. folic acid, purine and pyrimidine analogues)

Solvents (e.g. benzene, dimethylsulfoxide, propylene glycol)

Pesticides (e.g. 2,4,5-T, carbaryl, captan, folpet)

Industrial effluents (e.g. some compounds of Hg, Pb, As, Li, Cd)

Miscellaneous (e.g. trypan blue, triparanol, diamox, etc.)

[a]Teratogenic effects were usually seen only at doses well above therapeutic levels for the drugs, or above likely exposure levels for the environmental chemicals.

[b]From Wilson, J.G. 1972. Environmental effects on development——teratology. In *Pathophysiology of Gestation*, ed. N. S. Assali, Vol. 2. New York: Academic; 1973. *Environment and Birth Defects.* New York: Academic.

There is not always close correlation between the chemical structure or pharmacological action of a drug and its teratogenic potential. A few classes such as the polyfunctional alkylating agents have been found to be teratogenic in every instance in which they have been adequately tested. By the nature of their biological effects, antibiotics also would be expected to interfere with embryonic development, and many have been shown to do so. Those bacteriocidal agents that act by interference with protein biosynthesis, however, seem to be exceptional, for they have not been found to cause malformations per se (unpublished data), probably owing to the essentiality of protein synthesis in all aspects of development, although they do cause early embryonic death. The diazo dyes, of which trypan blue is the best-known example, show highly variable teratogenicity despite being closely related in chemical structure (8, 9); a similar situation holds for the substances related to meclizine (10) and thalidomide (11). Although acetazolamide is highly teratogenic in several rodent species, other carbonic anhydrase inhibitors and related sulfonamides are much less effective (12, 13).

Even though drugs are usually if not universally teratogenic when tested at high dosage at known times of high embryonic vulnerability in susceptible species, it is surprising that so few drugs are known or suspected to be teratogenic in man, particularly considering their extensive use during human pregnancy (14). The teratogenicity of specific drugs has recently been reviewed in some detail (15, 16) and is only briefly summarized here. Only three types of drugs have been positively implicated in man: androgenic hormones, thalidomide, and the folic acid antagonists. To produce persistent developmental alterations in the genital organs of genetic females, male hormones must be administered prior to the twelfth week of gestation when the normal differentiation of these organs is completed. The thalidomide syndrome is so well known as to require no further characterization. The folate antagonists are more embryolethal than teratogenic, in the sense of causing irreversible structural or functional defects, but about 30% of surviving infants show a variety of anatomic or physiologic abnormalities. It now seems likely that another group of drugs will be added to these established as human teratogens, as indicated below.

A second category of drugs included those only suspected of some teratogenic potential in man. Although the percentage of total cases is small, the persistence of associations between the taking of these drugs during early pregnancy and reports of prenatal death or the birth of defective infants suggests the possibility of causal relationship. Most noteworthy in this group are the anticonvulsant drugs used in the treatment of epilepsy (15, 16). Since the earlier reviews, a spate of additional reports have left little doubt that a higher percentage of defective infants are born to epileptic women on anticonvulsant therapy during the first trimester of pregnancy than would be expected from births in the general population (17–31). Several important questions must be answered, however, before this effect can be attributed to the drugs used. The case reports and surveys have involved use of several different anticonvulsants and, of course, many of the women were on more than one of these drugs during all or part of their pregnancies. Furthermore, there has been no clear segregation of the effects of taking the drugs and of the physiologic imbalances that accompany and follow convulsive seizures occurring during pregnancy. Finally, whichever genetic factors may predispose to epilepsy may introduce an additional element of instability into embryonic development. Until these questions are nearer resolution, it seems more prudent to leave the anticonvulsant drugs in the "probable" category than to move them to the "proven" category as regards teratogenesis in man. Of incidental interest are the observations that diphenylhydantoin appears to have a low level of embryotoxicity in rhesus monkeys (32) and is unquestionably teratogenic in rodents (33–36).

There is less compelling evidence that certain neurotropic anorexogenic drugs, oral hypoglycemics, and perhaps all alkylating agents should also be suspected of some degree of teratogenic potential in man (15, 16).

A third category consists of drugs thought to have teratogenic potential under some conditions because of infrequently reported associations between their use during human pregnancy and the birth of defective children and/or of demonstrated teratogenicity in laboratory mammals (15, 16). This list includes the following: (a) aspirin and other salicylates, none of which has been directly implicated in man, are known to be embryotoxic at high dosage in rhesus monkeys and laboratory rodents; (b) antibiotics, some of which have been questionably associated with increased rates of abortion, stillbirth, and the birth of defective children and others of which have been clearly shown to be teratogenic in rodents; (c) antituberculous drugs about which the reports are meager and conflicting; (d) quinine, which, when used in high doses as an abortifacient in man, may have been responsible for a few visual and auditory defects but which in animals has mainly caused death and growth retardation; and (e) insulin as used in psychiatric therapy which, if applied during pregnancy, may occasionally lead to death in utero or to the birth of defective children. Imipramine, reported early in 1972 to have been associated with the birth of infants with reduction defects of the limbs (37), now seems very doubtful as a human teratogen. The earlier claims were not substantiated in more than 220 subsequent case reports in which only six malformed children were found, none with reduction defects of the limbs.

Until very recently, female sex hormones applied during pregnancy have rarely been associated with human developmental abnormality (38). A few cases of malformed newborns were attributed to maternal treatment with large doses of estrogen early in pregnancy (39), but no instances of feminization of genetic males with estrogenic steroids is known. In the last three years, however, smaller doses of combined estrogen and progestins have raised some questions. Unsuccessful attempts to induce abortion by taking a number of contraceptive pills containing synthetic progestins and estrogen have been associated with the birth of defective infants in a few instances (40, 41), but arguments against such causation have also been presented (42). Questions have been raised about the possibility of teratogenic effects following use of hormonal pregnancy tests involving pills containing estrogenic and progestational hormones, although two well-controlled studies have found no significant association between such tests and specific malformations (43, 44). However, other recent reports of uses of female hormones during pregnancy have noted some associations with the birth of a number of defective infants (45–48). One study on reduction deformities of the limbs found a higher than expected number of contraceptive pill failures and of the birth of twins among the mothers of the deformed babies, but the authors (49) tended to relate both occurrences to maternal endocrine dysfunction. The teratogenic status of these hormones will depend upon the collection of further data, but their widespread use would suggest that if any appreciable teratogenic potential existed, it would already have been detected.

A puzzling reaction to maternal treatment with the nonsteroidal estrogenic substance, diethylstilbestrol, during pregnancy has been noted. Approximately 100 girls and young women between ages 8 and 25 years have been diagnosed as having vaginal or cervical adenocarcinoma, and a majority of the histories revealed that their mothers had been given stilbestrol, related drugs, or unidentified drugs for bleeding during pregnancy (50–52). Although these neoplasms do not appear to represent deviations of normal developmental processes, and accordingly are not strictly teratic in origin, they seem to have been induced during early differentiation of the mullerian ducts, possibly as a somatic mutation. In any event, they raise interesting questions about the relationship between carcinogenesis and teratogenesis.

As already noted, there is some basis for assuming that all drugs are embryotoxic if given under optimal conditions to laboratory animals. Nevertheless, there is ample reason to regard some drugs as safe for use during human pregnancy at recommended therapeutic levels. This opinion is supported by the fact that many drugs have been widely used during pregnancy and have not been associated with adverse effects on the conceptus. A few drugs have for one reason or another at some time been suspect, but have been found after further investigation to pose little risk for therapeutic or other use during pregnancy. This group includes LSD, sulfonamides, meclizine, adrenocortical steroids, and tranquilizers and antiemetics generally (15, 16). The possibility that these and other seemingly safe drugs may have undesirable effects during pregnancy under conditions of overdosage, individual sensitivity, or potentiative interaction with other drugs or environmental factors cannot be ruled out.

Before leaving the subject of the types of drug and causation of embryotoxicity, it should be recalled that chemical composition is the major factor in determining mechanisms of action, whether teratologic or pharmacologic. Mechanisms of teratogenic action are as yet poorly understood, although attempts have been made to enumerate several that appear to be supported by experimental evidence or logical presumption (15). As will be noted below, the type of drug also determines the rate and manner in which it is absorbed, metabolized, excreted, and transferred to the conceptus.

LEVEL AND DURATION OF EXPOSURE

That the level of dosage determines the degree and type of response above the no-effect level is as firmly established in teratology as in other aspects of toxicology. The existence of a threshold below which no embryotoxic effects can be demonstrated for a given substance has on occasion been questioned, probably because of uncertainties about thresholds as regards mutagenic and carcinogenic effects. Actually most teratologists accept the concept of threshold, owing to the vast accumulation of experimental studies on multiple dosage levels in which one or more doses caused no developmental deviations greater than those seen in controls. Nevertheless, the argument can be raised that because the lower end of the dose-response curve may be extremely flat, very large numbers of offspring would be necessary to rule out a low level of embryotoxicity at low dosage. This argument has logical validity, but in practice two facts mitigate against it, in addition to the large volume of contrary data: (a) the dose-response curve for embryotoxic effects tends to have a steep slope, and (b) highly integrated systems such as embryos are well known to have appreciable regulatory and regenerative powers. The latter fact is significant because it would permit recovery from effects such as a slowed proliferative rate or a modest amount of cell death, assuming that these occurred at small doses. Until such time as experiments involving thousands of animals are able to demonstrate otherwise, it seems justifiable on pragmatic grounds to accept the existence of a threshold for teratogenic effects (15).

The period of time over which drug treatment is given can influence embryotoxicity under two conditions: (a) when the drug is capable of inducing or inhibiting its own enzymatic metabolism, and (b) when continued use of the drug would interfere with the function of the maternal liver, kidneys, or other organs essential for homeostasis, including the elimination of other potentially embryotoxic substances. Because of such considerations, single doses are sometimes more effective than multiple doses of equivalent or greater total amount. Using a number of pesticides, Robens (53) provided an experimental example of the fact that repeated dosage may produce different embryotoxic results than a single treatment. Groups of pregnant hamsters were treated on days 6 through 10 with the test compounds, while other groups were treated with smaller total amounts of the same compounds as a single dose on gestation day 7 or 8. Multiple treatments caused few developmental defects even at high doses but did cause some resorption and maternal death. The single treatments produced numerous defects in liveborn young. A similar phenomenon was observed by King et al (10) who gave chlorcyclizine to pregnant rats at 50 mg/kg/day from days 10 to 15 of gestation and produced a high incidence of cleft palate. However, when other rats were given the same daily dosage from days 1 through 15 of gestation, malformations were greatly reduced. The possible explanation in both instances is that repeated treatments induced metabolizing enzymes that were able to lower maternal plasma levels of the test substance before the embryo's most sensitive period was reached. In this and several other ways (Table 3) a potential embryotoxic effect could be masked by repeated dosage prior to the peak of the susceptible period of the embryo. These possibilities are of obvious importance in teratogenicity testing.

MATERNAL MODULATION OF DOSAGE

The dosage of a drug reaching the embryo or fetus in part depends on maternal plasma levels, particularly of free drug and metabolites. Concentration in maternal blood is the differential between rate of absorption and rate of dispersal by the maternal homeostatic and other factors that tend to reduce the plasma level. Dispersal is used here in the collective sense of all factors that reduce concentration: placental transfer as well as metabolism, excretion, storage, etc. Aside from the role of the placenta, which is discussed below, the subject of removal of drugs from the maternal blood stream is generally the same in the pregnant as in the nonpregnant individual and needs no particular consideration here. Figure 1 is a diagrammatic

Table 3 Ways in which repeated treatment prior to the peak susceptible period of the embryo may produce misleading results[a]

Time of treatment	Primary effect	Secondary effect capable of altering test results
1. Before implantation	Interference with implantation	No issue
2. Early organogenesis	Early embryonic death	No issue
3. Before peak susceptibility	Induction of catabolizing enzymes	Reduced blood level during susceptible period
4. Before peak susceptibility	Inhibition of catabolizing enzymes	Increased blood level during susceptible period
5. Before peak susceptibility	Liver pathology or reduced function	Increased blood level during susceptible period
6. Before peak susceptibility	Kidney pathology or reduced function[b]	Increased blood level during susceptible period
7. Before peak susceptibility	Saturation of protein binding sites[b]	Increased blood level during susceptible period

[a]From Wilson, J. G. 1973. *Environment and Birth Defects.* New York: Academic.

[b]These effects have not been demonstrated in experimental teratology but their existence in other toxicological situations makes their applicability to teratology likely.

representation of the fact that plasma concentration and secondarily embryo dose are influenced by the several maternal homeostatic functions that tend to reduce them.

ACCESS TO THE CONCEPTUS

Aside from being trite, the term "placental barrier," is inaccurate in the sense that the placenta probably does not totally exclude any chemical present in more than negligible amounts in maternal plasma. Certainly this applies to drugs, most of which have molecular weights of less than 600 (53). There is now abundant evidence that a variety of chemicals cross the placenta and are present in the conceptus in measurable amounts in both man (54–58) and in laboratory animals (59–61). Aside from the protein-type hormones such as glucagon (62), reports of failure of therapeutic agents to traverse the placenta in some fraction of maternal plasma concentration are virtually unknown; even some immune proteins are known to reach the conceptus in effective amounts. Thus the critical question would seem to be not whether, but at what rate, drugs taken by pregnant women reach their concepti.

Much remains to be learned about the dynamics of placental transfer, particularly at developmental stages that correspond to times of high teratogenic susceptiblity in the early embryo. Most studies to date have been done on rodent or near-term human placentas. Although human material obtained at surgical abortion is being used increasingly to study placental transfer (63–65), the substances studied to date

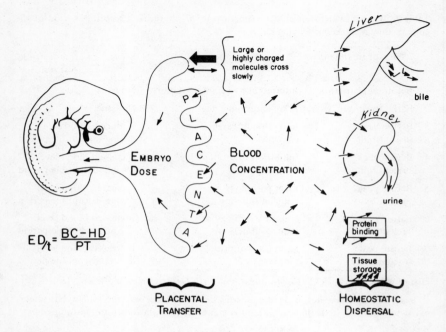

$$ED_{/t} = \frac{BC-HD}{PT}$$

Figure 1 Diagram of the factors that influence embryo dose of a foreign chemical present in the maternal blood stream. The maternal blood concentration under usual conditions of exposure is subject to considerable change, representing as it does the differential between maternal absorption and the several routes for dispersal, including the maternal homeostatic processes of metabolism, excretion, protein binding, and tissue storage, as well as passage across the placenta to the embryo. These various biological processes are all functions of time; therefore the embryo dose depends on the duration as well as the level of a chemical in maternal blood. Embryo dose is proportional to maternal blood concentration, however, only for substances that traverse the placenta by simple diffusion. Otherwise the placenta imposes various rates of transfer depending on the nature of the substance being transferred. The formulation $ED/t = BC - HD/PT$ is in no sense a precise mathematical one, but does attempt to state the basic fact that embryo dose (ED) over a given period of time (t) depends on the maternal blood concentration (BC) which tends constantly to be reduced by homeostatic dispersal (HD) and by placental transfer (PT). From Wilson, J. G. 1973. *Environment and Birth Defects.* New York: Academic.

have been largely medications of therapeutic benefit to the mother that were given after the period of highest embryonic susceptibility, estimated to occur between 3 to 7 weeks of gestation. Both the thickness and the area of the membrane across which transfer occurs are known to vary markedly during development (59, 66, 67), conditions that would inevitably influence rate of transfer. Studies using rodents and rabbits to investigate placental transfer functions in relation to teratogenicity are of doubtful significance for man because the atypical yolk sac placenta, on which these animals depend during early organogenesis, is thought to transfer many chemicals differently from that seen in higher mammals (68–71). A concentration gradient, with fetal tissues and fluid compartments having lower levels than maternal plasma, have usually been observed during middle and late pregnancy in animals and man (61, 63, 65, 72). This could be attributed to any of three factors postulated to reduce the amount of foreign chemicals that reach and are retained by the conceptus. The first has to do with the dynamics of simple diffusion, by which most drugs are thought to be transferred, and relates to the probability that concentration in maternal plasma would begin to fall as a result of homeostatic dispersal before fetal concentration would have time to reach equilibrium. The second possibility is that the placenta, by biotransformation of foreign chemicals, can catabolize a part of the dosage during transfer or conjugate them so that the rate of transfer would be slowed, as is discussed below. A third possibility is that a part of the dose reaching the conceptus would be metabolized in situ, thereby reducing the likelihood of appreciable concentration in the embryo or fetus, as will also be discussed below. Before considering the evidence concerning the latter two possibilities, however, it should be noted that embryonic or fetal concentration is not always less than that in maternal plasma. For example, hydroxyurea level in the 12-day rat embryo became and remained higher than the level in maternal plasma for several hours after ip dosage of the pregnant female (73), probably as a result of binding within the embryo. Incorporation of pyrimidine analogs in appreciable amounts into the DNA and RNA of rapidly growing rodent embryos has been repeatedly demonstrated (74, 75).

Much interest has recently centered on the possibility that the placenta may afford some protection to the embryo or fetus by metabolizing foreign chemicals before they are transferred to the intrauterine occupant. There is no longer any doubt that the placenta at term contains the enzymatic equipment to transform chemicals by all of the standard metabolic pathways, oxidation, reduction, hydrolysis, and conjugation (76–78). Some of these reactions have also been demonstrated in homogenates of fetal placentas from early in the second trimester (79) but, regardless of the gestational age when examined, such metabolic activity in vitro does not necessarily reflect activity in the intact placenta in vivo. In fact there seems little reason to believe that the placenta of any age contains more catabolizing enzymes than are needed in support of its own maintenance and extensive biosynthetic activities. Certainly there is no reason to regard the placenta as capable of protecting the embryo or fetus from exposure to drugs by virtue of its ability to degrade them metabolically.

DEVELOPMENTAL STAGE WHEN EXPOSURE OCCURS

That the degree and type of reaction shown by a developing organism depend on the stage in development when exposure to an adverse influence occurs is one of the most basic principles of teratology. The subject has been extensively discussed elsewhere (80), and the present purpose only requires a brief summary. Susceptibility to developmental deviation in man is thought to be low from fertilization until the embryonic germ layers begin differentiation on about day 17; it then abruptly rises during early organogenesis and probably reaches a peak between days 25 and 35. It gradually subsides during later organogenesis and throughout the fetal period, and continues at a low level in certain tissues (nervous and endocrine systems) until about puberty. The time of exposure not only governs the severity of the reaction but also the type of developmental toxicity, i.e. death, malformation, growth retardation, or functional deficiency. During the embryonic period when proliferation and differentiation of tissues and organs is predominant, gross malformation or embryonic death is the usual response to an adequate dosage. During the fetal period when overall growth and functional maturation are in progress, adverse influences are more likely to result in growth retardation or functional deficiency, although high dosage may still lead to abnormal histogenesis or even to death. After birth only those organs which remain functionally incomplete, mainly brain and some endocrine glands, are likely to be vulnerable to impairment of final functional maturation, although unfavorable factors can still interfere with overall growth to mature stature.

DISPOSITION OF DRUGS WITHIN THE CONCEPTUS

This subject has recently been the focus of considerable attention. Data are virtually nonexistent on the capacity of the early mammalian embryo to carry out any type of catabolic metabolism of foreign chemicals. It is a safe assumption that embryos do not metabolize drugs until such organs as the liver, lungs, and kidneys have completed organogenesis, or at least have accumulated some parenchymatous tissue with a degree of functional competence resembling that in postnatal animals. This degree of organ maturation does not occur in rodents and rabbits until approximately term, and the situation may be only moderately more advanced in carnivores and ungulates at birth. It is not surprising, therefore, that newborn animals of these types generally have little or no capacity to metabolize drugs (81–84). In contrast, the histogenesis of the human liver is relatively advanced at birth. An appreciable accumulation of agranular endoplasmic reticulum (microsomes) is apparent by electron microscopy as early as the third month of gestation (85). The liver of the human newborn is able to carry out several enzymatic biotransformations (58), although the possibility exists that some of the necessary enzymes were induced by maternal drug therapy a few days before delivery, and some induction may even occur before surgical abortion at midpregnancy (86). Limited capacity to carry out certain drug metabolizing reactions has been repeatedly shown by the liver and other organs of fetuses removed at abortion during the second trimester (63, 64, 87, 88), but these have been quite weak and altogether lacking in some pathways, e.g. conjugation, as compared with adult liver (89, 90).

Whole-body autoradiography after treatment of pregnant mice with radiolabeled drugs has generally shown concentrations in fetal organs to be much lower than in maternal organs (61, 72) with the exception of such substances as steroids, vitamin B_{12}, and iron. The observation of appreciable amounts of labeled compounds in the uterine lumen has led one investigator (61) to suggest that the inverted yolk sac epithelium may be able to concentrate and excrete drugs directly into the lumen of the genital tract where they could be eliminated directly without passage back across the chorioallantoic placenta to the maternal blood stream. This is an interesting possibility but it is so far supported only by circumstantial evidence. In any event, it would only apply to drug elimination in rodents and rabbits, the principal mammals possessing this unique accessory placental structure.

In sum the drug-metabolizing capacity of the embryo, except for incorporation of certain analogs in biosynthesis, is thought to be negligible for want of parenchymatous tissue with any degree of functional maturity, in the postnatal sense. This is the time that major teratogenesis has its inception; therefore, it is highly unlikely that the embryo has intrinsic defenses against foreign chemicals at the time they are most needed. This period of presumed high vulnerability extends only through the seventh or eighth week of human gestation; however, it occupies a much greater proportion of intrauterine development in rodents, in which tissue maturation is not appreciable until near term. The considerably longer fetal period of man is undoubtedly associated with significantly more functional development in such organs as liver, lungs, and kidneys; indeed, these organs have been shown to possess some capacity for enzymatic transformation of drugs as early as midgestation. Whether this capacity has significance in protecting against an adverse effect of drugs, however, can be questioned on two bases. First, the enzymatic activity in these fetal organs has generally been found to be quite low by postnatal standards; second, by the time appreciable drug-metabolizing competence is achieved by fetal tissues, most organs have reached advanced developmental stages that would render them immune from most structural and many functional deviations. Exceptions may be the brain and some endocrine glands.

SUSCEPTIBILITY OF THE SPECIES (AND INDIVIDUAL)

This subject has received much attention in experimental teratology and has been extensively reviewed elsewhere (15, 91). Of particular interest here are the factors that determine susceptibility to teratogenesis and their relation to the extrapolation of safety evaluation data from animal to man. As indicated in the foregoing discussions, the ultimate reaction of the conceptus to a given drug or foreign chemical in the maternal blood stream depends on three questions: 1. Can maternal homeostatic functions reduce the plasma level soon enough to avert an embryotoxic dose to the conceptus? 2. Are the structural and functional characteristics of the placenta such as to favor or impede transfer of an embryotoxic dose? 3. To what extent is the embryo or fetus inherently vulnerable to the chemical in question? The answers to these questions are in large measure determined by the genetic makeup of both the mother and the conceptus and, of course, in a broader sense to the genetic makeup of the species. Interspecies differences in the conditions that relate to all of these questions, possibly excepting the third, are now known, but they must be much more fully understood before test results in an animal species can be applied to safety predictions in man with a high degree of assurance. Thus, the preclinical evaluation of drugs for teratogenic potential in man will remain largely empirical until much more data have accumulated on the mechanisms of actions of drugs in the conceptus, the dynamics of their placental transport, and the factors governing their disposition in the maternal organism, both in man and the test species.

Literature Cited

1. Cahen, R. L. 1966. *Advances in Pharmacology,* ed. S. Garottini, P. A. Shore, 263–334. New York: Academic
2. Kalter, H., Warkany, J. 1959. *Physiol. Rev.* 39:69–115
3. Karnofsky, D. A. 1965. *Ann. Rev. Pharmacol.* 5:447–72
4. Nishimura, H. 1964. *Chemistry and Prevention of Congenital Anomalies.* Springfield: Thomas
5. Tuchmann-Duplessis, H., Mercier-Parot, L. 1964. *Bull. Schweiz. Akad. Med. Wiss.* 35:490–526
6. Karnofsky, D. A. 1965. *Teratology, Principles and Techniques,* ed. J. G. Wilson, J. Warkany, 185–213. Chicago: Univ. Chicago Press
7. Wilson, J. G. 1964. *Am. J. Obstet. Gynecol.* 90:1181–92
8. Wilson, J. G. 1955. *Anat. Rec.* 123: 313–34
9. Beaudoin, A. R., Pickering, M. J. 1960. *Anat. Rec.* 137:297–306
10. King, C. T. G., Weaver, S. A., Narrod, S. A. 1965. *J. Pharmacol. Exp. Ther.* 147:391–98
11. Smith, R. L., Fabro, S., Schumacher, H., Williams, R. T. 1965. *Embryopathic Activity of Drugs,* ed. J. M. Robson, F. M. Sullivan, R. L. Smith. Boston: Little, Brown
12. Wilson, J. G., Maren, T. H., Takano, K., Ellison, A. 1968. *Teratology* 1:51–61
13. Maren, T. H., Ellison, A. C. 1972. *Johns Hopkins Med. J.* 130:95–104
14. Forfar, J. O., Nelson, M. M. 1973. *Clin. Pharmacol. Ther.* 14:632–42
15. Wilson, J. G. 1973. *Environment and Birth Defects.* New York: Academic
16. Wilson, J. G. 1973. *Teratology* 7:3–16
17. Crombie, D. L., Pinsent, R. J. F. H., Slater, B. C., Fleming, D., Cross, K. W. 1970. *Brit. Med. J.* 4:178–79
18. Elshove, J., van Eck, J. H. M. 1971. *Ned. Tijdschr. Geneesk.* 115:1371–75
19. Fedrick, J. 1973. *Brit. Med. J.* 2:442–48
20. Grosse, K. P., Schwanitz, G., Rotl, H. D., Wissmüller, H. F. 1972. *Humangenetik* 16:209–16
21. Hill, R. M., Horning, M. G., Horning, E. C. 1973. *Fetal Pharmacology,* ed. L. O. Boréus, 375–380. New York: Raven
22. Kuenssberg, E. V., Knox, J. D. E. 1973. *Lancet* 1:198
23. Lewin, P. 1973. *Lancet* 1:559
24. Loughnan, P. M., Gold, H., Vance, J. C. 1973. *Lancet* 1:70–72
25. Lowe, C. R. 1973. *Lancet* 1:9–10

26. Melchoir, J. C., Svensmark, O., Trolle, D. 1967. *Lancet* 2:860–61
27. Niswander, J. D., Wertelecki, W. 1973. *Lancet* 1:1062
28. South, J. 1972. *Lancet* 2:1154
29. Speidel, B. D., Meadow, S. R. 1972. *Lancet* 2:839
30. Starreveld-Zimmerman, A. A. E., van der Kolt, W. J., Meinardi, H., Elshove, J. 1973. *Lancet* 2:48–49
31. Watson, J. D., Spellacy, W. N. 1971. *Obstet. Gynecol.* 37:881–85
32. Wilson, J. G. Teratogenic causation in man and its evaluation in non-human primates, *Proc. Int. Conf. Birth Defects, 4th, Vienna, Sept. 2–8, 1973.* Amsterdam: Excerpta Med. Found. Submitted
33. Elshove, J. 1969. *Lancet* 2:1074
34. Gabler, W. L. 1968. *Arch. Int. Pharmacodyn.* 175:141–52
35. Harbison, R. D., Becker, B. A. 1969. *Teratology* 2:305–12
36. Harbison, R. D., Becker, B. A. 1972. *Toxicol. Appl. Pharmacol.* 22:193–200
37. McBride, W. G. 1972. *Teratology* 5:262
38. Bacic, M., Wesselius de Casparis, A., Diczfalusy, E. 1970. *Am. J. Obstet. Gynecol.* 107:531–34
39. Uhlig, H. 1959. *Geburtsh. Frauenheilk.* 19:346–52
40. Gardner, L. I., Assemany, S. R., Neu, R. L. 1970. *Lancet* 2:667–68
41. Papp, L., Gardo, S. 1971. *Lancet* 1:753
42. Neumann, F., Elger, W., Steinback, H. 1970. *Lancet* 2:1258–59
43. Laurence, M., Miller, M., Vowles, M., Evans, K., Carter, C. 1971. *Nature* 233: 495–96
44. Center for Disease Control. June 1973. *Congenital Malformations Surveillance, March–April 1973*
45. Gal, I., Kirman, B., Stern, J. 1967. *Nature* 216:83
46. Kaufman, R. L. 1973. *Lancet* 1:1396
47. Levy, E. P., Cohen, A., Fraser, F. C. 1973. *Lancet* 1:611
48. Nora, J. J., Nora, A. H. 1973. *Lancet* 1:941–42
49. Janerich, D. T., Piper, J. M., Glebatis, D. M. 1973. *Lancet* 2:96–97
50. Greenwald, P., Barlow, J. J., Nasca, P. C., Burnett, W. S. 1971. *N. Engl. J. Med.* 285:390–92
51. Herbst, A. L., Ulfelder, H., Poskanzer, D. C. 1971. *N. Engl. J. Med.* 284:878–81
52. Herbst, A. L., Kurman, R. J., Scully, R. E., Poskanzer, D. C. 1972. *N. Engl. J. Med.* 287:1259–64

53. Robens, J. F. 1969. *Toxicol. Appl. Pharmacol.* 15:152–63
54. Mirkin, B. L. 1973. *Clin. Pharmacol. Ther.* 14:643–47
55. Adamsons, K. 1965. *Symposium on the Placenta,* ed. D. Bergsma, 1:27–34. Nat. Found.–March of Dimes
56. Dancis, J., Money, W. L., Springer, D., Levitz, M. 1968. *Am. J. Obstet. Gynecol.* 101:820–29
57. Ginsburg, J. 1971. *Ann. Rev. Pharmacol.* 11:387–408
58. Horning, M. G. et al. See Ref. 21, pp. 355–73
59. Panigel, M. 1971. *Malformations Congenitales des Mammiferes,* ed. H. Tuchmann-Duplessis, 27–48. Paris: Masson
60. Villee, C. A. 1965. *Ann. NY Acad. Sci.* 123:237–44
61. Waddell, W. J. 1972. *Fed. Proc.* 31:52–61
62. Johnston, D. I., Bloom, S. R., Greene, K. R. Beard, R. W. 1973. *Biol. Neonate* 21:375–80
63. Idänpään-Heikkilä, J. E., Jouppila, P. I., Puolakka, J. O., Vorne, M. S. 1971. *Am. J. Obstet. Gynecol.* 109:1011–16
64. Juchau, M. R. et al. See Ref. 21, pp. 321–34
65. Nishimura, H. 1973. See Ref. 21, pp. 47–53
66. Aladjem, S. 1970. *Congenital Malformations,* 117–46. Amsterdam: Excerpta Med.
67. Boyd, J. D., Hamilton, W. J. 1970. *The Human Placenta.* Cambridge: Heffer
68. Beck, F., Lloyd, J. B., Griffiths, A. 1967. *J. Anat.* 101:461–78
69. Brent, R. L., Johnson, A. J., Jensen, M. 1971. *Teratology* 4:255–75
70. Payne, G. S., Deuchar, E. M. 1972. *J. Embryol. Exp. Morphol.* 27:533–42
71. Holson, J. F., Wilson, J. G. 1973. *Teratology* 7:A–17
72. Ullberg, S. 1973. See Ref. 21, pp. 57–73

73. Scott, W. J., Ritter, E. J., Wilson, J. G. 1971. *Develop. Biol.* 26:306–15
74. Dagg, C. P., Doerr, A., Offutt, C. 1966. *Biol. Neonate* 10:32–46
75. Schumacher, H. J., Wilson, J. G., Jordan, R. L. 1969. *Teratology* 2:99–106
76. Juchau, M. R. 1972. *Fed. Proc.* 31:48–51
77. Juchau, M. R., Dyer, D. C. 1972. *Pediatric Clinics of North America,* ed. S. J. Yaffe, 19:65–79. Philadelphia: Saunders
78. Kyegombe, D., Franklin, C. 1973. *Lancet* 1:405–6
79. Juchau, M. R., Pedersen, M. G., Fantel, A. G., Shepard, T. H. 1973. *Clin. Pharmacol. Ther.* 14:673–79
80. Wilson, J. G. 1973. *Pathobiology of Development,* ed. E. V. D. Perrin, M. J. Finegold, 11–30. Baltimore: Williams & Wilkins
81. Fouts, J. R. 1973. See Ref. 21, pp. 305–20
82. Jondorf, W. R., Maickel, R. T., Brodie, B. B. 1958. *Biochem. Pharmacol.* 1:352–54
83. Rane, A., Berggren, M., Yaffe, S. J., Ericsson, J. L. E. 1973. *Xenobiotica* 3: 37–48
84. Short, C. R., Davis, L. E. 1970. *J. Pharmacol. Exp. Ther.* 174:185–96
85. Zamboni, L. 1965. *J. Ultrastruct. Res.* 12:509–24
86. Kirby, L., Hahn, P. 1973. *Pediat. Res.* 7:75–81
87. Rane, A., Sjöqvist, F. 1972. *Pediat. Clin. N. Am.* 19:37–49
88. Rane, A., Von Bahr, C., Orrenius, S., Sjöqvist, F. See Ref. 21, pp. 287–303
89. Gillette, J. R., Menard, R. H., Stripp, B. 1973. *Clin. Pharmacol. Ther.* 14:680–92
90. Rane, A., Sjöqvist, F., Orrenius, S. 1973. *Clin. Pharmacol. Ther.* 14:666–72
91. Kalter, H. 1968. *Teratology of the Central Nervous System.* Chicago: Univ. Chicago Press

PERINATAL PHARMACOLOGY[1]   ❖6590

Sumner J. Yaffe

Department of Pediatrics, School of Medicine, State University of New York at Buffalo and Division of Pharmacology, Children's Hospital, Buffalo, New York

Mont R. Juchau

Department of Pharmacology, School of Medicine, University of Washington, Seattle, Washington

The perinatal period has been recognized as an identifiable area of pharmacological endeavor by reviews in Volumes 8, 10, and 12 of this series (1–3) and in Volumes 17 and 24 of the *Annual Review of Medicine* (4, 5). These reviews initially identified adverse effects in the fetus and newborn infant; however, as data accumulated, the importance of the influence of the developmental stage of the host upon pharmacologic responses was emphasized.

The purpose of this paper is to discuss drug disposition in the perinatal organism with major emphasis on the human fetus and newborn infant. The specific areas that have been singled out for discussion include placental transfer, distribution of drugs within the feto-placental unit, fetal drug metabolism and absorption, protein binding, metabolism, and excretion in the neonate. Awareness of the differences that exist in the prenatal host in these important parameters may minimize the adverse effects previously seen at this age.

DRUG DISPOSITION IN THE FETUS

Until recently, drugs were rarely administered for the treatment of fetal disorders. However, rapid progress in the diagnosis of such disorders has led an increasing number of physicians to consider the various possibilities for intrauterine treatment with medicinal chemicals (6). Nevertheless, the present lack of knowledge concerning the pharmacologic-toxicologic effects of drugs on the human fetus and newborn infant would greatly hamper the physician in his attempts to evaluate intelligently the risk-benefit ratios of various drug regimens. Of even greater concern is the

[1]This work was supported in part by grants from the National Institute for Child Health and Human Development (HD 04287 and HD 06611).

219

exposure of unborn and newborn children to drugs administered for treatment of the maternal organism rather than the fetus or neonate. In addition, a large number of foreign chemicals of no therapeutic value either to the mother or her child enter into the maternal circulation, and subsequently into the fetal or neonatal circulation (via placental transfer or the maternal milk respectively). Such chemicals may enter unintentionally as a result of contact with an ever-increasing chemical contamination of the environment, including contaminants in food and water, or as a result of intentional drug abuse.

One of the greatest challenges to modern pharmacologists is to increase understanding of the pharmacology of human development to the extent that rational guidelines for risk-benefit ratios during pregnancy might be developed for a wide range of specific chemical agents, particularly therapeutic agents and other foreign chemicals to which pregnant and lactating women are, or may be, frequently exposed. Observations of the effects of drugs on the fetus or offspring represents a necessary empirical approach toward the resolution of these problems; however, research into basic mechanistic aspects will provide a much more satisfactory long-range approach. In particular, studies of the mechanisms regulating the rates of access to and egress from fetal and neonatal pharmacologic-toxicologic receptors seem to be of prominent importance.

Transplacental Drug Movement

Recent studies on the transplacental passage of drugs have begun to question earlier concepts that suggested a direct relationship between the physicochemical properties of drug molecules and their rates of transfer between maternal and fetal circulations (7). Experimental evidence has been provided for the participation of a number of previously neglected factors that may regulate the rate and extent of placental drug transfer. These include the following:

1. Binding of drugs to placental macromolecules. Experiments performed by Tjalve et al (8) tended to indicate that such an effect could occur with nicotine. Even though such drug binding could markedly retard transplacental drug movement, systematic studies of this phenomenon appear to be nonexistent.

2. Active transport of drug molecules from the fetal to maternal circulation. McNay & Dayton (9) administered triamterene, a substituted pteridine diuretic agent, intravenously into the circulation of fetal lambs as well as into the maternal systemic circulation during the last month of pregnancy. Although an active transport mechanism was not verified, the rate of transfer from the fetal to maternal circulation was calculated to be 150 times the rate of transfer from the maternal to fetal circulation. A recent report (10) has provided evidence for the presence of a Mg^{2+}-dependent $Na^+ + K^+$-activated ATPase (ouabain sensitive) as well as a Ca^{2+}-ATPase (ouabain insensitive) in human term placentas. Ouabain, dinitrophenol, and Na^+-free media also reduced the uptake of α-aminoisobutyric acid into placental tissue slices of rabbits and humans (11). These studies are highly interesting from the viewpoint of transplacental drug movement because of the apparent involvement of ATPase enzymes in the active transport of organic ions.

3. Differences in affinity for adult vs fetal blood proteins. Evidence is now plentiful that drugs can bind to fetal or neonatal plasma proteins to different extents and

with different affinity constants as compared with their binding to analogous maternal plasma proteins (12–15). The implications of these phenomena with respect to maternal-fetal drug distribution are obvious.

4. Biotransformation of drugs during transplacental passage. Morgan et al (16) have provided experimental evidence that both placental monoamine oxidase and catechol-O-methyltransferase could influence the rate of transfer of norepinephrine and isoproterenol between the fetal and maternal circulations. It is increasingly recognized that the placenta contains enzymes capable of catalyzing the biotransformation of drug substrates and that such reactions could play a role in the determination of rates of the transplacental movement of certain drugs. This subject has been reviewed recently by Juchau (17).

5. Biotransformation of drugs in fetal tissues. This topic has been reviewed recently by Rane et al (18). Fetal tissues, particularly in primates, contain enzyme systems that can catalyze the biotransformations of a variety of drug substrates. As one example, various studies indicated that newborn infants (and therefore presumably the human fetus at term) could metabolize lidocaine quite rapidly and that, as might be expected, the maternal fetal lidocaine plasma concentration ratio was well above unity, even following repeated administrations of the drug (19, 20).

6. The ability of various vasoactive drugs to exert effects on the utero-placental-umbilical vascular systems that in turn may result in changes in placental perfusion. This topic also has been the subject of a recent review (21). Since rates of placental drug exchange are strongly related to rates of placental perfusion, pronounced effects on drug transfer rates could be expected with vasoactive drugs. Thus, by virtue of the drug's own pharmacologic effect, its rate of transfer from maternal to fetal circulations may be disproportional to its physicochemical properties. Although many drugs are known to exhibit profound effects on this vascular system, no specific examples of such an effect on drug transfer have been reported. Mirkin, however, has alluded to such a phenomenon in a recent review (22).

In addition to the above considerations, Oh & Mirkin (23) found that, whereas certain drugs that are nearly 100% ionized at pH 7.4 (eg. salicylates) would pass into brain tissues with considerable difficulty, their rates of transplacental passage were quite rapid. Even bis-quaternary ammonium compounds are capable of entering the fetal circulation (24), albeit at extremely slow rates. Thus it seems imperative that the question once commonly posed as to whether a given drug would enter the fetal circulation must now be replaced by the questions, "At what rate? What is the extent and time course of its accumulation on the fetal side? What is the relative exposure and distribution of the drug in the fetus vs mother?" It also seems apparent that the many factors governing the kinetics of drug disposition in utero now require a systematic evaluation.

Drug Distribution In Utero

Rapid advances in the study of fetal drug distribution have been made with the aid of autoradiographic techniques. Studies with whole body autoradiography have led Ullberg (25) to the conclusion that the more "unphysiological" a compound is, the more is its fetal-maternal distribution determined by purely physicochemical properties, whereas the distribution of "physiological" substances such as vitamins, hormones, amino acids, minerals, etc are strongly influenced by specific mechanisms including active transport, facilitated diffusion, specific binding to endogenous macromolecules, etc. Ullberg also pointed out that even though many drugs cross the placental barrier more readily than they cross the blood-brain barrier, some drugs, such as certain tertiary amines, accumulate much more readily in the brain than in fetal tissues. Ullberg also presented additional evidence to indicate that various amino acid analogs may be actively transported by the placenta from the maternal to the fetal circulation.

The intrauterine distribution of a large number of specific chemical agents have been studied in experimental animals (for recent reviews see 22, 25) with whole body autoradiographic techniques that allow comparisons of the distribution of drugs in fetal vs maternal tissues. These studies have indicated that the relative distribution of most drugs in fetal organs tend to parallel that observed in the corresponding maternal organs except that the maternal liver appears to be much more capable than the fetal liver of sequestering drugs. As expected, organs with high lipid content, such as the liver, lungs, intestines, and adrenal glands, tend to concentrate fat-soluble drugs. It has frequently been found that drugs will accumulate selectively and strongly in a single type of fetal tissue. Tetracycline accumulation in the fetal skeleton, thiouracil in the fetal thyroid, chloroquine and chlorpromazine in the pigment of the fetal eye, and diphenylhydantoin and progesterone in the fetal adrenal gland (22, 25) represent examples of the phenomenon. It was found that Vitamin B_{12} accumulated more than a hundredfold in the fetus if a low dose was administered.

A recent study of the maternal-fetal distribution of trans-Δ^9-tetrahydrocannabinol (THC) indicated that even though THC distributed to the fetus in only very low concentrations, the drug exhibited a definite affinity for the fetal central nervous system (26). Although it is now apparent that certain drugs distribute in fetal tissues with fairly uniform pattern and others distribute with a more selective affinity for given organs or tissues, sufficient data are not yet available to allow broad generalizations or predictions of fetal distribution from a knowledge of the chemical structure of the drug molecule.

Studies of the passage of drugs from the maternal circulation to the uterine fluid and subsequently into the preimplantation blastocyst also have been reviewed recently (27, 28). A large number of drugs and chemicals now are known to penetrate the blastocyst and alter or arrest the normal developmental process. Particularly interesting were some of the studies by Fabro (28) which indicated that the pregnant state could modify the degree to which drugs pass from the maternal circulation into the uterine fluid. In nonpregnant rabbits the uterine fluid/plasma radioactivity ratio ranged between 0.78 and 1.75 following the administration of ^{3}H-nicotine. In 6 day pregnant does, however, there was 5–10 times more radioactivity in the uterine fluid than in the plasma. This increase in accumulation also could be effected by treatment of nonpregnant does either with human chorionic gonadotrophin or progesterone. Cotinine, a more polar metabolite of nicotine, did not appear to pass into the uterine fluid as readily as unchanged nicotine. Thus, it would seem possible that active transport of certain drugs from the maternal circulation into the uterine fluid can occur and that such processes could be influenced markedly by the hormonal status of the host. Concentrations of drugs in human Fallopian tubular fluid have not been measured. They are urgently required because of their clinical importance.

Fetal (and Neonatal) Drug Biotransformation

Chemical alterations of drugs and other foreign compounds in tissues of the fetus and placenta have received increasing attention during the past few years. A significant stimulus for this research was the recent observation of Yaffe et al (29) that human fetal liver microsomes contained necessary electron transport components (NADPH-specific cytochrome c reductase and cytochrome P-450) for drug hydroxylation reactions. These investigators were able to demonstrate significant rates of mixed-function oxidation of endogenous substrates such as testosterone or laurate, but variable results were obtained with drug substrates. Positive results were later obtained for the oxidative N-demethylation of desmethyl imipramine and ethyl morphine and p-hydroxylation of aniline in human fetal liver preparations in vitro (18, 30, 31).

These findings were somewhat surprising in view of the inability of a large number of investigators to detect significant quantities of cytochrome P-450 or P-450-dependent drug hydroxylation reactions in liver microsomes from fetuses of a wide variety of animal species, even at comparatively late stages of gestation (32–39). The possibility remains, however, that such phenomena do not represent a genetically determined species difference but rather a difference in the extent of exposure of humans vs experimental animals to chemicals that can induce or stimulate these systems in the fetus. The bulk of the currently available evidence, nevertheless, does not support this idea.

Prior to the report of Yaffe et al (29) other investigators had reported the oxidative biotransformation of several drug substrates in post mitochrondrial supernatant fractions of human fetal liver homogenates (40) but were unable to detect cytochrome P-450 in the microsomal fractions (41). This possibly was due to the fact that the human fetal liver homogenates were centrifuged at 12,000 X g for 20 min prior to the sedimentation of the microsomal fraction at 100,000 X g. From the experiments of Ackermann et al (42) and Chatterjee et al (43) it would be expected that recoveries of endoplasmic reticulum elements in those microsomal pellets would be very low and that detection of cytochrome P-450 therefore would be quite difficult. Electron microscopic studies of various human fetal hepatic homogenate subfractions revealed (42) that the endoplasmic reticulum appeared to be converted partly to long, slender cisternae and partly to uniform microsomes during homogenization. This led to a substantial loss of microsomal marker enzyme activity into the low speed subfractions. Later, Pelkonen & Karki (44) confirmed the presence of significant quantities of cytochrome P-450 in human fetal liver microsomal fractions.

It should be pointed out that various investigators also have reported negative results with respect to the mixed-function oxidation of several xenobiotic substrates in human fetal liver preparations: N-demethylation of N-monomethyl p-nitroaniline (45), O-demethylation of p-nitroanisole (45), N-demethylation of aminopyrine

(46), and hydroxylation of 3,4-benzpyrene (29, 31). Several subsequent investigations, however, indicated that hydroxylation of 3,4-benzpyrene would be catalyzed in human fetal hepatic tissues as well as a large number of other human fetal tissues at several stages of gestation (46, 49). Specific activities were one to two orders of magnitude lower as compared with analogous preparations of rat liver microsomes under similar reaction conditions. [Transplacental induction of the fetal benzpyrene hydroxylating system did not appear to occur readily, as judged both from animal experiments (50, 51) as well as from studies in humans (46–49, 52)]. Thus far, positive results have been reported for the N-demethylation of aminopyrine (29), hydroxylation of 3,4-benzpyrene (46, 49), N-demethylations of ethylmorphine (18, 31), and desmethylimipramine (53) and p-hydroxylation of aniline (31, 46). Again, enzyme induction in certain cases could account for some of the apparently conflicting data. Another explanation may be found in methodological differences when using indirect measurements of activity.

The human fetal adrenal gland also has attracted attention as a site of drug biotransformation. Following the observation that this organ appeared to be much more active than other human fetal tissues with respect to aromatic nitro group reduction (54), Juchau & Pedersen (46) showed that microsomal fractions of fetal adrenal homogenates contained exceptionally high concentrations of cytochrome P-450 and were active with respect to catalysis of hydroxylations of 3,4-benzpyrene and aniline as well as the reductions of aromatic nitro groups and azo linkages. Specific concentrations of cytochrome P-450 as well as specific activities of the drug metabolic reactions were considerably higher than those observed in the fetal liver under the reaction conditions used. A very similar pattern of fetal drug biotransformation was observed in a subhuman primate species. In spite of these observations, however, significant catalysis of the N-demethylation of aminopyrine or the $\omega(\omega-1)$ oxidation of laurate could not be detected in the human fetal adrenal gland (55). Such studies are of considerable interest because of the comparatively very large size of the human fetal adrenal gland and the extremely important role it plays in steroid biosynthesis and biotransformation during fetal development. The similarities between drug and steroid hydroxylation reactions suggest that drugs could act as alternative substrates for at least some of the many steroid hydroxylases present in that organ.

The first fetal tissue to be encountered by drugs circulating in the maternal plasma of humans is the syncitial trophoblast of the placenta. It is possibly for that reason that several investigators have studied drug biotransformation reactions in various preparations of human placental tissues in recent years. Evidence has accumulated that the placenta is capable of catalyzing the biotransformation of various types of drug substrates (55). The types of reactions catalyzed indicate that this tissue exhibits a much higher degree of substrate specificity than the extremely versatile hepatic tissues. Most of the reactions also appear to occur at considerably slower rates, although hydroxylation of 3,4-benzpyrene can occur at rates approaching those observed in analogous rat liver preparations (56). This appears to occur in genetically susceptible individuals who have been exposed to relatively large quantities of polycyclic aromatic hydrocarbons present in the environment, particularly in tobacco smoke (52, 57–59). Pretreatment of experimental animals with such hydrocarbons markedly increases rates of placental hydroxylation of 3,4-benzpyrene and a limited number of other xenobiotic substrates, presumably via induction of the components of the hydroxylase systems in a large number of tissues. Studies on the placental hydroxylase have indicated that induction of the enzyme system in this organ occurs much more readily near term than during the early stages of gestation. This appears to apply to humans (52, 59) as well as to experimental animals (60, 61). The higher growth rate of the placenta during early gestation may be responsible for such observations, for many studies have shown that drug hydroxylation reactions tend to occur at very slow rates in such rapidly growing tissues as regenerating liver, fetal and neonatal liver, and liver tumors. However, hepatic drug hydroxylating enzymes appear to be more responsive to enzyme induction in younger animals (38).

As compared with drug oxidation-reduction reactions, the study of conjugation reactions in fetal tissues have received only slight attention. Earlier reports (62, 63) indicated that the human fetal kidney was more active than the fetal liver with respect to the catalysis of glucuronide formation using O-aminophenol or 4-methylumbelliferone as substrates. The activities observed were, however, very low as compared with human adult liver. Recent studies, however, have reported negative results with respect to the capacity of the human fetal liver to exhibit significant glucuronyl transferase activity during early gestation (18, 64). 4-Methylumbelliferone, α-naphthol, and p-nitrophenol were tested as aglycone acceptors.

It has been demonstrated that pre-exposure to certain drugs, notably phenobarbital, can enhance glucuronyl transferase activity in fetal livers near term (65–67) and by this mechanism contribute to an observed decrease in jaundice by increasing the rate of bilirubin glucuronidation. Other effects of phenobarbital such as an increase in bile flow and increase in anion acceptor protein also play a role. Recently, evidence that heroin addiction may exert a similar effect in humans has appeared in the literature (68).

The fetal liver and adrenal glands are extremely active with respect to the catalysis of sulfate transfer and, although no specific examples have been given, sulfurylation of foreign phenolic compounds (e.g. morphine, diethylstilbesterol, etc) could be an important factor in fetal drug distribution as well as in transplacental drug movement and modification of drug actions on the fetus. The highly active sulfatase enzymes present in the placenta also may be significant in this regard.

Some preliminary investigations have indicated that human fetal tissues may catalyze various other drug conjugation reactions including acetylation and glycine conjugation (69). Uher (70) was able to demonstrate significant rates of acetylation of sulfamethoxypyrimidine in cultures of human trophoblast.

Investigators also have continued to search for an explanation for the low rates of mixed-function oxidation and glucuronidation observed with xenobiotic substrates in fetal or neonatal hepatic tissues. Fouts (71) noted that most studies have indicated that hepatic parenchymal cells are the principal sites of most drug hydroxylation reactions and that the proportion of parenchymal cells to reticuloendothelial cells is quite low in fetal livers. In addition, the studies of Leskes et al (72,

73) indicated that the smooth-surfaced endoplasmic reticulum (SER) was essentially absent before birth and developed asynchronously in hepatocytes after birth. Koga, however, was able to show the presence of SER as early as 6 weeks of fetal age in human hepatocytes (74), an observation that coincides with the reported capacity of human fetal livers to catalyze mixed-function oxidation of drug substrates as measurable rates during early gestation.

Feuer & Liscio (75) postulated that the low levels of drug hydroxylating activity observed in newborn animals was due to the presence of relatively high levels of maternal inhibitory factors (female gonadal hormones) in the fetal and neonatal circulation. This postulate was based on the following observations: 1. Pregnant female rats exhibited longer hexobarbital sleeping times than nonpregnant females. 2. Early weaning accelerated the development of drug metabolic activities in rats. 3. There was a rapid increase in drug metabolic activity postpartum. Although such studies suggest that female sex hormones inhibit drug metabolic activity (several previous studies, in vitro and in vivo have shown this to be the case) they do not indicate to what extent the gonadal hormones contribute to the low activities observed. However, certain metabolites of progesterone were shown to be extremely potent inhibitors of drug biotransformation in vitro (76). The fact that inducing agents can markedly increase rates of drug hydroxylation reactions in tissue culture systems but appear to be much less effective in intact pregnant animals (or humans) also leads one to suspect that maternal factors may be responsible.

Because the hepatic content of cytochrome P-450 and the capacity of fetal and neonatal livers to catalyze drug hydroxylation seem to increase in parallel during development, Woods & Dixon (77) investigated aspects of the hepatic capacity of prenatal rats, rabbits, and guinea pigs to synthesize hemoproteins. They found that the activity of the enzyme that catalyzes the rate limiting step of heme biosynthesis (δ-aminolevulinic acid synthetase) was four to eight times higher in the livers of prenatal animals than in those of corresponding adult animals. The fetal enzyme, however, appeared to be much less susceptible to induction or repression, and it was postulated that this resistance to regulatory control might in some way account for the decreased cytochrome P-450 concentrations and drug hydroxylating activity observed in immature hepatic cells.

A number of other factors have been proposed to explain the low rates of mixed-function oxidation, reduction, and glucuronidation of xenobiotic substrates in the fetus and neonate. These include the following: 1. Inability of inducing agents to reach fetal hepatic tissues in quantities sufficient to yield adequate induction due to clearance of the inducer by other maternal, placental, or fetal tissues (46). 2. Inability of inducing agents to bind to critical proteins in fetal hepatic tissues (71). 3. Presence of repressors (or possibly other inhibitors) in the fetal livers (78). 4. The influence of growth hormone (STH) on rapidly growing tissues (79). Various aspects of these possibilities have been discussed in recent reviews (71, 80). It would seem likely that none of the above items can be viewed as the sole explanation but that each may act as a single contributing factor in decreased microsomal drug biotransformation in the prenatal and perinatal periods.

DRUG DISPOSITION IN THE NEONATE

During intrauterine existence the fetus has at its disposal the metabolic and excretory capabilities of the maternal organism. Once the umbilical cord is severed the neonate must use his own mechanisms to distribute and then eliminate xenobiotic substances. In contrast to the fetus, drug concentration at receptors is governed by the traditional process of absorption, distribution, metabolism, and excretion. These will be discussed in the following sections, although it must not be forgotten that drugs may also be present in the neonate as a consequence of medications administered to the mother prior to or during delivery.

Absorption

The gastrointestinal tract of the neonate undergoes a marked change in function shortly after birth, e.g. transit time is prolonged, gastric pH decreased, and permeability increased. In addition, the gastrointestinal tract represents a relatively larger portion of the body in the newborn than in later life. Therefore, it is not surprising that the bioavailability of drugs given orally differs from that seen in the adult organism. One of the first investigations of drug absorption in the newborn infant demonstrated that triple sulfa-suspension (mixture of equal weights of sulfadizaine, sulfamerazine, and sulfamethazine) was absorbed less well in the low birthweight (premature) infant than in the full term infant (81). The hypoglycemic effect of orally administered insulin in newborn infants was observed only during the first few minutes after birth. Insulin is absorbed intact at this time. After several hours, gastric pH decreases and hydrolyzes the insulin in the gastrointestinal lumen (82). The absorption of riboflavin is found to be much lower in the neonate than in the older infant (83). The same percentage of dose was absorbed. The absorptive process lasted 16 hr in the newborn in contrast to only 3–4 hr in the older organism. The authors hypothesize that the specialized intestinal transport process for riboflavin is much less active in the newborn and that the slow absorption is accounted for by passive diffusion over a much longer segment of the gastrointestinal tract. Prolonged transit time mentioned above would also support this view. Another possibility is that because riboflavin was administered as a phosphate salt, the phosphatase-mediated conversion to riboflavin in the intestine was rate limiting in the neonate and delayed the absorption.

No systematic studies of the absorption of pharmacologic agents in newborn infant have been conducted. The available data deals mainly with the absorption of antibiotics because these are used so frequently in the newborn infant. When the intramuscular route has been compared with the oral route, higher serum concentrations as anticipated have been achieved following parenteral administration. O'Connor et al (84) compared serum levels of sodium nafcillin achieved after oral administration in newborn infants and adults. A significantly higher concentration was reached in the newborn. The area under the serum concentration curve was five times greater in the newborn than in adults given equivalent doses on the basis of body weight. While the more prolonged serum concentrations are undoubtedly due to decreased renal excretion, there is no question that the absorptive process from the GI tract is functioning at a greater rate. Silverio & Poole (85) have recently compared ampicillin absorption in newborn infants and adults. The results are in agreement with those found with nafcillin with the area under the curve approximately three times greater in the newborn infant. They also contrasted two dosage forms, anhydrous and trihydrate, and found that the anhydrous was absorbed to a greater extent than the trihydrate in a ratio similar to that seen in adults. Thus, the ionized form of the penicillin, monobasic nafcillin, or amphoteric ampicillin, does not appear to affect its absorption in the neonate. Jusko (86) has analyzed, kinetically, data available in the literature and has contrasted the availability of ampicillin in the newborn infant when administered by mouth or by intramuscular injection. About two thirds of the oral dose was absorbed in the newborn, and this can be compared with about 30% availability of ampicillin from capsules in adults. A new antimycotic agent, chlortrimazole, has been found to be well absorbed in neonates including premature infants with serum concentrations achieved sufficient to effect systemic Candida infections (87).

Digoxin is another drug frequently used in the newborn. When absorption by oral and intramuscular routes was compared after the administration of labeled digoxin (88) to infants with severe congenital cardiac malformations who required digitalization, absorption was a rapid and in the same range as that seen in adults. Digoxin could be detected in blood 5 min after oral administration, reaching a peak concentration in 1–3 hr. The intramuscular route delivered the drug into the circulation 1 min after injection, and peak levels were achieved 15–30 min later.

The parenteral route is also used frequently to administer drugs in the sick neonate. In general, drugs injected into skeletal muscles or subcutaneous tissues are absorbed rapidly. Comparative studies between these two sites in newborn infants are not available and are needed because, under hypoxic conditions, newborns may selectively curtail circulation in muscles and skin, hindering absorption of drugs given by these two routes. Kupferberg & Way (89) found no difference in the rate of disappearance of morphine from its injection site after subcutaneous administration of the alkaloid in a dosage of 50 mg/kg to 16 and 32 day old rats. These investigators directly analyzed the amount of free morphine remaining at the injection site (right hind limb) at various time intervals following administration. Mention should be made of absorption via the skin. While no studies have been carried out, the toxicity of hexachlorphene when used in the routine bathing of newborn infants has recently attracted considerable attention in the United States at large. Consideration of the histology of the infants' skin in contrast to the adults' clearly indicates less impediment to absorption, particularly of lipophilic compounds. The tragic results with hexachlorophene are therefore not surprising.

Recently Kandall et al (90) measured the activities of the enzymes β-glucuronidase and UDP-glucuronal transferase in the gastrointestinal tract during the perinatal period. Both of these enzymes are concerned with the deconjugation of bilirubin. Activity of β-glucuronidase before birth was relatively high while transferase activity was barely detectable. During the first 4 days after birth, β-glucuronidase reached a level nearly seven times that of adult activity, whereas glucuronyl transferase activity approximated adult activity. β-Glucuronidase activity in the perinatal period was predominantly located in lysosomes in contrast to a microsomal location later in development. The authors speculate that the excess capacity of the intestine for deconjugation of bilirubin, over that of conjugation, favors the active reabsorption of bilirubin and therefore contributes significantly to the hyperbilirubinemia seen in the neonate. While this relationship remains to be more clearly demonstrated by kinetic studies, the data do serve to exemplify the changing biochemistry of the developing gastrointestinal tract and the potential role that this may have in drug absorption.

Distribution and Drug Plasma Protein Binding

Differences in the distribution of pharmacologic agents in the neonate as compared with the adult may be attributable to variations in membrane permeability or in protein binding. Changes in body composition in the young subject may also result in quantitative alterations in drug distribution. Body water content is higher in the newborn than in the adult and in the newborn infant varies from 85% of body weight in small prematures to 70% in the full-term infant. Fat content is likewise altered with a marked decrease being found in the infant born prematurely. These variations in body composition were associated with increases in the volume of distribution of sulfonamides and bromsulphalein (91). Several studies have shown a differential permeability from blood to brain as a function of the age of the host. This is of particular importance for psychopharmacologic agents whose action in the newborn may also be modified because of differences in brain receptors at this age. The distributional aspects have been reviewed previously (4). Preliminary experiments in our laboratories have shown that the malnourished preweanling rodent is more susceptible to the action of hexobarbital, presumably because of variations in distribution and binding to brain receptors.

The plasma protein binding of diphenylhydantoin has been studied in mixed cord plasma by means of an ultrafiltration technique using carbon-14 labeled diphenylhydantoin (92) at concentrations of 16 mμg/ml (mean therapeutic concentration). The unbound fraction of diphenylhydantoin in 13 normal infants was 10.6 $\pm$ 1.4%. The corresponding value in adult plasma was 7.4 $\pm$ 0.7%. In addition to the lower degree of binding noted in cord plasma, the range of values in individual samples was much greater than in adult plasma. Binding of diphenylhydantoin was also investigated in 20 hyperbilirubinemic infants in whom the concentration of total bilirubin (mainly unconjugated) varied from 4.5–24.5 mg/ml of serum. There was a definite correlation between the size of the unbound fraction of diphenylhydantoin and the total concentration of bilirubin. At concentrations of bilirubin greater than 20 mg/100 ml, the unbound fraction of diphenylhydantoin was twice as high as in plasma from nonhyperbilirubinemic infants. Correlation became even greater when the bilirubin/albumin ratio was plotted against the percentage of unbound diphenylhydantoin. This strengthens the hypothesis that diphenylhydantion and bilirubin may compete for the same binding site on the albumin molecule. This difference in binding may account for the greater adverse effects often seen in the newborns when diphenylhydantoin is administered, even though the dose is reduced to take the size of the patient into consideration.

The binding of salicylate to albumin fractionated from pooled neonatal cord serum was found to be quite different from that seen with adult serum (93). The apparent association constant of $1.7 \times 10^5 M^{-1}$ in the infant was one third of the adult value of $4.0 \times 10^5 M^{-1}$. Nafcillin binding to pooled cord serum was also studied by the same investigators using the technique of equilibrium dialysis. The percentage of the drug bound increased from 16% at a low antibiotic concentration (5 μg/ml) up to 28% and 200 μg/ml. This represents a considerable difference from adult values reported in the literature (94) of 86% of the antibiotic bound. Furthermore, examination of the Scatchard plots of nafcillin binding in newborn cord serum suggested that binding occurred to some protein fraction other than albumin. Electrophoresis on acetate membranes of cord serum incubated with nafcillin and subsequent biological assay of each band, showed that α-1-globulin had a greater affinity for nafcillin than albumin. This contrasts with the reported binding to adult serum for penicillins (94).

Many drugs have been suspected of displacing bilirubin from its binding to albumin. This has serious clinical consequences (neurotoxicity) in the newborn infant whose capacity to metabolize bilirubin is limited and whose blood-brain barrier is more permeable than in the adult. The physicochemical properties of bilirubin have hampered examination of its binding to albumin in aqueous systems. Krasner (95) was able to circumvent this problem by using dimethylsulfoxide as the solvent. Association constants for the interaction of bilirubin with albumin were obtained at varying dimethylsulfoxide concentrations, and these were plotted as a function of the concentration of the solvent. This resultant curve was then extrapolated from 10% dimethylsulfoxide to 0% to obtain the apparent association constant for the binding of bilirubin to albumin. Albumin purified from cord serum appeared to bind bilirubin with a greater affinity than adult albumin with apparent k values of $5.2 \times 10^7 M^{-1}$ and $2.4 \times 10^7 M^{-1}$ respectively. Because large quantities of serum were required in the equilibrium dialysis method, the same author developed a fluorometric assay that measured the direct interaction of bilirubin with albumin in microliter quantities (96). He was able to measure bilirubin binding capacity and to determine whether or not other pharmacologic agents could displace bilirubin from its binding to albumin. Sodium salicylate displaced bilirubin from its binding to albumin at high concentrations (200 mg/100 ml), but at usual therapeutic concentrations of 20 mg/100 ml it was without effect. Sodium benzoate at high concentrations (144 mg/100 ml) caused approximately 30% reduction of bilirubin binding capacity, but lower concentrations were without effect. This is in contrast to the recently described phenomenon in which two drugs, caffeine and injectible diazepam, commonly used in the treatment of newborn infants, were shown to displace bilirubin from its binding to albumin (97). By using a combination of gel filtration and bilirubin spectral curves to assess the displacement, it was shown that the responsible agent was the added preservative sodium benzoate. The discrepancy between investigators is probably due to methodologies.

These data regarding drug-protein interaction in newborn serum clearly demonstrate that plasma protein binding differs in the newborn infant from that seen in the adult. Should these observations be operative in vivo, they would explain in part why drugs administered to the newborn often are associated with side effects, even though the dose used takes into consideration the smaller size of the patient. The changes in binding may be due to lower concentrations of plasma proteins (particularly albumin) seen in the newborn infant. However, the methods employed in the formulation of the Scatchard plot normalize for the amount of protein present. It is more likely that the binding characteristics reported by these several investigators are due to variations in the neonatal plasma proteins themselves. In addition, endogenous substances during the first few days of life, especially hormones transferred across the placenta and/or fatty acids, may occupy binding sites and thus reduce binding capacity.

Metabolism

In general, studies of drug metabolism in perinatal organisms of many species have shown low activity. During the postnatal and suckling period, drug metabolic capability increases quite rapidly and reaches maximum activity at varied ages according to the pathway being studied. Some pathways, for example glucuronidation and sulfation, reach peak values during the perinatal period which are much higher than later in life. Details regarding in vitro studies have been discussed in previous reviews (1–5). However, exceptions to the general concept that all newborn animals have low drug metabolizing capacity can be found for reduction (98) and sulfation (99). Both reactions are well developed at birth with in vitro activites in the adult range. One of the major questions which immediately arises concerns the regulation of drug metabolic activity and what initiates the increase that is noted soon after birth. This has been discussed in some detail in the previous section under drug metabolism in the fetus. Weaning appears to affect drug metabolism, which suggests that the maternal organism plays a role in limiting drug metabolic activity. Rats weaned early, and therefore removed from the influence of their mother, had a high 4-methylcoumarin hydroxylase activity than their unweaned counterparts. However, prolongation of weaning did not affect the development of aminopyrine demethylation (100). We have found similar results with hexobarbital oxidation in the mouse, namely a marked increase in in vitro activity and concomitant decrease in sleeping time associated with early weaning. In contrast to Henderson's findings (100), prolongation of weaning from 21–28 days delayed the increase in activity of hexobarbital oxidase (101). No explanation for this discrepancy other than species specificity is available. The effect of weaning may be mediated by hormones because profound hormonal changes take place at birth and at weaning. This hypothesis has received considerable attention with emphasis on progesterone and growth hormone. These aspects are discussed in detail in our previous review (5) and earlier in this article. It is also possible that separation from the mother via some neuroendocrine mechanism can trigger drug metabolic enzyme activity. Other environmental influences such as food, temperature, and space should also be considered, as these undergo marked changes at weaning.

In contrast to studies in the human fetus, only one in vitro study has been reported in newborn infants (102). NADPH cytochrome *c* reductase activity and cytochrome

b_5 content were found to be similar to those of adult rats in hepatic tissue obtained postmortum from one premature and one full-term newborn infant.

A number of in vivo studies of drug metabolism in newborn infants have recently been reported. The development of sensitive analytic techniques such as mass fragmentography (combination of mass spectroscopy with gas chromotography) has permitted identification of metabolites in small biologic samples. The urine of newborn infants whose mothers received therapeutic doses of chlorpromazine, pethidine, and promazine during labor contained conjugated metabolites other than those normally excreted in adults (103). This was considered an indication of a different metabolic pathway in the newborn infant. No kinetic studies were performed. A proglonged half-life of nortryptiline was found in a newborn infant whose mother took a suicidal overdose of the drug one day prior to delivery (104). Newborns of mothers taking diphenylhydantoin as an anticonvulsant were shown to excrete the drug in a significant amount only on the third day of life. This gave a half-life of 60 hr compared with 12 hr in the adult (105). It should be pointed out that this estimation of half-life is based upon a smaller number of samples. In contrast to this, it was surprising to find lower concentrations of diphenylhydantoin in the plasma of neonates given the drug for convulsive disorders than in adults (106). Both groups received the same relative dose per unit of body weight. It is conceivable that chronic administration has led to induction of hydroxlyase activity in the newborn infant. More specific investigations of this phenomenon, including measurement of hydroxylated derivatives in urine, are necessary before this decrepancy with the results reported following transplacental passage can be resolved. Analysis of the urinary metabolites following administration of digoxin to the newborn revealed a greater proportion of unchanged glycoside as compared with the older child. This was considered evidence for decreased metabolic activity in the newborn (88). The frequent administration of ethanol to women during labor has been used to determine its elimination in the infant who received the drug via transplacental passage (107). The half-life was twice as long in the newborn as in the mother.

Conjugating activity has been studied extensively because of the frequent occurrence of jaundice in the newborn infant and the demonstration, many years ago in the guinea pig, that the enzymes in the last two steps of glucuronide formation, glucuronyl transferase, and UDPG dehydrogenase, were deficient in activity when tested in vitro (108). Bilirubin conjugation, itself, was analyzed in great detail following its intravenous administration (109). The plasma half-life in infants up to 30 days of age was significantly longer than in children 4 months to 14 years of age. While this prolongation of half-life was ascribed to a diminished capacity to eliminate the bilirubin via glucuronidation, it should be emphasized that elimination also involves hepatic uptake and secretion into bile. Both of these processes have also been shown to be limited in capacity in the young animal. The plasma half-life of sulfobromophthalein, which is conjugated with different amino acids and glutathione, was studied in a large number of healthy full-terms and premature, newborn infants as well as in older children. Half-lives were twice as long during the neonatal period as in the older infants and children. Half-lives were longer in age, although these differences disappeared by four months of age. It was concluded from a comparison of the developmental course that exogenous factors were more important than endogenous ones for maturation of the process (110). The reason for the delayed elimination of sulfobromophthalein in the newborn is unknown, although it has been suggested (111) that secretion of the test substance into bile is insufficient. There might be other contributing factors such as low concentration of hepatic carrier protein. p-Aminobenzoic acid, which is coupled to glucuronic acid, and glycine and N-acetyl-p-aminophenol, which is glucuronidated before excretion, were both eliminated more slowly in newborn and premature infants (112, 113). Besides the finding that the rate of disappearance of p-aminobenzoic acid increased with age, there was a qualitative difference in the pattern of metabolites between newborn infants and older children. The former excreted p-aminobenzoic acid mainly in the form of acetyl-p-aminobenzoic acid, while the latter formed mainly glycine conjugates (p-aminohippuric acid). In contrast to these findings the ability to acetylate sulfadiazine was found to be decreased in young children (114).

Oxidative capacity has been studied using several drugs and has generally been shown to be deficient in the neonate. When acetanalid was given to 10 newborn infants, the peak concentration of the oxidative product, paraaminophenol, appeared later than in older children (113). Tolbutamide administered orally or intravenously to 10 normal full-term infants had a prolonged plasma retention during the first two days of life (115). The plasma disappearance of the drug showed an inverse correlation with the appearance of the oxidized metabolite, carboxytolbutamide, in the urine. Further evidence for a decrease in oxidative ability was gathered when aminopyrine half-lives were measured on the first and eighth days of life in 15 normal full-term infants (116). There was a successive increase with age of aminopyrine elimination rate from plasma. The metabolism of diazepam was studied in premature, newborn infants and older children, following intramuscular administration of the drug for the management of convulsive disorders (117). Premature and newborn infants had higher and longer lasting concentrations of the drug in plasma as contrasted with older children. N-Demethyldiazepam was formed in the young infant and could be detected in the blood and urine 4 hr after administration of the parent drug. However, conjugated forms of the oxidized derivatives, N-methyloxazepam and oxazepam, could be found only in children, suggesting that the young infant cannot oxidize the drug.

More precise and quantitative investigations of the ability of human newborn infants to handle drugs are needed. For example, we assessed glucuronide formation in 14 newborn infants by administering salicylamide orally in a single dose of 20 mg/kg of body weight and determining the amount of salicylamide glucuronide in the urine. This showed an extemely wide variation among the 14 infants in whom this parameter was investigated on the fifth day of life (118). The variation ranged from as high as 45% of the dose excreted as the glucuronide (normal for adults) to as little as 8% of the dose. Furthermore, there was an inverse relationship between the serum indirect bilirubin concentration on the fifth day of life and the urinary percentage of the dose of salicylamide appearing in the urine as a glucuronide. This five- to sixfold variation in glucuronide forming capacity is striking and suggests that interplay of environmental and genetic factors are responsible.

A wide variety of drugs and environmental chemicals are known that can induce the synthesis or inhibit the activity of drug metabolizing enzymes. This subject has been extensively reviewed in 1967 (119) and again in 1973 (120). It seemed logical to determine whether this mechanism could be used to alter the low microsomal enzyme activity in the newborn. Inscoe & Axelrod (121) demonstrated that benzpyrene injected into newborn rats caused a significant increase in hepatic glucuronyl transferase activity (with ortho-aminophenol as aglycone acceptor) when compared with untreated litter mates. No increase occurred in the newborn following administration to the pregnant female just prior to term, although activity was enhanced in the mother. We were able to demonstrate a two- to threefold increase in bilirubin glucuronide conjugating activity in the newborn mouse after pretreatment of the pregnant female with sodium barbital for 4–6 days prior to delivery (122). Striking increases in the activity of this enzyme were produced on the fourth day following administration of the barbiturate directly to the newborn mouse for the first 3 days after birth. Both oxidative and reductive pathways were increased following pretreatment of newborn rabbits with phenobarbital for 3–4 days (123). The extent of enhancement of enzyme activity was not uniform and varied with the drug metabolic pathway being studied. Induction also occurred following phenobarbital administration to the pregnant doe at term, but of great importance was the observation that there was no increase in enzyme activity when treatment occurred earlier in gestation (1–2 weeks prior to term). This implied the absence of a responsive enzyme synthesizing system. Exposure of newborn animals to phenobarbital excreted into breast milk is sufficient to induce an increase in hepatic drug metabolism (124). The increased metabolism induced by treatment of the mother one week prenatally, can still be observed at 3–4 weeks of age in the young rat, while in adult animals induction lasted only 5–7 days following discontinuation of phenobarbital (125). The molecular events responsible for the inductive effect of phenobarbital and other drugs during the perinatal period have not been completely elucidated. In addition to its effect upon glucuronidation in the neonate, phenobarbital also results in increased hepatic uptake of bilirubin as well as an increase in biliary flow (122). It also results in an increase in the amount of Y protein, one of the hepatic cytoplasmic anion binding fractions shown to be low in the perinatal period (126).

This first clinical application of enzyme induction was in several infants with unconjugated hyperbilirubinemia (127, 128). Phenobarbital treatment caused a rapid decrease in serum bilirubin concentrations accompanied in one patient by an increased output of salicylamide glucuronide in the urine (127) and in the other by an increased plasma disappearance of labeled bilirubin (128). Following these observations, attention was focused on the use of phenobarbital to modulate neonatal hyperbilirubinemia. Retrospectively, it was demonstrated that infants born to epileptic mothers treated with phenobarbital throughout pregnancy had a low serum bilirubin during the neonatal period (129). In several studies, phenobarbital has been given to the mother several days prior to delivery or to the newborn infant directly, and as a result significant lower serum bilirubin concentrations were found when compared with untreated control groups (118, 130, 131). Enhancement of glucuronide formation was demonstrated, albeit indirectly, by recording an increase in the excretion of salicylamide glucuronide in infants treated with phenobarbital (118).

As mentioned previously, the mechanisms underlying the lower concentrations of bilirubin are probably complex. Other drugs such as phenobutazine, diethylnicotinamide, and ethanol have been used to decrease neonatal hyperbilirubinemia with somewhat lesser effect than with phenobarbital (116, 132, 133). In contrast to animal studies (123) induction seems to take place even during early pregnancy as judged by in vitro assay (134). This again emphasizes the marked species differences that exist particularly with respect to fetal drug metabolism.

Excretion

The final common pathway for the removal of xenobiotic substances whether unchanged or metabolized is via the kidney. It has long been known that renal function in the newborn infant is much less than that of the adult even when corrected for differences in body size (135). Adult values are not achieved until usually the latter half of the first year of life. There is usually no functional impairment noted in the normal neonate because of the high rates of body growth and of biosynthetic functions (particularly that of protein) that are physiologically present. Drugs, which are not significantly metabolized and depend upon renal excretion for termination of their action, will have a noticeably longer effect in the newborn infant. Antibiotics are the major prototype of this class of pharmacologic agent, and because of their frequent use during the neonatal period they have been studied extensively. The clearance of penicillin G (136), which is mainly dependent upon tubular secretion for elimination, was decreased in the neonate to 17% of that found in a group of 2 year old children (calculated on a surface area basis). Three other penicillins, ampicillin, methacillin, and oxacillin, also had a prolonged half-life following intramuscular injection in premature infants (137).

Despite marked differences in birth weight associated with differences in intrauterine gestational age, all of the serum half-lives approached adult values at 3 weeks of postnatal development. This suggests that the maturation of renal function, which is responsible for the decrease in serum half-life, is a postnatal phenomenon. Aminoglycoside antibiotics such as kanamycin, neomycin, and streptomycin, which are mainly excreted by glomerular filtration, had a developmental pattern in premature infants similar to that observed for the penicillins (138). This has also been demonstrated in the full-term neonate for gentamycin (139). An interesting finding involved the antibiotic, colistin, another member of the aminoglycoside group, which, although dependent upon glomerular filtration for excretion, showed no difference in serum half-lives between the very young infants and the adult (137). This suggests that colistin is handled differently by the neonatal kidney. Further investigations concerning the role of renal excretion in modifying pharmacologic effects during the neonatal period are urgently needed, particularly because renal function at this age may be seriously compromised during systemic disease.

CONCLUDING REMARKS

In this review we have attempted to summarize what is known concerning drug disposition in the fetus and newborn. Despite the extensive bibliography, more questions have been asked than have been answered. The marked differences that exist between the human fetus and that of experimental animals in so far as drug metabolism is concerned have far-reaching implications concerning the teratogenicity of drugs administered to the pregnant woman and their preclinical evaluation. The formation of highly reactive epoxides during the hydroxylation of double bonds and the N-oxygenation of amines has great potential significance for the production of congenital malformations. Of greater importance is the need for knowledge regarding drug disposition in the human fetus as a requisite to fetal therapy. In contrast to the historical secondary adverse effects of drugs upon the fetus following administration to the mother, the future will witness drug administration to treat fetal disease. Drug disposition in the sick, newborn infant is a *sine qua non* for the establishment of sound guidelines for drug therapy in this important age. The aggressive intervention in the management of the sick newborn through the establishment of intensive care centers requires rational pharmacologic intervention as well. Despite the caution urged in extrapolating animal data to the immature organism, continued basic research is required if basic questions regarding the influence of environment upon drug disposition are to be answered. Finally, continued investigations into the phenomenon of enzyme induction in the perinatal period should prove most helpful, not only in elucidating the mechanism of action of inducing agents but also in affording a better understanding of the developmental process itself and its regulation.

Literature Cited

1. Sereni, F., Principi, N. 1966. *Ann. Rev. Pharmacol.* 8:453–66
2. Mirkin, B. L. 1970. *Ann. Rev. Pharmacol.* 10:255–72
3. Wilson, J. T. 1972. *Ann. Rev. Pharmacol.* 12:423–50
4. Yaffe, S. J. 1966. *Ann. Rev. Med.* 17: 213–34
5. Eriksson, M., Yaffe, S. J. 1973. *Ann. Rev. Med.* 24:29–40
6. Fuchs, F. 1973. *Fetal Pharmacology.* New York: Raven. 463 pp.
7. Moyer, F., Thorndike, V. 1962. *Am. J. Obstet. Gynecol.* 84:1778–92
8. Tjälve, H., Hannsson, E., Schmiterlöw, C. G. 1968. *Acta Pharmacol. Toxicol.* 26:539–55
9. McNay, J. L., Dayton, P. G. 1970. *Science* 167:988–90
10. Miller, R. K., Berndt, W. O. 1973. *Proc. Soc. Exp. Biol. Med.* 143:118–22
11. Miller, R. K., Berndt, W. O. 1972. *Fed. Proc.* 31:595(Abstr.)
12. Shoeman, D. W., Kauffman, R. E., Azarnoff, D., Boulos, B. M. 1972. *Biochem. Pharmacol.* 21:1237–46
13. Krasner, J., Giacoia, G. P., Yaffe, S. J. 1973. *Ann. NY Acad. Sci.* 7:317
14. Boulos, B. M., Almond, C. H., Davis, L. E., Hammer, M. 1972. *Arch. Int. Pharmacodyn. Ther.* 196:357–62
15. Ehrnebo, M., Agurell, S., Jalling, B., Boréus, L. O. 1971. *Eur. J. Clin. Pharmacol.* 3:189–98
16. Morgan, C. D., Sandler, M., Panigel, M. 1972. *Am. J. Obstet. Gynecol.* 112: 1068–75
17. Juchau, M. R. 1974. *CRC Crit. Rev. Toxicol.* In press
18. Rane, A., Sjöqvist, F., Orrenius, S. 1974. *Clin. Pharmacol. Ther.* In press
19. Shnider, S. M., Way, E. L. 1968. *Anesthesiology* 29:944–50
20. Fox, G. S., Houle, G. L., Desjardins, P. D., Mercier, G. 1971. *Am. J. Gynecol.* 110:896–99
21. Juchau, M. R., Dyer, D. C. 1972. *Pediat. Clin. No. Am.* 19:65–79
22. Mirkin, B. L. See Ref. 6, p. 1
23. Oh, Y., Mirkin, B. L. 1971. *Fed. Proc.* 30:2034
24. Speirs, I., Sim, A. W. 1972. *Brit. J. Anaesth.* 44:370–73
25. Ullberg, S. See Ref. 6, p. 55
26. Kennedy, J. S., Waddell, W. J. 1972. *Toxicol. Appl. Pharmacol.* 22:252–58
27. Lutwak-Mann, C. See Ref. 6, p. 419
28. Fabro, S. See Ref. 6, p. 443
29. Yaffe, S. J., Rane, A., Sjöqvist, F., Boreus, L. O., Orrenius, S. 1970. *Life Sci.* 9:1189–1200

30. Rane, A., Sjöqvist, F., Orrenius, S. 1971. *Chem. Biol. Interact.* 3:305-7
31. Rane, A., Ackermann, E. 1972. *Clin. Pharmacol. Ther.* 13:663-70
32. Jondorf, W. R., Maickel, R. P., Brodie, B. B. 1958. *Biochem. Pharmacol.* 1: 352-54
33. Fouts, J. R., Adamson, R. H. 1959. *Science* 129:897-98
34. Hart, L. G., Adamson, R. H., Dixon, R. L., Fouts, J. R. 1962. *J. Pharmacol. Exp. Ther.* 137:103-6
35. Kato, R., Vassanelli, P., Fontino, G., Chiesara, E. 1964. *Biochem. Pharmacol.* 13:1037-51
36. Dallner, G., Siekevitz, P., Palade, G. E. 1966. *J. Cell Biol.* 30:73-97
37. Short, C. R., Davis, L. E. 1970. *J. Pharmacol. Exp. Ther.* 174:185-96
38. Basu, T. K., Dickerson, J. W. T., Parke, D. V. 1971. *Biochem. J.* 124:19-24
39. Rane, A., Berggren, M., Yaffe, S., Ericsson, J. L. E. 1973. *Xenobiotica* 3:37-48
40. Pelkonen, O., Vorne, M., Kärki, N. T. 1969. *Acta Physiol. Scand. Suppl.* 330: 69-74
41. Pelkonen, O., Vorne, M., Jouppila, P., Kärki, N. T. 1971. *Acta Pharmacol. Toxicol.* 29:284-94
42. Ackermann, E., Rane, A., Ericsson, J. L. E. 1972. *Clin. Pharmacol. Ther.* 13: 652-62
43. Chatterjee, I. B., Price, Z. H., McKee, R. W. 1965. *Nature* 207:1168-70
44. Pelkonon, O., Kärki, N. T. 1971. *Acta Pharmacol. Toxicol.* 30:158-60
45. Pomp, H., Schnoor, M., Netter, K. J. 1969. *Deut. Med. Wochenschr.* 94: 1232-40
46. Juchau, M. R., Pedersen, M. G. 1973. *Life Sci.* 12:193-204
47. Juchau, M. R., Pedersen, M. G., Symms, K. G. 1972. *Biochem. Pharmacol.* 21:2269-72
48. Pelkonen, O. 1973. *Arch. Int. Pharmacodyn. Ther.* 200:259-65
49. Pelkonen, O., Arvela, P., Kärki, N. T. 1971. *Acta Pharmacol. Toxicol.* 30: 385-95
50. Welch, R. M., Gomni, B., Alvares, A. P., Conney, A. H. 1972. *Cancer Res.* 32:973-78
51. Nebert, D. W., Gelboin, H. V. 1969. *Arch. Biochem. Biophys.* 134:76-89
52. Pelkonen, O., Jouppila, P., Kärki, N. T. 1972. *Toxicol. Appl. Pharmacol.* 23: 399-412
53. Rane, A., Von Bahr, C., Orrenius, S., Sjöqvist, F. See Ref. 6, p. 287
54. Juchau, M. R. 1971. *Arch. Int. Pharmacodyn. Ther.* 194:346-58
55. Juchau, M. R., Pedersen, M. G., Fantel, A. G., Shepard, T. H. 1974. *Clin. Pharmacol. Ther.* In press
56. Juchau, M. R., Symms, K. G. 1972. *Biochem. Pharmacol.* 21:2053-65
57. Welch, R. M. et al 1968. *Clin. Pharmacol. Ther.* 10:100-9
58. Nebert, D. W., Winker, J., Gelboin, H. V. 1969. *Cancer Res.* 29:1763-69
59. Juchau, M. R. 1971. *Toxicol Appl. Pharmacol.* 18:665-75
60. Schlede, E., Merker, H. J. 1972. *Naunyn Schmiedebergs Arch. Pharmakol.* 272:89-100
61. Schlede, E., Kasper, C., Merker, H. J. 1972. *Int. Congr. Pharmacol. Abstr., 5th,* p. 204
62. Dutton, G. J. 1959. *Biochem. J.* 71: 141-48
63. Hirvonen, T. 1966. *Biologica-Geographica,* Turku, Sarja. Ser. A 11
64. Chakraborty, J., Hopkins, R., Parke, D. V. 1971. *Biochem. J.* 125:15P
65. Yaffe, S. J., Levy, G., Matsuzawa, T., Baliah, T. 1966. *N. Engl. J. Med.* 275: 1461-66
66. Ramboer, C., Thompson, R. P. H., Williams, R. 1969. *Lancet* 1:966-68
67. Stern, L., Khanna, N. N., Levy, G., Yaffe, S. J. 1970. *Am. J. Dis. Child.* 120:26-31
68. Nathenson, G., Cohen, M. I., Litt, I. F., McNamara, H. 1972. *J. Pediat.* 81:899-903
69. Juchau, M. R., Yaffe, S. J. 1969. *The Foeto-Placental Unit.* Amsterdam: Exerpta Med. Found. 260 pp.
70. Uher, J. See Ref. 69, p. 240
71. Fouts, J. R. See Ref. 6, p. 305
72. Leskes, A., Siekevitz, P., Palade, G. E. 1971. *J. Cell Biol.* 49:264-87
73. Leskes, A., Siekevitz, P., Palade, G. E. 1971. *J. Cell Biol.* 49:288-302
74. Koga, A. 1971. *Z. Analyt. Entwickl. Gesch.* 135:156-61
75. Feuer, G., Liscio, A. 1969. *Nature* 223: 68-70
76. Soyka, L. F., Long, R. J. 1972. *J. Pharmacol. Exp. Ther.* 182:320-31
77. Woods, J. S., Dixon, R. L. 1972. *Biochem. Pharmacol.* 21:1735-44
78. Klinger, W., Zwacka, G., Ankermann, H. 1968. *Acta Biol. Med. Ger.* 20: 137-45
79. Wilson, J. T. 1970. *Nature* 225:861-63
80. Netter, K. J. 1971. *Arch. Gynaekol.* 211:112-33
81. Fichter, E. G., Curtis, J. A. 1956. *Pediatrics* 18:50-58
82. Znamenacek, K., Pribylova, H. 1963. *Cesk. Pediat.* 18:104-14

83. Jusko, W. J., Khanna, N., Levy, G., Stern, L., Yaffe, S. J. 1970. *Pediatrics* 45:945–49
84. O'Connor, W. J., Warren, G. H., Mandala, P. S., Edrada, L. S., Rosenman, S. B. 1964. *Antimicrob. Ag. Chemother.*, 188–91
85. Silverio, J., Poole, J. W. 1973. *Pediatrics* 51:578–80
86. Jusko, W. J. 1973. *Pediat. Clin. N. Am.* 19:81–100
87. Weingärtner, L., Sitka, V., Ratsch, R., Gründig, C. 1972. *Int. J. Clin. Pharmacol.* 6:358–63
88. Hernandez, A. 1969. *Pediatrics* 44: 418–28
89. Kupferberg, H. J., Way, E. L. 1963. *J. Pharmacol. Exp. Ther.* 141:105–12
90. Kandall, S. R., Thaler, M. M., Erickson, R. P. 1973. *J. Pediat.* 82:1013–19
91. Burmeister, W. 1970. *Int. Z. Klin. Pharmakol. Ther. Toxicol.* 4:32–36
92. Rane, A., Lunde, P. K. M., Jalling, B., Yaffe, S. J., Sjöqvist, F. 1971. *J. Pediat.* 78:877–82
93. Yaffe, S. J., Krasner, J. 1973. *Ann. NY Acad. Sci. Conf., January*
94. Kunin, C. M. 1967. *Ann. NY Acad. Sci.* 145:282–90
95. Krasner, J., Stern, L. J., Yaffe, S. J. 1972. *Pediat. Res.* 6:405
96. Krasner, J. 1973. *Biochem. Med.* 7: 135–44
97. Schiff, D. G., Chan, G., Stern, L. 1971. *Pediatrics* 48:139–41
98. Short, C. R., Davis, L. E. 1971. *J. Pharmacol. Exp. Ther.* 174:185–96
99. Percy, A. K., Yaffe, S. J. 1964. *Pediatrics* 33:965–68
100. Henderson, P. T. 1971. *Biochem. Pharmacol.* 20:1225–32
101. Yaffe, S. J. 1968. *Ross Conf. Pediat. Res.* 58–65
102. Soyka, L. F. 1970. *Biochem. Pharmacol.* 19:945–51
103. O'Donoghue, L. E. J. 1971. *Nature* 229:125–26
104. Sjöqvist, F., Bergfors, F. G., Borga, O., Lind, M., Ygge, H. 1972. *J. Pediat.* 80: 496–600
105. Mirkin, B. L. 1971. Ibid 78:329–37
106. Jalling, B., Boréus, L. O., Rane, A., Sjöqvist, F. 1970. *Pharmacol. Clin.* 2: 200–2
107. Idapa, J. 1972. *Am. J. Obstet. Gynecol.* 112:387–93
108. Brown, A. K., Zuelzer, W. W., Burnett, H. H. 1958. *J. Clin. Invest.* 37:332–40
109. Gladtke, E., Rud, H. 1967. *Monstsschr. Kinderheilk.* 115:231–33
110. Wichmann, H. M., Rind, H., Gladtke, E. 1968. *Z. Kinderheik.* 103:262–76
111. Vest, M. F. 1962. *J. Clin. Invest.* 41: 1013–20
112. Vest, M. F., Salzberg, R. 1965. *Arch. Dis. Childhood* 40:97–105
113. Vest, M. F., Streiff, R. R. 1949. *Am. J. Dis. Child.* 98:688–93
114. Fichter, G., Curtiss, J. I. 1955. *Am. J. Dis. Child.* 90:596–97
115. Nitowsky, H. M., Matz, L., Berzofsky, J. A. 1966. *J. Pediat.* 69:1139–49
116. Reinicke, C., Rogner, G., Frenzel, Y., Maak, B., Klinger, W. 1970. *Pharmacol. Clin.* 2:167–72
117. Garattini, S. *Pharmacol. Toxicol. Program Symp., Washington DC, May 17–19, 1971*
118. Stern, L., Khanna, N. N., Levy, G., Yaffe, S. J. 1970. *Am. J. Dis. Child.* 120:26–31
119. Conney, A. H., 1967. *Pharmacol. Rev.* 19:317–66
120. Conney, A. H., Levin, M. S., Jacobsen, M., Kuntzman, R. 1973. *Clin. Pharmacol. Ther.* 14:727–41
121. Inscoe, J. K., Axelrod, J. 1960. *J. Pharmacol. Exp. Ther.* 129:128–31
122. Catz, C., Yaffe, S. J. 1968. *Pediat. Res.* 2:361–70
123. Hart, L. G., Adamson, R. H., Dixon, R. L., Fouts, J. R. 1962. *J. Pharmacol. Exp. Ther.* 137:103–6
124. Fouts, J. R., Hart, L. G. 1965. *Ann. NY Acad. Sci.* 123:245–51
125. Mitoma, C., LeValley, S. E. 1970. *Arch. Int. Pharmacodyn. Ther.* 187:155–62
126. Reyes, H., Levi, A. J., Gatmaitan, Z., Arias, I. M. 1969. *Proc. Nat. Acad. Sci. USA* 64:168–70
127. Yaffe, S. J., Levy, G., Matsuzawa, T., Baliah, T. 1966. *N. Engl. J. Med.* 275: 1461–66
128. Crigler, J., Gold, N. I. 1966. *J. Clin. Invest.* 45:998–99
129. Trolle, D. 1968. *Lancet* 1:251–52
130. Maurer, H. M. et al 1968. *Lancet* 2: 122–24
131. Ramboer, C., Thompson, R. P. H., Williams, R. 1969. *Lancet* 1:966–68
132. Sereni, F., Perletti, L., Marini, A. 1967. *Pediatrics* 40:446–49
133. Waltman, R., Bonura, F., Nigrin, G., Pipat, C. 1969. *Lancet* 2:108–10
134. Pelkonen, O., Karki, N. T. 1972. *Int. Congr. Pharmacol., 5th*, p. 179
135. West, J. R., Smith, H. W., Chasis, H., 1948. *J. Pediat.* 32:10–18
136. Barnett, H. L., McNamara, H., Schultz, S., Tompsett, R. 1949. *Pediatrics* 3: 418–22
137. Axline, S. G., Yaffe, S. J., Simon, H. J. 1967. *Pediatrics* 39:97–107
138. Simon, H. J., Yaffe, S. J. 1970. *Proc. Int. Congr. Chemother., 6th*, 11:761–67
139. McCracken, G. H., West, N. R., Horton, L. J. 1971. *J. Infec. Dis.* 123: 257–62

BLOOD-BRAIN BARRIER PERMEABILITY TO DRUGS

❖6591

William H. Oldendorf

Research and Neurology Services, V. A. Wadsworth Hospital Center, Los Angeles,
California and Department of Neurology, School of Medicine, University of California,
Los Angeles, California

To affect central nervous system (CNS) cells directly, a drug must appear in the
extracellular fluid (ECF) of the CNS. How much of an administered drug distributes
to CNS ECF is determined by a number of interdependent factors. If taken orally,
a molecule of drug must survive in the gut lumen, penetrate the intestinal wall,
traverse the liver, resist degradation by enzymes in blood plasma and other organs,
remain unionized in solution unattached to plasma proteins, and ultimately penetrate the blood-brain barrier (BBB). In this review it is assumed a drug is in the
peripheral blood, and only those factors directly related to its entry into brain are
discussed.

Many of the characteristics of BBB permeability to drugs referred to in this review
have been long established and well described previously in this series (1) and in
other reviews (2, 3). These well-established areas will be discussed briefly here but
emphasis will be placed on what probably are the most interesting relevant developments during the past decade: the demonstration that the brain capillary cell wall
almost certainly is the site of the BBB; the discovery that the brain has an appreciable extracellular space; the characterization of carrier-mediated BBB permeability;
the development of reversibly lipophilic derivatives of drugs to promote BBB penetration; and the modification by capillary endothelial cell cytoplasm of some substances entering the brain.

RELATION OF CNS ECF TO GENERAL ECF

Since the last review of BBB permeability in this series (1), certain relationships of
the CNS fluid compartments to each other and to fluid compartments outside the
nervous system have been clarified. These compartments outside the CNS are here
referred to as general compartments.

239

The blood plasma is a moving subcompartment of the general ECF that serves, through its bulk flow through the microcirculation, to produce short effective diffusion distances between all body cells. It is effective in this role because of the permeability of general capillary walls to all small molecules (4, 5). When injected intravenously all polar molecules with molecular weights less than 20,000–30,000 distribute to a fluid compartment (the general ECF) of about 4 times greater volume than the plasma. This distribution has an equilibration $T_{1/2}$ of considerably less than 1 min in small animals (6). Nonpolar molecules of any size distribute in an even shorter time to a space 10–15 times greater than the plasma volume (7). Polar molecules larger than about 30,000 mol wt remain for some time confined to the plasma compartment distributing to an anatomically undefined larger space with a $T_{1/2}$ of several hours (8).

The permeability of general capillaries to polar molecules is nonspecific other than being a function of molecular size. The cutoff appears to be at a molecular diameter of 70–90 Å. Larger molecules pass through general capillary walls inefficiently but nearly independently of molecular size once their diameter exceeds about 100 Å (9). In the CNS there is no such nonspecific capillary permeability, and most polar solutes in plasma exchange very slowly with brain ECF. This observed failure of many solutes to enter the brain is the basis of the concept of a BBB. Although many solutes fail to enter the brain, it is obvious that the BBB must be permeable to the brain's metabolic substrates and perhaps to some metabolic endproducts. In view of the instantaneous effects of some drugs, the BBB must also be reasonably permeable to them as well. Rather than being a completely impermeable barrier, the BBB is more like a selectively permeable barrier exercising criteria other than simple molecular size. It is through this selectively permeable barrier that exchanges take place between CNS ECF and the general ECF.

On the CNS side of the BBB, diffusional exchange readily takes place between various areas of brain and with the cerebrospinal fluid (CSF). The CSF is currently conceived as an aggregation of fluid in the ventricles and subarachnoid space which is an extension of the CNS interstitial ECF, because tracers introduced into CSF diffuse readily throughout the interstitial ECF of brain (10, 11). Similarly, plasma tracers that enter CNS ECF at the site of an induced lesion, where the BBB is not functioning, diffuse readily into the ECF of the surrounding healthy brain tissue (12).

In view of this concept of CSF as an extension of brain ECF, the term "blood-CSF barrier" is probably of limited usefulness because it refers to an empirical rate of exchange from blood to CSF. This exchange can occur at many sites such as the BBB, the ependymal layer of the choroid plexus, or at the arachnoidal membrane. These sites are of such divergent structure and function that it is impossible to establish an anatomical substrate for a blood-CSF barrier. For most substances it probably reflects predominantly the permeability of the BBB.

Because many drugs cannot penetrate the BBB, they have little effect on the CNS when administered systemically but since drugs in CSF diffuse readily into the brain interstitial ECF, the same drug that was without effect when administered systemically may evoke striking effects after ventricular injection (13).

The CSF acts as a "sink" for solutes in CNS ECF (14–16). The term "sink" refers to the net movement of solute from one region to another by diffusion down a concentration gradient for that solute existing between these regions. The concentration gradient removing solutes from the brain's ECF probably is maintained by constant dilution of the CSF by fresh choroidal secretion which is probably virtually free of all but those osmotically important solutes required to make it isotonic with the brain (17–19). Most (20, 21) but probably not all (22) of the CSF is formed in the choroid plexus. How much of the CSF originates from the choroid plexus and how much from the brain parenchyma is controversial and will probably continue to defy experimental clarification. Water moves so freely through living systems in response to slight osmotic and hydrostatic pressure gradients that results obtained under necessarily abnormal experimental conditions cannot accurately represent related processes taking place in the intact animal.

By virtue of this sink action, any solutes that are in higher concentration in the interstitial ECF than in the CSF move toward the ependymal or pial surfaces where they mix with CSF and are carried into blood by bulk flow through the arachnoidal villi. These and other aspects of CSF physiology are described in lucid depth in the 1967 monograph by Davson (23).

In addition to this sink removing solutes nonselectively from brain ECF into blood, certain anions such as iodide (24), thiocyanate (25), and pertechnetate (26), as well as diodrast (27), phenosulfonthalein (27), serotonin, and epinephrine (28), appear to be actively transported out of the ventricle into blood by the choroid plexus. Iodide (29) and potassium (30) probably are excreted from brain ECF into blood against a concentration gradient at the BBB.

The controversy about whether or not there is appreciable ECF in the CNS has been settled. Brain tissue that is allowed to expire in situ shows essentially no ECF by electron microscopy (31). That this observation is artifactual is supported by the demonstration of an abrupt increase in electrical impedance of brain several minutes after circulatory arrest (32), and by the relatively large amount of extracellular space observed by electron microscopy when the brain is frozen rapidly in life and lyophylized (33, 34). These observations and recent tracer distribution studies (15) indicate that the CNS has an extracellular space of 10–20% (35), of the same order as the mean extracellular space for the entire body (36). The virtual absence of ECF noted during routine electron microscopy is the result of postmortem movement of ECF into cells, probably in response to the high sodium gradient which can no longer be maintained when cellular membrane energy reserves are depleted.

ANATOMIC BASIS OF THE BBB

In the past decade considerable clarification of the structural basis of the BBB has been achieved by the electron microscopic definition of the distribution of horseradish peroxidase (mol wt $\sim$ 40,000) after intravenous (10, 37) or intraventricular injection (38, 39). Hydrolyzed horseradish peroxidase (mol wt 1900) retains sufficient peroxidase activity to allow its use as an electron microscopic marker (40). It has been used to demonstrate BBB tight junctions to this relatively small molecule.

The histologic site of the BBB has in the past been variously located at the capillary endothelial cell, its basement membrane, or the investing layer of astrocytic membrane. It is now generally believed that the barrier is based upon the continuous layer of tight-junctioned endothelial cells (10, 37, 41). These flattened cells are joined together about the complete periphery of each cell to the periphery of adjoining endothelial cells. They are bound together by what might be considered a "strip weld," whereas general capillaries are "spot welded" together. Implicit in this analogy is the absence of physically open narrow clefts between brain capillary endothelial cells. These clefts between general capillary cells are probably responsible for the passage of small polar molecules through general capillary walls such as found in skin and muscle. Such lipophobic molecules are incapable of penetrating lipid cell membranes, and their passage through the general capillary wall must be between cells rather than directly through the endothelial cell membranes and cytoplasm. The intercellular cleft is, logically, a likely site of passage of small molecules, and this is confirmed by electron microscopy of the general capillary using tracer substances (42).

The BBB is almost completely impermeable to macromolecules (43), and this may be related to the virtual absence of pinocytotic vesicles from brain capillary cytoplasm (37). These vesicles are a prominent feature of general capillary cell cytoplasm (44) and may account for the slight, but real, permeability of the general capillary to macromolecules (5).

The two structural features of CNS capillaries that seem to explain their impermeability to most hydrophilic molecules are the tight endothelial cell junctions and the absence of pinocytosis. The physiological basis for these unique characteristics of CNS endothelial cells is unknown but it has been speculated to be a function of the production of a humoral agent by the astrocytic membranes which affects the apposed capillary cell membrane causing it to form tight junctions and stop pinocytosis (45).

Neither the brain capillary basement nor surrounding astrocytic membrane contribute to the BBB according to electron microscopic observations that the electron-dense protein ferritin (39) and horseradish peroxidase (10) introduced into the ventricle diffuse readily through the ECF into the pericapillary space between astrocytic membrane and capillary cell. These tracers then freely pass through the capillary basement membrane, enter the intercellular cleft, and stop at the tight junctions (10).

Thus, if a molecule is to pass through the CNS capillary wall, it must pass directly through the lumenal endothelial cell membrane, the thin layer of cytoplasm, and the outer cell membrane (41). It presumably is the permeability of these two membranes that determines the permeability of the BBB. In 1946 August Krogh stated that the BBB had the permeability characteristics of a biological membrane (46). The membrane of the brain capillary endothelial cell apparently fulfills this prediction. In this review, the term "BBB" refers to this structural complex of two endothelial cell membranes and interposed cytoplasm. The monograph by Crone & Lassen (47) is an excellent compilation of recent thinking on capillary permeability.

MEASUREMENT OF BBB PERMEABILITY

BBB permeability to a solute is usually defined as an all or none phenomenon. All statements regarding BBB permeability to a substance should be quantitated because the BBB is measurably, though sometimes only slightly, permeable to all small molecules.

BBB permeability for many substances can be easily determined by the simultaneous carotid injection of a labeled test substance and a highly diffusible internal reference substance (48, 49). By measuring the amounts of the injected substances remaining in the brain 15 sec after carotid injection, the amount of test substance lost to brain in a single passage through the microcirculation can be measured. A surprisingly large percentage of many drugs and metabolites are taken up by brain in a single passage (48, 49). For instance nicotine, ethanol, imipramine, caffeine, heroin, procaine, and antipyrine are all nearly completely deposited in brain (49). This route of administration and method of measurement is useful, however, only for substances which penetrate BBB rapidly. For many solutes no measurable uptake occurs in a single brain passage after carotid injection.

Because drugs are seldom administered into the carotid system, a clinically more relevant estimate can be made by measuring brain concentrations after systemic administration. The usual routes of administration are intravenous, subcutaneous, intramuscular, or intraperitoneal. In most instances only the intravenous route should be used, as the rates of absorption into blood from other routes are often much slower than the rate of BBB penetration, and brain concentrations accordingly reflect rate of absorption rather than BBB permeability. The literature concerning BBB permeability to drugs describing measurements of brain concentration after systemic administration is so voluminous and involves so many diverse substances and techniques that individual review here is impossible.

In addition to BBB permeability, brain concentrations of a drug after systemic administration will be affected by retention of the drug at the injection site, plasma protein binding, accumulation of drug by liver, kidney or other tissues, the rate of systemic degradation of the drug, and the degree of brain tissue binding. These factors must be considered before a firm relationship can be established between a systemically administered dose and the intrinsic BBB permeability to the drug.

Molecular Criteria for BBB Permeability

To penetrate the endothelial cell membranes, a molecule must escape the polar environment of the blood plasma and enter the nonpolar environment of the lipid of the plasma membrane. It must subsequently escape this plasma membrane, enter the cytoplasmic water and repeat these transitions at the outer plasma cell membrane.

The transition from blood plasma to inner plasma membrane is largely predictable on the basis of the molecule's relative affinities for plasma proteins, water, and membrane lipid. If strongly bound to plasma protein, this macromolecular complex cannot escape into the lumenal membrane because it is unlikely it will ever achieve the energy level required to make a water-lipid phase transition.

Plasma Protein Binding

Plasma protein binding has been adequately discussed in other reviews (50, 51). The review by Mayer & Guttman contains an exhaustive review of the literature relating to specific studies of drug binding. For our purposes the important result of protein binding is the establishment of the concentration of free drug in plasma, because it is this unbound fraction that may possibly traverse the BBB. It is assumed the protein molecule, by virtue of its size and hydrophilic character, will not penetrate the BBB. Thyroxin (T_4) is an example of penetration of only the unbound plasma fraction. Unbound plasma T_4 represents much less than 1% of the total plasma T_4. Although CSF T_4 is very much lower than total plasma T_4, its absolute concentration is approximately equal to the unbound plasma concentration (52). This suggests that unbound T_4 readily equilibrates between plasma and brain ECF.

Competition for protein binding sites may result in displacement of one substance by another, raising its unbound plasma concentration and consequently its CNS concentration. Christensen (53) has suggested that displacement of T_4 from its protein binding sites by another drug could explain some of the observed drug effects on metabolic rate. Such a displacement, with a rise in free plasma T_4, could be expected to result in a rapid rise in CNS T_4.

Bilirubin is neurotoxic but there is little CNS effect even when jaundice is severe because of protein binding and removal of bilirubin from free solution. The CSF concentration, our only clinical index of CNS bilirubin, is much lower than in plasma (54), and brain staining at necropsy is minimal. Administration of sulfadiazine may displace bilirubin and, in the newborn, result in significant neurotoxicity (55).

Lipid Versus Water Affinity

Although protein binding is the dominant factor affecting BBB permeability to many solutes, the most important relationship for most solutes is their relative affinities for water and lipid because these establish the ease with which a solute molecule can escape plasma or cytoplasmic water and enter membrane lipid. This relative affinity can be established in vitro by measuring the lipid/water partition coefficient. Many nonpolar substitutes for plasma membrane lipid have been used with similar results, but none can precisely substitute for the living membrane lipid and for its carrier transport systems that confer upon the living membrane highly specific affinities.

Ionization greatly influences BBB penetration by a drug making it more hydrophilic and lipophobic thus favoring its retention by the water phase. The charge-dipole interaction between an ion and its surrounding water molecules is much stronger than the dipole-dipole interaction between a molecule hydrogen-bonded to water. An ion is, by virtue of this interaction, surrounded by a shell of several water molecules each of which, by hydrogen bonding, is anchored in the water phase (56). The state of ionization of a drug may also alter its affinity for plasma protein binding sites. Accordingly, the degree of dissociation at blood pH is a major determinant of permeability to a drug. If a drug is largely unionized at pH 7.4, its entry into brain is favored (57, 58). It is generally believed that only the unionized fraction penetrates the BBB (58). Because the blood pH is quite stable and can shift in life only about ± 0.5, changes in blood pH are not nearly as important for most drugs in altering penetration of BBB as are gut pH changes because a very great range of pH is encountered in the gut. Drugs such as thiopental having a pK near 7.4 could, however, undergo a considerable change in ionization with the slight shifts in blood pH encountered in respiratory and metabolic acid-base imbalances.

Whereas the hydrophilic character of an ionized molecule is dominated by its electrical charge, the relative lipid versus water affinity of the unionized molecule is largely determined by its hydrogen bonding capability. For most large organic molecules, water affinity is dominated by their hydrogen bonding capability.

The lipid/water partition coefficient of a substance can be estimated by examining its structure and adding up the total number and relative hydrogen-bonding capabilities of polar groups. Stein (56) has classified the apparent strength of hydrogen bonding by various common organic groups and related them to Collander's earlier observations (59) of membrane permeability. To define the apparent strength of hydrogen bonding by organic groups, Stein assigned a weighted numerical value (N) proportional to apparent hydrogen bonding strength. $N = 2$ was attributed to the –OH group of alcohols, sugars, glycols, carboxylic acids and to the –NH$_2$ group of primary amines. $N = 1$ was attributed to the –N(R)H of secondary amines and to the –CO group of carboxylic acids, amides, and aldehydes, $N = 1/2$ was attributed to the –CO– of esters, and $N = 0$ to the –O– of ethers. Knowledge of the bonding strengths of these and other groups is vital for predicting membrane permeability. Stein estimated that (56) each additional full-strength hydrogen bond to water decreased the likelihood of a water-membrane transition by a factor of 6–10.

Latentiation

The BBB is responsible for a very restricted distribution of many lipid-insoluble drugs to the brain. The penetration of BBB can be greatly increased by shielding hydrogen bond-forming sites by substituting relatively lipophilic groups. If the brain has the enzymatic capability of removing these added lipophilic groups, the original compound is regenerated and has in effect penetrated the BBB. This process of adding lipophilic groups that can be removed in the body with regeneration of the original compound has been termed "latentiation" (60) and will probably be widely applied to cause drugs to enter the brain. This is one form of a more general pharmacological strategy in which the body is caused to generate a drug in a given location by providing a suitable precursor. The first, although inadvertent, application of a lipid-soluble, reversible drug derivative to promote brain effects was the synthesis of heroin by acetylating the two hydroxyl groups of morphine (61). This greatly increases the amount of the drug entering the brain (49) and, once in the brain, it is deacetylated through 6-monoacetyl morphine to morphine, in which form it probably is most pharmacologically active (62).

The BBB is quite impermeable to all known CNS transmitter substances (48), and this has prevented raising CNS dopamine levels in parkinsonism by the systemic administration of dopamine. Its precursor, L-dopa, despite its great total hydrogen bonding capability, freely penetrates the BBB by virtue of its affinity for the large neutral amino acid carrier system (48). Cells of the brain's dopaminergic system can then decarboxylate it to dopamine. Lipophilic derivatives of dopamine should freely penetrate the BBB and, if brain cells can remove these lipophilic groups, dopamine should be regenerated. Various 3,4-O-derivatives of dopamine have been synthesized (63, 64), and some have been shown to activate dopamine receptors (65). Whether or not this approach will prove therapeutically useful remains to be established. Such a ploy for raising brain dopamine levels is unphysiological in that lipid-mediated BBB penetration would result in a distribution to the entire brain. Because deacetylases are ubiquitous, dopamine levels probably would be raised throughout the brain. This is quite different from forcing an increased output from deficient dopaminergic cells by introducing an excess of precursor because such dopamine presumably would be distributed specifically to its usual receptor areas (largely in basal ganglia), creating a quite different distribution from that likely to be found after administration of lipophilic derivatives. Conversely, latentiation of dopamine may be effective in some cases in which the dopaminergic cells are so deficient that they have essentially completely lost their decarboxylating function. In such cases raised brain tissue dopamine levels might still be created by reversible lipophilic derivates.

Similar attempts have been made to develop reversible lipophilic derivatives of norepinephrine (66) and various other amines (67). Using this general approach, many possibilities of raising brain concentrations of central transmitter substances, neurohumoral agents, antibiotics, and other drugs remain to be explored.

Biotransformation Within the Endothelial Cell

In addition to penetration of the inner and outer endothelial cell membranes, a drug must traverse the intervening thin layer of cytoplasm. That biotransformation can occur within this cytoplasm is indicated by the presence of monoamine oxidase (68) and the demonstration of dopamine fluorescence (69) in this cytoplasm. This cytoplasmic action may serve to enhance the effectiveness of the BBB in blocking the entry into the brain of systemic amines that might otherwise exert a CNS effect when blood concentrations change. This capability of brain capillary endothelial cytoplasm may bring about biotransformation of certain drugs before they enter brain ECF where they can affect neuronal activity.

Carrier Mediated BBB Transport

Although the BBB is impermeable to many polar small molecules, it is permeable to some metabolic subtrates such as glucose (70, 71), despite their extremely lipophobic character. Several specific BBB carrier systems have been demonstrated, and these exhibit sufficient affinity that they can, for their transported substances, compete successfully against even strong hydrogen bonding to water. Although many such carrier systems probably exist in the BBB, four independent carriers have been clearly defined. There is one carrier for D-glucose and related hexoses (48), one for large neutral amino acids, one for basic amino acids (48, 72), and one for short-chain monocarboxylic acids (73). The presence of these carrier sites, presumably located in the endothelial cell membranes, creates membrane affinities not predictable from simple lipid/water partition coefficients. Such carrier sites, being of restricted number, are saturable. They also exhibit stereospecificity (74). Although little attention has been directed to this area, the BBB penetration of some drugs may be accelerated by these carriers beyond that which would have been predicted by examination of the molecular structure for hydrophilic sites. The BBB penetration of amphetamine, for example, is partially saturable (75).

In general, BBB selective permeability for a large number of substrates resembles that of the red cell plasma membrane (48).

ACKNOWLEDGMENTS

I wish to express my sincere appreciation to Victoria Millet, M.S. and to Stella Z. Oldendorf, M.S. for their valuable support in the preparation of this review.

Literature Cited

1. Rall, D. P., Zubrod, C. G. 1962. *Ann. Rev. Pharmacol.* 2:109–28
2. Barlow, C. F., Lorenzo, A. V. 1971. *Radionuclides in Pharmacology,* ed. Y. Cohen, 2:539–64. New York: Pergamon. 962 pp.
3. Schanker, L. S. 1965. *Antimicrob. Ag. Chemother.* 5:1044–50
4. Landis, E. M., Pappenheimer, J. R. 1963. *Handb. Physiol.,* 2:961–1074
5. Renkin, E. M. 1964. *The Physiologist* 7:13–28
6. Oldendorf, W. H., Kitano, M. 1972. *Proc. Soc. Exp. Biol. Med.* 141:940–43
7. Oldendorf, W. H. 1972. *J. Nucl. Med.* 13:681–85
8. Gitlin, D. 1957. *Ann. N. Y. Acad. Sci.* 70:122–36
9. Areskog, N. H., Artuson, G., Grotto, G., Wallenius, G. 1964. *Acta Physiol. Scand.* 62:218–23
10. Brightman, M. W. 1968. *Progr. Brain Res.* 29:19–40
11. Brightman, M. W., Klatzo, I., Osson, Y. 1970. *J. Neurolog. Sci.* 10:215–39
12. Klatzo, I., Wisniewski, H., Steinwall, O., Streicher, E. 1967. *Brain Edema,* ed. I. Klatzo, F. Seitelberger, 554–59. New York: Springer-Verlag
13. Feldberg, W. 1963. *A Pharmacological Approach To Brain.* London: Arnold 128 pp.
14. Davson, H., Segal, M. D. 1969. *Brain* 92:131–36
15. Oldendorf, W. H., Davson, H. 1967. *Arch. Neurol.* 17:196–205
16. Davson, H., Bradbury, M. 1965. *Progr. Brain Res.* 15:124–34
17. De Rougemont, J., Ames, A., Nesbett, F. B., Hofmann, H. F. 1960. *J. Neurophysiol.* 23:483–95
18. Ames, A., Sakanove, M., Endo, S. 1964. *J. Neurophysiol.* 27:672–81
19. Ames, A., Higashi, K., Nesbitt, F. B. 1965. *J. Physiol.* 181:506–15
20. Welch, K. 1965. *Am. J. Physiol.* 205:617–24
21. Welch, K. 1966. *Am. J. Physiol.* 210:232–36
22. Milhorat, T. M. 1971. *Science* 173:330–32
23. Davson, H. 1967. *Physiology of the Cerebrospinal Fluid.* Boston: Little, Brown. 445 pp.
24. Welch, K. 1962. *Am. J. Physiol.* 202:757–60
25. Pollay, M., Davson, H. 1963. *Brain* 86:137–50
26. Oldendorf, W. H., Sisson, W. B. 1970. *J. Nucl. Med.* 11:85–88
27. Pappenheimer, J. R., Heisey, S. R., Jordan, E. F. 1961. *Am. J. Physiol.* 200:1–10
28. Tochino, Y., Schanker, L. S. 1965. *Biochem. Pharmacol.* 14:1557–66
29. Ahmed, V., Van Harreveld, A. 1969. *J. Physiol.* 204:31–50
30. Bradbury, M., Segal, M. B., Wilson, J. 1971. *J. Physiol.* 221:617–32
31. Wycoff, R. W. S., Young, J. Z. 1956. *Proc. Roy. Soc. Biol.* 144:440–50
32. Van Harreveld, A., Ochs, S. 1956. *Am. J. Physiol.* 198:180–92
33. Van Harreveld, A., Crowell, J., Malhotra, S. K. 1965. *J. Cell. Biol.* 25:117–37
34. Van Harreveld, A., Steiner, J. 1970. *Anat. Rec.* 166:117–29

35. Levin, V. A., Fenstermacher, J. D., Patlak, C. 1970. *Am. J. Physiol.* 219: 1528–33
36. White, H. L., Rolfe, D. 1951. *Am. J. Physiol.* 188:151–55
37. Reese, T. S., Karnovsky, M. J. 1967. *J. Cell. Biol.* 34:207–17
38. Brightman, M. W. 1965. *J. Cell. Biol.* 26:99–123
39. Brightman, M. W. 1965. *Am. J. Anat.* 117:193–330
40. Feder, N. 1971. *J. Cell. Biol.* 51:339–343
41. Crone, C., Thompson, A. M. 1970. *Capillary Permeability,* ed. C. Crone, N. Lassen, 447–53. New York: Academic. 681 pp.
42. Reese, T. S., Feder, N., Brightman, M. W. 1971. *J. Neuropath. Exp. Neurol.* 30:137–38
43. Sisson, W. B., Oldendorf, W. H. 1971. *Amer. J. Physiol.* 221:214–17
44. Palade, G. E. 1953. *J. Appl. Physiol.* 24: 1424
45. Davson, H., Oldendorf, W. H. 1967. *Proc. Roy Soc. Med.* 60:10–12
46. Krogh, A. 1946. *Proc. Roy. Soc. Med.* 133:140–220
47. Crone, C., Lassen, N. A., eds. 1970. *Capillary Permeability,* New York: Academic. 681 pp.
48. Oldendorf, W. H. 1971. *Am. J. Physiol.* 221:1629–39
49. Oldendorf, W. H., Hyman, S., Braun, L., Oldendorf, S. Z. 1972. *Science* 178: 984–98
50. Mayer, M. C., Guttman, D. E. 1968. *J. Pharm. Sci.* 57:895–918
51. Cohen, Y. See Ref. 2, 2:241–73
52. Molholm, H. J., Sierbaek-Nielsen, K. 1969. *J. Clin. Endocrinol.* 29:1023–26
53. Christensen, K. 1959. *Acta Pharmacol. Toxicol.* 16:129–35
54. Nasralla, M., Gawronska, E., Hsia, D. Y. Y. 1958. *J. Clin. Invest.* 37:1403–12
55. Odell, G. B. 1959. *J. Pediat.* 55:268–79
56. Stein, W. D. 1971. *The Movement of Molecules Across Cell Membranes.* New York: Academic. 369 pp.
57. Goldsworthy, P. D., Aird, R. B., Becker, R. A. 1954. *J. Cell. Comp. Physiol.* 44: 519–26
58. Brodie, B. B., Kurze, H., Schanker, L. S. 1960. *J. Pharmacol. Exp. Ther.* 130: 20–25
59. Collander, R., Barlund, H. 1933. *Acta Botan. Fenn.* 11:1–14
60. Harper, N. J. 1959. *J. Med. Pharm. Chem.* 1:467–500
61. Wright, C. R. A. 1874. *J. Chem. Soc. London* 24:1031–43
62. Way, E. L. 1968. In *The Addictive States,* ed. A. Wickler, 13–31. Baltimore: Williams and Wilkins
63. Casagrande, C., Ferrari, G. 1972. *Il Farmaco* 28:143–48
64. Pinder, R. M. 1970. *Nature* 228:358
65. Borgman, R. J. 1973. *J. Med. Chem.* 16: 630–33
66. Creveling, C. R., Daly, J. W., Tokuyama, T., Witkop, B. 1969. *Experentia* 25: 26–27
67. Verbiscar, J. A., Abood, L. G. 1970. *J. Med. Chem.* 13:1176–79
68. Bertler, A., Falck, B., Owman, C. H., Rosengren, E. 1966. *Pharmacol. Rev.* 18:369–85
69. Owman, C., Rosengren, E. 1967. *J. Neurochem.* 14:547–50
70. Crone, C. 1965. *J. Physiol.* 181:103–13
71. Fishman, R. A. 1964. *Am. J. Physiol.* 206:836–44
72. Richter, J. J., Wainer, A. 1971. *J. Neurochem.* 18:613–20
73. Oldendorf, W. H. 1973. *Am. J. Physiol.* 224:1450–53
74. Oldendorf, W. H. 1973. *Am. J. Physiol.* 224:967–69
75. Pardridge, W. M., Connor, J. D. 1973. *Experentia* 29:302–3

RELATIONSHIP BETWEEN DRUG DISTRIBUTION AND THERAPEUTIC EFFECTS IN MAN

❖6592

Elliot S. Vesell

Department of Pharmacology, Milton S. Hershey Medical Center, Pennsylvania State University College of Medicine, Hershey, Pennsylvania

INTRODUCTION

The intensity and duration of therapeutic effects derived from drugs other than those exerting an immediate, irreversible action depend theoretically on maintaining adequate concentrations of the active form of the drug at receptor sites. For the purposes of this review receptor sites may be considered to be molecules located anywhere in the body that combine with a drug or its metabolite to produce a pharmacological effect. It follows that the distribution of drugs must be carefully considered in selecting an appropriate dose, dosage form, dosage interval, and route of administration; judicious modification of these parameters permits attainment of effective concentrations of the active form of drugs at receptor sites. Quantitative measurement of the pharmacological response is often difficult or impossible. Furthermore, in man and most experimental animals, concentrations of the free active form of drugs at many receptor sites cannot be conveniently determined. Instead, drug concentrations in more accessible locations, such as plasma and urine, have had to suffice. These technical problems in quantitating precisely the pharmacological responses and receptor site concentrations of many drugs have seriously impaired efforts to define the relationship between drug distribution and therapeutic effects in man. Unfortunately, most assays of drug concentrations in plasma do not distinguish between the free active and the protein-bound inactive forms of a drug. Some assays fail to separate the parent drug from its metabolites. This flaw is serious because if only the parent drug or its metabolites possess pharmacological activity, an assay combining both cannot satisfactorily serve as the basis for gaining a true picture of the relationship between drug concentrations and pharmacological effect.

Distribution of a drug mainly depends upon such physical properties as its lipid solubility and degree of ionization. The degree of ionization is determined by the $pK\alpha$ of a drug and the pH of the fluid in which it is dissolved. For example, the

249

nonionized form of a drug is much more lipid soluble than the ionized form and hence much more capable of penetrating lipid cell membranes such as line the gastrointestinal tract.

Distribution refers to the various body fluid compartments a drug enters after its administration. Conceptually, body water exists as three functionally distinct compartments: the vascular, the extracellular (interstitial), and the intracellular fluids. The apparent volume of distribution (Vd) of a drug is the fluid volume in which the drug seems to be dissolved. Gillette (1) defines the kinetic Vd as the total amount of drug in the body at any given time after the distribution phase is completed divided by the plasma concentration of drug at that time. The distribution of some drugs, like dicumarol, phenylbutazone, and diphenylhydantoin, is largely limited to the space occupied by plasma protein, because these compounds bind avidly to albumin (the circulating plasma volume is approximately 3 liters in normal 70 kg subjects). Other drugs, such as bromide salts, thiocyanate, iodide, sucrose, and inulin, do not readily penetrate cell membranes and are therefore distributed mainly in the extracellular fluid compartment (12 liters in normal 70 kg subjects). Antipyrine passes through cell membranes without difficulty and thus distributes in the total body water (41 liters in normal 70 kg subjects), which antipyrine has been employed to quantitate (2). As a result of macromolecular binding, fat solubility, or active transport, some compounds such as phenoxybenzamine, thiopental, and quinacrine accumulate in certain tissues of the body that may or may not contain the receptor sites through which the drugs produce their therapeutic effects. In a two-compartment model, the Vd is frequently approximated by extrapolation to the y-intercept of the straight terminal portion (β-phase) of the curve relating the log of the plasma concentration of drug to time after its administration and dividing the total amount of drug in the body at time 0 by this y-intercept value. Certain apparent anomalies can arise. For example, if a drug such as thiopental or cyclopropane is sequestered by tissue binding to extravascular sites, so much of the drug can be withdrawn from the circulation that the apparent Vd of the drug may greatly exceed the entire fluid volume of the body.

The distribution of a drug is generally rapid as evidenced by the steep initial component of the curve relating the log of drug concentration in plasma to time. For a drug that is rapidly metabolized or localized in tissues, only this portion of the curve may be observed after a single dose; continuous infusion of drug can be used to test whether this single phase is due mainly to distribution or elimination. Appropriate treatment of the infusion data can yield a biphasic curve, indicating that distribution is followed by metabolism and elimination (1). Initial distribution of a drug is influenced by such factors as blood flow (bone and adipose tissue, being poorly supplied with blood, require a much longer time for drugs to attain equilibrium concentrations), the availability of and the drug's avidity for binding sites on albumin and tissue proteins, and finally the degree of ionization and lipid solubility of the drug. During or after this initial distribution of the drug in the body, processes of drug metabolism and excretion ensue.

A sharp break appears in the curve relating the log of plasma drug concentration to time after most of the drug has been distributed and drug metabolism and elimination have begun. This terminal portion of the curve is called the β-phase. Because metabolism and elimination can proceed prior to the β-phase, extrapolation of the β-phase portion of the curve to the y-intercept may constitute an underestimate of the total amount of drug in the body at the time of drug administration. Other approaches can be employed; in small laboratory animals the Vd can be directly measured by determining, simultaneously in tissue and plasma, drug concentrations at various times. In humans, mathematical models have been developed to avoid the underestimation of the y-intercept if metabolism is rapid (1, 3, 4).

During the β-phase certain tissues may undergo drug redistribution, through which process drug concentrations in tissues may shift dramatically. Redistribution may generate additional inflections or phases in the curves relating drug concentrations in plasma to time and is often encountered in tissues such as bone or fat where affinity for the drug may be great; however, blood flow is insufficient to allow for rapid accumulation. The classical example of the key role played by drug redistribution in modifying the therapeutic effects of a drug is that of thiopental (5). A small intravenous dose of thiopental produces anesthesia of rapid onset but short duration. Because of its high lipid to water partition coefficient, thiopental gains extremely quick access to the brain, but blood concentrations of thiopental decline rapidly, mainly due to its distribution into other tissues (not its metabolism). Consequently the drug moves rapidly out of the brain to remain in equilibrium with blood concentrations, and the subject awakens. Much later, thiopental becomes highly localized in fat depots. Elegant pharmacokinetic analyses of the relationship between drug distribution and pharmacologic effects have been published by Levy (6–9).

Because the topic of the influence of drug distribution on therapeutic effects is broad, many different aspects could be reviewed; for example, in this series last year, autoradiographic methods for investigating tissue distribution of drugs were discussed (10). Additional aspects in drug distribution include physiocochemical mechanisms of passage into or through tissues, membranes, and subcellular particles; physiocochemical mechanisms of drug binding to proteins (now being illuminated by extremely sensitive electron spin resonance and nuclear magnetic resonance techniques); analysis of dose response curves; pharmacokinetic and pharmacogenetic influences; effects of acidosis, alkalosis, fever, starvation, blood flow, and of cardiovascular, hepatic, renal or hormonal status. Exploration of these topics would provide interesting interrelationships between drug distribution and therapeutic effects, but could not all be summarized satisfactorily in a single article. Instead, attention here is focused on an area of current controversy in pharmacology: the relationship of drug blood levels to therapeutic effects. Much discussion of this topic has taken place; a recent conference was held to help define the underlying pharmacological significance of drug blood levels and to place them into better perspective (11). In describing the relationship of drug blood levels to the therapeutic effects of drugs, this review dwells on those pharmacologic principles that offer insight into the rational use of blood concentrations and that make some drugs more suitable than others for its application.

HISTORICAL BACKGROUND

The relationships between drug distribution and pharmacological effects were ill defined until sensitive, accurate methods were developed for measuring drug concentrations in the blood, urine, and tissues of an organism. Such techniques became available in the early 1950s, mainly as a result of work by Brodie and associates (12–16), who based their methods on the differential polarity and hence lipid solubility of drugs and their metabolites. It was recognized previously that for most drugs a poor correlation exists between dose and pharmacological effects. Introduction of spectrophometric, fluorimetric, and, more recently, gas-liquid chromotographic, mass spectrographic, and radioimmunologic techniques for assay of drugs and their metabolites permitted investigations of the correlation between drug concentrations in various body compartments and tissues and pharmacological effects.

Studies by Brodie and associates revealed a close relationship between the blood concentrations of certain drugs and their effects. Even among different species, similar pharmacological effects were observed when similar blood concentrations of a drug were achieved. For example, Quinn et al (17) showed that the same hypnotic dose of hexobarbital (100 mg/kg for mouse, rabbit, and rat) produced markedly different durations of action in these species; an inverse relationship existed between the duration of action of the drug and the enzyme activity in liver microsomes responsible for metabolizing hexobarbital (Table 1) (17). Thus species variations in the duration of action of hexobarbital could be traced to species differences in enzymatic capacity to metabolize the drug. However, once the same blood drug level was attained in different species, pharmacological response was similar as indicated by the observation that all species awakened at similar blood concentrations of hexobarbital. From these and other studies, several concepts emerged. First, pharmacologic effects relate more closely to blood concentrations of certain agents than to the dose of drug administered. Second, as a corollary, large interindividual variations exist in the dose of drug required to achieve the same blood concentration in various subjects. Third, normal experimental animals of the same species or even of different species exhibit great similarity in certain drug receptor sites.

CURRENT VIEWS ON DRUG DISTRIBUTION AND PHARMACOLOGICAL EFFECTS

Concentrations of a drug and its metabolites in biological fluids now constitute fundamental facts from which such critical properties of a drug as its absorption, distribution, biotransformation and excretion can be partially deduced. Therefore, it is understandable that data on blood levels are gathered during phase one studies and that assessment of dosage forms, dose intervals, and routes of administration rests largely on comparisons of blood levels. Blood levels of drugs have also become widely used in checking on patient compliance, since several studies revealed that a large segment of patients fail to take medicines as directed or, unknown to their physician, may consume other agents that interfere with the pharmacological actions of prescribed drugs (18).

Table 1 Species difference in duration of action and in metabolism of hexobarbitone[a]
(Dose of barbiturate: 100 mg/kg for mouse, rabbit, and rat, and 50 mg/kg for dog)

Species	Duration of action	Biologic half-life	Plasma level of hexobarbitone on awakening	Relative enzyme activity
	min	min	$\mu g/ml$	$\mu g/g/hr$
Mouse (12)[c]	12 ± 8	19 ± 7	89 ± 31[b]	598 ± 184
Rabbit (9)	49 ± 12	60 ± 11	57 ± 12	196 ± 28
Rat (10)	90 ± 15	140 ± 54	64 ± 8	134 ± 51
Dog (8)	315 ± 105	260 ± 20	19 ± 4	36 ± 30
Man[d]	—	360	20	—

[a]Reproduced by permission from Quinn et al 1958 (17).

[b]Micrograms per gram of tissue. Tissue levels are about 50% higher than plasma levels.

[c]Figures in brackets refer to number of animals.

[d]Unpublished data (J.J. Burns and E.M. Papper).

A major difficulty in relating drug blood levels to pharmacological effects has been the tendency to generalize too broadly. With few exceptions (19–21) most treatments of the subject have failed to identify which drugs are amenable to this technique and to define those situations in which drug blood levels are particularly useful. There are several distinguishing characteristics that render a drug suitable for blood level analysis as a basis for monitoring pharmacological effects.

For drug blood levels to correlate with pharmacological effects, the free concentration of the drug in blood must be in equilibrium with the concentration of drug bound to the receptor site through which it produces its actions. Furthermore, the pharmacological responses being investigated must bear a direct relationship to the drug's concentration at receptor sites. Certain drugs, such as monoamine oxidase and cholinesterase inhibitors, must accumulate at receptor sites until a certain level is attained before pharmacological effects will ensue. During this initial period of drug accumulation at receptor sites, no direct relationship between the drug blood level and pharmacological effects is discerned. Similarly, although appreciable blood levels of various coumadin anticoagulants may be obtained shortly after their administration, the pharmacological effect, prolongation of prothrombin time, may be delayed by many hours due to persistence in the blood of previously synthesized clotting factors. Brodie has referred to a group of drugs that continue to produce their pharmacological actions on receptor sites long after they disappear from plasma as "hit-and-run" drugs (17); alkylating agents that form irreversible covalent bonds exemplify this group of drugs whose blood levels bear no direct relationship to their pharmacologic effects.

If a drug exerts easily quantifiable therapeutic effects, such as changes in blood pressure, prothrombin time, or heart rate, the appropriate dose of drug may be determined by titration against changes in these parameters. In the absence of easily measured endpoints, other methods must be used to relate the dose of drug to therapeutic effect; in such situations drug blood levels may be useful as a guide to selecting appropriate drug dosage.

For drugs whose blood levels do correlate with their pharmacological actions, several additional properties of the drug make blood level measurements of clinical value in selecting appropriate dosage to insure therapeutic effects while avoiding toxicity. The ideal drug for this approach is one that possesses a low therapeutic index but has clearly separable ineffective, therapeutic, and toxic regions of drug concentration in the blood. The agent should be potent and exhibit large interindividual variations in rates of elimination from the body, so that the same dose could conceivably yield ineffective, therapeutic, or toxic blood concentrations in different subjects. Only a few therapeutic agents have been described in which certain clearly defined blood concentrations have the desired therapeutic effects, above which toxicity may occur, and below which little therapeutic benefit is obtained. Koch-Weser (21) cites the following ten drugs with their usual therapeutic ranges of serum concentrations: digitoxin (14–30 μg/liter), digoxin (0.9–2 μg/liter,) diphenylhydantoin (10–20 mg/liter), lidocaine (1.5–4 mg/liter), lithium (0.5–1.3 meq/liter), nortriptyline (50–140 μg/liter), procainamide (4–8 mg/liter), propranolol (20–50 μg/liter), quinidine (2–5 mg/liter), and salicylates (150–300 mg/liter).

It should be stressed that, like all other clinical chemical determinations, drug concentrations are maximally useful when placed in the broad context of a particular patient's problem; taken out of this context, such measurements may prove misleading. Presently, the availability of drug level measurements constitutes a major advance in avoiding therapeutic accidents with an important group of commonly used potent drugs with low therapeutic indices. However, even for a small group of carefully selected drugs this approach carries significant drawbacks; and an occasional patient may experience toxic reactions at therapeutic drug blood levels. One possible explanation for these anomalies is that in several disease states receptor sites on which drugs act may be aberrant. The clinical utility of drug blood levels is predicated on the usually safe assumption that the responsiveness of drug receptor sites does not exhibit large interindividual variations. Numerous environmental perturbations as well as supervention of several diseases may render this assumption invalid. A second cause of apparent dissociation between drug blood levels and drug effects involves the drug assay. For example, radioimmunoassays of digoxin are so specific that they fail to detect digitoxin. Patients with digitalis toxicity may take both drugs. Thus a normal digoxin blood level may be reported in patients with digitalis toxicity; unless blood digitoxin levels are also determined, anomalous dissociations of drug blood levels and effects may occur.

Drugs such as salicylates and certain antibiotics have high therapeutic indices that permit wide latitude in dosage; large amounts of these agents can be administered with low risk of severe toxicity. Normally, no major advantage may be obtained from precise quantitative data on the concentrations of these drugs in biological fluids. However, when continuously high blood levels of salicylates are desirable, as in the therapy of rheumatoid arthritis or the carditis of rheumatic fever, blood level measurements of salicylates become useful, because they serve as checks on the bioavailability of different commercial preparations, on patient compliance, and on the normal function of the processes of drug absorption, distribution, metabolism, and excretion.

BIOLOGICAL BASIS FOR THE NEED TO MEASURE DRUG BLOOD LEVELS

The need to measure drug blood levels in clinical medicine and in pharmacological studies on outbred species arises from the large interindividual variations that occur after administration of the same dose of an agent to different subjects of the same species. For example, Figure 1 shows threefold variations in the plasma half-lives of phenylbutazone after a single intramuscular dose of 800 mg in six unrelated cirrhotic subjects (22). Figure 2 shows that tenfold variations in the plasma decay of the anticoagulant ethyl biscoumacetate occurred in eight unrelated normal individuals after a single intravenous dose of this drug (23). Tenfold differences in plasma half-life are impressive compared with the much smaller range of variation for other biochemical parameters in normal subjects. Moreover, if blood concentrations of the anticoagulant 3 hr after its administration are compared, the range of interindividual variation becomes twentyfold. If chronic administration of such an agent were contemplated for individuals at the extremes, the magnitude of this variation expands considerably beyond twentyfold.

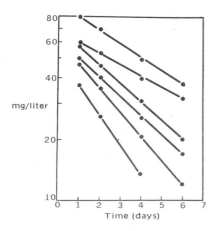

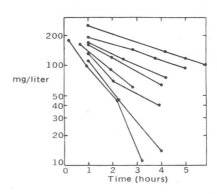

Figure 1 Decay of phenylbutazone in the plasma of six cirrhotic subjects after a single intramuscular dose of 800 mg. Reproduced by permission from Burns et al (22).

Figure 2 Decay of ethyl biscoumacetate in the plasma of eight normal volunteers after a single intravenous dose of 20 mg/kg. Reproduced by permission from Brodie et al (23).

With respect to switching from single to multiple doses, the pharmacokinetic relationship between the plasma half-life ($t\frac{1}{2}$) of a drug after a single dose and the steady-state blood concentration (C) of that drug is given by the equation of van Rossum & Tomey (24):

$$C = 1.44 \ (Q \cdot t\frac{1}{2} / Vd \cdot \Delta t)$$

where Q is the maintenance dose, Vd is the apparent volume of distribution, and Δt is the dosage interval. For completely absorbed drugs and for situations where the maintenance dose and dosage interval do not change, this formula indicates that alterations in the steady-state plasma concentrations arise from differences in $t\frac{1}{2}$, Vd, or both.

Studies in animals revealed that numerous factors can alter drug blood levels under certain conditions (25–29). Such factors include exposure to agents that stimulate or depress rates of drug metabolism; agents that alter the binding of a drug to plasma or tissue proteins; agents that alter rates of drug excretion in urine, saliva, sweat, bile or milk; and changes in hepatic blood flow, gastrointestinal absorption, and hormonal or nutritional status. In mice, responsiveness to a drug such as hexobarbital depends upon age, strain, sex, litter, painful stimuli, ambient temperature, degree of crowding, time of day of drug administration, type of bedding, and even the frequency with which this bedding is changed (28). Numerous compounds (30), including antipyrine (31), will on repeated administration enhance their own metabolism by induction of hepatic microsomal enzyme systems; thus, shifting from a single dose to chronic administration of some agents can substantially decrease the blood levels. Other drugs, such as diphenylhydantoin, produce metabolites that inhibit biotransformation of the parent drug, thereby tending to augment drug levels of the parent compound after chronic administration (32, 33).

The dose of a drug can affect blood concentrations in several other ways. For example, when the dose is small, the drug can be so strongly bound to plasma or tissue proteins that only a small proportion is available for metabolism and elimination. At higher doses, the protein binding capacity may be exceeded so that more of the drug is present in the free form, the form available for metabolism. At still higher doses, the biotransforming capacity of the body may become saturated, causing sustained elevations in drug blood levels. The mathematical treatment of the influence of different degrees of drug binding on drug elimination has been ingeniously described by Gillette (29), who also developed a mathematical model for the influence of the rate of hepatic blood flow on the biological half-life of a drug.

The multiple factors affecting drug blood levels can be divided into genetic and environmental subgroups. Such a division has broad implications in understanding the mechanisms that underlie interindividual variations and in attempting to translate such observations into practical clinical measures to improve therapy. Earlier passages in this review might suggest that in humans an important reason for variations among individuals in drug blood levels would be environmental. As we shall see, this prediction is incorrect in healthy, otherwise nonmedicated, normal volunteers.

Study of human twins permits separation of the control of a trait into hereditary and environmental components. This method, introduced in 1875 by Francis Galton

(34), has the advantage of comparing age- and sex-matched individuals and depends on the fact that identical twins have identical genomes, whereas fraternal twins share, on the average, only half their genes. The major assumption implicit in all twin studies is that identical and fraternal twins live within similar environments; this assumption has been challenged on the grounds that adult identical twins living in different households tend to create more similar environments for themselves than do fraternal twins under the same circumstances.

The twin method has been employed to identify the relative contribution of genetic and environmental factors to large interindividual differences in rates of decay of commonly used drugs. Healthy, adult, nonmedicated twins were studied pharmacokinetically for rates of elimination of the following drugs after a single oral or intravenous dose: phenylbutazone (35), antipyrine (36), bishydroxycoumarin (37), ethanol (38), and halothane (39). Steady-state blood levels of nortriptyline were measured in twins after 8 days of nortriptyline administration (40). Large interindividual differences in half-life or steady-state blood level tended to vanish within a set of identical twins, but to be preserved within a set of fraternal twins. Table 2 shows data for three drugs investigated at different times in seven sets of identical and seven sets of fraternal twins.

Several methods exist for estimating the relative contributions of environmental and genetic factors to the control of a trait (41); most of these are too complex to consider here. A rough estimate of the hereditary component of variation can be made by determination of the mean variance within sets of identical and fraternal twins; these variances are then treated according to the following formula for heritability (42, 43):

$$\frac{\text{variance within pairs of fraternal twins} - \text{variance within pairs of identical twins}}{\text{variance within pairs of fraternal twins}}$$

This expression yields values from 0, indicating negligible hereditary and complete environmental control, to 1, indicating virtually complete hereditary influence. For phenylbutazone, antipyrine, bishydroxycoumarin, and ethanol, values for the contribution of heredity were 0.99, 0.98, 0.97, and 0.99, respectively. Our studies on twins yielded intraclass correlation coefficients close to theoretical expectation solely on the basis of genetic control, according to which fraternal twins, having in common approximately half of their total number of genes, should have a value of 0.5, whereas identical twins should have a value of 1. For rates of metabolism of phenylbutazone, antipyrine, bishydroxycoumarin, and ethanol the intraclass correlation coefficients of identical twins were 0.83, 0.85, 0.85, and 0.82, respectively; and for fraternal twins, 0.33, 0.47, 0.66, and 0.38, respectively. Evidently for these drugs and for these subjects, large interindividual differences in rates of drug elimination from plasma are surprisingly free of environmental influence. As shown by repeated plasma drug half-life determinations, normal subjects have remarkably reproducible plasma half-lives for these drugs. Because phenylbutazone (22) and bishydroxycoumarin (44) are 98% bound to plasma proteins, differences among individuals in plasma elimination rates might involve variability in the binding of the drug to albumin. However, antipyrine is not appreciably bound to plasma proteins (45). Therefore, it seems reasonable to conclude that for antipyrine, if not also for phenyl-

Table 2 Dicumarol, antipyrine, and phenylbutazone half-lives with smoking and coffee history in 28 twins[a]

Twin	Age, sex	Half-life Dicumarol (hr)	Antipyrine (hr)	Phenylbutazone (days)	Smoking (pack/day)	Coffee (cups/day)
Identical twins						
Ho. M.	48,M	25.0	11.3	1.9	0.5	2
Ho. M	48,M	25.0	11.3	2.1	1	3
D. T.	43,F	55.5	10.3	2.8	0	5–6
V. W.	43,F	55.5	9.6	2.9	2	8–10
J. G.	22,M	36.0	11.5	2.8	1	1–2
P. G.	22,M	34.0	11.5	2.8	1	1–2
Ja. T.	44,M	74.0	14.9	4.0	0	6
Ja. T.	44,M	72.0	14.9	4.0	0	2–3
C. J.	55,F	41.0	6.9	3.2	0	2
F. J.	55,F	42.5	7.1	2.9	0	2
Ge. L.	45,M	72.0	12.3	3.9	0	4
Gu. L.	45,M	69.0	12.8	4.1	0	4
D. H.	26,F	46.0	11.0	2.6	0	0–1
D. W.	26,F	44.0	11.0	2.6	0	3–4
Fraternal twins						
A. M.	21,F	45.0	15.1	7.3	1.5	2
S. M.	21,M	22.0	6.3	3.6	0	0
D. L.	36,F	46.5	7.2	2.3	0	2–3
D. S.	36,F	51.0	15.0	3.3	2	3–4
S. A.	33,F	34.5	5.1	2.1	1	2
P. M.	33,F	27.5	12.5	1.2	0.5	2
Ja. H.	24,F	7.0	12.0	2.6	0	10–15
Je. H.	24,F	19.0	6.0	2.3	1.5	10
F. D.	48,M	24.5	14.7	2.8	0	1
P. D.	48,M	38.0	9.3	3.5	1.5	8
L. D.	21,F	67.0	8.2	2.9	1	6
L. W.	21,F	72.0	6.9	3.0	1	2–3
E. K.	31,F	40.5	7.7	1.9	0	0
R. K.	31,M	35.0	7.3	2.1	1	0

[a]The difference between identical and fraternal twins in intrapair variance is significant: $P < 0.005$ (F = 36.0, $N_1 = N_2 = 7$). Reproduced by permission from Vessell and Page, 1968 (37).

butazone and bishydroxycoumarin, interindividual variability in plasma half-life arises from genetic differences in drug metabolism rather than in drug distribution. That appreciable variations do exist in rates of metabolism of these drugs is indicated by ranges for the plasma half-lives of ethanol, antipyrine, phenylbutazone, and bishydroxycoumarin of twofold, threefold, sixfold, and tenfold, respectively, among the 28 individuals in the study (Table 2).

Family studies using pharmacokinetic measurements tend to support the results of the twin experiments; the family studies disclosed predominantly genetic control over large interindividual variations in plasma half-lives of bishydroxycoumarin (46), phenylbutazone (47), and nortriptyline (48). Furthermore, the results of all three studies suggest polygenic control.

There also exist in man at least a dozen monogenically controlled conditions that produce unusual responses to drugs (41, 49). These include acatalasia, atypical plasma pseudocholinesterase, slow acetylation of isoniazid, deficient parahydroxylation of diphenylhydantoin, sensitivity to bishydroxycoumarin, glucose-6-phosphate dehydrogenase deficiency, resistance to warfarin, and drug-sensitive abnormal hemoglobins. The first five conditions are hereditary abnormalities that affect enzymes directly involved in drug metabolism. These conditions may result in drug toxicity attributable to elevated blood levels from drug accumulation after continuous administration of even a low dose. By contrast, the last three conditions represent genetically transmitted aberrations, not of drug metabolism, but of sites of drug action. In these disorders toxicity or failure to elicit a therapeutic response can occur at what are generally considered therapeutic drug blood levels. Some structural alteration in a protein with which the drug or drug metabolite can interact causes these blood levels, safe in most subjects, to be either toxic or ineffective. For example, O'Reilly (50, 51) described two extensive pedigrees of warfarin resistance, an autosomal dominant trait; the normal mean daily dose of warfarin (6.8 ± 2.8 mg) was completely ineffective in anticoagulating these subjects although their warfarin blood levels were within normal range. A daily 20 mg dose of warfarin was required in affected individuals; resistance was attributed to a structurally altered hepatic receptor site with greater affinity than normal for Vitamin K (50, 51).

ROLE OF ENVIRONMENTAL FACTORS

Despite the abundant evidence described in the preceding section indicating predominantly genetic control over large interindividual differences in rates of drug metabolism for normal, nonmedicated subjects living in relatively uninduced environments, nongenetic factors can also significantly alter both drug distribution and therapeutic response. Many drugs, or environmental agents such as insecticides (26, 52, 53), can accelerate rates of drug metabolism and elimination from the body; other drugs and environmental agents can retard these rates (54). However, recognition of the numerous factors that accelerate or retard drug metabolism and elimination is insufficient to permit adequate adjustment of drug dosage, because individuals vary greatly in their quantitative response to inducing (31, 55, 56) or inhibiting (54, 57–62) agents. A twin study revealed that phenobarbital administered for two weeks

(2 mg/kg qd po) produced a wide range of responses, as estimated by the degree of shortening of plasma antipyrine half-lives (55). The extremes were total failure to alter antipyrine half-life and a shortening of antipyrine half-life from 18 to 6 hr. These variations in response to phenobarbital were shown to be predominantly under genetic control (55). Furthermore, the extent to which phenobarbital shortened antipyrine half-lives was related to the control value for plasma antipyrine half-life; subjects with relatively long antipyrine half-lives before phenobarbital administration reduced their half-lives much more than did subjects with initially short values (Figure 3) (55). In harmony with these observations, genetic control of the induction of aryl hydrocarbon hydroxylase activity in cultured human lymphocytes by 3-methylcholanthrene was demonstrated (56); this study of cells from 353 healthy subjects from 67 families revealed hereditary control by a single genetic locus with gene frequencies of the alleles for low and high inducibility being 0.717 and 0.283, respectively (56).

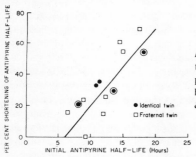

Figure 3 Positive correlation (0.84) between the initial antipyrine half-life in plasma and the phenobarbital-induced shortening of antipyrine half-life. Reproduced by permission from Vesell & Page (55).

As mentioned previously, large interindividual variations also exist in response to compounds that inhibit drug metabolism (57–62), but these differences appear from twin studies (63) to be more under environmental than genetic control. Inhibition of drug metabolism presumably arises from binding of compounds to hepatic microsomal proteins (64, 65) and does not involve protein synthesis, whereas induction requires protein synthesis that is under direct genetic control. For these reasons, predominantly environmental control of interindividual differences in response to inhibiting drugs, and underlying genetic control of large interindividual differences in drug metabolism, drug blood levels, and induction of drug metabolizing enzymes could have been predicted. On the other hand, the numerous, previously described environmental factors capable of altering drug blood levels by affecting processes of drug absorption, distribution, metabolism, interaction at receptor sites, and/or excretion might have been expected to obscure the fundamental genetic control. In this connection, several disease states should be mentioned as examples of altered environments capable of changing both drug blood levels and receptor site sensitivity. In hyperthyroidism, antipyrine metabolism is accelerated, whereas it is retarded in myxedema (54). However, in myxedema, decreased sensitivity of warfarin receptor sites has also been described (66). In myasthenia gravis, decreased sensitivity of the acetycholine receptors in the postjunctional membrane may be the principal mechanism for skeletal muscle weakness, although it may develop only after prolonged deficiency of acetylcholine (67). Thus, for myasthenia gravis, the interrelationship between acetylcholine distribution and therapeutic response is complex and as yet not completely resolved. After injury or section of peripheral nerve to skeletal muscle, supersensitivity of the acetylcholine receptor sites on the muscle develops as a compensatory mechanism for decreased availability of acetyl-choline. Here an inverse relationship exists between acetylcholine distribution and receptor site response.

Large interindividual differences in drug blood levels after exposure to inducing or inhibiting compounds render hazardous predictions of the extent to which any particular therapeutic agent will affect the blood level of another drug in any given patient. The most direct solution to this problem lies in measuring drug blood levels in each subject to whom such inducing or inhibiting agents have been administered. Drug blood level determinations will reveal directly the degree to which each subject responds to an inducing or inhibiting agent. Nevertheless, problems arise if too much faith is placed in drug blood levels. Specific information is required on each drug whose blood level is being measured to insure a direct correlation between drug blood level and therapeutic effect. For example, a recent experimental study in dogs contrasted serum and interstitial levels of various antibiotics administered chronically or acutely (68). The results revealed that after a single dose the concentrations of certain antibiotics, including ampicillin, were much lower in the tissue fluid, where they normally act, than in serum (68). Furthermore, the shape of the curve relating antibiotic levels to time differed in serum and tissue fluid. For several antibiotics the peaks of the curves did not occur simultaneously. On chronic administration, higher tissue concentrations of antibiotics could be produced. These data suggest that reliance on blood levels as indicators of antibiotic concentrations in interstitial fluid may be invalid for several antibiotics after a single dose and that for certain rapidly excreted antibiotics frequent administration of high doses is required to achieve effective tissue concentrations.

Another possible misinterpretation that could arise from too literal a reading of drug blood levels is exemplified by the patient who fails to take his medication for several weeks or even months but decides to resume the prescribed drug several days prior to visiting his physician. High drug blood levels at the time of the visit without much therapeutic effect could mislead the physician into believing that either this particular patient was resistant to the drug or that poor correlation exists between blood levels of the drug and therapeutic effects.

Three diverse drug interactions are pertinent to this discussion. Although the literature on drug interactions is vast, few studies have succeeded in defining systematically whether a drug interaction occurs during drug absorption, distribution, biotransformation, binding at receptor sites, excretion or a combination of these. Too often a drug interaction is described without elucidation of its mechanism, or else a mechanism is proposed with insufficient supporting evidence. To illustrate how a drug interaction having profound therapeutic effects can occur without changing the drug blood level, the interaction between warfarin and Vitamin K is cited. In a patient taking warfarin, administration of Vitamin K does not alter the blood level or plasma half-life of warfarin. However, through competition with warfarin at sites in the liver where certain clotting factors are synthesized, Vitamin K restores prothrombin times toward normal. Frequently, after a drug interaction has been documented, its precise clinical significance is unclear. The following three examples illustrate aspects of these and related problems in drug interactions.

One study with cyclophosphamide revealed that patients before and after exposure to microsomal enzyme-inducing drugs exhibited marked changes in their plasma cyclophosphamide half-lives and in the peak plasma alkylating concentrations (69). However, no significant alteration in clinical response occurred; this lack of interference was attributed by the authors to the relative constancy of the product of the total drug concentration and time (69).

The second example concerns displacement of one drug from albumin by administration of another drug that binds to albumin more avidly. Because only the unbound portion of a drug is considered available to produce therapeutic effects, this type of drug interaction has the potential for changing therapeutic effects by changing the ratio of bound, pharmacologically inactive drug to unbound, pharmacologically active drug. However, few reports contain quantitative data on the degree to which such drug displacements actually intensify therapeutic effects; as a result much confusion on this point has been generated. Gillette (29) has clarified the situation by developing a formula to describe the relationship between the biological half-life of a drug and its binding to albumin and muscle under specified conditions. According to these formulas, 50% binding of a drug to albumin increases the drug half-life by only 11% when the unbound drug is distributed in the total body water; if 75% of the drug is bound to albumin, the drug half-life is prolonged by only 33% (29). Reduction in drug binding to albumin from 95 to 90% would decrease the biologic half-life by only 50%, but reduction from 99 to 98% binding would diminish it by 86%. Greater effects would occur for drugs whose unbound portions are distributed in the extracellular, rather than the total body, fluids; for example, if 75% of such a drug were bound to albumin, its biological half-life would be prolonged by 111% (29). Furthermore, Gillette demonstrated that variations in binding of a drug to albumin would produce little effect if the drug were also highly bound to skeletal muscle. In instances of changes in the extent of binding of a drug to skeletal muscle, marked alterations in the biologic half-life of a drug could result because the volume of skeletal muscle greatly exceeds the plasma albumin volume. Thus more attention should be devoted to drug binding to tissues with large volumes such as skeletal muscle (29).

The third example concerns oversimplification in classification of drugs that alter rates of hepatic microsomal drug metabolism. It has become popular to distribute lists separating those drugs that increase from those that retard or produce no change in the rates of biotransformation of other drugs. This approach stems from the trend in studies on drug interactions to investigate the effect on drug metabolism only at a single time after chronic administration of a compound. While technical problems prevent the clinical pharmacologist from investigating effects on drug metabolism at multiple time points in his patients, restriction of such studies to a single time point can yield erroneous conclusions if results are generalized too broadly. Many so-called inducing drugs exhibit biphasic effects; 2 to 10 hr after their administration certain inducing agents can inhibit drug metabolism by binding to hepatic microsomal proteins (30). For example, a recent study in rats on the effects of an experimental anti-inflammatory agent revealed that 2 hr after its oral administration hepatic microsomal aniline hydroxylase and ethylmorphine N-demethylase activities were inhibited, but 24 hr after oral administration of the same dose analine hydroxylase activity and cytochrome P-450 content were enhanced (70). After 4 daily doses of this experimental anti-inflammatory drug no significant change occurred in either enzyme activity, but cytochrome P-450 content remained slightly elevated (70). These studies suggest that interactions affecting rates of drug metabolism may be more complex than previously recognized and that the same agent can produce polyphasic alterations depending on the experimental conditions. From the point of view of this review, such investigations illustrate that the same dose of a drug can affect drug blood level and therapeutic response in markedly different, even opposite, ways depending on the time selected to examine the effects. In this connection changes in the dose of a drug or its route of administration (71, 72) can alter drug blood levels, metabolism and therapeutic effects.

This discussion of the role of environmental factors in altering drug blood levels will be concluded with two examples in which actual measurement of drug blood levels helped to identify the factors affecting drug blood levels and to develop safer, more effective ways of administering the drug in man. The first example concerns the use of procainamide in prophylaxis of antiarrhythmias after myocardial infarction (73). Until recently the usual dosage interval for procainamide was 6 hr. Koch-Weser et al (73) demonstrated that when the compound was administered in the usual dose every 6 hr, large fluctuations occurred in the serum concentrations of the drug (Figure 4) such that both the peak and lowest serum concentrations were out of the optimal therapeutic range (4–8 mg/liter). By changing the administration interval from 6 hr to 3 hr, they observed that the amplitude of these fluctuations was reduced and that patients could be maintained more consistently within therapeutic serum concentrations (Figure 4).

The second example involves biological availability of a dosage form. Lindenbaum et al (74) reported wide differences of serum digoxin levels in patients receiving various proprietary preparations of the drug. Each tablet contained equal

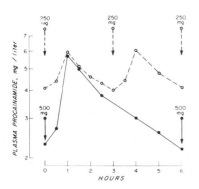

Figure 4 Fluctuation of plasma procainamide concentrations on two dosage schedules in the same patient. Reproduced by permission from Koch-Weser et al (73).

Table 3 Relationships between drug blood concentrations and therapeutic effects

Drug	Method (Ref.)	Drug Concentration in Serum	Reported Pharmacologic Effect
Acetaminophen	spectrophotometry (85)	10-20 μg/ml	analgesia
Acetohexamide	spectrophotometry (86)	20-55 μg/ml	hypoglycemia
Aminopterin	spectrophotofluorometry (87)	0.2-1 μg/ml	carcinostatic action
Amitriptyline	spectrophotometry (88)	0.3-0.9 μg/ml	antidepressant
Amphetamines	gas chromotography (89, 90)	1-2 μg/ml	analepsis
Antihistamines	gas chromatography (91)	0.008-0.016 μg/ml	antihistaminic
Barbiturates	spectrophotometry (92) & gas chromatography (93, 94)		sedation
Phenobarbital		20 μg/ml	
Amobarbital		5 μg/ml	
Pentobarbital		1 μg/ml	
Secobarbital		1 μg/ml	
Bishydroxycoumarin	spectrophotometry (95)	18-26 μg/ml	anticoagulant
Bretylium	gas chromatography (96)	0.5-1.3 μg/ml	antiarrhythmic
Bromide	spectrophotometry (97)	40-50 μg/ml	sedation
Brompheniramine	gas chromatography (98)	0.008-0.016 μg/ml	antihistaminic
Bromural	gas chromatography (99)	1-3 μg/ml	sedation - hypnosis
Butaperazine	spectrophotofluorometry (100)	4-6 μg/ml	antipsychotic
Captodiamine	spectrophotometry (101)	2-4 μg/ml	sedation, anti-spasmotic
Carbamazepine	gas chromatography (102)	2-10 μg/ml	anticonvulsive
Carbromal	gas chromatography (99)	1-3 μg/ml	sedation - hypnosis
Carisoprodal	gas chromatography (99, 103)	10-40 μg/ml	muscle relaxant
Chloral hydrate	gas chromatography (104)	5-10 μg/ml	hypnosis
Chlordiazepoxide	spectrophotofluorometry (105)	1-2 μg/ml	tranquilizer
Chlorpheniramine	gas chromatography (98)	0.008-0.016 μg/ml	antihistaminic
Chlorpromazine	gas chromatography (106)	0.5-0.7 μg/ml	tranquilizer, antiemitic
Chlorpropamide	spectrophotometry (86)	30-140 μg/ml	hypoglycemia
Chlorothiazide	spectrophotometry (107)	2-2.5 μg/ml	natriuretic action
Chlorprothixene	spectrophotofluorometry (105, 108, 109)	0.04 μg/ml	antipsychotic, antiemitic
Desipramine	spectrophotofluorometry (110)	0.6-1.4 μg/ml	antidepressant
Digoxin	radioimmunoassay (111)	0.0003-0.003 μg/ml	stabilize sinus rhythm & antiarrhythmic
Diphenylhydantoin	spectrophotometry (112)	6-17 μg/ml	anticonvulsive
	gas chromatography (113)	4-24 μg/ml	antiarrhythmic (Ventricular premature systoles)
		12-23 μg/ml	antiarrhythmic (Supraventricular tachycardia)
Ethchloroynol	gas chromatography (103)	4-6 μg/ml	sedation
Ethinamate	gas chromatography (99)	5-10 μg/ml	sedation
Ethyl ether	gas chromatography (97)	900-1000 μg/ml	anesthesia

Table 3 Continued

Drug	Method (Ref.)	Drug Concentration in Serum	Reported Pharmacologic Effect
Glutethimide	spectrophotometry (114, 115)	0.2-0.4 μg/ml	sedation
Griseofulvin	spectrophotofluorometry (87)	0.3-1.3 μg/ml	antifungal
Halofenate	gas chromatography (116)	150-250 μg/ml	hypolipidemic
Hydroxyphenamate	gas chromatography (99)	5-10 μg/ml	muscle relaxant, tranquilizer
Imipramine	spectrophotofluorometry (117)	2-6 μg/ml	antidepressant
Lidocaine	gas chromatography (118)	1.0-2.0 μg/ml	local anesthesia
Lithium	flame emission spectrometry (119)	1.0-2.0 mEq/liter	antidepressant
Meperidine	spectrophotometry (120)	0.6-0.75 μg/ml	sedation
Meprobamate	gas chromatography (103)	10-20 μg/ml	tranquilizer
Methaqualone	spectrophotometry (121)	2-5 μg/ml	sedation
Methohexitone	gas chromatography (122)	1-4 μg/ml	anesthesia
Methyprylon	gas chromatography (99)	10 μg/ml	sedation
Methapyrilene	spectrophotometry (123)	2-4 μg/ml	antihistaminic
Nitrofurantoin	spectrophotometry (124)	1-2 μg/ml	antibiotic
Nortriptyline	spectrophotometry (88) & gas chromatography	0.015-0.035 μg/ml	antidepressant
Oxazepam	gas chromatography (97)	1-2 μg/ml	antidepressant
Paracetamol	spectrophotometry (121)	4.5-25 μg/ml	analgesia
Paraldehyde	gas chromatography (103)	30-150 μg/ml	hypnosis
Pentazocine	spectrophotofluorometry (125)	0.14-0.16 μg/ml	analgesia
Phenylbutazone	spectrophotometry (22)	40-60 μg/ml	analgesia
Prilocaine	gas chromatography (118)	less than 2 μg/ml	local anesthesia
Probenecid	spectrophotometry (126)	100-200 μg/ml	uricosuric
Procainamide	spectrophotofluorometry (127)	4-8 μg/ml	antiarrhythmic
Propranolol	spectrophotofluorometry (128)	0.035-0.200 μg/ml	β-adrenergic blockade
Propoxyphene	gas chromatography (129)	0.1-0.2 μg/ml	analgesia
Quinacrine	spectrophotofluorometry (87)	0.005-0.05 μg/ml	antimalarial
Quinidine	spectrophotofluorometry (87)	3-6 μg/ml	antiarrhythmic
Quinine	spectrophotofluorometry (87)	2-5 μg/ml	antimalarial
Salicylate	spectrophotometry (130)	50-100 μg/ml	analgesia (therapeutic)
		350-400 μg/ml	antiarthritic
		$>$ 250 μg/ml	rheumatic fever therapy
Sulfonamides	spectrophotofluorometry (105)	50-100 μg/ml	bacteriostatic
Tetracycline	spectrophotofluorometry (117)	1.2-1.9 μg/ml	antibiotic
Thiobarbiturate	spectrophotometry (131)		hypnosis
Thiopental		30 μg/ml	
Thiamylal		30 μg/ml	
Thioridazine	spectrophotofluorometry (109)	0.04-0.3 μg/ml	tranquilizer
Tolbutamide	spectrophotometry (86, 132)	50-95 μg/ml	hypoglycemia
Trimethobenzamide	spectrophotofluorometry (105)	1-2 μg/ml	antivertigo
Zoxazolamine	spectrophotometry (133)	3-12 μg/ml	muscle relaxant

amounts of digoxin as measured in vitro. Wide differences in serum digoxin levels, ranging from four- to sevenfold, occurred not only between preparations from different companies but even between different lots from the same company (74). Previously there had been reported similar differences in the bioavailability of other drugs, including diphenylhydantoin (75, 76), bishydroxycoumarin (77), phenylbutazone (78), prednisone (79), thyroid (80), tolbutamide (81), chloramphenicol (82), and oxytetracycline (83, 84). Thus differences in bioavailability of dosage forms can contribute to intraindividual and interindividual variations in drug blood levels and therapeutic response.

Gathered from the current literature, Table 3 summarizes the correlation between drug blood levels and therapeutic effects. It is presented with the recognition that certain of these drug levels represent approximations, that many change under various environmental circumstances and are not invariably associated with the therapeutic effects listed. The diverse causes for such limitations in the use of drug blood levels have been the topic of this review.

CONCLUSION

Certain pharmacological principles governing relationships between drug distribution and therapeutic effects have been described. A major obstacle to a clear understanding of the subject and a principal cause for the controversy surrounding it are tendencies to generalize too broadly rather than to recognize that the individual properties of a drug define the relationship between its distribution and therapeutic effects. Genetic and environmental factors represent important determinants of the relationship between the distribution and therapeutic effects of specific drugs. The close relationship that applies for certain drugs between blood levels and pharmacologic effects is exemplified by diphenylhydantoin. Administration of the usual doses of diphenylhydantoin produces serum concentrations from 2 to 50 mg/liter due to large interindividual differences in rates of hepatic diphenylhydantoin metabolism (134); however, the therapeutically effective range of serum concentration (10–20 mg/liter) is comparatively quite narrow. Progressive increments in diphenylhydantoin toxicity are associated with progressive elevations of blood concentrations above the therapeutic serum levels, as shown in Figure 5 (135).

In certain disease states or after administration of avidly bound compounds, the free, pharmacologically active fraction of a drug may be increased; thus, correlations between pharmacodynamic effects should be attempted with the unbound rather than with the total plasma drug concentration. For example, in renal failure with uremia the capacity of plasma albumin to bind drugs is decreased; and the apparent volume of distribution of such highly bound drugs as digitoxin and diphenylhydantoin is increased (136, 137). In addition to actual drug concentrations at the receptor sites for cardiac glycosides, many other environmental factors, such as potassium concentration, anoxia, and acidosis, influence the pharmacodynamic effects of the cardiac glycosides. Limitations exist in the precision and accuracy with which many pharmacodynamic effects can be measured. If correlations are to be sought, only plasma drug levels should be used that produce a pharmacodynamic response on linear, rather than the plateau, portion of the dose-response curve. Although methodology for measuring drug blood levels has developed tremendously, many problems remain. One difficulty involves the distinction between the free and the bound forms of a drug. For drugs administered as racemic mixtures, such as warfarin (138), hexobarbital (139), methadone (140), propranolol (141), and amphetamine (142), problems exist in establishing the distinction between the pharmacologically active and inactive isomers and between potentially different rates of metabolism and hence different blood levels of the isomers.

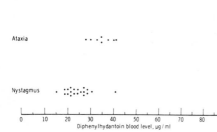

Figure 5 Progression from nystagmus to ataxia to mental changes in relationship to diphenylhydantoin blood concentrations. Each circle represents the blood diphenylhydantoin concentration and toxic clinical manifestation of a single patient. Reproduced by permission from Kutt et al (134).

ACKNOWLEDGMENTS

Dr. G. Thomas Passananti of this department prepared Table 3. This study was supported in part by grant No. MH21327 from the National Institute of Mental Health.

Note added in proof: A high correlation between drug toxicity and plasma drug concentrations has actually been observed for relatively few therapeutic agents in clinical practise; Prescott et al (143) documents this conclusion for thiopental, α-methyldopa, methaqualone, glutethimide, salicylates, and paracetamol (143).

Literature Cited

1. Gillette, J. R. 1974. In *Pharmacokinetics, Fogarty International Center Proceedings No. 20*, ed. T. Teorell, R. Dietrich, P. Condliffe. New York: Plenum
2. Soberman, R. et al. 1949. *J. Biol. Chem.* 179:31–42
3. Riegelman, S., Loo, J., Rowland, M. 1968. *J. Pharm. Sci.* 57:128–33
4. Gibaldi, M., Nagashima, R., Levy, G. 1969. *J. Pharm. Sci.* 58:193–97
5. Brodie, B. B., Mark, L. C., Papper, E. M., Lief, P. S. 1950. *J. Pharmacol. Exp. Ther.* 98:85–96
6. Gibaldi, M., Levy, G., Weintraub, H. 1971. *Clin. Pharmacol. Ther.* 12:734–42
7. Levy, G., Gibaldi, M., Jusko, W. J. 1969. *J. Pharm. Sci.* 58:422–24
8. Levy, G., Nelson, E. 1965. *J. Pharm. Sci.* 54:812
9. Levy, G. 1966. *Clin. Pharmacol. Ther.* 7:362–72
10. *Second Deer Lodge Conference on Implications of Blood Level Assays of Therapeutic Agents.* To be published in 1974 as a supplementary volume in *Clin. Pharmacol. Ther.*
11. Waddell, W. J. 1973. *Ann. Rev. Pharmacol.* 13:153–68
12. Brodie, B. B., Udenfriend, S., Baer, J. E. 1947. *J. Biol. Chem.* 168:299–310
13. Brodie, B. B., Udenfriend, S., Dill, W., Downing, G. 1947. *J. Biol. Chem.* 168:311–18

14. Brodie, B. B., Udenfriend, S., Dill, W., Chenkin, T. 1947. *J. Biol. Chem.* 168: 319–26
15. Brodie, B. B., Udenfriend, S., Taggart, J. V. 1947. *J. Biol. Chem.* 168:327–34
16. Brodie, B. B., Udenfriend, S., Dill, W. 1947. *J. Biol. Chem.* 168:335–40
17. Quinn, G. P., Axelrod, J., Brodie, B. B. 1958. *Biochem. Pharmacol.* 1:152–59
18. Bourne, H. R. 1972. In *Clinical Pharmacology,* ed. K. L. Melmon, H. F. Morrelli. 555–57. New York: Macmillan
19. Brodie, B. B. 1967. *J. Am. Med. Assoc.* 202:600–9
20. Vesell, E. S., Passananti, G. T. 1971. *Clin. Chem.* 17:851–66
21. Koch-Weser, J. 1972. *N. Engl. J. Med.* 287:227–31
22. Burns, J. J. et al. 1953. *J. Pharmacol. Exp. Ther.* 109:346–57
23. Brodie, B. B., Weiner, J., Burns, J. J., Simson, G., Yale, E. K. 1952. *J. Pharmacol. Exp. Ther.* 106:453–63
24. van Rossum, J. M., Tomey, A. H. W. 1968. *J. Pharm. Pharmacol.* 20:390–92
25. Conney, A. H., Burns, J. J. 1972. *Science* 178:576–86
26. Fouts, J. R. 1970. *Toxicol. Appl. Pharmacol.* 16:48–65
27. Koch-Weser, J., Sellers, E. M. 1971. *N. Engl. J. Med.* 285:487–98, 547–58
28. Vesell, E. S. 1968. *Pharmacology* 1: 81–97
29. Gillette, J. R. 1971. *Ann. NY Acad. Sci.* 179:43–66
30. Conney, A. H. 1967. *Pharmacol. Rev.* 19:317–66
31. Breckenridge, A., Orme, M. 1971. *Ann. NY Acad. Sci.* 179:421–31
32. Borondy, P., Chang, T., Glazko, A. J. 1972. *Fed. Proc.* 31:582
33. Levy. G., Ashley, J. J. 1973. *J. Pharm. Sci* 62:161–62
34. Galton, F. 1875. *J. Brit. Anthropol. Inst.* 5:391–406
35. Vesell, E. S., Page, J. G. 1968. *Science* 159:1479–80
36. Vesell, E. S., Page, J. G. 1968. *Science* 161:72–73
37. Vesell, E. S., Page, J. G. 1968. *J. Clin. Invest.* 47:2657–63
38. Vesell, E. S., Page, J. G., Passananti, G. T. 1971. *Clin. Pharmacol. Ther.* 12: 192–201
39. Cascorbi, H. F., Vesell, E. S., Blake, D. A., Helrich, M. 1971. *Clin. Pharmacol. Ther.* 12:50–55
40. Alexanderson, B., Evans, D. A., Sjöqvist, F. 1969. *Brit. Med. J.* 4: 764–68
41. Vesell, E. S. 1973. *Progr. Med. Genet.* 9:291–367
42. Neel, J. V., Schull, W. J. 1954. *Human Heredity.* p. 280. Chicago: Univ. Chicago Press
43. Osborne, R. H., DeGeorge, F. V. 1959. *Genetic Basis of Morphological Variation, an Evaluation and Application of the Twin Study Method.* Cambridge, Mass.: Harvard Univ. Press
44. Weiner, M., Shapiro, S., Axelrod, J., Cooper, J. R., Brodie, B. B. 1950. *J. Pharmacol. Exp. Ther.* 99:409–20
45. Brodie, B. B., Axelrod, J. 1950. *J. Pharmacol. Exp. Ther.* 98:97–104
46. Motulsky, A. 1964. *Progr. Med. Genet.* 3:49–74
47. Whittaker, J. A., Evans, D. A. 1970. *Brit. Med. J.* 4:323–28
48. Åsberg, M., Evans, D. A., Sjöqvist, F. 1971. *J. Med. Genet.* 8:129–35
49. Vesell, E. S. 1969. *Advan. Pharmacol. Chemother.* 7:1–52
50. O'Reilly, R. A., Aggeler, P. M., Hoag, M. S., Leong, L. S., Kropatkin, M. L. 1964. *New Engl. J. Med.* 271:809–15
51. O'Reilly, R. A. 1970. *New Engl. J. Med.* 282: 1448–51
52. Kolmodin, B., Azarnoff, D. L., Sjöqvist, F. 1969. *Clin. Pharmacol. Ther.* 10: 638–42
53. Poland, A., Smith, D., Kuntzman, R., Jacobson, M., Conney, A. H. 1970. *Clin. Pharmacol. Ther.* 11:724–32
54. Vesell, E. S., Passananti, G. T. 1973. *Drug Metab. Disp.* 1:402–10
55. Vesell, E. S., Page, J. G. 1969. *J. Clin. Invest.* 48:2202–2209
56. Kellermann, G., Luyten-Kellermann, M., Shaw, C. R. 1973. *Am. J. Hum. Genet.* 25:327–31
57. Vesell, E. S., Passananti, G. T., Greene, F. E. 1970. *New Engl. J. Med.* 283: 1484–88
58. Vesell, E. S., Passananti, G. T., Lee, C. H. 1971. *Clin. Pharmacol. Ther.* 12: 785–92
59. Vesell, E. S., Ng, L., Passananti, G. T. 1971. *Lancet* 2:370
60. Vesell, E. S., Passananti, G. T., Viau, J.-P., Epps, J. E., DiCarlo, F. J. 1972. *Pharmacology* 7:197–206
61. O'Reilly, R. A. 1973. *Ann. Intern. Med.* 78:73–76
62. O'Malley, K., Stevenson, I. H., Crooks, J. 1972. *Clin. Pharmacol. Ther.* 13: 552–57
63. Andreasen, P. B., Froland, A., Skovsted, L., Andersen, S. A., Hauge, M. 1973. *Acta Med. Scand.* 193:561–64

64. Netter, K. J. 1973. *Drug Metab. Dist.* 1:162–63
65. Gillette, J. R., Sasame, H., Stripp, B. 1973. *Drug Metab. Dist.* 1:164–73
66. Rice, A. J., McIntosh, T. J., Fouts, J. R., Brunk, S. F., Wilson, W. R. 1971. *Am. J. Med. Sci.* 262:211–15
67. Koelle, G. B. 1970. In *The Pharmacological Basis of Therapeutics,* ed. L. S. Goodman, A. Gilman, p. 460. New York: Macmillan
68. Chisholm, G. D., Waterworth, P. M., Calnan, J. S., Garrod, L. P. 1973. *Brit. Med. J.* 1:569–73
69. Bagley, C. M., Bostick, F. W., DeVita, V. T. 1973. *Cancer Res.* 33:226–33
70. Vesell, E. S., Lee, C. H., Passananti, G. T., Shively, C. A. 1972. *Pharmacology.* 8: 217–21
71. Dollery, C. T., Davies, D. S., Conolly, M. E. 1971. *Ann. NY Acad. Sci.* 179: 108–14
72. Williams, R. T. 1971. *Ann. NY Acad. Sci.* 179:141–54
73. Koch-Weser, J., Klein, S. W., Foo-Canto, L. L., Kastor, J. A., Descantis, R. W. 1969. *New Engl. J. Med.* 281: 1253–60
74. Lindenbaum, J., Mellow, M. H., Blackstone, M. O., Butler, V. P. 1971. *New Engl. J. Med.* 285:1344–47
75. Martin, C. M., Rubin, M., O'Malley, W. E., Garagusi, V. S., McCauley, C. E. 1968. *Pharmacologist* 10:167
76. Tyrer, J. H., Eadie, M. J., Sutherland, J. M., Hooper, W. D. 1970. *Brit. Med. J.* 4:271–73
77. Lozinski, E. 1960. *Can. Med. Assoc. J.* 83:177–78
78. Searl, R. O., Pernarowski, M. 1967. *Can. Med. Assoc. J.* 96:1513–20
79. Campagna, F., Cureton, G., Mirigian, R. A., Nelson, E. 1963. *J. Pharm. Sci.* 52:605–6
80. Catz, B., Ginsburg, E., Salenger, S. 1962. *New Engl. J. Med.* 266:136–37
81. Varley, A. B. 1968. *J. Am. Med. Assoc.* 206:1745–48
82. Glazko, A. J., Kinkel, A. W., Alegnani, W. C., Holmes, E. L. 1968. *Clin. Pharmacol. Ther.* 9:472–83
83. Brice, G. W., Hammer, H. F. 1969. *J. Am. Med. Assoc.* 208:1189–90
84. Blair, D. C., Barnes, R. W., Wildner, E. L., Murray, W. J. 1971. *J. Am. Med. Assoc.* 215:251–54
85. Gwilt, J. R., Robertson, A., McChesney, E. W. 1963. *J. Pharm. Pharmacol.* 15:440–44
86. Sheldon, J., Anderson, J., Stoner, L. 1965. *Diabetes* 14:362–67

87. Udenfriend, S. 1962. *Fluorescence Assay in Biology and Medicine.* New York: Academic
88. Wallace, J. E., Dahl, E. V. 1967. *J. Forsenic Sci.* 12:484–96
89. Beckett, A. H., Rowland, M. A. 1964. *J. Pharm. Pharmacol.* 16:27T–30T
90. Beckett, A. H., Rowland, M. 1965. *J. Pharm. Pharmacol.* 17:59–60
91. Jain, N. C., Kirk, P. L. 1967. *Microchem. J.* 12:242–48
92. Goldbaum, L. R. 1952. *Anal. Chem.* 24:1604–7
93. Parker, K. D., Kirk, P. L. 1961. *Anal. Chem.* 33:1378–81
94. Jain, N. C., Kirk, P. L. 1967. *Microchem. J.* 12:249–55
95. Axelrod, J., Cooper, J. R., Brodie, B. B. 1949. *Proc. Soc. Exp. Biol. Med.* 70: 693–95
96. Kuntzman, R., Tsai, I., Chang, R., Conney, A. H. 1970. *Clin. Pharmacol. Ther.* 11:829–37
97. Winek, C. L. 1970. *Clin. Toxicol.* 3: 541–49
98. Bruce, R. B., Pitts, J. E., Pinchbeck, F. M. 1968. *Anal. Chem.* 40:1246–50
99. Goldbaum, L. R., Domanski, T. J. 1966. *J. Forensic Sci.* 11:233–42
100. Simpson, G. M., Lament, R., Cooper, T. B., Lee, J. H., Bruce, R. B. 1973. *J. Clin. Pharmacol.* 13:288–97
101. McBay, A. J., Algeri, E. J. 1963. In *Progress in Chemical Toxicology,* I. ed. A. Stolman. New York: Academic
102. Roger, J. C., Rodgers, G., Soo, A. 1973. *Clin. Chem.* 19:590–92
103. Maes, R. et al. 1969. *J. Forensic Sci.* 14:235–54
104. Jain, N. C., Kaplan, H. L., Forney, R. B., Hughes, F. W. 1967. *J. Forensic Sci.* 12:497–508
105. deSilva, J. A. F., D'Arconte, L. 1969. *J. Forensic Sci.* 14:184–204
106. Curry, S. H. 1968. *Anal. Chem.* 40: 1251–55
107. Baer, J. E., Leidy, H. L., Brooks, A. V., Beyer, K. H. 1959. *J. Pharmacol. Exp. Ther.* 125:295–302
108. Mellinger, T. J., Mellinger, E. M., Smith, W. T. 1964. *Am. J. Psychiat.* 120:1111–14
109. Mellinger, T. J., Keeler, C. E. 1964. *Anal. Chem.* 36:1840–47
110. Yates, C. M., Todrick, A., Tait, A. C. 1963. *J. Pharm. Pharmacol.* 15:432–39
111. Smith, T. W., Butler, V. P., Haber, E. 1969. *New Engl. J. Med.* 281:1212–16

112. Wallace, J. E. 1966. *J. Forensic Sci.* 11: 552–59
113. Bigger, J. T., Schmidt, D. H., Kutt, H. 1968. *Circulation* 38:363–74
114. Goldbaum, L. R., Williams, M. A. 1960. *Anal. Chem.* 32:81–84
115. Knowlton, M., Goldbaum, L. R. 1969. *J. Forensic Sci.* 14:129–35
116. Hucker, H. B. et al. 1971. *J. Pharmacol. Exp. Ther.* 179:359–71
117. Udenfriend, S. 1969. *Fluorescence Assay in Biology and Medicine.* Vol. II. New York: Academic
118. Keenaghan, J. B. 1968. *Anesthesiology* 29:110–12
119. *Lithium in the Treatment of Mood Disorders.* 1970. Nat. Inst. Ment. Health, U.S. Dep. Health, Educ., Welfare, Public Health Ser. Publ. No. 2143
120. Fochtman, F. W., Winek, C. L. 1969. *J. Forensic Sci.* 14:213–18
121. Curry, A. 1969. *Poison Detection in Human Organs.* Springfield, Ill.: Thomas. 2nd ed.
122. Sunshine, I., Whitwam, J. G., Fike, W. W., LeBeau, J. 1966. *Brit. J. Anaesth.* 38:23–28
123. O'Dea, A. E., Liss, M. 1953. *New Engl. J. Med.* 249:566–67
124. Loughridge, L. W. 1962. *Lancet* 2: 1133–38
125. Berkowitz, B. A., Asling, J. H., Shnider, S. M., Way, E. L. 1969. *Clin. Pharmacol. Ther.* 10:320–28
126. Dayton, P. G. et al. 1963. *J. Pharmacol. Exp. Ther.* 140:278–86
127. Koch-Weser, J., Klein, S. W. 1971. *J. Am. Med. Assoc.* 215:1454–60
128. Shand, D. G., Nuckolls, E. M., Oates, J. A. 1970. *Clin. Pharmacol. Ther.* 11: 112–20
129. Wolen, R. L., Gruber, C. M. 1968. *Anal. Chem.* 40:1243–46
130. Williams, L. A., Linn, R. A., Zak, B. 1959. *J. Lab. Clin. Med.* 53:156–62
131. Williams, L. A., Hardy, A. T., Cohen, J. S., Zak, B. 1960. *J. Med. Pharm. Chem.* 2:609–14
132. Forist, A. A., Miller, M. L., Krake, J., Struck, W. A. 1957. *Proc. Soc. Exp. Biol. Med.* 96:180–83
133. Burns, J. J., Yu, T. F., Berger, L., Gutman, A. B. 1958. *Am. J. Med.* 25:401–8
134. Kutt, H. 1971. *Ann NY Acad. Sci.* 179:704–22
135. Kutt, H., Winters, W., Kokenge, R., McDowell, F. 1964. *Arch. Neurol.* 11: 642–48
136. Reidenberg, M. M., Odar-Cederlöf, I., Von Bahr, C., Borga, O., Sjöqvist, F. 1971. *New. Engl. J. Med.* 285:264–67
137. Shoeman, D. W., Azarnoff, D. L. 1972. *Pharmacology.* 7:169–77
138. West, B. D., Preis, S., Schroeder, C. H., Link, K. P. 1961. *J. Am. Chem. Soc.* 83:2676–79
139. Furner, R. L., McCarthy, J. S., Stitzel, R. E., Anders, M. W. 1969. *J. Pharmacol. Exp. Ther.* 169:153–58 •
140. Elison, C., Elliott, H. W., Look, M., Rapoport, H. 1963. *J. Med. Chem.* 6:237–46
141. George, C. F., Fenyvesi, T., Conolly, M. E., Dollery, C. T. 1972. *Eur. J. Clin. Pharmacol.* 4:74–76
142. Debackere, M., Massart-Lëen, A. M. 1965. *Arch. Int. Pharmacodyn.* 155:459–62
143. Prescott, L. F., Roscoe, P., Forrest, J. A. H. 1973. In *Biological Effects of Drugs in Relation to their Plasma Concentration,* ed. D. S. Dazies, B. N. C. Prichard. Baltimore: University Park Press

BIOCHEMICAL MECHANISMS OF DRUG TOXICITY[1]

❖6593

James R. Gillette, Jerry R. Mitchell, and Bernard B. Brodie
Laboratory of Chemical Pharmacology, National Heart and Lung Institute,
National Institutes of Health, Bethesda, Maryland
and the Department of Pharmacology, The University of Arizona
College of Medicine, Tucson, Arizona

INTRODUCTION

It has long been known that many drugs can be converted in the body to various metabolites that evoke therapeutic and toxicologic responses. In most instances these metabolites are chemically inert and bring about their effects by combining reversibly with action sites in tissues. In some instances, however, drugs and other foreign compounds can be converted in the body to chemically reactive metabolites which either uncouple integrated biochemical processes in cells or combine covalently with various tissue macromolecules, such as DNA, RNA, protein, and glycogen. During the past several years it has become increasingly evident that chemically reactive metabolites mediate many different kinds of serious toxicity, including carcinogenesis, mutagenesis, cellular necrosis, hypersensitivity reactions, methemoglobinemia, hemolytic anemia, blood dyscrasias, and fetotoxicities. This review is devoted mainly to the mechanisms by which various kinds of toxicities are mediated by chemically reactive metabolites of drugs and the factors that affect the severity of the toxicities.

Since the pioneering work of the Millers in Wisconsin and of Magee and co-workers in England, it has become increasingly evident that most if not all chemical carcinogens bring about their effects by combining covalently with DNA and other tissue macromolecules or by being transformed to chemically reactive metabolites that in turn combine covalently with tissue macromolecules (1–4).

The many studies on the mechanism of formation of carcinogenic metabolites in the body have revealed that chemically inert substances can be converted to chemically reactive metabolites by a variety of different reactions (Figure 1). For example,

[1] The following abbreviations are used: SKF 525-A, β-diethylaminoethyl diphenylpropylacetate; ANIT, α-naphthylisothiocyanate; DDT, 1,1,1-trichloro-2,2-bis (*p*-chlorophenylethane); GSH, glutathione; CCl_4, carbon tetrachloride; $CHCl_3$, chloroform.

271

secondary amines, such as N-methyl-4-aminoazobenzene, primary amines including β-naphthylamine and aminobiphenyl, and acetylated primary amines including 2-acetylaminofluorene are N-hydroxylated by either cytochrome P-450 enzymes or amine N-oxidase. In some instances the metabolites are further activated by being converted to N-O-sulfate esters (1, 2, 4). Dialkylnitrosamines are N-demethylated by cytochrome P-450 enzymes to monoalkylnitrosamines, which in turn spontaneously rearrange to unknown active metabolites, possibly alkyl carbonium ions (3).

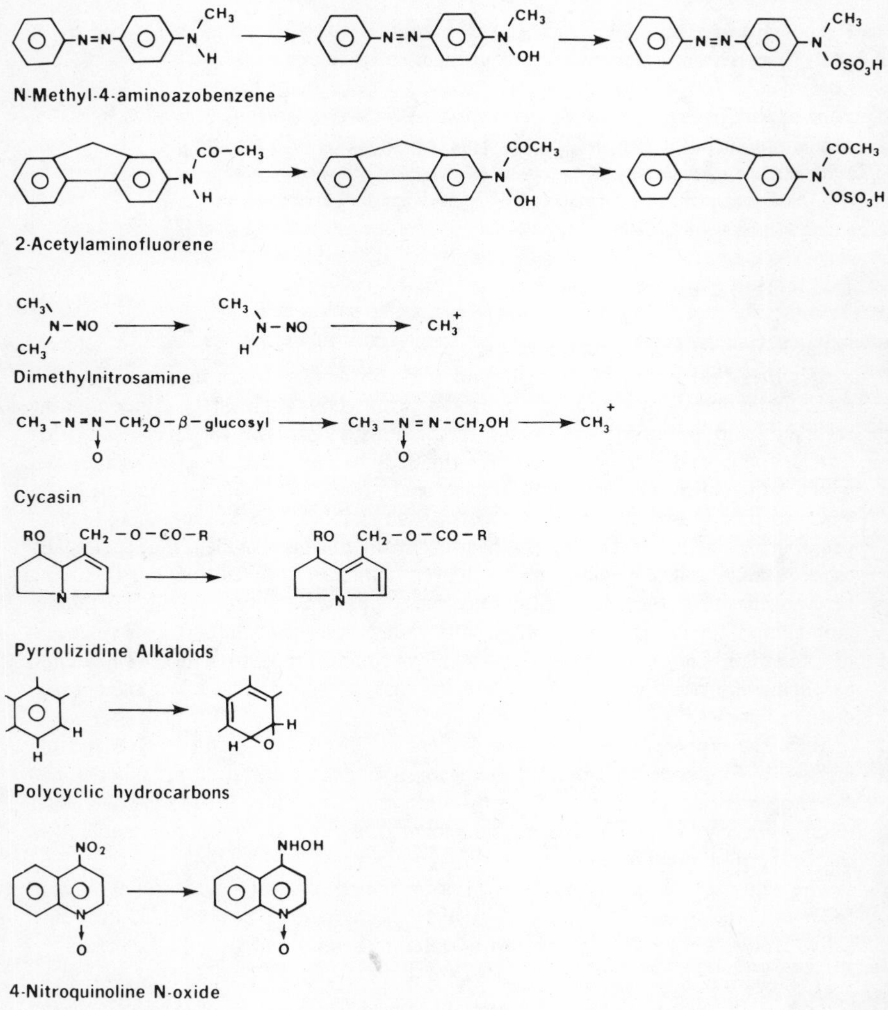

N-Methyl-4-aminoazobenzene

2-Acetylaminofluorene

Dimethylnitrosamine

$$CH_3-N=N-CH_2O-\beta-glucosyl \longrightarrow CH_3-N=N-CH_2OH \longrightarrow CH_3^+$$

Cycasin

Pyrrolizidine Alkaloids

Polycyclic hydrocarbons

4-Nitroquinoline N-oxide

Figure 1 Biochemical mechanisms for the formation of chemically reactive metabolites.

Cycasin is hydrolyzed in the intestine by bacterial β-glucosidase to methylazoxyme-thanol which acts as a methylating agent (5). Urethan may undergo an N-hydroxy-lation before it is converted to an ethylating agent (6). Pyrrolizidine alkaloids are thought to be dehydrogenated to chemically reactive pyrrole derivatives (7, 8). Polycyclic hydrocarbons undergo epoxidation by cytochrome P-450 enzymes to form potent arylating agents (9). Nitroaryl compounds, such as 4-nitroquinoline N-oxide, may act either as arylating agents per se or be converted to chemically reactive hydroxylamine derivatives (10). Similar reactions have also been implicated in the formation of chemically reactive metabolites that effect other kinds of toxicity rather than carcinogenesis or mutagenesis. Presumably these metabolites bring about their effects by combining with macromolecules other than DNA or RNA.

TOXICITIES BY THERAPEUTIC AGENTS

The possibility that therapeutic agents as well as environmental agents cause various kinds of pathological lesions in addition to maligant tumors through the formation of active metabolites occurred to us several years ago (11). The evaluation of this possibility, however, has been difficult because potential therapeutic agents that cause pathological lesions reproducibly in animals are usually eliminated from consideration by carefully performed animal toxicity tests. For the rational develop-ment of nontoxic therapeutic agents, therefore, the factors that control the severity of the lesions need to be better understood. In this regard there are two sets of factors to the problem: in one set are those factors that control the formation and reactivity of the active metabolite and in the other set are those factors that affect the severity of the lesion after the active metabolite reacts with its action sites. Although for most drug-induced toxicities little is known of the latter set of factors, considerable progress has been made in elucidating those factors that control the formation and fate of active metabolites.

For many years it has been realized that the effects of an active metabolite that acts by combining reversibly with action sites can be frequently related to its plasma level. But when the response is tissue damage caused by the covalent binding of chemically reactive metabolites to tissue macromolecules, it would not be logical to expect a relationship between the plasma level of the active metabolite and the severity of the lesions. Indeed, with highly reactive metabolites, little or none would reach the plasma. Nevertheless, for any particular compound there should be a relationship between the severity of the lesion and the amount of covalently bound active metabolite.

Hepatic Necrosis

Many of the ways by which the severity of drug-induced tissue damage can be affected by changes in either the formation or fate of chemically reactive metabolites can be illustrated by studies on the mechanism of liver necrosis induced by haloben-zenes. Although these compounds are chemically inert, they can be converted by a cytochrome P-450 enzyme in liver microsomes to their epoxides, some of which become covalently bound to macromolecules. Recently it was found that the magnitude of the covalent binding of radiolabeled metabolites caused by these compounds paralleled their toxic effects; at doses of 1.0 mmol/kg administered to rats, chlorobenzene, bromobenzene, iodobenzene, and o-dichlorobenzene lead to liver necrosis and considerable covalent binding of reactive metabolites to liver protein, whereas fluorobenzene and p-dichlorobenzene do not cause liver necrosis and are not appreciably bound (12–14). Moreover, studies with ^{14}C-bromobenzene revealed that the covalent binding of its chemically reactive metabolite occurs predominately in the centrilobular necrotic areas of liver. Pretreatment of rats with phenobarbital, a compound that stimulates the activity of the cytochrome P-450 drug-metabolizing enzymes in liver, also increases the rate of disappearance of bromobenzene from the body, the covalent binding of radiolabeled bromobenzene in liver, and the severity of liver necrosis (13, 15, 16). In contrast, SKF 525-A (β-diethylaminoethyl diphenylpropylacetate) and piperonyl butoxide (27), compounds that decrease the activity of drug-metabolizing enzymes in liver, also decrease the rate of disappearance of bromobenzene, the covalent binding of radiolabeled bromobenzene, and the severity of the liver necrosis (13, 15–18). Thus, the necrosis is caused by the covalent binding of a metabolite and not by bromobenzene itself, and the severity of the necrosis apparently depends on the rate at which the active metabolite is formed.

The nature of the active intermediate was confirmed in vitro by studies using liver microsomes, labeled substrate and glutathione (GSH) (12, 18, 19). The results showed that bromobenzene in the presence of TPNH and O_2 is activated by microsomes to a substance that reacts covalently with GSH, thereby trapping the active intermediate. The amount of this complex is increased in microsomes from rats pretreated with phenobarbital. In addition, carbon monoxide, which lowers the activity of the cytochrome P-450 enzymes, decreases the formation of the complex. Thus, the reactive metabolite is formed by a cytochrome P-450 enzyme.

Dose response studies with bromobenzene in rats have revealed that the proportion of the dose that becomes covalently bound to liver microsomes remains low until a critical dose between 1.20 and 2.15 mmol/kg is used (13, 14). Above this critical dose the proportion of the dose that becomes covalently bound is nearly doubled, and the necrosis is manifested. Moreover, the effects of phenobarbital pretreatment depend on the dose of bromobenzene used; with subtoxic doses of bromobenzene, pretreatment with phenobarbital decreased the covalent binding in rats, whereas with high doses of the toxicant, the pretreatment increased the covalent binding.

The reason for the threshold dose of bromobenzene and the dichotomous effects of phenobarbital was clarified by studies on the pathways of bromobenzene metabolism. The major route of metabolism of bromobenzene is through the formation of 3,4-bromobenzene epoxide (9, 19, 20). Liver cells, however, have a number of ways of converting the epoxide to chemically inert metabolites. The epoxide can rearrange to form p-bromophenol (9, 19). An enzyme in the soluble fraction of liver can catalyze a reaction between the epoxide and GSH to form a GSH conjugate (12) that ultimately is excreted in urine as a mercapturic acid (21, 22). Another enzyme present in the endoplasmic reticulum of liver can catalyze the addition of water to the epoxide to form a dihydrodiol which in turn can be oxidized to a catechol (20). The steady-state concentration of the epoxide in liver thus depends on the rate of formation of the epoxide on the one hand and the rates at which the epoxide is converted to the phenol, the GSH conjugate, and the dihydrodiol on the other hand. When the concentration of the epoxide is high, it presumably would react with macromolecules in liver and thus lead to liver necrosis.

As bromobenzene is converted to its GSH conjugate, however, the GSH levels are decreased until the rate of formation of the conjugate is limited by the rate of GSH synthesis. Covalent binding and the severity of the necrosis would be expected to increase after the GSH stores in the liver had been depleted. This view was confirmed (19, 23) by taking advantage of the fact that large doses of bromobenzene administered intraperitoneally are slowly absorbed, and thus the liver levels of the toxicant are maintained for several hr (16), whereas, small doses of bromobenzene administered intravenously are rapidly metabolized with a half-life of about 9 min (16). Thus by administering a large dose of unlabeled bromobenzene intraperitoneally and then injecting radiolabeled bromobenzene intravenously at various times thereafter the magnitude of the covalent binding of the radiolabeled metabolites could be determined while the GSH levels were decreasing, were at their nadir levels, and were returning to normal. Little covalent binding of the radiolabeled bromobenzene occurred when GSH levels were high, but considerable binding occurred when they were low (19, 23). Thus, the degree of covalent binding of bromobenzene and the severity of necrosis depends on the liver levels of GSH, which in turn depend on the relative rates at which GSH is being synthesized and being consumed in the formation of the GSH conjugate.

Pretreatment of animals with phenobarbital increases the rate of bromobenzene epoxide formation and thus hastens the depletion of liver GSH. In addition, it may also increase the activity of GSH transferase as well as the epoxide hydrase in rats (9, 19), because it decreases the covalent binding of subtoxic doses of bromobenzene in this species (14). At toxic doses, however, pretreatment with phenobarbital increases both the amount of covalent binding of bromobenzene metabolites and the severity of the bromobenzene-induced liver necrosis (13) presumably because the increase in rate of bromobenzene epoxide formation exceeds the increase in hydrase activity and the rate of GSH conjugate formation is limited by GSH synthesis (19). By contrast, SKF 525-A inhibits the formation of bromobenzene epoxide and thus slows the depletion of liver GSH to such an extent that the liver levels of GSH are never severely depleted. As a consequence, the covalent binding (13) is markedly decreased and the toxicity almost completely prevented.

On the other hand, pretreatment of rats with 3-methylcholanthrene decreases the severity of bromobenzene necrosis (16, 116) by changing the relative proportions of the kinds of epoxide that are formed; very little 2,3-bromobenzene epoxide is formed in untreated rats, whereas considerable amounts of this epoxide is formed in 3-methylcholanthrene pretreated rats (16, 18). In addition, the protection by 3-methylcholanthrene may be due in part to an induction of epoxide hydrase (9, 19).

The concept that the pattern of metabolism can change with the dose also accounts for the finding that drugs may not be toxic unless a certain threshold dose is exceeded. For example, acetaminophen is among the safest of all minor analgesics when taken in normal therapeutic doses. But large overdoses of acetaminophen can produce fatal hepatic necrosis in man (24), rats (25, 26), and mice (26).

In unpretreated mice, acetaminophen does not cause centrilobular necrosis in the liver unless the dose is greater than about 300 mg/kg (26). Pretreatment of the mice with phenobarbital, however, markedly increases the severity of the toxicity (26), whereas pretreatment of mice with piperonyl butoxide, cobaltous chloride or α-naphthylisothiocyanate (ANIT), which decrease the activities of the microsomal cytochrome P-450 enzymes (27–29), decrease the severity of the necrosis (26, 30).

As with the halobenzene derivatives, the severity of the necrosis parallels the magnitude of the covalent binding of radiolabeled acetaminophen to liver proteins and the decrease in liver GSH levels (31, 32, 34). For example, little covalent binding and no liver necrosis occurs at doses of acetaminophen that deplete liver GSH less than 85%. But considerable binding and liver necrosis occurs with doses that deplete liver GSH more than 85%. Moreover, pretreatment of mice with phenobarbital increases the covalent binding, the rate at which acetaminophen depletes the liver GSH and the severity of the necrosis, whereas pretreatment with cobaltous chloride, piperonyl butoxide or ANIT decreases them (30, 31, 34).

These findings suggest that GSH in liver prevents the necrosis and the covalent binding by reacting with an active metabolite of acetaminophen, presumably N-hydroxy-N-acetyl-p-hydroxyaniline (32, 32a). In accord with this view, the prior administration of diethyl maleate, which depletes liver GSH (33) without causing necrosis, increases the covalent binding of acetaminophen metabolites to liver protein and the severity of acetaminophen-induced liver necrosis (34). But the prior administration of cysteine, which leads to the synthesis of GSH, or of cysteamine or dimercaprol, which presumably react chemically with the reactive metabolite, decreases both the covalent binding of the acetaminophen metabolite and the severity of liver necrosis (34, 35). Thus, a fundamental role of GSH may be to protect essential thiol and other nucleophilic groups in tissue macromolecules from electrophilic reactants formed in animals.

The significance of GSH in protecting man from acetaminophen and other drug-induced hepatic damage is still uncertain, but it probably is responsible for the remarkable safety of the drug after usual therapeutic doses. For example, the toxic metabolite of acetaminophen can be shown to combine preferentially with GSH in animals to form a nontoxic conjugate that is ultimately excreted as a mercapturic acid (34–37). As the dose of acetaminophen is increased to levels that deplete hepatic GSH and cause significant covalent binding and liver necrosis, the proportion of the dose excreted as a mercapturic acid decreases (38). The measurement of acetaminophenmercapturic acid in urine has been used to estimate the formation of the toxic metabolite of acetaminophen in humans. In 12 patients the amount of mercapturate formed was always about 2% of the administered dose over a dose range from 600 to 1800 mg, demonstrating that the availability of GSH was never limiting after these therapeutic doses (35, 38). In addition, phenobarbital pretreatment of these patients for 5 days increased the amount of acetaminophen excreted as a mercapturate from 2% to about 4.5% of the therapeutic doses, suggesting an increased formation of the toxic metabolite after phenobarbital induction but again without exceeding the availability of GSH at these doses. These data suggest that the hepatic toxicity after acetaminophen overdosage might be increased in humans receiving inducers such as phenobarbital. In fact, a retrospective study of patients suffering from acetaminophen-induced hepatic necrosis has confirmed this view (39).

Because acetaminophen-induced hepatic damage and covalent binding in animals are prevented, but not reversed, by a variety of exogenously administered nucleophiles, such as cysteamine and dimercaprol (34, 35), these substances may provide a possible rationale for treatment of overdosed patients seen early after poisoning.

The formation of the chemically reactive metabolite of acetaminophen represents a relatively minor pathway of the metabolism of the drug in mice and hamsters as well as in man. Indeed, most of the drug in animals is excreted as its glucuronide and sulfate conjugates (40), which are not formed by cytochrome P-450 enzymes. As a result, pretreatment of mice with phenobarbital or cobaltous chloride do not alter the biological half-life of the drug even though these treatments markedly affect its toxicity (26). Moreover, although these treatments cause statistically significant changes in the pattern of urinary metabolites (38), the changes may not appear impressive and could have been easily overlooked. These findings illustrate the problem of finding an animal species which mimics humans in the metabolism and toxicity of drugs when the toxicity is mediated by metabolites formed along minor pathways.

Another commonly used drug, furosemide, is also safe at the usual therapeutic doses but at high doses produces a dose-dependent hepatic necrosis in male mice (35, 41). The necrosis is restricted to midzonal and centrilobular hepatocytes after doses of 150 mg/kg, ip. Larger doses (400 mg/kg) produce a massive necrosis in which confluent zones of anuclear and eosinophilic cells bridge adjacent hepatic lobules. Inhibitors of cytochrome P-450 enzymes, such as piperonyl butoxide, cobaltous chloride and ANIT, prevent furosemide-induced hepatic necrosis, which suggests that furosemide-induced hepatotoxicity may also be mediated by toxic metabolites (35, 41).

As with the toxic halobenzenes and acetaminophen, the severity of necrosis after these pretreatments parallels the amounts of furosemide metabolites that are covalently bound to liver macromolecules (42). In addition, dose response curves have revealed that little covalent binding occurs below a critical dose of 150 mg/kg. But furosemide, unlike the halobenzenes and acetaminophen, does not deplete the liver of GSH. Thus, the reason for the threshold is unclear, but preliminary evidence suggests that it may be due to saturation by the drug of the reversible binding sites of plasma proteins either alone or in combination with the saturation of the active secretory systems in the kidney (38).

In the past CCl_4 has been used as an anthelmintic, and $CHCl_3$ has been used as an anesthetic gas. But the well-known toxicities caused by these substances soon led to their disuse in man. Indeed, the mechanism of CCl_4-induced liver necrosis has become the subject of numerous studies and reviews (43–46). Only during the past few years, however, has the mechanism by which CCl_4 and $CHCl_3$ been clarified.

A number of studies have provided indirect evidence that the toxic actions of CCl_4 and $CHCl_3$ are mediated through an active metabolite. For example, the lethal effects of CCl_4 were increased by prior administration of phenobarbital (47), 1,1,1,-trichloro-2,2-bis (p-chlorophenylethane) (DDT) (47), or isopropyl alcohol (48).

Moreover, the toxic effects were diminished by the administration of dibenamine (49) or cobaltous chloride (50) or by feeding the animals protein-deficient diets (47). Similarly the liver necrosis caused by chloroform is also increased by pretreatment of rats with phenobarbital (43). Moreover, the finding that radiolabeled CCl_4 became irreversibly bound to proteins (51–53) and to lipids (52, 54) led to the concept that the active metabolite of CCl_4 combines covalently with proteins and lipids and thereby causes centrilobular necrosis, presumably by promoting lipid peroxidation (43–46). In accord with this view, pretreatment of rats with dibenamine prevents the toxic effects of CCl_4 and decreases the covalent binding of CCl_4 metabolites to lipids presumably by impairing the liver enzyme system that catalyzes the formation of the reactive metabolite (49). On the other hand, pretreatment of rats with phenobarbital or isopropyl alcohol increases not only the toxic effects but also the covalent binding of CCl_4 in vivo (23, 55, 56).

Many years ago, Butler raised the possibility that CCl_4 was homolytically split to form the free radicals, $CCl_3\cdot$ and $Cl\cdot$, in the body (57). It now appears, however, that the formation of the chemically reactive metabolite occurs by reductive cleavage of CCl_4 to $CCl_3\cdot$ and chloride ion. Covalent binding of CCl_4 metabolites occurs in incubation mixtures consisting of liver microsomes, NADPH and $^{14}CCl_4$ (58–60). The binding is inhibited by CO (58–60) and by an antibody against liver microsomal NADPH cytochrome c reductase (61); thus the enzyme that catalyzes the formation of the free radical is probably a cytochrome P-450 enzyme system. Moreover, covalent binding of CCl_4 occurs to a greater extent under anaerobic conditions than in air (60, 61), indicating that the reaction is reductive rather than oxidative. On the other hand, the covalent binding of $^{14}CHCl_3$, which is also mediated by a cytochrome P-450 system in liver microsomes, does not occur under anaerobic conditions (62), indicating that the activation is oxidative rather than reductive. It is also noteworthy that the covalent binding of CCl_4 by liver microsomal preparations in the presence of NADPH is also decreased by pretreating rats with dibenamine (63) and increased by pretreating them with phenobarbital (61) or isopropyl alcohol (64).

Although GSH does not appreciably decrease the in vitro covalent binding of CCl_4 metabolite to rabbit liver microsomes (60), it markedly inhibits the covalent binding of CCl_4 to rat liver microsomes (58, 59). Thus it seemed possible that GSH may also tend to protect the liver against the toxic effects of CCl_4, even though the liver levels of GSH are not depleted after the administration of CCl_4 to rats. In accord with this view, prior administration of diethyl maleate, which depletes liver GSH (33) without causing toxicity, increases both the toxicity of CCl_4 and the covalent binding of CCl_4 metabolites in vivo (23, 56). The mechanism by which GSH diminishes covalent binding, however, remains to be clarified.

In addition to causing centrilobular necrosis and fatty infiltration of liver, CCl_4 also causes the destruction of liver microsomal cytochrome P-450. As a consequence, the toxic effects of CCl_4 may be self-limiting. Indeed, the administration of sublethal doses of CCl_4 to animals protects them from the lethal effects of high doses of CCl_4 (65). The mechanisms by which CCl_4 causes the destruction are not yet clear. Studies in vitro have shown that the CCl_4-induced destruction of cytochrome

P-450 may be mediated by lipid peroxidation, because EDTA added to liver microsomal systems blocks both the NADPH-dependent lipid peroxidation and the cytochrome P-450 destruction caused by CCl_4 (66). However, the finding that the administration of the antioxidants, α-tocopherol or diphenylphenylenediamine, does not affect the CCl_4-induced destruction of cytochrome P-450 seemed to contradict this view (67). But this interpretation of the in vivo results may have been incorrect because it was recently found that the antioxidants have little effect on lipid peroxidation induced by CCl_4 in vivo as measured by diene conjugation of liver microsomal lipids (68).

A mechanism similar to that of CCl_4 may play an etiologic role in the clinical hepatitis seen after halothane anesthesia, because microsomes isolated from the livers of rats pretreated with phenobarbital followed by halothane had elevated lipid diene conjugates and decreased cytochrome P-450 content (69). In spite of these interesting preliminary results, however, final conclusions must await more definitive experiments.

Liver damage caused by other kinds of foreign compounds may also be mediated by chemically reactive metabolites. For example, there is considerable evidence that the hepatic necrosis caused by pyrrolizidine alkaloids is mediated by a chemically reactive intermediate that becomes covalently bound to liver macromolecules (70–72). There is also evidence that the toxic effects of sesquiterpenes (73), ANIT (29), and the toxins in amanita toadstools (74, 75) are also mediated through active metabolites, because either stimulators of drug metabolism increase their toxic effects or inhibitors prevent the toxicities.

Lung Necrosis

Although a number of compounds are known to cause lung toxicities, including carcinoma and necrosis, the mechanisms by which these toxicities occur is poorly understood. However, a recent study shows that bromobenzene causes lung necrosis apparently by being covalently bound to lung macromolecules (76), which suggests the possibility that at least some substances, including drugs, might evoke their toxic effects by being converted to chemically reactive metabolites. In mice, bromobenzene causes necrosis of bronchiolar and bronchial cells but does not cause any specific alterations in alveolar morphology. In rats, bromobenzene caused similar but less severe pathological changes. After the administration of ^{14}C-bromobenzene, autoradiograms revealed a preferential accumulation of covalently bound bromobenzene metabolite in the bronchi and bronchioles in both rats and mice. In vitro studies revealed that lung microsomes contain a cytochrome P-450 enzyme system that converts bromobenzene to a reactive intermediate that becomes covalently bound to lung microsomal proteins and that the system is more active in mice than in rats. But pretreatment with phenobarbital does not increase the activity of the enzyme system in lung of either species. With subtoxic doses of bromobenzene, pretreatment with phenobarbital did not affect the in vivo covalent binding of ^{14}C-bromobenzene metabolites to liver and lung protein in mice and decreased it in rats. But with toxic doses, pretreatment of mice with phenobarbital increased the covalent binding in both liver and lung. The finding that phenobarbital increases the covalent binding of bromobenzene in the lung without inducing the lung enzyme suggests that the chemically reactive metabolite of bromobenzene can escape the liver after depletion of GSH and can be carried to the lung where it becomes covalently bound to proteins in the lung. In accord with this view, phenobarbital pretreatment increases the small amounts of ^{14}C-bromobenzene covalently bound to heart muscle in vivo, a tissue that does not metabolize bromobenzene.

Not all chemically induced toxicities in the lung are caused by covalent binding of chemically reactive metabolites, however. For example, paraquat causes hemorrhage, edema, and fibrosis in rat lung (77), but does not become covalently bound to lung macromolecules (78). Indeed, the mechanism by which paraquat evokes these pathological changes is not clear. The realization that paraquat, also called methyl viologen, is a well-known redox dye, raised the possibility that paraquat might act by promoting the formation of hydrogen peroxide and thereby cause tissue damage (79). Indeed in vitro experiments have shown that paraquat at high concentrations does stimulate NADPH oxidation and hydrogen peroxide formation (78, 79). But these reactions are insignificant at the concentrations of paraquat found in vivo (78).

Renal Toxicity

Low doses of chloroform (2.5 mmol/kg) cause necrosis of the epithelial cells of the proximal convoluted tubules of kidney in male C-57 Black mice but not in females. In accord with the view that the toxicity is mediated by covalent binding of chloroform metabolites, the in vivo covalent binding of ^{14}C-CHCl$_3$ was only about one-tenth as much in kidneys of females as it was in those of males (80). Moreover, pretreatment of male mice with either phenobarbital or piperonyl butoxide decreased both the covalent binding of the reactive chloroform metabolite and the toxicity.

Kidney toxicities, however, are not always mediated by covalent binding of metabolites. For example, the polyuric, vasopressin-resistant renal insufficiency associated with the administration of methoxyflurane anesthesia appears to be dose-related in man and can be correlated with high levels of serum inorganic fluoride, a metabolite of methoxyflurane (81). The lesion can be reproduced in rats either by administration of methoxyflurane or a comparable dose of the fluoride ion. As might be expected, sensitive rat strains metabolize methoxyflurane to a greater extent than do insensitive strains (82). Moreover, pretreatment of the animals with phenobarbital increased the severity of the toxicity, whereas the administration of SKF 525-A decreased it (83).

Testes Toxicity

Although spironolactone induces cytochrome P-450 enzymes in liver (84–86), it causes a selective destruction of testicular cytochrome P-450 and thereby decreases the synthesis of testosterone (87). Since NADPH is required for the destruction of testicular cytochrome P-450 by spironolactone in vitro, the effect probably is mediated by an active metabolite (88). But neither the identity of the active metabolite nor its mechanism of action is known. The impairment in testicular cytochrome

P-450 is not due to cellular necrosis and is fully reversible within 5 days after withdrawal of the drug (87). Experiments in vivo in male dogs demonstrate that spironolactone not only decreases testicular cytochrome P-450 but also decreases the release of both testosterone and estradiol into the plasma (89). As in animals, spironolactone also caused decreases in the plasma levels of testosterone in patients (90, 90a). But whether the decrease is due mainly to decreased synthesis in testis or increased catabolism in liver is not known. It is also not known whether these effects of spironolactone on the metabolism of sex steroids account for the gynecomastia and decreased libido observed in humans receiving the drug.

Nitrofurazone, a compound used as a topical antibacterial agent, is known to cause mammary tumors in rats (91). Moreover, it also causes a decrease in testicular cytochrome P-450, and impairs testosterone synthesis in mice (92). In addition, it causes aspermatogenesis (92, 93) as manifested by a decrease in spermatozoa, increased vacuolization of the spermatocytes and an increase in polynucleated spermatotides. Aspermatogenesis also occurs with furadroxyl, an analog of nitrofurazone (94). Because nitrofurazone can be reduced to its hydroxylamine derivative by xanthine oxidase (95) and aldehyde oxidase (96) as well as by liver microsomal NADPH cytochrome c reductase (97), it is not surprising that it becomes covalently bound to proteins of various tissues in vivo including liver, kidney, and either testis or mammary glands (92). Strangely, nitrofurazone causes a decrease of GSH in liver but not in testes even though the toxicity occurs in testes but not in liver. The possible relationship between the toxic effects of the drug and covalent binding thus remains obscure.

In rats, testicular damage is also caused by high doses of the carcinogen, 7,12-dimenthylbenzanthracene (98). But again the mechanism by which the toxicity occurs is unknown.

Bone Marrow Aplasia

Studies on the toxic effects of chloramphenicol have been hampered by the inability of the drug to produce aplastic anemia in laboratory animals. Nevertheless, it may be important that chloramphenicol in rats becomes covalently bound to both bone marrow (100 pmoles/mg) and to liver (450 pmoles/mg) and that phenobarbital pretreatment increases the covalent binding in both tissues by about 2–3-fold (99).

Most studies on bone marrow aplasia have been carried out with model compounds. For example, it is well known that 7,12-dimethylbenzanthracene causes leukopenia, thrombocytopenia, and bone marrow aplasia (98). Recent studies have shown that the severity of the syndrome produced by 7,12-dimethylbenzanthracene could be reduced by inhibitors of cytochrome P-450, SKF 525-A, or 7,8-benzoflavone (100). Because 7,12-dimethylbenzanthracene is not metabolized by bone marrow preparations of rats, it seems likely that a metabolite formed in the liver mediates the toxicity.

Repeated injections of benzene also produce bone marrow aplasia in rats. The lesion is prevented when the metabolism of benzene is altered by a variety of pretreatments (SKF 525-A, piperonyl butoxide, phenobarbital) (101). Although the finding that phenobarbital pretreatment protects against benzene-induced bone marrow damage has led investigators to propose that benzene itself is the toxic agent (102), this seems unlikely because pretreatments such as cobaltous chloride and aminotriazole, which inhibit the synthesis of cytochrome P-450 in rats, block the metabolism of benzene and markedly reduce the bone marrow damage (103). Thus, it seems likely the bone marrow aplasia caused by benzene is mediated by an unknown active metabolite.

Methemoglobinemia and Hemolytic Anemia

It has been well established that aromatic amines including aniline cause methemoglobinemia by being converted to phenylhydroxylamines which on oxidation to their nitroso derivatives and subsequent reduction back to the phenylhydroxylamines promote the formation of methemoglobin (104, 105). In addition, certain drugs including aniline derivatives also cause hemolysis, especially in patients having a genetic deficiency in erythrocyte glucose-6-phosphate dehydrogenase (106). Because both kinds of toxicity can be caused by various aniline derivatives, it has not been clear whether they are mediated by the same or different metabolites of any given drug. In order to evaluate the severity of hemolysis, ^{51}Cr-labeled rat erythrocytes injected intravenously into rats have been used to measure the effects of drugs on the turnover rate of erythrocytes (35, 107, 108). After the intraperitoneal administration of aromatic amines, such as aniline, p-phenetidine and p-chloroaniline the rate at which ^{51}Cr declined in blood was greatly increased, confirming that these drugs induced hemolysis in rats. These drugs when added to incubation mixtures had no effect on erythrocyte survival, and the pretreatment of rats with CCl_4, which decreased the metabolism of the drugs prevented the hemolysis by the aromatic amines. Thus, the hemolysis is probably caused by metabolites rather than by the parent amines.

The corresponding N-acetylated derivatives, namely acetanilide, phenacetin, and p-chloroacetanilide, also caused hemolysis in this sytem, although to a lesser degree than did the free amines. The hemolysis produced by the acetylated amines was prevented by pretreatment of the rats with CCl_4 and by pretreatment with bis-p-nitrophenyl phosphate, which inhibits deacetylation (109). In contrast, the administration of the deacetylase inhibitor did not prevent the hemolysis induced by the free amines. These results suggest that these analgesic drugs require metabolic transformation in two steps in order to cause hemolysis, presumably deacetylation and N-hydroxylation (35, 107, 108).

Because methemoglobinemia caused in rats by phenacetin or acetanilide also is prevented by pretreatment with piperonyl butoxide and by bis-p-nitrophenyl phosphate, it might seem possible that the same active intermediate causes both hemolysis and methemoglobinemia. However, phenobarbital pretreatment of rats increases the methemoglobinemia but decreases the hemolysis caused by acetanilide and aniline, whereas pretreatment with an inhibitor of metabolism, piperonyl butoxide, brings about exactly the opposite effects (35, 107, 108). Although the identity of the metabolite that induces hemolysis remains obscure, the results clearly demonstrate that methemoglobinemia and drug-induced hemolysis are mediated by different active metabolites and suggest that methemoglobinemia is not a prerequisite for hemolysis.

Porphyria

At least three different types of experimental porphyria can be induced by drugs and other foreign compounds (110): 1. That produced by allyl ureide and allyl acetamide compounds, such as sedormid, allylisopropylacetamide, and secobarbital; 2. that caused by hexachlorobenzene; 3. that caused by dicarbethoxydihydrocollidine and related compounds. In addition to causing porphyria and increasing the synthesis of δ-aminolevulinic acid, the allyl compounds, such as allylisopropylacetamide (111, 112), secobarbital, allobarbital and aprobarbital (112) that produce porphyria, also catalyze the destruction of the various heme compounds in liver, especially cytochrome P-450. Recently, it was shown that a number of other allyl compounds, including allyl alcohol, acrylamide, and the anesthetic gas, fluoroxene, also cause a selective destruction of liver microsomal cytochrome P-450 (23). The finding that these effects are markedly increased after pretreatment of rats with phenobarbital suggest that they are caused by active metabolites of the foreign compounds. In support of this view, secobarbital decreases the cytochrome P-450 in liver microsomes only when NADPH is present in the incubation system (112). In contrast to the destructive effects of compounds such as CCl_4 (66) on cytochrome P-450, the effects of secobarbital are not blocked by EDTA (112). Thus, the effects probably are not mediated by lipid peroxidation. Because allyl compounds are converted to epoxides, it seems possible that these might be the active metabolites. However, this possibility has not been confirmed, and it is not known whether the active metabolites bring about their action by becoming covalently bound to cytochrome P-450 or to other macromolecules.

The destruction of heme compounds in liver may be an initial event in the development of porphyria (111). Because heme is known to exert a negative feedback control on the conversion of succinyl-CoA to δ-aminolevulinic acid, the rate-limiting step in heme synthesis, any mechanism that decreases the level of the intracellular heme pool that exerts the feed-back control would be expected to increase the rate of porphyrin synthesis. However, the rate-controlling pool of heme probably is not cytochrome P-450, because the heme in cytochrome P-450 does not exchange with free heme (113). The finding that heme in the mitochondrial and the soluble fractions of liver is also destroyed by allylisopropylacetamide (111) raises the possibility that a heme pool in these fractions may serve to control porphyrin synthesis.

Hypersensitivity Reactions

The mechanisms by which drugs cause allergic responses remains largely unexplored. Since the classic work of Landsteiner and his colleagues during the 1920s (114), it has been shown by many investigators that small molecules can serve as antigens only after they become covalently bound to macromolecules, such as plasma albumin (115). Consequently, the finding that drugs can be converted to chemically reactive metabolites that combine covalently to macromolecules raised the possibility that the formation of chemically reactive metabolites might be an initial event in drug-induced hypersensitivity reactions. Indeed the failure to demonstrate covalent binding of drugs to macromolecules either in vivo or in vitro might suggest that the drug would not evoke hypersensitivity reactions in man. On the other hand, it has become evident that covalent binding of the drug does not always lead to antibody formation or an immunologic response. Indeed, investigators rarely are able to find antibodies to a given drug either in patients manifesting hypersensitivity reactions or in animals receiving a drug that is known to be covalently bound to macromolecules.

PHARMACOKINETICS AND OTHER CONSIDERATIONS

Inhibitors and inducers of drug metabolizing enzymes have obviously played an important role in determining whether a compound evokes its pharmacologic and toxic responses by itself or through the formation of an active metabolite. It is not always realized, however, that the finding that inhibitors such as SKF 525-A increase the response or that inducers such as phenobarbital decrease the response does not preclude the possibility that a toxin exerts its effect through the formation of a chemically reactive metabolite (23). Moreover, if the rate of metabolic activation of a toxin is kinetically a first order reaction, increasing or decreasing the rate of formation theoretically should not change the total amount of toxin produced, assuming that the elimination of the compound from the body is primarily dependent on its metabolism through the toxic pathway. Most substances, however, are eliminated by competing or coupled metabolic reactions in the liver as well as by elimination via the kidneys, lungs, or biliary system. Thus, with drugs that are eliminated from the body largely unchanged, treatments that change the rate of conversion of the parent drug to the chemically reactive metabolite would be expected to alter the amount of metabolite formed even though the treatments do not affect the biological half-life of the drug. On the other hand, with drugs that are largely metabolized along a number of different pathways, the effect of the treatments on the total amount of chemically reactive metabolite formed would depend on whether the treatments changed the relative importance of the different pathways of metabolism. When the treatments increase or decrease the rates of metabolism along the different pathways to the same extent, the total amount of chemically reactive metabolite formed would not be changed. It is also important to realize that treatments can alter the fate of the chemically reactive metabolites and thereby affect the amounts of the metabolites that become covalently bound.

These principles may be illustrated by a number of examples of the covalent binding of drugs to liver macromolecules; 1. Although pretreatment of mice with phenobarbital markedly increases the rate of bromobenzene metabolism both in vivo and in vitro, it does not appreciably affect the amount of a subtoxic dose that becomes covalently bound to liver proteins (76), because almost all of the toxicant is converted to 3,4-bromobenzene epoxide in both untreated and pretreated animals. 2. In contrast, pretreatment of rats with 3-methylcholanthrene prevents the hepatic damage produced by bromobenzene (16, 116) and 2-acetylaminofluorene (117) apparently by stimulating detoxifying metabolic pathways more than toxifying ones. 3. The major pathways by which acetaminophen is eliminated is not through the formation of its chemically reactive metabolite but through the formation of its conjugates with glucuronic acid and sulfate (40). Consequently, the covalent binding and hepatotoxicity of acetaminophen in mice is increased by phenobarbital and decreased by cobaltous chloride, even though these treatments have no significant effect on the half-life of the drug in mice (26). 4. Dibenamine decreases the toxicity of CCl_4 by preventing its conversion to the free radical and chloroform, yet dibenamine has no effect on the half-life of CCl_4 (49), because most of the toxicant is eliminated via the lungs. 5. The proportion of the dose of furosemide that becomes covalently bound to liver protein increases as the dose is increased above a threshold, apparently because the clearance of the drug from the body is decreased as the dose is increased (38). 6. When doses of bromobenzene or acetaminophen that deplete the liver of GSH are used, pretreatment of animals with phenobarbital increases the covalent binding (13, 14, 23, 34) because the rate of formation of the GSH conjugate is limited by the rate of formation of GSH rather than by that of the epoxide. 7. Depletion of sulfate decreases the toxicity of 2-acetylaminofluorene because the formation of the chemically reactive N-hydroxy sulfate conjugate of the carcinogen is decreased (3, 4) relative to the other pathways of elimination of the toxicant. On the other hand, depletion of hepatic GSH by diethyl maleate increases the toxicity of the halobenzenes and acetaminophen (13, 14, 19, 23, 34) by decreasing the formation of the nontoxic GSH conjugates of these substances. In addition, diethyl maleate increases the covalent binding and toxicity of CCl_4 and furosemide even though these compounds themselves do not decrease GSH levels in liver. Thus, nontoxic substances can affect the severity of the injury caused by toxicants even through the nontoxic substance is neither an "inducer" nor an "inhibitor" in the usual sense of these words.

The kinetic aspects of chemically reactive metabolites are even more complex when the metabolites are formed in extrahepatic tissues as well as in the liver. They depend on whether the chemically reactive metabolite can escape the liver and then be carried to the extrahepatic tissue by the blood. If the metabolite is so chemically reactive that it cannot escape the hepatocyte in which it is formed, then pretreatment of animals with substances that induce the liver enzymes but not the extrahepatic tissues would be expected to decrease toxicity in the extrahepatic tissues. Moreover, substances that specifically inhibit the extrahepatic enzymes but not the liver enzymes would also be expected to decrease toxicity in the extrahepatic tissues. However, inducers and inhibitors of drug metabolizing enzymes are seldom specific, and their effects on extrahepatic enzymes are incompletely understood. For these reasons, it often is not possible to obtain unequivocal information that would differentiate among the various mechanisms for the toxicity of drugs in extrahepatic tissues.

CONCLUSIONS

In most studies of the mechanisms of chemical toxicity, emphasis has been placed on the use of toxic substances as metabolic probes of cellular function (118). When the toxin brings about its effect by interacting with a specific biochemical system, such studies are useful approaches to an understanding of how the biological system responds to such metabolic rearrangements. But when the toxins interact with a number of biochemical systems simultaneously, as chemically reactive metabolites

286   GILLETTE, MITCHELL & BRODIE

frequently do, it is difficult to determine whether changes in cell function result from a sequence of changes originating from a single initial biochemical alteration or from the concerted action of a number of different initial biochemical alterations. In any event, such studies frequently fail to provide any practical information about the nature of the active form of the toxin or any clues to methods for preventing the toxicity.

From studies with liver microsomes in vitro, it is now clear that many drugs can be converted to chemically reactive metabolites because they become covalently bound to microsomal protein in incubation systems containing liver microsomes, NADPH, and the drug. But it is not clear to what extent the covalent binding can be used to predict the incidence of various kinds of toxicity in animals or man. Nevertheless, such in vitro studies might be useful in choosing which of a series of analogs having similar pharmacologic activity should receive the highest priority in the development of drugs, particularly when the members of the series also lead to widely different amounts of covalently bound metabolites in vivo.

Literature Cited

1. Miller, E. C., Miller, J. A. 1966. *Pharmacol. Rev.* 18:805–38
2. Miller, J. A. 1970. *Cancer Res.* 30:559–76
3. Magee, P. N., Barnes, J. M. 1967. *Advan. Cancer Res.* 10:163–256
4. Weisburger, J. H., Weisburger, E. K. 1973. *Pharmacol. Rev.* 25:1–66
5. Laqueur, G. L. 1964. *Fed. Proc.* 23:1386–87
6. Mirvish, S. S. 1968. *Advan. Cancer Res.* 11:1–42
7. Mattocks, A. R. 1973. *Proc. Int. Congr. Pharmacol., 5th,* 2:114–23. Basel: Karger
8. McLean, E. K. 1970. *Pharmacol. Rev.* 22:429–83
9. Daly, J. W., Jerina, D. M., Witkop, B. 1972. *Experientia* 28:1129–49
10. Endo, H., Kume, F. 1965. *Gann* 56:261–65
11. Brodie, B. B. 1967. *Drug Responses in Man,* 188–213. London: Churchill
12. Brodie, B. B. et al 1971. *Proc. Nat. Acad. Sci. USA* 68:160–64
13. Reid, W. D., Krishna, G. 1973. *Exp. Mol. Pathol.* 18:80–99
14. Reid, W. D. 1973. *Proc. Int. Congr. Pharmacol., 5th,* 2:62–74. Basel: Karger
15. Reid, W. D. et al 1971. *Pharmacology* 6:41–55
16. Zampaglione, N. et al 1973. *J. Pharmacol. Exp. Ther.* 187:218–27
17. Mitchell, J. R. et al 1971. *Res. Commun. Chem. Pathol. Pharmacol.* 2:877–88
18. Jollow, D., Mitchell, J. R., Zampaglione, N., Gillette, J. R. 1972. *5th Int. Congr. Pharmacol. Abstr. Vol. Papers,* 117
19. Jollow, D. J., Mitchell, J. R., Zampaglione, N., Gillette, J. R. *Pharmacology.* In press
20. Azouz, W. M., Parke, D. V., Williams, R. T. 1953. *Biochem. J.* 55:146–51
21. Knight, R. H., Young, L. 1958. *Biochem. J.* 70:111–19
22. Baumann, E., Preusse, C. 1879. *Ber. Deut. Chem. Ges.* 12:806–10
23. Gillette, J. R. 1973. *Proc. Int. Congr. Pharmacol., 5th* 2:187–202
24. Prescott, L. F., Wright, N., Roscoe, P., Brown, S. S. 1971. *Lancet* i:519–22
25. Boyd, E. M., Bereczky, G. M. 1966. *Brit. J. Pharmacol.* 26:606–14
26. Mitchell, J. R. et al 1973. *J. Pharmacol. Exp. Ther.* 187:185–94
27. Anders, M. W. 1968. *Biochem. Pharmacol.* 17:2367–71
28. Tephly, T. R., Hibbeln, P. 1971. *Biochem. Biophys. Res. Commun.* 42:589–95
29. Plaa, G. L. 1970. *Essays Toxicol.* 2:137–52
30. Mitchell, J. R., Jollow, D. J. *Int. Symp. Drug Interactions, Milan, Italy.* In press
31. Jollow, D. J. et al 1973. *J. Pharmacol. Exp. Ther.* 187:195–201
32. Potter, W. Z. et al 1973. *J. Pharmacol. Exp. Ther.* 187:202–10

32a. Thorgeirsson, S. S., Jollow, D. J., Sasame, H. A., Green, I., Mitchell, J. R. 1973. *Mol. Pharmacol.* 9:398–404
33. Boyland, E., Chasseaud, L. F., 1970. *Biochem. Pharmacol.* 19:1526–28
34. Mitchell, J. R., Jollow, D. J., Potter, W. Z., Gillette, J. R., Brodie, B. B. 1973. *J. Pharmacol. Exp. Ther.* 187:211–17
35. Mitchell, J. R., Jollow, D. J., Gillette, J. R., Brodie, B. B. 1973. *Drug Metab. Disposition* 1:418–23
36. Jollow, D. J. et al 1973. *Fed. Proc.* 32:305
37. Jagenburg, O. R., Toczko, K. 1964. *Biochem. J.* 92:639–43
38. Mitchell, J. R., Thorgeirsson, S. S., Jollow, D. J., Keiser, H. *Int. Symp. Hepatotoxicity, 1973, Tel Aviv, Israel.* In press
39. Wright, N., Prescott, L. F. 1973. *Scot. Med. J.* 18:56–58
40. Brodie, B. B., Axelrod, J. 1948. *J. Pharmacol. Exp. Ther.* 94:22–28
41. Mitchell, J. R., Potter, W. Z., Jollow, D. J. 1973. *Fed. Proc.* 32:305
42. Potter, W. Z. et al 1973. *Fed. Proc.* 32:305
43. Judah, J. D., McLean, A. E. M., McLean, E. K. 1970. *Am. J. Med.* 49:609–17
44. Recknagel, R. O. 1967. *Pharmacol. Rev.* 19:145–207
45. Slater, T. F. 1966. *Nature* 209:36–40
46. Plaa, G. L., Larson, R. E. 1964. *Arch. Environ. Health* 9:536–43
47. McLean, A. E. M., McLean, E. K. 1969. *Brit. Med. Bull.* 25:278–81
48. Traiger, G. J., Plaa, G. L. 1971. *Toxicol. Appl. Pharmacol.* 20:105–12
49. Maling, H. M. et al 1972. *Proc. 5th Int. Congr. Pharmacol. Abst. Vol. Papers,* 147
50. Suarez, K. A. 1973. *Pharmacologist* 15:582
51. Cessi, C., Colombini, C., Mameli, L. 1966. *Biochem. J.* 101:46c–47c
52. Reynolds, E. 1967. *J. Pharmacol. Exp. Ther.* 155:117–26
53. Rao, K. S., Recknagel, R. O. 1968. *Exp. Mol. Pathol.* 9:271–78
54. Gordis, E. 1969. *J. Clin. Invest.* 48:203–9
55. Reynolds, E. S., Ree, H. J., Moslen, M. T. 1972. *Lab. Invest.* 26:290–99
56. Maling, H. M. et al 1974. *Biochem. Pharmacol.* In press
57. Butler, T. C. 1961. *J. Pharmacol. Exp. Ther.* 134:311–19
58. Corsini, G., Sipes, I. G., Krishna, G., Brodie, B. B. 1972. *Fed. Proc.* 31:1882
59. Sipes, I. G., Corsini, G., Krishna, G., Gillette, J. R. 1972. *Proc. 5th Int. Congr. Pharmacol. Abst. Vol. Papers,* 215
60. Uehleke, H., Hellmer, K. H., Tabarelli, S. 1973. *Xenobiotica* 3:1–11
61. Krishna, G., Sipes, I. G., Gillette, J. R. 1973. *Pharmacologist* 15:260
62. Sipes, I. G. et al. In preparation
63. Stripp, B. et al 1972. *Proc. 5th Int. Congr. Pharmacol. Abst. Vol. Papers,* 223
64. Sipes, I. G., Stripp, B., Krishna, G., Maling, H. M., Gillette, J. R. 1973. *Proc. Soc. Exp. Biol. Med.* 142:237–40
65. Glende, E. A. 1972. *Biochem. Pharmacol.* 21:169–72
66. Reiner, O., Athanassopoulos, S., Hellmer, K. H., Murray, R. E., Uehleke, H. 1972. *Arch. Toxikol.* 29:219–33
67. Castro, J., Sasame, H., Sussman, H., Gillette, J. R. 1968. *Life Sci.* 7:129–36
68. Maling, H. M., Gillette, J. R. In preparation
69. Reynolds, E. S., Moslen, M. T. 1973. *Fed. Proc.* 32:306
70. Mattocks, A. R. 1972. *Chem.-Biol. Interactions* 5:227–42
71. White, I. N. H., Mattocks, A. R., Butler, W. H. 1973. *Chem. Biol. Interact.* 6:207–18
72. Mattocks, A. R., White, I. N. H. 1971. *Chem. Biol. Interact.* 3:383–96
73. Seawright, A. A., Hrdlicka, J. 1972. *Brit. J. Exp. Pathol.* 53:242–52
74. Floersheim, G. L. 1966. *Biochem. Pharmacol.* 15:1589–93
75. Floersheim, G. L. 1966. *Helv. Physiol. Acta* 24:219–28
76. Reid, W. D., Ilett, K. F., Glick, J. M., Krishna, G. 1973. *Am. Rev. Resp. Dis.* 107:539–51
77. Clark, D. G., McElligott, T. F., Hurst, E. W. 1966. *Brit. J. Ind. Med.* 23:126–32
78. Ilett, K. F., Stripp, B., Menard, R. H., Reid, W. D., Gillette, J. R. 1974. *Toxicol. Appl. Pharmacol.* In press
79. Gage, J. C. 1968. *Biochem. J.* 109:757–61
80. Krishna, G., Ilett, K, Sipes, I. G., Reid, W. D. In preparation
81. Cousins, M. J., Mazze, R. I. 1973. *J. Am. Med. Assoc.* In press
82. Mazze, R. I., Cousins, M. J., Kosek, J. C. 1973. *J. Pharmacol. Exp. Ther.* 184:481–88
83. Cousins, M. J., Mazze, R. I., Kosek, J. C., Love, F. V., Hitt, B. A. *Proc. Sci.*

Meet. Am. Soc. Anesthesiol., San Francisco, October 1973
84. Solymoss, B., Varga, S., Classen, H. G. 1970. *Eur. J. Pharmacol.* 10:127–30
85. Solymoss, B., Classen, H. G., Varga, S. 1969. *Proc. Soc. Exp. Biol. Med.* 132: 940–42
86. Stripp, B., Hamrick, M. E., Zampaglione, N. G., Gillette, J. R. 1971. *J. Pharmacol. Exp. Ther.* 176:766–71
87. Stripp, B., Menard, R. H., Zampaglione, N. G., Hamrick, M. E., Gillette, J. R. 1973. *Drug Metab. Disposition* 1: 216–23
88. Menard, R. H., Stripp, B., Gillette, J. R. In preparation
89. Menard, R. H., Stripp, B., Loriaux, D. L. In preparation
90. Pentikainen, P. J., Pentikainen, L. A., Huffman, D. H., Azarnoff, D. L. 1973. *Clin. Res.* XXI:472
90a. Dymling, J., Nilsson, K. O., Hokfelt, B. 1972. *Acta Endocrinol.* 70(1):104–12
91. Cohen, S. M., Bryan, G. T. 1973. *Proc. 5th Int. Congr. Pharmacol.* 2:164–70
92. Stripp, B., Menard, R. H., Gillette, J. R. 1973. *Pharmacologist* 15:190
93. Nelson, W. D., Patanelli, D. J. 1961. *Fed. Proc.* 20:418
94. Prior, J. T., Ferguson, J. 1950. *Cancer* 3:1062–72
95. Morita, M., Feller, D. R., Gillette, J. R. 1971. *Biochem. Pharmacol.* 20:217–26
96. Wolpert, M. K., Althaus, J. R., Johns, D. G. 1973. *J. Pharmacol. Exp. Ther.* 185:202–13
97. Feller, D. R., Morita, M., Gillette, J. R. 1971. *Proc. Soc. Exp. Biol. Med.* 137: 433–37
98. Phillips, F. S., Sternberg, S. S., Marquardt, H. 1973. *Proc. Int. Congr. Pharmacol, 5th* 2:75–88
99. Krishna, G. 1974. *Postgrad. Med. J.* In press

100. Suria, A., Mitchell, J. R., Stripp, B., Jollow, D., Gillette, J. R. 1971. *Pharmacologist* 13:241
101. Mitchell, J. R. 1971. *Fed. Proc.* 20:2044
102. Ikeda, M., Ohtsuji, H. 1971. *Toxicol. Appl. Pharmacol.* 20:30–43
103. Mitchell, J. R., Jollow, D. J., Gillette, J. R. In preparation
104. Kiese, M. 1966. *Pharmacol. Rev.* 18: 1091–1161
105. Uehleke, H. 1973. *Proc. Int. Congr. Pharmacol, 5th* 2:124–36
106. Beutler, E. 1969. *Pharmacol. Rev.* 21: 73–103
107. DiChiara, G., Hinson, J. A., Potter, W. Z., Jollow, D. J., Mitchell, J. R. 1973. *Fed. Proc.* 32:305
108. DiChiara, G., Jollow, D. J., Mitchell, J. R. Submitted for publication
109. Heymann, E., Krisch, K., Buch, H., Buzello, W. 1969. *Biochem. Pharmacol.* 18:801–11
110. Onisawa, J., Labbe, R. F. 1963. *J. Biol. Chem.* 238:724–27
111. DeMatteis, F. 1973. *Drug Metab. Disposition* 1:267–74
112. Levin, W., Jacobson, M., Sernatinger, E., Kuntzman, R. 1973. *Drug Metab. Disposition* 1:275–85
113. Maines, M. D., Anders, M. W. 1973. *Drug Metab. Disposition* 1:293–98
114. Landsteiner, K. 1945. *The specificity of serological reactions.* Cambridge, Mass.: Harvard Univ. Press
115. Erlanger, B. F. 1973. *Pharmacol. Rev.* 25:271–80
116. Reid, W. D., Christie, B., Eichelbaum, M., Krishna, G. 1971. *Exp. Mol. Pathol.* 15:363–72
117. Cramer, J. W., Miller, J. A., Miller, E. C. 1960. *J. Biol. Chem.* 235:250–56
118. Farber, E. 1971. *Ann. Rev. Pharmacol.* 11:71–96

EFFECTS OF CHEMICALS ON ❖6594
EGG SHELL FORMATION

W. J. Mueller and R. M. Leach Jr.
Department of Poultry Science, The Pennsylvania State University,
University Park, Pennsylvania

The recent decline in certain species of wild birds, which is often accompanied by a decrease in shell thickness, has led to an increased interest in shell formation and the effects of pesticides and other chemicals on this process. In addition, there is a growing awareness among investigators that the intense and rapid mineral metabolism during shell formation offers unique opportunities for studying basic aspects of calcification, ion transport, and skeletal metabolism. The purpose of this review is to gather the widely scattered information on the effects of chemicals on shell strength and to relate these effects, wherever possible, to the processes involved in shell formation. The ability of birds to form strong shells has been assessed with a variety of different measurements (1), including shell thickness, specific gravity of the egg, and shell weight as percentage of egg weight. Since the correlation among these three methods is relatively high, we will use the general term "shell thickness" in most of our discussion. An effort has been made to deal with all avian species. However, because of the economic importance of egg breakage to the poultry industry, much of the research has been carried out with *Gallus domesticus* and, unless mentioned otherwise, the studies summarized below have been carried out with this species.

Current knowledge of shell formation and structure has been described in detail elsewhere (2–4). Nevertheless, it seems essential to begin with a summary of those aspects that are needed for an understanding of the mechanisms of action of different substances. In this summary, references to original papers will only be given if they can not be found in the reviews or if necessary for clarity.

EGG SHELL FORMATION AND STRUCTURE

General

Although there are some differences in shell structure among species, all avian egg shells contain the following layers from the inside to the outside: (*a*) two mem-

289

branes, containing a keratin-like protein, (*b*) the true shell, and (*c*) a proteinaceous cuticle. The true shell, which is the subject of this review, accounts for about 80% of the thickness of the shell in the chicken. It consists of about 98% crystalline calcium carbonate (calcite) and is permeated by an organic matrix. The matrix is a glycoprotein with an amino acid composition similar to that of cartilage; the polysaccharide moiety contains 35% chondroitin sulfate. Because the calcium, carbonate, and matrix content of the true shell is relatively constant and because a defect in the deposition of any of these three components results in thin shells, it seems that all three components are essential for shell formation.

The nuclei of the calcite crystals are deposited on the outer shell membrane in the isthmus region of the oviduct (5). The remainder of the shell is formed in the next section, the shell gland, where the egg remains for about 20 hr in chickens. During the first 5 hr, the egg is "plumped" by diffusion of water and certain electrolytes through the shell membranes into the albumen. Initially, calcium carbonate deposition is slow, but then it increases gradually to a rate of 330 mg/hr that remains constant during the last 15 hr of shell formation.

Calcium Deposition

Because the shell gland does not store significant quantities of calcium, this ion has to be extracted continuously from blood. The mechanisms by which calcium is translocated across the shell gland mucosa are not clear, although active transport may be involved (for review see 6). In the laying hen, the total amount of blood calcium is about 20–30 mg, so that with an extraction rate of 130 mg/hr, calcium would be cleared in 9 to 14 min. Thus, blood calcium has to be replenished continuously. It has been shown that intestinal calcium absorption increases nearly twofold during shell formation (7). Another important source is medullary bone (for review see 4) which supplies 30–40% of the egg shell calcium in chickens, even if calcium intake is adequate. This bone occurs naturally only in female birds and derives its name from the fact that it is most easily observed in the medulla of the femur and tibia. Medullary bone formation, which begins about 10 days before the first ovulation, as well as its maintenance are controlled primarily by the synergistic action of estrogens and androgens. Its mobilization during shell formation is accompanied by an increase in osteoclastic activity and increased phosphate excretion.

Carbonate Deposition

It has not been proven conclusively in what form the carbonate radical of the egg shell mineral is secreted into the shell gland lumen and what mechanisms are involved in its synthesis and/or transport (for a discussion of different models see 8–10). Experiments with ^{14}C-bicarbonate have shown that the arteriovenous bicarbonate gradient across the shell gland is practically zero during shell calcification (11). Thus it is likely that, similarly to the mammalian pancreas (12), most of the bicarbonate is derived from metabolic CO_2 produced by the shell gland, rather than from serum bicarbonate. The hydration of metabolic CO_2 to bicarbonate is probably catalyzed by carbonic anhydrase which has been localized in the shell gland mucosa by histochemical (13), autoradiographic (14), and fluorescent antibody techniques

(15). From the rate of shell formation it can be estimated that the rate of bicarbonate formation is about 56 μmol/min. Maximum inhibition of carbonic anhydrase in the hen with 12 to 25 mg/kg acetazolamide causes a reduction in shell weight of about 80% (16), yielding an uncatalyzed rate of 11 μmol/min. Because the bicarbonate concentration of shell gland fluid is three to four times greater than that of serum (16, 17) and because the potential gradient from the serosal side to the shell gland lumen is negative or zero (6, 18) it seems possible that bicarbonate is secreted by an active process. Precipitation of calcium carbonate on the shell may be facilitated by release of NH_3 gas from the forming egg (19) and/or the high affinity of the organic matrix for cations (20).

The formation of calcium carbonate, either from metabolic CO_2 or from bicarbonate, results in the release of two protons. Egg shell formation in laying hens is accompanied by metabolic acidosis which reaches a maximum when the egg has been in the shell gland for about 16 hr (21). The acidosis is partially compensated for by an increase in respiratory rate (22) and urinary acidity (23). That the shell gland is the source of at least part of the acid is indicated by the finding of Hodges (24) that the arteriovenous pH gradient across the shell gland increases during the first 15 hr of shell formation. This is accompanied by a decrease in the intracellular pH of shell gland tissue, which is abolished if carbonic anhydrase is inhibited with acetazolamide (25). Other investigators (26) have been unable to find any difference in systemic pH between laying and nonlaying quail and have concluded that the pattern is diurnal and not associated with shell formation.

Oviposition

The expulsion of the egg from the shell gland seems to be under both neural and hormonal control, although other factors may also be involved (for reviews see 2, 27). Premature oviposition can be induced by stimulation of the preoptic hypothalamus and administration of substances such as anesthetics, acetylcholine, histamine, oxytocin, and arginine vasotocin. Oviposition is delayed by stimulation of the telencephalon and by epinephrine, ephedrine, spironolactone (28), and possibly certain sex hormones and desoxycorticosterone. Shell-less or thin-shelled eggs may be due to either premature expulsion of the egg from the shell gland or a decreased rate of shell deposition. Unfortunately, many investigators have failed to consider the first possibility.

SUBSTANCES THAT MAY AFFECT MATRIX FORMATION

Lathrogens

Interest in lathrogens is related to the fact that these substances produce skeletal defects in many species. Inclusion of 0.03 to 0.06% of the lathrogen β-aminoproprionitrile (BAPN) in the diet of hens resulted in reduced egg production, hatchability, and the laying of many shell-less and malformed eggs (29). The malformed eggs were wrinkled, checked, and ridged. Although it has been demonstrated that there is an interaction between calcium and BAPN (30), the primary effect of lathrogens appears to be on the crosslinking of connective tissue proteins such as collagen and elastin (31). The protein of the shell membranes resembles collagen in that it contains the unique amino acid hydroxylysine (32). In another study (33), feeding the lathrogen semicarbazide to laying hens had no effect on shell thickness, but the shell membranes were thicker and less pigmented.

Manganese

Shortly after the discovery that manganese prevents a skeletal abnormality called perosis in young chicks (34), it was reported that manganese-deficient hens produce thin, rough, and translucent shells (35). More recent studies (36) confirmed this observation and showed that there was a decrease in shell matrix hexosamine content. These results are consistent with the effects of manganese deficiency on the mucopolysaccharide content of cartilage (37). Thus, the effect of manganese on shell formation is probably related to the role of this element in the synthesis of the polysaccharide component of the shell matrix.

SUBSTANCES THAT AFFECT CALCIFICATION

Calcium

In view of the high calcium requirement for shell formation, it is not surprising that egg shells become thinner when calcium intake is inadequate (for references on this and the effects of different calcium salts see 38). What is unexpected is that hens fed calcium-free diets stop laying after producing about six shells of decreasing thickness rather than continuing to lay eggs with uncalcified shells. The cessation of egg production is apparently due to inadequate gonadotrophin secretion, because hens continue to lay on calcium-deficient diets if they are injected daily with extracts of the avian anterior pituitary (39).

Phosphorus

Egg shell thinning, decreased breaking strength, and an increase in the number of shell-less eggs are some of the effects noted when hens receive an inadequate supply of phosphorus (40–43). Because the phosphorus content of the shell is very low (44), it is likely that phosphorus exerts its effect on shell formation by affecting bone mineral metabolism. Excessive levels of phosphorus have also been observed to cause a reduction in shell thickness (45, 46). Although it seemed likely that excess phosphorus was interfering with calcium metabolism, little evidence was obtained to support this hypothesis.

Magnesium

Magnesium might be expected to influence shell formation because it is second in abundance among the cations found in the shell mineral. However, the magnesium content of the shell is low (0.59%) relative to calcium (44). Severe magnesium deficiency in the laying hen results in reduced egg production and blood magnesium content. The thickness and magnesium content of the shell are also reduced under these conditions (47). Because some dolomitic limestones contain substantial quantities of magnesium, interest has also been shown in the effects of high dietary levels of this element. Studies of magnesium tolerance by the laying hen indicate that egg production, egg weight, and shell thickness are reduced if the diet contains more than 1.2% magnesium (48).

Strontium

The feeding of strontium to laying hens at levels up to 5% of the diet resulted in a progressive increase in strontium content of the shell (49). There was a concomitant decrease in shell calcium content. The chemical form of strontium in the shell could not be identified, but it did not appear to be either $SrCO_3$ or $Sr_3(PO_4)_2$. Levels of strontium above 3% resulted in a significant decrease in shell thickness.

Vitamin D

In view of the well-known effects of Vitamin D on calcium metabolism it is not surprising that thin egg shells are one of the symptoms of vitamin D deficiency in laying hens (50, 51). Vitamin D is necessary for the production of a calcium-binding protein in the intestinal (52) and shell gland (53) mucosa. Studies with laying hens have shown that the amount of intestinal binding protein is responsive to physiological needs, while the amount of shell gland protein remains relatively constant (54). From these findings and other experimental evidence, it was concluded that the vitamin D-dependent calcium-binding protein was not playing a key role in the transfer of calcium across the shell gland mucosa.

SUBSTANCES THAT MAY AFFECT CARBONATE DEPOSITION

Carbonic Anhydrase Inhibitors

Hinshaw & McNeil's observation (55) that turkeys and chickens lay soft-shelled eggs after sulfanilamide administration has been confirmed in a number of studies (56–61). Benesch et al (57) were the first to ascribe this effect to carbonic anhydrase inhibition. This conclusion was based on the finding that sulfapyridine, in which substitution of the sulfonamide group abolishes inhibition, was without effect. Furthermore, the laying of shell-less or thin-shelled eggs coincided with the time when sulfanilamide (80% in the acetylated form) was present in the egg contents. Subsequent studies (58) showed that diets containing 0.3 to 0.5% unsubstituted sulfonamides, such as Soluseptazine and Neoprontosil, caused thin shells, while similar levels of the substituted sulfonamides, sulfathiazole, sulfaguanidine, sulfamerazine, and sulfadiazine had negligible effects on shell thickness. The only exception was sulfapyridine which, in contrast to the previous study (57), caused thin shells for 3 days after a single oral dose of 200 mg/kg. A single intramuscular injection of 12 to 25 mg/kg acetazolamide causes a decrease in shell weight of 70 to 80% (16); oral administration seems less effective, with a reduction in shell thickness of 32 and 43% for dosages of 50 and 100 mg, respectively (62). On an $-SO_2NH_2$ basis, benzenesulfonamide is about as effective as acetazolamide (62).

The relationship between the percentage of decrease in shell thickness and the sulfanilamide content of the diet is linear for concentrations from 0.02 to 0.50%, with a maximum reduction of about 40% (56). A similar relationship was found if

2 to 12 mg/kg acetazolamide was injected before the egg reached the shell gland (unpublished data). Higher dosages caused no further reduction if the egg was laid at the expected time. However about 45 and 70% of the eggs laid after injection of 50 or 100 mg/kg acetazolamide were expelled prematurely, while lower dosages only rarely had this effect. Premature oviposition has also been observed in turkeys (55) and hens (55, 56) fed diets containing 60 to 357 mg/kg sulfanilamide.

The best evidence for a direct effect of sulfonamides on the secretory activity of the shell gland seems to be provided by the changes in intracellular pH (63) and acid-base balance of shell gland fluid (16) after acetazolamide administration. However, carbonic anhydrase inhibitors have a number of effects, besides premature oviposition, whose contribution to egg shell thinning is uncertain. Oral doses of 60 but not of 30 mg acetazolamide per hen per day reduce serum calcium levels (64), and intravenous injection of 300 or 600 mg inhibits the hypercalcemic response to parathyroid hormone (65). An effect on calcium metabolism is also suggested by the finding that hens are in negative calcium balance for about 5 weeks after a diet containing 0.03% sulfanilamide has been withdrawn and shell thickness has returned to normal (66). Since avian osteoclasts contain significant amounts of carbonic anhydrase (67), it is possible that some of these effects are due to inhibition of bone resorption. Acetazolamide also decreases the excretion of ammonia and titrable acidity in laying hens (68), but because the acid-base balance of blood is not affected (16, 69) it is unlikely that this factor plays a major role.

Zinc

This element might be expected to affect shell formation because carbonic anhydrase is a zinc-containing enzyme. Although zinc deficiency reduced the carbonic anhydrase activity of blood in the calf (70) and decreased egg production in laying hens, it had no effect on shell formation (71).

Alterations of Acid-Base Balance

Much of the interest in the relationship between acid-base balance and egg shell formation dates back to the report of Hall & Helbacka (72) that inclusion of 2% ammonium chloride or of 0.74% HCl in the diet of laying hens decreases shell thickness by about 10%. Later studies have confirmed this finding (16, 73) and also indicate that 1% NH_4Cl is only marginally effective (72, 73). It is likely that the inhibition of shell formation by NH_4Cl is due in large part to metabolic acidosis (16, 73, 74) which may reduce the bicarbonate concentration in the secretory cells of the shell gland by proton capture (12) and/or counteract the uptake into blood of protons released during carbonate deposition. It has been shown that NH_4Cl causes a significant reduction in the pH and bicarbonate content of shell gland fluid (16) as well as changes in the Na, K, Ca, and Cl content of the fluid which is added to the albumen in the shell gland (75). The effect of acidifying substances on shell formation may be modified by the accompanying anion. Dietary $(NH_4)_2SO_4$ and H_2SO_4 cause a smaller decrease in shell thickness and a less severe acidosis than equivalent quantities of H^+ in the form of NH_4Cl or HCl, possibly because the anion influences the renal excretion of H^+ (74). If the dietary chloride concentration is increased from 0.5 to 3.0% by addition of NaCl and KCl (Na/K = 0.2), shell thickness and strength decrease progressively (76). This effect may be due to a concomitant reduction of plasma bicarbonate, although the authors (76) ascribe it to carbonic anhydrase inhibition.

Attempts to increase shell thickness through feeding of sodium bicarbonate have had variable results (77–79), although metabolic alkalosis should promote shell formation by increasing the intracellular concentration of hydroxyl and bicarbonate ions (12). The variable results have been attributed to differences in dietary chloride (80), but further investigation is needed.

The effects of respiratory disturbances on shell formation are more consistent and shed additional light on the importance of acid-base balance in this process. Exposure to high environmental temperatures causes respiratory alkalosis and shifts in the acid-base balance of shell gland fluid accompanied by a reduction in shell thickness (16). A rather complete analysis of the effects of hypercapnia on shell formation in the hen has been carried out by Simkiss & Hunt (81, 82) and Sauveur & Mongin (83). Exposing hens to 7 or 20% CO_2 for about 12 hr (82) or to 2–5% for 12 to 54 hr (84), i.e. acute hypercapnia, caused a decrease in the base excess of serum (82) and formation of thin shells. If the exposure to CO_2 was prolonged for several weeks (chronic hypercapnia) blood bicarbonate increased, while blood pH decreased (85) and the egg shells became thicker than normal (77, 86). Similar changes in the acid-base balance of blood during hypercapnia have been observed in mammals (87) and were attributed to a delayed increase in renal bicarbonate reabsorption.

Hunt & Simkiss (82) suggested that the CO_3^{2-} concentration of plasma should be considered as an index for the ability of the shell gland to form $CaCO_3$, an idea further elaborated by Sauveur & Mongin (83). This concept seems particularly useful at the level of the shell gland, because it can be calculated from earlier data (16) that the thinning of egg shells after administration of NH_4Cl, acetazolamide, spironolactone, and exposure to high temperature was always accompanied by a decrease in the CO_3^{2-} concentration of shell gland fluid. The only substance for which this relationship did not hold was theophylline ethylenediamine which decreased shell thickness but caused an increase in CO_3^{2-} concentration.

PESTICIDES

Only the effects of pesticides on shell thickness and the processes involved in shell formation will be discussed; the general effects on birds (88) and chickens (89) have been reviewed earlier.

DDT

The argument that pesticides, particularly DDT and its metabolites, cause egg shell thinning and thereby interfere with the reproductive success of certain species of wild birds is based on three lines of evidence. First, an examination of museum eggs in Britain (90) and the U.S. (91) indicates a marked decrease in shell thickness of raptor eggs between 1940 and 1950. Second, studies show a negative correlation

Table 1 Effect of DDT on shell thickness

Species[1]	Pesticide	Dosage[2]	Percent change in shell quality[3]	Significance[4]	Ref.
Ringdove	p,p'-DDT	10 ppm	10–12[a]	5	102
Ringdove	p,p'-DDE	150 mg/kg i.p.	23[a]	1	102
Bobwhite quail	DDT (tech)	10 or 20 ppm	(2)–4[b]	nt	103
Mallard duck	DDT (tech)	10 or 20 ppm	1–6[b]	nt	103
Mallard duck	DDT (tech)	1000 mg/kg o	18–28[b]	nt	103
Mallard duck	p,p'-DDT	2.5 ppm	5[b]	ns	104
Mallard duck	p,p'-DDT	10 ppm	8[b]	ns	104
Mallard duck	p,p'-DDT	25 ppm	13[b]	1	104
Mallard duck	p,p'-DDE	10 or 40 ppm	8–13[b]	5	104
Mallard duck	DDD	10 or 40 ppm	3–5[b]	ns	104
Bengalese finch	p,p'-DDT	0–300 µg/day o	(7)[c]	1	105
Japanese quail	o,p'-DDT	100 ppm[a]	4[b]	0.1	106
Japanese quail	p,p'-DDT	100 ppm[a]	6[b]	0.1	106
Japanese quail	p,p'-DDT	100 ppm[b]	0[b]	ns	107
Japanese quail	p,p'-DDE	100 ppm[b]	2[b]	ns	107
Chicken[a]	DDT (tech)	10 or 50 ppm	increase[b]	5	108
Chicken[b]	DDT (tech)	10 or 50 ppm	decrease[b]	5	108
Chicken[a]	p,p'-DDT	5 to 300 ppm	no effect[b]		109
Chicken[a]	o,p'-DDT	5 to 300 ppm	no effect[b]		109
Chicken[a]	p,p'-DDE	5 to 300 ppm	no effect[b]		109
Chicken[a]	p,p'-DDT	100 or 200 ppm	0[b]		110
Chicken[a]	DDT (tech)	0.1 to 10 ppm	6[b]	5	111
Chicken[b]	DDT (tech)	1 to 7.5 ppm	3–6[b]	ns	112
Chicken[b]	DDT (tech)	10 ppm	9[b]	5	112

[1] Letter superscripts indicate age of hens: [a]: first year of egg production; [b]: second year of egg production.

[2] i.p.: single intraperitoneal injection. o: oral dose. In all other experiments the pesticide was added to the feed. Superscripts indicate diet concentration of calcium [a]: 0.56% Ca; [b]: 2.7% Ca.

[3] Changes relative to control group(s). Numbers in parentheses indicate an increase; all other values are either a decrease or no change. When the results were presented as graphs, the words increase, decrease, and no effect are used to describe the effect of DDT. Superscripts show the method used to measure shell quality: [a]: shell weight; [b]: shell thickness; [c]: shell weight as percentage of egg weight.

[4] Figures indicate level of significance for differences between control and treatment in percent. nt: significance not tested; ns: difference not significant at 5% level.

Table 2 Identity of pesticides mentioned in this review

Common name	Chemical name
p,p'-DDT	1,1,1-trichloro-2,2-bis (p-chlorophenyl) ethane
o,p'-DDT	1,1,1-trichloro-2-(p-chlorophenyl)-2-(o-chlorophenyl) ethane
p,p'-DDE	1,1-dichloro-2,2-bis (p-chlorophenyl) ethylene
o,p'-DDE	1,1-dichloro-2-(p-chlorophenyl)-2-(o-chlorophenyl) ethylene
DDD	2,2-bis (p-chlorophenyl) ethane
Methoxychlor	1,1,1-trichloro-2,2-bis (p-methoxy-phenyl)-1,1-dichloroethane
Lindane	99.5% Υ-isomer of 1,2,3,4,5,6-hexachlorocyclohexane
Aroclors®	mixtures of polychlorinated biphenyl isomers
Dieldrin	1,2,3,4,10,10-hexachloro-exo-6,7-epoxy-1,4,4a,5,6,7,8,8a-octahydro-1,4-endo-exo-5,8-dimethanonaphthalene
Parathion	O,O-diethyl-O-p-nitrophenyl phosphorothioate
Malathion	O,O-dimethyl S-(1,2-dicarbethoxyethyl) dithiophosphate
Chlordecone	decachloro-octahydro-1,3,4-metheno-2H-cyclobuta (cd) pentalen-2-one

between the concentration of DDT residues in eggs and various measures of shell thickness for herring gulls (91), peregrine falcons (92), prairie falcons (93, 94), double crested cormorants (95), and brown pelicans (96). The only exception seems to be a study with common terns in Alberta, where no correlation was found, despite low reproductive success of the colony and high DDE concentrations relative to other aquatic species of the area (97). The validity of both types of studies has been questioned, primarily with respect to sampling procedures. A good summary of the principal criticisms and their rebuttal can be found in a series of papers and letters (96, 98–101).

The third line of evidence is based on controlled studies of the effect of DDT on shell thickness (Table 1) and shell formation. These experiments were carried out with different isomers of DDT or DDE (Table 2) and with technical DDT. The isomer p,p'-DDE is the principal metabolite of DDT and accounts for 50 to 100% of the DDT residues in body tissues and eggs of wild birds (109). Technical DDT contains about 80% p,p'-DDT and 15–20% o,p'-DDT as well as other isomers and related compounds.

In general, the decrease in shell thickness is greater in wild populations, where thinning in excess of 50% has occurred (103), than in controlled experiments, even if the concentration of DDT residues is similar. The degree of shell thinning caused by DDT varies considerably among species (Table 1). Ringdoves (102) and mallard ducks (103, 104) seem to be relatively sensitive, while Japanese quail (106, 107), bobwhite quail (103), and particularly chickens (108–112) are relatively resistant. In an experiment with Bengålese finches (105) and in one experiment with chickens during their first year of lay (108) DDT caused a significant increase in shell thickness.

There is some evidence that the effect of DDT depends on the method of administration. In Japanese quail, 100 ppm p,p'-DDT caused significant shell thinning if the diet was deficient in calcium (106) but not if the calcium level was adequate (107). Tucker & Haegele (103) concluded that a single dose of DDT was more effective than continuous administration, a conclusion that could also be drawn from data obtained for ringdoves (102). However, in both instances the single dose was rather massive, so that the difference in response may have been due to the larger amount of DDT rather than to the method of administration. The response to DDT may also depend on the age of the bird. With one exception (111), administration of DDT to chickens during their first year of lay caused no change (109, 110) or increased shell thickness (108), while during the second year of production, levels in excess of 10 ppm caused shell thinning (108, 112). Another factor may be the position of the egg in the clutch, where a clutch is a sequence of eggs laid on successive days and two clutches are separated by one or more days when no egg is laid. In Japanese quail fed 0.56% calcium, DDT had little effect on the shell of the first egg in the clutch, while later eggs showed a progressive decline in shell calcium (106). Susceptibility may also vary among individual birds. When Japanese quail were fed DDT, about 80% of the broken eggs were produced by one quarter of the birds (107).

Other Pesticides

Feeding of 25 to 5000 ppm methoxychlor, a pesticide whose use has increased since the banning of DDT, had no effect on shell thickness in laying hens (113). Similar results have been obtained for lindane at a concentration of 100 ppm (114).

Although polychlorinated biphenyls may affect a number of reproductive traits, shell formation is usually not inhibited. Negative results have been obtained in studies with ringdoves (115), Japanese quail (116), mallards (117), bobwhite quail (117), and chickens (118, 119).

A number of experiments have also been carried out with dieldrin. Feeding 20 ppm (110) or administering 6 oral doses of 3 mg each over an 11 day period (120) had no effect on shell thickness in laying hens. In one study with mallard ducks, dietary levels of 1.6, 4, and 10 ppm dieldrin caused significant shell thinning (121), while in another experiment 4 ppm had no such effect (122). Prairie falcons that ate starlings fed a diet containing 10 ppm dieldrin showed a significant reduction of shell thickness, if the dieldrin content of their eggs was more than 20 ppm, but not if it was less (94).

Parathion at a concentration of 10 ppm caused significant shell thinning when it was fed to mallard ducks (122).

Effect of Pesticides on Processes Involved in Shell Formation

The similarity in configuration of DDT to the synthetic estrogen diethylstilbestrol has stimulated investigation of the estrogenic activity of DDT in mammals and birds (for references see papers cited below). The isomer o,p'-DDT was found to be estrogenic in chickens and quail, stimulating growth and glycogen deposition in the oviduct, while *p,p'*-DDT was only weakly estrogenic (123). There are a number of other effects of DDT which suggest that it may interfere with the reproductive endocrinology of birds. DDT delayed sexual maturity and ovulation in Bengalese finches (105), Japanese quail (106, 107), and ringdoves (102). Both technical DDT (10 ppm) and dieldrin (2 ppm) increased the breakdown of testosterone and progesterone by liver microsomes to polar metabolites in king pigeons (124), and *p,p'*-DDT (10 ppm) reduced the concentration of estradiol in the blood of ringdoves (102). One mechanism through which these effects might interfere with shell formation is by inhibition of medullary bone formation. Such inhibition was observed when 100 ppm *p,p'*-DDT was fed to king pigeons (125). It has also been reported that 10 ppm *p,p'*-DDTdecreased the accumulation of ^{45}Ca in bone during the prelaying period of ringdoves (102). Other investigators (106) found no effect of DDT on medullary bone. It can also be argued that any decrease in bone calcium stores would be compensated for by increased utilization of dietary calcium, particularly in raptorial birds that have a relatively high calcium intake. On the other hand, it is possible that the greater sensitivity of Japanese quail on low calcium diets (106, 107) is due to increased dependence on medullary bone calcium.

Jefferies and co-workers have suggested that the effect of DDT on shell thickness may be due to altered thyroid function. In Bengalese finches, *p,p'*-DDT caused hyperthyroidism and increased shell thickness (105, 126), while pigeons became hypothyroid at dose rates in excess of 3 mg/kg/day (126, 127) and produced shells of lower weight (102). Besides accounting for one species difference in the response to DDT, these findings are also in concert with some studies on the effect of thyroid function on shell thickness (see below).

A number of recent investigations have focused on the effects of pesticides on the shell-forming process itself. Studies with the scanning electron microscope (128) have shown that feeding technical DDT (225 ppm) or Chlordecone (5 to 225 ppm) causes marked changes of shell structure in Japanese quail that cannot be explained completely by shell thinning alone.

There is controversy with regard to the effects of DDT on carbonic anhydrase. In one study with Japanese quail, diets containing 100 ppm *p,p'*-DDT or *p,p'*-DDE reduced the carbonic anhydrase activity of blood by 22 and 44% (129), while in another experiment with 100 ppm technical DDT there was no such effect (130). Inhibition of carbonic anhydrase has also been reported for quail shell glands after feeding of *p,p'*-DDT or *o,p'*-DDT (129) and for the oviduct of ringdoves after a single injection of 150 mg/kg *p,p'*-DDE but not of dieldrin (102).

Several authors have claimed that these results may be artifacts. Dvorchick et al (131) found no inhibition of human red cell or purified bovine carbonic anhydrase in vitro at *p,p'*-DDT or *p,p'*-DDE concentrations of 50 to 100 µg/ml. Pocker et al (132) confirmed these results and suggested that the reduction of catalytic efficiency by DDT may be due to precipitation of carbonic anhydrase. However, Serine & Schraer (133) have shown that both *o,p'*-DDT and *p,p'*-DDT inhibit purified chicken carbonic anhydrase in buffers containing 34% dimethylformamide which prevents coprecipitation of the enzyme and DDT (132).

OTHER SUBSTANCES

Mercury

The interest in environmental contamination from mercury has led to two investigations of the effect of this element on egg shell thickness. In experiments with Japanese quail (134), feeding from 1 to 8 ppm mercury as mercuric chloride produced a progressive decrease in egg shell thickness. Tissue mercury content was proportional to dosage. Methyl mercury was not detected in the tissues of this species. Contrasting results were obtained with methylmercury administration to ringdoves and American kestrels (135). This form is thought to be an important source of mercury for predatory birds. In these studies, injection or oral dosing with amounts equivalent to a dietary intake of 10 ppm had no significant effect on egg shell thickness.

Lithium

Inclusion of lithium carbonate at levels of 282 to 685 ppm lithium in the diet produced diarrhea, excessive salivation, regurgitation, and shell-less eggs as early as 24 hr after initiation of treatment (136). The mode of action of lithium on shell formation is unknown. Although lithium resulted in reduced serum calcium levels, soft-shelled eggs were produced before this change took place.

Hormones

The endocrine control of shell formation is poorly understood. Administration of hormones to laying hens often reduces egg production and egg size, resulting in a decreased need for calcium which may indirectly increase shell thickness.

It has been shown that medullary bone formation and maintenance depend on the synergistic action of estrogens and androgens, but other endocrine glands such as the thyroids and adrenals may also be involved (4). Little is known about the mechanisms that synchronize the metabolic activity of bone with the different stages of egg formation, although it has been proposed that either parathyroid hormone or estrogen is the regulatory factor (4). Administration of female sex hormones to laying hens has no effect on shell thickness, while testosterone may cause a slight improvement (for references see 38).

The calcemic and phosphatemic response of laying hens to parathyroid hormone is considerably larger, more rapid, and more transient than that of mammals (137), while administration of calcitonin has generally no effect (138). To our knowledge the effect of parathyroid hormone on shell formation has not been studied. When 10 MRC units/kg porcine calcitonin was injected intramuscularly at the onset of shell calcification, shell thickness was not affected although the interval between successive ovipositions was significantly shortened (139).

The effects of thyroprotein (iodinated casein) and of thiouracil have been studied rather extensively in laying hens (for references see 38). Although the results are conflicting, taken together, they suggest that shell thickness may be improved by iodinated casein and decreased by thiouracil, at least under certain conditions.

Thyroidectomy decreased egg production, egg weight, and shell thickness in chickens (140).

Cortisone, which is not known to occur in the fowl, increased shell thickness in one experiment (141) but not in another (142). When the aldosterone anatagonist spironolactone was injected daily at dosages of 4 to 9 mg per hen, shell weight decreased initially by 12 to 24% but then returned gradually to control values (28).

Injection of 0.8 mg/kg glucagon (138), 300 mg/kg imidazole (138), or 6 mg/hen theophylline ethylenediamine (16) at the onset of shell calcification reduced shell thickness without affecting the time of oviposition.

Literature Cited

1. Tyler, C. 1961. *Brit. Poult. Sci.* 2:3–19
2. Sturkie, P. D. 1965. *Avian Physiology.* Ithaca, NY: Cornell Univ. Press. 766 pp.
3. Simkiss, K., Taylor, T. G. 1971. *Physiology and Biochemistry of the Domestic Fowl,* ed. D. J. Bell, B. M. Freeman, 3:1331–43. New York: Academic
4. Taylor, T. G., Simkiss, K., Stringer, D. A. See Ref. 3, 2:621–40
5. Stemberger, B. 1971. *Microscopic examination of the avian egg membrane from the posterior oviduct to study the formation of the mammillae.* MS thesis. Pennsylvania State Univ., Univ. Park, Pa. 51 pp.
6. Schraer, R., Schraer, H. 1970. *Biological Calcification: Cellular and Molecular Aspects,* ed. H. Schraer, 347–73. New York: Appleton. 462 pp.
7. Hurwitz, S. 1970. *Ann. Biol. Anim. Biochim. Biophys.* 10 (no. hors-ser. 2): 69–76
8. Mongin, P. 1967. *World's Poult. Sci. J.* 24:200–30
9. Hodges, R. D., Lörcher, K. 1967. *Nature* 216:609–10
10. Simkiss, K. 1968. *Egg Quality – A Study of the Hen's Egg,* ed. T. C. Carter, 3–25. Edinburgh: Oliver & Boyd. 336 pp.
11. Lörcher, K., Zscheile, C., Bronsch, K. 1970. *Ann. Biol. Anim. Biochim. Biophys.* 10 (no. hors-ser. 2):193–98
12. Maren, T. H. 1967. *Physiol. Rev.* 47: 595–781
13. Diamantstein, T., Schluns, J. 1964. *Acta Histochem.* 19:296–302
14. Gay, C. V., Mueller, W. J. 1973. *J. Histochem. Cytochem.* 21:693–702
15. Faleski, E. J., Gay, C. V., Schraer, R. 1973. *Fed. Proc.* 32:898
16. Mueller, W. J., Brubaker, R. L., Caplan, M. D. 1969. *Fed. Proc.* 28: 1851–56

17. el Jack, M. H., Lake, P. E. 1967. *J. Reprod. Fert.* 13:127–32
18. Leonard, E. 1969. *J. Physiol. London* 203:83P–84P
19. Reddy, G., Campbell, J. W. 1972. *Experientia* 28:530–32
20. Simkiss, K., Tyler, C. 1958. *Quart. J. Microsc. Sci.* 99:5–13
21. Mongin, P., Lacassagne, L. 1964. *C. R. Acad. Sci. Paris* 258:3093–94
22. Mongin, P., Lacassagne, L. 1966. *Ann. Biol. Anim. Biochim. Biophys.* 6: 101–11
23. Anderson, R. S. 1967. *Vet. Rec.* 80: 314–15
24. Hodges, R. D. 1970. *Ann. Biol. Anim. Biochim. Biophys.* 10 (no. hors-ser. 2): 199–213
25. Simkiss, K. 1970. *J. Physiol. London* 207:63P–64P
26. Dacke, C. G., Musacchia, X. J., Volkert, W. A., Kenny, A. D. 1973. *Comp. Biochem. Physiol.* 44A:1267–75
27. Gilbert, A. B. 1971. See Ref. 3, 3: 1345–52
28. Mueller, W. J. 1967. *Poult. Sci.* 46: 743–49
29. Barnett, B. D., Richey, D. J., Morgan, C. L. 1957. *Proc. Soc. Exp. Biol. Med.* 95:101–4
30. Naber, E. C., Scott, K., Johnson, R. M. 1965. *Poult. Sci.* 44:1540–44
31. Piez, K. A. 1968. *Ann. Rev. Biochem.* 37:547–70
32. Candlish, J. K., Scougall, R. K. 1969. *Int. J. Protein Chem.* 1:299–302
33. Bannister, D. W., Candlish, J. K., Freeman, H. 1971. *Brit. Poult. Sci.* 12: 129–36
34. Wilgus, H. S., Norris, L. C., Heuser, G. F. 1936. *Science* 84:252–53
35. Lyons, M. 1939. *Bull. Ark. Agr. Exp. Sta.* No. 374. 18 pp.
36. Longstaff, M., Hill, R. 1972. *Brit. Poult. Sci.* 13:377–85

37. Leach, R. M. Jr. 1971. *Fed. Proc.* 30: 991–94
38. Wolford, J. H., Tanaka, K. 1970. *World's Poultry Sci. J.* 26:763–80
39. Taylor, T. G., Morris, T. R., Hertelendy, F. 1962. *Vet. Rec.* 74:123–25
40. Norris, L. C., Heuser, G. F., Wilgus, H. S. Jr., Ringrose, A. T. 1933. *NY State Coll. Agr. 46th Ann. Rep.* 137–38
41. Evans, R. J., Carver, J. S., Brant, A. W. 1944. *Poult. Sci.* 21:9–15
42. Gillis, M. B., Norris, L. C., Heuser, G. F. 1953. *Poult. Sci.* 32:977–84
43. Crowley, T. A., Kurnich, A. A., Reid, B. L. 1963. *Poult. Sci.* 42:758–65
44. Tyler, C., Geake, F. H. 1953. *J. Sci. Food Agr.* 4:587–96
45. Arscott, G. H., Rachapaetayakom, P., Bernier, P. E., Adams, F. W. 1962. *Poult. Sci.* 41:485–88
46. Taylor, T. G. 1965. *Brit. Poult. Sci.* 6: 79–87
47. Cox, A. C., Sell, J. L. 1967. *Poult. Sci.* 46:675–80
48. McWard, G. W. 1967. *Brit. Poult. Sci.* 8:91–99
49. Doberenz, A. R., Weber, C. W., Reid, B. L. 1969. *Calcif. Tissue Res.* 4:180–84
50. Hughes, J. S., Payne, L. F., Latshaw, W. L. 1925. *Poult. Sci.* 4:151–56
51. Hart, E. B. et al 1925. *J. Biol. Chem.* 65:579–95
52. Wasserman, R. H., Taylor, A. N. 1966. *Science* 152:791–93
53. Corradino, R. A., Wasserman, R. H., Pubols, M. H., Chang, S. I. 1968. *Arch. Biochem. Biophys.* 125:378–80
54. Bar, A., Hurwitz, S. 1973. *Comp. Biochem. Physiol.* 45A:579–86
55. Hinshaw, W. R., McNeil, E. 1943. *Poult. Sci.* 22:291–94
56. Scott, H. M., Jungherr, E., Matterson, L. D. 1944. *Poult. Sci.* 23:446–53
57. Benesch, R., Barron, N. S., Mawson, C. A. 1944. *Nature* 153:138–39
58. Bernard, R., Genest, P. 1945. *Science* 101:617–18
59. Tyler, C. 1950. *Brit. J. Nutr.* 4:112–28
60. Gutowska, M. S., Mitchell, C. A. 1945. *Poult. Sci.* 24:159–67
61. Becker, W. A., Bearse, G. E. 1962. *Poult. Sci.* 41:198–200
62. Mehring, A. L., Titus, H. W., Brumbaugh, J. H. 1955. *Poult. Sci.* 34: 1385–89
63. Simkiss, K. 1969. *Biochem. J.* 111: 647–52
64. Siegmund, P., Dulce, H. J. 1960. *Hoppe-Seyler's Z. Physiol. Chem.* 320: 149–67
65. Siegmund, P., Bauditz, W. 1966. *Naunyn Schmiedebergs Arch. Exp. Pathol. Pharmakol.* 251:288–94
66. Tyler, C. 1954. *J. Agr. Sci.* 45:156–63
67. Gay, C. V., Mueller, W. J. 1972. *Fed. Proc.* 31:708
68. Wolbach, R. A. 1955. *Am. J. Physiol.* 181:149–56
69. Mongin, P. 1970. *Ann. Biol. Anim. Biochim. Biophys.* 10:119–30
70. Miller, J. K., Miller, W. J. 1960. *J. Dairy Sci.* 43:1854–56
71. Kienholz, E. W., Turk, D. E., Sunde, M. L., Hoekstra, W. G. 1961. *J. Nutr.* 75:211–21
72. Hall, K. N., Helbacka, N. V. 1959. *Poult. Sci.* 38:111–14
73. Hunt, J. R., Aitken, J. R. 1962. *Poult. Sci.* 41:434–38
74. Sauveur, B. 1969. *Ann. Biol. Anim. Biochim. Biophys.* 9:379–91
75. Sauveur, B. 1970. *Ann. Biol. Anim. Biochim. Biophys.* 10 (no. hors-ser. 2): 215–27
76. Lörcher, K., Diamantstein, T., Kobow, J. 1964. *Z. Tierphysiol. Tierernaehr. Futtermittelk.* 19:218–36
77. Frank, F. R., Burger, R. E. 1965. *Poult. Sci.* 44:1604–6
78. Cox, A. C., Balloun, S. L. 1968. *Poult. Sci.* 47:1370–74
79. Howes, J. R. 1967. *Distill. Feed Conf., 22nd,* 32–35
80. Mongin, P. 1970. *Proc. Cornell Nutr. Conf.,* 99–102
81. Simkiss, K. 1967. *Nature* 214:84–86
82. Hunt, J. R., Simkiss, K. 1967. *Comp. Biochem. Physiol.* 21:223–30
83. Sauveur, B., Mongin, P. 1972. *Comp. Biochem. Physiol.* 41A:869–75
84. Helbacka, N. V., Casterline, J. L., Smith, C. J. 1963. *Poult. Sci.* 42: 1082–84
85. Mongin, P., Sauveur, B. 1970. *Ann. Biol. Anim. Biochim. Biophys.* 10 (no. hors-ser. 2):141–50
86. Mongin, P. 1968. *Proc. Eur. Poult. Congr., 3rd, Work Group Nb7,* 565
87. Schwartz, M. B., Brackett, N. C., Cohen, J. J. 1965. *J. Clin. Invest.* 44:291–301
88. Pimentel, D. 1971. *Ecological Effects of Pesticides on Non-Target Species.* Washington DC: GPO. 220 pp.
89. Vogt, H. 1972. *Arch. Gefluegelk.* 36: 137–58
90. Ratcliffe, D. A. 1967. *Nature* 215: 208–10
91. Hickey, J. J., Anderson, D. W. 1968. *Science* 162:271–73

92. Cade, T. J., Lincer, J. L., White, C. M. 1971. *Science* 172:955–57
93. Fyfe, R. W., Campbell, J., Hayson, B., Hodson, K. 1969. *Can. Field-Natur.* 83:191–200
94. Enderson, J. H., Berger, D. D. 1970. *BioScience* 20:355–56
95. Anderson, D. W., Hickey, J. J., Risebrough, R. W., Hughes, D. F., Christensen, R. E. 1969. *Can. Field-Natur.* 83:91–112
96. Blus, L. J., Gish, C. D., Belisle, A. A., Prouty, R. M. 1972. *Nature* 235:376–77
97. Switzer, B., Lewin, V. Wolfe, F. H. 1971. *Can. J. Zool.* 49:69–73
98. Hazeltine, W. 1972. *Nature* 239:410–11
99. Switzer, B. C., Wolfe, F. H. 1972. *Nature* 240:162–63
100. Wiemeyer, S. N., Porter, R. D. 1972. *Nature* 240:163
101. Risebrough, R. W. 1972. *Nature* 240:164
102. Peakall, D. B. 1970. *Science* 168:592–94
103. Tucker, R. K., Haegele, H. A. 1970. *Bull. Environ. Contam. Toxicol.* 5:191–94
104. Heath, R. G., Spann, J. W., Kreitzer, J. F. 1969. *Nature* 224:47–48
105. Jefferies, D. J. 1969. *Nature* 222:578–79
106. Bitman, J., Cecil, H. C., Harris, S. J., Fries, G. F. 1969. *Nature* 224:44–46
107. Cecil, H. C., Bitman, J., Harris, S. J. 1971. *Poult. Sci.* 50:657–59
108. Cecil, H. C., Bitman, J., Fries, G. F., Harris, S. J., Lillie, R. J. 1973. *Poult. Sci.* 52:648–53
109. Cecil, H. C. et al 1972. *Poult. Sci.* 51:130–39
110. Davidson, K. L., Sell, J. L. 1972. *Bull. Environ. Contam. Toxicol.* 7:9–18
111. Sauter, E. A., Steele, E. E. 1972. *Poult. Sci.* 51:71–76
112. Smith, S. I., Weber, C. W., Reid, B. L. 1970. *Poult. Sci.* 49:233–37
113. Lillie, R. J., Cecil, H. C., Bitman, J. 1973. *Poult. Sci.* 52:1134–38
114. Whitehead, C. C., Downing, A. G., Pettigrew, R. J. 1972. *Brit. Poult. Sci.* 13:293–99
115. Peakall, D. B. 1971. *Bull. Environ. Contamin. Toxicol.* 6:100–1
116. Cecil, H. C., Harris, S. J., Bitman, J., Fries, G. F. 1973. *Bull. Environ. Contamin. Toxicol.* 9:179–85
117. Heath, R. G., Spann, J. W., Kreitzer, J. F., Vance, C. 1970. *Proc. Int. Ornithol. Congr., XVth,* 20 pp.
118. Scott, M. L., Vandehra, D. V., Mullenhoff, P. A., Rumsey, G. L., Rice, R. W. 1971. *Proc. Cornell Nutr. Conf.* 56–64
119. Whitehead, C. C., Downie, J. N., Phillips, J. A. 1972. *Nature* 239:411–12
120. Mick, D. L., Long, K. R., Aldinger, S. M. 1973. *Bull. Environ. Contamin. Toxicol.* 9:197–203
121. Lehner, P. N., Egbert, A. 1969. *Nature* 224:1218–19
122. Muller, H. D. 1971. *Poult. Sci.* 51:239–41
123. Bitman, J., Cecil, H. C., Harris, S. J., Fries, G. F. 1968. *Science* 162:371–72
124. Peakall, D. B. 1967. *Nature* 216:505–6
125. Oestreicher, M. I., Shuman, D. H., Wurster, C. F. 1971. *Nature* 229:571
126. Jefferies, D. J., French, M. C., Osborne, B. E. 1971. *Brit. Poult. Sci.* 12:387–99
127. Jefferies, D. J., French, M. C. 1969. *Science* 166:1278–80
128. McFarland, L. Z., Garrett, R. L., Nowell, J. A. 1971. *Proc. Ann. Scanning Elec. Microsc. Symp., 4th,* 377–84
129. Bitman, J., Cecil, H. C., Fries, G. F. 1970. *Science* 168:594–96
130. Gadhok, R. S., Kenny, A. D. 1973. *Symp. Trace Subst. Environ. Health, 6th,* 166–72
131. Dvorchik, B. H., Istin, M., Maren, T. H. 1971. *Science* 172:728–29
132. Pocker, Y., Beug, M. W., Ainardi, V. R. 1971. *Science* 174:1336–38
133. Serine, E. A., Schraer, R. 1972. *Fed. Proc.* 31:726
134. Stoewsand, G. S., Anderson, J. L., Gutenmann, W. H., Bache, C. A., Lisk, D. J. 1971. *Science* 173:1030–31
135. Peakall, D. B., Linger, J. L. 1972. *Bull. Environ. Contam. Toxicol.* 8:89–90
136. Creek, R. D., Lund, P., Thomas, O. P., Pollard, W. O. 1971. *Poult. Sci.* 50:577–80
137. Mueller, W. J., Hall, K. L., Maurer, C. A. Jr., Joshua, I. G. 1973. *Endocrinology* 92:853–56
138. Simkiss, K., Dacke, C. G. See Ref. 3, 1:481–88
139. Joshua, I. G. 1972. *Effect of hypocalcemic agents on shell formation and plasma calcium, inorganic phosphate and protein in the laying hen.* MS thesis. Pennsylvania State Univ., Univ. Park, Pa. 59 pp.
140. Taylor, L. W., Burmester, B. R. 1940. *Poult. Sci.* 19:326–31
141. Howes, J. R. 1969. *Poult. Sci.* 48:1822
142. Gabuten, A. R., Shaffner, C. S. 1954. *Poult. Sci.* 33:47–53

THE USE OF NEUROPOISONS IN THE STUDY OF CHOLINERGIC TRANSMISSION

❖6595

Lance L. Simpson

College of Physicians & Surgeons of Columbia University, New York, New York

INTRODUCTION

Poisons are useful investigational tools for the obvious reason that a truly poisonous substance must be active in minuscule quantities and therefore highly selective in its site of action. Furthermore, that site must be crucial to the function of an isolated tissue or to an entire organism. Poisons, by their very nature, are substances whose sites and mechanisms of action are highly specific.

Poisons are valuable investigational tools because they modify their target organs in ways that are both reliable and predictable. Hence, poisons have been used to analyze innumerable physiological processes. This review will focus on the mechanism of cholinergic transmission. There is probably no area of research that has relied more upon poisons than has the study of synaptic and neuromuscular transmission. In deference to their longstanding importance (and existence), poisons of biological origin are the main topics of discussion in this review.

ACETYLCHOLINE AND AXONAL TRANSMISSION

Acetylcholine (ACh) is believed to be a transmitter at numerous central and peripheral synapses. Another hypothesis, but one that has few advocates, is that ACh is involved in axonal transmission. The major advocate of this hypothesis has been Nachmansohn (1, 2). According to this investigator, ACh is stored in an inactive form (bound or sequestered) within conducting membranes. Following nerve stimulation, ACh is released and diffuses to a receptor, which is also within membranes. The interaction between ACh and its receptor leads to conformational changes, and these in turn initiate the sequence of events that culminate in a propagated action potential. The role of ACh at synaptic and neuromuscular junctions is hypothesized to be analogous to that in conducting membranes.

To be accepted as an essential component of axonal transmission, ACh must satisfy certain minimal criteria. In all likelihood, the criteria used to identify putative transmitter substances (3–6) are equally germane in identifying putative agents that regulate axonal transmission. In brief, it is expected that a substance be present and releasable in sufficient amounts to exert its supposed action, and that there be means both for generating the substance and for removing it from its site of action. In addition, an exogenous substance of known identity must mimic the action of the putative endogenous substance. All known components of the cholinergic system have been studied with these criteria in mind. If nerves of the lobster walking leg are deemed representative, ACh is present in axons (7, 8). Axonal and nerve terminal ACh are both released into perfusing medium which contains an esterase inhibitor, and that release is affected by local concentrations of calcium (9). Axons and nerve terminals are also similar in that choline acetylase (ChA) is primarily a cytoplasmic enzyme (8, 10), and acetylcholinesterase (AChE) is partially membrane bound (8).

While it is true that axons contain components of the cholinergic system, it is not certain that their presence is related to electrical excitability. A more widely held belief is that these components are merely in transit from the soma to the nerve terminal. Because of the differing opinions on the reasons for the presence of the cholinergic system in axons, many workers have studied the action of ACh applied exogenously to axons. Early studies demonstrated that ACh could depolarize the nerve trunk (11). However, the amount of ACh needed to produce effects on axons was far greater than that needed to elicit effects at junctional regions. There was, and is, a valid explanation. There are permeability barriers around the axon that limit diffusion of ACh and other drugs to potentially reactive sites. Any test of whether ACh is equiactive at junctional and axonal sites must contend with differences in diffusion rates.

The claim that axons are protected by permeability barriers was substantiated by the use of snake venoms (for review and tabulation of data, see 12). An acid-boiled fraction of cottonmouth venom substantially decreased permeability barriers to ACh and other quarternary agonists and antagonists (13). Thus, axons treated with venom became more sensitive to exogenous ACh. The mechanism by which venoms increase permeability is not clear, because venoms contain so many pharmacologically active substances (14). An earlier notion that phospholipase A is the active component that sensitizes axons appears untenable (15, 16). Yet, regardless of the mechanism by which venoms decrease barriers to penetration, they do not render axons as sensitive to ACh as are junctional regions and isolated electroplax (12).

Research utilizing snake venoms has not generated compelling evidence that axons require ACh for conduction. However, the work has renewed interest in axonal ChA and AChE. That interest has resulted in two noteworthy studies. The first (10) demonstrated that 80% inhibition of squid giant axon ChA did not alter nerve excitability. The other (17) showed that 98–99% inhibition of squid axon AChE did not affect electrical activity. Neither report encourages the belief that cholinergic activity and electrical excitability are interrelated.

TRANSMITTER STORES

According to theory, ACh is stored inside synaptic vesicles. During synaptic transmission, vesicles discharge their contents into the cleft. This theory, although widely accepted, is based mainly on indirect evidence. Several attempts have been made to provide direct evidence that vesicles are essential to transmission. The main approach has been to stimulate neuromuscular preparations repetitively in an effort to deplete nerve terminals of their synaptic vesicles. Early work along these lines was not particularly successful (18). However, more recent studies have demonstrated that intense stimulation can influence vesicle turnover (19–23).

Almost simultaneously with the stimulation research, a new technique for studying vesicles and transmission was developed. The technique is based on the finding that a variety of pharmacological agents will deplete nerve terminals of their vesicles. Among these agents are ammonium (24), lanthanum (25), β-bungarotoxin (26, but see 27), and black widow spider venom (28, 29). Black widow spider venom has been most widely used, so it can be considered a prototype for the group.

Most spiders are not venomous. Notable exceptions are members of the genus *Latrodectus. Latrodectus mactans,* more commonly known as the black widow spider, is of particular interest. When frightened or perturbed, it will bite and envenomate man. Of a variety of pathophysiological effects that result from envenomation, the more prominent are spreading pain, hypertension, and spasmodic muscular contractions. The toxic effects of the venom can be reversed by appropriate antibodies. Death from envenomation is rare.

Initial studies (30) on the cellular pharmacology of black widow spider venom indicated that the substance does not block nerve propagation or muscle contracture, whereas it does block synaptic and neuromuscular transmission. Detailed studies (28, 29) on the venom have shown that it produces two profound effects. Electrophysiologically, the venom evokes an extraordinary increase in the rate of spontaneous miniature endplate potentials. The increase in rate is not antagonized by an absence of calcium or an excess of magnesium. Apparently the venom changes the properties of the nerve terminal in such a way as to promote explosive release of ACh. Morphologically, the substance causes the disappearance of synaptic vesicles. Concomitantly with the loss of vesicles, there is an increase in the mass of presynaptic membrane (31). It may be that venom-induced disappearance of vesicles is due to coalescence of synaptic membrane with nerve terminal membrane. It has been reported that morphological changes in the frog are reversible (31). In contrast, it has been reported that mammalian motor nerve terminals are destroyed (32). The venom acts both peripherally and centrally on cholinergic terminals (33). Also, the substance acts to deplete catecholamine containing nerve fibers of their transmitter stores (34).

Black widow spider venom has aided in several aspects of the study of cholinergic transmission. First, it has provided reasonable evidence that vesicles and transmission are interrelated. This conclusion follows from the observation that venom-induced vesicle depletion stops both transmission and spontaneous ACh release (29,

31). Second, the venom has provided a means for quantitating the number of transmitter packets in nerve terminals (28). During the period of explosive ACh release, the number of spontaneous potentials can be monitored. The number of quanta that were present originally may be determined by calculation of the number of spontaneous potentials. Such calculations have produced estimates of the number of vesicles that are comparable to estimates made by other techniques (35). Finally, the venom has provided a means for determining the residual stores of transmitter in terminals that have been subjected to other forms of experimental treatment (36). For example, venom will evoke release of ACh from nerves that have been tetanically stimulated. Quantitation of venom-induced ACh release permits estimation of residual stores of transmitter that withstood tetanization.

RELEASE OF TRANSMITTER

We know little about the mechanism by which nerve terminals discharge their stores of transmitter substance (37). Nevertheless, it has been established that calcium plays an essential role. Although preceded by other studies, the work of Harvey & MacIntosh (38) was instrumental in linking calcium to ACh release. They demonstrated that sympathetic ganglia of the cat did not release ACh when perfused with calcium-free medium. During the years since that report, there have been hundreds of studies dealing with calcium and exitation-secretion coupling (39).

Several research strategies can be used to study calcium and cholinergic transmission. The simplest is to modify the concentration of calcium in the perfusate bathing isolated tissues. Such studies have indicated a quantitative relationship between transmitter release and extracellular calcium concentration (40–42). In addition, there is cooperativity in the release phenomenon; that is, more than one calcium ion is necessary to evoke quantal release of transmitter (43–45, but see 46). A more sophisticated strategy is to omit calcium from the bathing medium and then apply it iontophoretically to suspected sites of action. A representative study of this nature was conducted by Katz & Miledi (47). They demonstrated that calcium promotes ACh release by acting at the junctional region, and not remotely on the axon. In a similar type study, Miledi & Slater (48) showed that calcium must cross the nerve membrane to be active, because direct injection of calcium into the nerve terminal does not cause transmitter release.

Because other ions are known to interact or compete with calcium, it would be useful to minimize their effects. Sodium is one of the ions whose presence complicates interpretation of calcium studies. The most direct of several approaches that have been used to diminish the effects of sodium has been to suspend tissues in medium in which sodium is replaced by calcium (49, 50). Tissues bathed in high calcium release ACh spontaneously, and depolarizing currents will evoke additional transmitter release. A limitation of this approach is that prolonged exposure to high calcium will cause morphological changes and irreversible losses of function (50). It would be more desirable to have all ions present at physiological concentrations, under conditions in which calcium, but not sodium, can affect excitation-secretion coupling. Tetrodotoxin makes this possible.

Tetrodotoxin is a biological substance that can be extracted from the tissues of two unrelated creatures: the puffer fish and the newt. The active substance is an amino perhydroquinazoline ($C_{11}H_{17}N_3O_8$). The structure of tetrodotoxin is known (51), but factors such as relative insolubility in water, nonvolatility, and instability at high or low pH, made structural studies laborious. Intuitive leads were hampered by the fact that tetrodotoxin was unrelated to any other biological product known at the time. The molecule is a highly polar zwitterion, and it contains a guanidinium group. Most investigators agree that the guanidinium group contributes to the neurotoxicity of the substance (52, 53). In view of the similarity in the dimensions of guanidinium and sodium, the proposal seems reasonable. However, the guanidinium group alone does not account for neurotoxicity because slight alterations of the molecule that leave the guanidinium group intact cause marked losses in activity (51, 54).

Tetrodotoxin is neurotoxic by virtue of its ability to block sodium permeability associated with action potentials (55–58). It does this without altering the resting membrane potential or the flux of other ions. Understandably, tetrodotoxin has been used in many experimental settings to study the relation between sodium (or sodium channels) and tissue excitability. Nearly a decade ago the substance had been used in so many studies that it was the subject of an excellent review (59). Besides its obvious usefulness for investigating propagated potentials, tetrodotoxin has also been invaluable to the study of cholinergic transmission because it does not block the action of endogenous or exogenous ACh. Moreover, tetrodotoxin-treated preparations release ACh in response to locally applied depolarization (60, 61). Therefore, tetrodotoxin can be used to block propagated potentials and sodium flux, without affecting synaptic and neuromuscular transmission. (Needless to say, the existence of a drug that differentially affects axonal transmission and synaptic transmission does not support the Nachmansohn model.)

Tetrodotoxin has been used to great advantage in studying the link between calcium and excitation-secretion coupling. Space does not permit consideration of the many fine studies that have appeared. As an alternative, two representative reports will be described. In one report, Katz & Miledi (62) used tetrodotoxin to study the timing of calcium action during neuromuscular transmission. Double-barreled micropipettes were inserted into the junctional region of tetrodotoxin-treated sartorius muscle. One barrel was used to apply depolarizing pulses, and the other was used to inject calcium. The interval between depolarizing pulses and iontophoretic discharge of calcium was varied. The data indicated that calcium was most effective in promoting transmitter release when it was present immediately prior to depolarization. Injection of calcium during synaptic delay did not facilitate ACh release. It was concluded that movement of calcium into nerve terminals is only the first step in a sequential process leading to transmitter release.

In another report, Weinreich (63) studied post-tetanic potentiation (PTP) in control and in tetrodotoxin-treated neuromuscular preparations. Previous work (64) had suggested that PTP might be caused by an intracellular accumulation of sodium. Tetrodotoxin was used to abolish sodium flux during repetitive stimulation associated with tetanus. It was found that PTP developed in tetrodotoxin-treated preparations just as it did in control preparations. In addition, PTP developed in muscles bathed in isotonic calcium chloride. It was concluded that PTP is dependent upon the movement of calcium rather than sodium into nerve terminals.

ACETYLCHOLINE RECEPTOR

Considerable progress has been made toward isolation and characterization of the ACh receptor. Much of this progress stems from research using α-bungarotoxin. This substance is one of several neurotoxins that can be isolated from elapid venoms. Alpha bungarotoxin is a polypeptide with 74 amino acid residues in a single chain (65). There is a remarkable degree of similarity between the structures of sea snake neurotoxins, cobra neurotoxins, and α-bungarotoxin (see references 14 and 15 for comparisons of amino acid sequence). All of these substances produce postsynaptic blockade of cholinergic transmission. This action is due to an irreversible, or only slowly reversible, binding of the toxins to the ACh receptor (66–69). The binding of α-bungarotoxin is least reversible, perhaps due to its relatively greater number of hydrophobic amino acids (14).

Generally speaking, there are two techniques that have been used in attempts to isolate the ACh receptor (70). One technique relies upon reversible agonists and antagonists, and the other relies upon irreversible antagonists. The rationale underlying the two approaches is somewhat different. With a reversible agent, an investigator can examine binding and dissociation of several drugs at each step during purification. With an irreversible agent, an investigator expedites receptor isolation. He need only monitor the whereabouts of a receptor ligand (radiolabeled) as purification proceeds.

Several biological products have been used as reversible agonists or antagonists in isolating the receptor, including ACh itself, atropine, muscarone, d-tubocurarine, and nicotine (70). There are two classes of irreversible antagonists. One class, the synthetic affinity label, has been used by Karlin and his associates (71, 72). Their technique involves the formation of a covalent bond between site-directed (affinity) compounds and the ACh receptor (73, 74). The second class of antagonists are the snake neurotoxins, of which α-bungarotoxin is the favored substance. The various methodologies are not necessarily incompatible. For example, one group has used reversible agents during isolation of the receptor and then used α-bungarotoxin to aid in confirming identity of the endproduct (75). Another group has used reversible agents as ligands in affinity chromatography, and then used α-bungarotoxin to assess purification of the chromatographically isolated receptor (76). Finally, a group has studied the interaction between snake neurotoxins and irreversible affinity labels (77). It was concluded that "neurotoxin and . . . affinity reagents have overlapping although not identical sites or modes of attachment to the receptor."

Localization of the Receptor

Because of the high specificity of α-bungarotoxin for the ACh receptor, it has proved valuable in both histochemical and biochemical research. Radiolabeled bungarotoxin has been used to localize ACh receptors autoradiographically at mouse

(78) and rat (79) neuromuscular junctions. Estimates of the number of receptors per endplate vary modestly, but the average is about 4×10^7. There is a one-to-one ratio between receptors per endplate and cholinesterase active sites per endplate (78). Similar findings have been noted for electric organs (68, 69). Comparative autoradiographs for the receptor ($^3H-\alpha$-bungarotoxin label) and for cholinesterase (^3H-diisopropylfluorophosphate label) indicate that the two molecules are different (78).

Isolation of the Receptor

Changeux et al (68) were the first to demonstrate binding of bungarotoxin to membrane fragments rich in cholinergic receptor protein. Their report was followed by studies on electric organs (69, 80–83), striated muscle (84, 85), and brain (82, 86). As might be predicted, the amount of bungarotoxin-binding protein varies from tissue to tissue, depending upon the richness of cholinergic innervation. There is also some variability in the reported molecular weight of the receptor protein, with most estimates being reasonably close to 30,000–50,000. Variability probably reflects both species differences and differences in isolation techniques.

Two surprising findings have emerged from the intense research on the ACh receptor: one deals with methodology, and the other with results. Levinson & Keynes (87) have published a report on the use of organic extraction procedures for isolation of receptor-ligand complexes. Their work was prompted by that of DeRobertis and associates, who routinely use chloroform-methanol extraction followed by column chromatography (see 88 for review). Levinson & Keynes found that ligands could be eluted from columns in a manner that suggested specific binding to a receptor, whereas binding was not in fact occurring. They concluded that earlier findings by the Argentine group (see 24) may have been artifactual.

O'Brien and associates have reported the surprising finding that the internal (89, 90) surface of axonal membranes from lobster nerves contains macromolecules that bind cholinergic drugs. Among the substances tested was α-bungarotoxin. The axonal "receptor" exhibited several properties characteristic of postsynaptic receptors. However, axonal receptors had a lower affinity than junctional receptors for ACh. It was proposed that the axonal protein that binds ACh may be a component of sodium and potassium gates. This is an important proposal, and one that should be further explored. Along this line, Raftery et al (81) did not detect significant binding of α-bungarotoxin to axons of either *Torpedo* or gar fish.

TROPHIC EFFECTS ON MUSCLE

Efferent nerves exert a variety of trophic effects on muscle (91). Among those aspects of muscle physiology that are regulated by nerve, the most important are degree of innervation, sensitivity to ACh, distribution of cholinesterases, speed of contracture, concentration of enzymes, and rate of metabolism. Typically, studies of trophic effects on muscle have involved sectioning of nerve trunks. Denervated muscles undergo profound changes, most of which are reversible following reinnervation. In such studies, muscle should preferably be pharmacologically disconnected without the trauma of nerve section. Botulinum toxin is ideally suited to this purpose.

Botulinum toxin is produced by *Clostridium botulinum,* an organism that is nearly ubiquitous in soil. The toxin is produced in several immunologically distinct forms designated types A, B, C_α and C_β, D, E, and F. The organisms are not totipotential in their ability to produce toxins; each strain produces but one type, this being true also for C_α and C_β. Type A botulinum toxin is the most potent of the group, and it has been the main subject of research. Type A toxin was originally crystallized by investigators at Camp Detrick (92, 93). The crystalline molecule has a molecular weight of approximately 1,000,000, and it is composed of at least two biologically active subunits. One of the subunits, referred to as botulinum hemagglutinin, causes agglutination of red blood cells. The other, known as botulinum neurotoxin, causes paralysis of cholinergic transmission. The two active components of type A botulinum toxin have been separated chromatographically (94). It appears that the neurotoxic fragment has a molecular weight of about 150,000 (94, 95). A claim (96) that the neurotoxin has a molecular weight in the range of 10,000 has not been confirmed (97–99).

The precise mechanism by which botulinum toxin blocks cholinergic transmission is not understood. It has been known for many years that the toxin acts at nerve terminals to prevent both nerve impulse transmission and spontaneous release of ACh (100, 101). The toxin does not act like magnesium, i.e. it is not a competitive antagonist of calcium-evoked transmitter release (102). The mechanism of action of the toxin appears to be much more complex. Recent studies (103, 104) indicate that the toxin binds rapidly and irreversibly to the neuromuscular junction, and that this binding occurs independently of transmitter release. Following binding, there is a second step that is dependent on transmitter release. In the absence of calcium, or in the presence of high magnesium concentrations, botulinum activity is greatly retarded. It may be that transmitter release exposes reactive sites in the nerve that are not otherwise available for interaction with toxin. It is interesting that another biological poison, β-bungarotoxin, has a similar dependence on transmitter release (27). It has been suggested that the active sites in botulinum toxin may be free amino groups (105, 106). This could account for the finding that botulinum toxin is inactivated by the sialic acid groups of gangliosides (107, 108). Gangliosides have frequently been suggested as important components of the transmitter releasing system (109, 110). The precise mechanism by which transmitter release is blocked by botulinum toxin is not known. Nevertheless, the certainty with which the substance paralyzes cholinergic transmission, plus the absence of any other known effects, make the toxin a highly suitable agent for functionally disconnecting nerve and muscle.

Degree of Innervation

In mammals there exists a one-to-one relationship between muscle fibers and the nerves that innervate them. Furthermore, innervated muscles will not develop additional neuromuscular contacts, even when accessory nerves are mechanically implanted. Only when a muscle has been denervated will it accept and make functional contacts with other nerves. Such findings suggest that intact nerves govern the receptivity of muscle to endplate formation. A likely candidate for the governing role is ACh. It has been demonstrated that botulinum-poisoned gastrocnemius muscle will accept implants of peroneal nerves (111). It has also been shown that new sprouts will generate from the terminal arborizations of poisoned nerves, and that these sprouts will develop contact with underlying muscle (112). The development of nerve sprouts and of muscle endplates proceeds more rapidly in slow muscle (soleus) than in fast muscle (gastrocnemius; 113, 114).

Because of the known action of botulinum toxin in blocking ACh release, the findings described above have been interpreted to mean that ACh release controls neurotization. While this is probably a valid conclusion, there is at least one limitation worth considering. It appears that a variety of substances are released from cholinergic nerves, including protein (115, 116), prostaglandin (117, 118), and ATP (119). The ability of botulinum toxin to block release of these substances has not been determined. Therefore, it is possible that an unidentified substance, by itself or in concert with ACh, regulates formation of neuromuscular contacts.

Sensitivity to Acetylcholine

The endplate region of normal muscle is highly sensitive to iontophoretically applied ACh. Sensitivity to the transmitter diminishes with distance from the junctional region. There is reason to believe that the nerve itself acts to restrict the area of maximum sensitivity. For example, following denervation there is a gradual spread of increased sensitivity (denervation supersensitivity) beyond the endplate region (120). Conversely, reinnervation causes a gradual loss of sensitivity in extra-junctional regions (121). It has been reported that supersensitivity will develop in skeletal muscle poisoned with botulinum toxin (122). In addition, spread of sensitivity appears greatest in fibers that have the lowest spontaneous release of ACh.

While it may be true that ACh release acts to restrict the chemosensitive zone, how it does this is unresolved. Spontaneous release of ACh alone is not sufficient to restrict development of denervation supersensitivity (123, 124). In fact, it may be that sensitivity is not even regulated by ACh per se, but instead by the consequence of ACh release, i.e. muscle activity. In an interesting report, Drachman & Witzke (125) studied ACh sensitivity in muscles that were electrically stimulated to mimic normal patterns of activity. They found that electrical stimulation greatly diminished the spread of supersensitivity in denervated diaphragms. The authors concluded that "muscle activity may account for neurotrophic regulation of the acetylcholine sensitivity."

Distribution of Cholinesterases

There is a complex relation between denervation and muscle cholinesterase activity. Factors such as species, duration of denervation, and muscle group under study, all contribute effects (91). Moreover, cholinesterases are both neural and muscular in origin. Thus, assays of denervated neuromuscular preparations must distinguish neural from muscular changes. Under the circumstances, the use of botulinum toxin is highly preferable to severing nerves. In studies utilizing the toxin, it has been shown that muscle cholinesterase does not depend upon ACh release. This has been demonstrated both biochemically (126) and histochemically (113). As there is evidence that muscle cholinesterase is partially under neural regulation (91), the regulatory factor must be something whose release or activity is not impaired by botulinum toxin.

Atrophy

Atrophy is a term that signifies gradual loss of metabolic and mechanical activity. It implies a deteriorative change that involves nearly the whole of muscle physiology. There is convincing evidence that ACh is the trophic factor that supports muscle integrity. The most important evidence is the repeated observation that botulinum toxin-induced neuromuscular blockade will produce atrophy (127–130). The possibility that some substance other than ACh may be implicated has been diminished by the work of Drachman (131). He has demonstrated that atrophy occurs in muscles treated with hemicholinium, d-tubocurarine, or botulinum toxin. These three drugs block ACh activity at three different sites. It is difficult to envision how they could have comparable effects on a substance other than ACh.

CONCLUDING REMARKS

The number of poisons that have been used to study cholinergic transmission, and the number of contexts in which they have been used, far exceeds the bounds of a single review. Suffice it to say, poisons are indispensable to the study of synaptic and neuromuscular transmission. Biological products that have been used range from the commonplace to the esoteric. Among the more commonly used substances, d-tubocurarine has become nearly an essential ingredient to research on postsynaptic potentials. Among those substances of unknown value are antibodies directed against specific protein and lipid components of pre- and postsynaptic membranes.

It is likely that the importance of poisons in neurobiology will increase. As our understanding of neural phenomena approaches molecular level, our need for drugs with well-defined mechanisms and sites of action increases. And thus poisons, whether biologic or synthetic in origin, will continue in a paramount role.

ACKNOWLEDGMENTS

The excellent assistance of Mrs. Ruby Hough in the literature search and in the preparation of the manuscript is gratefully acknowledged. The author is supported in part by a grant from the National Science Foundation.

Literature Cited

1. Nachmansohn, D. 1959. *Chemical and Molecular Basis of Nerve Activity.* New York: Academic. 235 pp.
2. Nachmansohn, D. 1971. *Proc. Nat. Acad. Sci. USA* 68:3170–74
3. Paton, W. D. M. 1958. *Ann. Rev. Physiol.* 20:431–70
4. Curtis, D. R. 1961. *Nervous Inhibition,* ed. E. Florey, 342–49. Oxford: Pergamon. 475 pp.
5. McLennan, H. 1963. *Synaptic Transmission.* London: Saunders. 134 pp.
6. Werman, R. 1966. *Comp. Biochem. Physiol.* 18:745–66
7. Keyl, M. J., Michaelson, J. A., Whittaker, V. P. 1957. *J. Physiol.* 139:434–54
8. Welsch, F., Dettbarn, W.-D. 1970. *J. Neurochem.* 17:927–40
9. Dettbarn, W.-D., Rosenberg, P. 1966. *J. Gen. Physiol.* 50:447–60
10. Rosenberg, P., Kremzner, L. T., McCreery, D., Willette, R. E. 1972. *Biochim. Biophys. Acta* 268:49–60

11. Rothenberg, M. A., Sprinson, D. B., Nachmansohn, D. 1948. *J. Neurophysiol.* 11:111–16
12. Rosenberg, P. 1971. *Neuropoisons: Their Pathophysiological Actions,* ed. L. L. Simpson, 111–37. New York-London: Plenum. 361 pp.
13. Rosenberg, P., Hoskin, F. C. G. 1963. *J. Gen. Physiol.* 46:1065–73
14. Lee, C. Y. 1972. *Ann. Rev. Pharmacol.* 12:265–86
15. Lee, C. Y. 1971. *Neuropoisons: Their Pathophysiological Actions,* ed. L. L. Simpson, 21–70. New York-London: Plenum. 361 pp.
16. Rosenberg, P. 1973. *Toxicon* 11:149–54
17. Kremzner, L. T., Rosenberg, P. 1971. *Biochem. Pharmacol.* 20:2953–58
18. Birks, R., Huxley, H. E., Katz, B. 1960. *J. Physiol.* 150:134–44
19. Atwood, H. L., Lang, F., Morin, W. A. 1972. *Science* 176:1353–55
20. Ceccarelli, B., Hurlbut, W. P., Mauro, A. 1972. *J. Cell. Biol.* 54:30–38
21. Heuser, J. E., Reese, T. S. 1972. *Anat. Rec.* 172:329–30
22. Perri, V., Sacchi, O., Raviola, E., Raviola, G. 1972. *Brain Res.* 39:526–29
23. Pysh, J. J., Wiley, R. G. 1972. *Science* 176:191–93
24. April, S. P. 1972. *The Effects of Divalent Cations on Spontaneous and Neurally Evoked Transmitter Release at the Crustacean NMJ.* PhD thesis. Columbia University, New York City. 203 pp.
25. Heuser, J., Miledi, R. 1971. *Proc. Roy. Soc. London B* 179:247–60
26. Chen, I.-L., Lee, C. Y. 1970. *Virchows Arch. Abt. B. Zellpath.* 6:318–25
27. Chang, C. C., Chen, T. F., Lee, C. Y. 1973. *J. Pharmacol. Exp. Ther.* 184:339–45
28. Longenecker, H. E., Hurlbut, W. P., Mauro, A., Clark, A. W. 1970. *Nature* 225:701–03
29. Clark, A. W., Mauro, A., Longenecker, H. E., Hurlbut, W. P. 1970. *Nature* 225:703–05
30. Sampayo, R. R. L. 1944. *J. Pharmacol.* 80:309–22
31. Clark, A. W., Hurlbut, W. P., Mauro, A. 1972. *J. Cell. Biol.* 52:1–14
32. Okamoto, M., Longenecker, H. E., Riker, W. F., Song, S. K. 1971. *Science* 172:733–36
33. Frontali, N., Granata, F., Parisi, P. 1972. *Biochem. Pharmacol.* 21:969–74
34. Frontali, N. 1972. *Brain Res.* 37:146–48
35. Elmqvist, S., Quastel, D. M. J. 1965. *J. Physiol.* 177:463–82
36. Ceccarelli, B., Hurlbut, W. P., Mauro, A. 1973. *J. Cell. Biol.* 57:499–524
37. Hubbard, J. I. 1970. *Progr. Biophys. Mol. Biol.* 21:33–124
38. Harvey, A. M., MacIntosh, F. C. 1940. *J. Physiol.* 97:408–16
39. Rubin, R. P. 1970. *Pharmacol. Rev.* 22:389–428
40. Del Castillo, J., Stark, L. 1952. *J. Physiol.* 116:507–15
41. Jenkinson, D. H. 1957. *J. Physiol.* 138:434–44
42. Birks, R., MacIntosh, F. C. 1961. *Can. J. Biochem. Physiol.* 39:787–827
43. Dodge, F. A., Rahamimoff, R. 1967. *J. Physiol.* 193:419–32
44. Landau, E. M. 1968. *J. Physiol.* 203:281–99
45. Hubbard, J. I., Jones, S. F., Landau, E. M. 1968. *J. Physiol.* 196:75–86
46. Cooke, J. D., Okamoto, K., Quastel, D. M. J. 1973. *J. Physiol.* 228:459–97
47. Katz, B., Miledi, R. 1965. *Proc. Roy. Soc. London B* 161:496–503
48. Miledi, R., Slater, C. R. 1966. *J. Physiol.* 184:473–98
49. Katz, B., Miledi, R. 1969. *J. Physiol.* 203:689–706
50. Heuser, J., Katz, B., Miledi, R. 1971. *Proc. Roy. Soc. London B* 178:407–15
51. Tsuda, K. et al 1964. *Chem. Pharm. Bull.* 12:642–45
52. Tsuda, K. et al 1964. *Chem. Pharm. Bull.* 12:1357–74
53. Kao, C. Y., Nishiyama, A. 1965. *J. Physiol.* 180:50–66
54. Narahashi, T., Moore, J. W., Poston, R. N. 1967. *Science* 156:976–78
55. Narahashi, T., Deguchi, T., Urakawa, N., Ohkubo, Y. 1960. *Am. J. Physiol.* 198:934–38
56. Nakajima, S., Iwasaki, S., Obata, K. 1962. *J. Gen. Physiol.* 46:97–115
57. Takata, M., Moore, J. W., Kao, C. Y., Fuhrman, F. A. 1966. *J. Gen. Physiol.* 49:977–88
58. Hille, B. 1968. *J. Gen. Physiol.* 51:199–219
59. Kao, C. Y. 1966. *Pharmacol. Rev.* 18:997–1049
60. Katz, B., Miledi, R. 1965. *Nature* 207:1097–98
61. Bloedel, J., Gage, P. W., Llinas, R., Quastel, D. M. J. 1966. *Nature* 212:49–50
62. Katz, B., Miledi, R. 1967. *J. Physiol.* 189:535–44
63. Weinreich, D. 1971. *J. Physiol.* 212:431–46
64. Birks, R. I., Cohen, M. W. 1968. *Proc. Roy. Soc. London B* 170:401–21
65. Mebs, D., Narita, K., Iwanaga, S., Samejima, Y., Lee, C. Y. 1971. *Biochem. Biophys. Res. Commun.* 44:711–16

66. Chang, C. C., Lee, C. Y. 1963. *Arch. Int. Pharmacodyn.* 144:241–57
67. Lee, C. Y., Tseng, L. F. 1966. *Toxicon* 3:281–90
68. Changeux, J.-P., Kasai, M., Lee, C. Y. 1970. *Proc. Nat. Acad. Sci. USA* 67:1241–47
69. Miledi, R., Molinoff, P., Potter, L. T. 1971. *Nature* 229:554–57
70. O'Brien, R. D., Eldefrawi, M. E., Eldefrawi, A. T. 1972. *Ann. Rev. Pharmacol.* 12:19–34
71. Karlin, A., Prives, J., Deal, W., Winnik, M. 1971. *J. Mol. Biol.* 61:175–88
72. Reiter, M. J., Cowburn, D. A., Prives, J. M., Karlin, A. 1972. *Proc. Nat. Acad. Sci. USA* 69:1168–72
73. Karlin, A., Winnik, M. 1968. *Proc. Nat. Acad. Sci. USA* 60:668–74
74. Silman, I., Karlin, A. 1969. *Science* 164:1420–21
75. Eldefrawi, M. E., Eldefrawi, A. T., Seifert, S., O'Brien, R. D. 1972. *Arch. Biochem. Biophys.* 150:210–18
76. Schmidt, J., Raftery, M. A. 1973. *Biochem.* 12:852–56
77. Prives, J. M., Reiter, M. J., Cowburn, D. A., Karlin, A. 1972. *Mol. Pharmacol.* 8:786–89
78. Barnard, E. A., Wieckowski, J., Chiu, T. H. 1971. *Nature* 234:207–9
79. Fambrough, D. M., Hartzell, H. C. 1972. *Science* 176:189–91
80. Changeux, J.-P., Meunier, J.-C., Huchet, M. 1971. *Mol. Pharmacol.* 7:538–53
81. Raftery, M. A., Schmidt, J., Clark, D. G., 1972. *Arch. Biochem. Biophys.* 152:882–86
82. Moore, W. J., Loy, N. J. 1972. *Biochem. Biophys. Res. Commun.* 46:2093–99
83. Raftery, M. A. 1973. *Arch. Biochem. Biophys.* 154:270–76
84. Miledi, R., Potter, L. T. 1971. *Nature* 233:599–603
85. Berg, D. K., Kelly, R. B., Sargent, P. B., Williamson, P., Hall, Z. W. 1972. *Proc. Nat. Acad. Sci. USA* 69:147–51
86. Bosmann, H. B. 1972. *J. Biol. Chem.* 247:130–45
87. Levinson, S. R., Keynes, R. D. 1972. *Biochim. Biophys. Acta* 288:241–47
88. DeRobertis, E. 1971. *Science* 171:963–71
89. Denburg, J. L., Eldefrawi, M. E., O'Brien, R. D. 1972. *Proc. Nat. Acad. Sci. USA* 69:177–81
90. Denburg, J. L., O'Brien, R. D. 1973. *J. Med. Chem.* 16:57–60
91. Guth, L. 1968. *Physiol. Rev.* 48:645–87
92. Abrams, A., Kegeles, G., Hottle, G. A. 1946. *J. Biol. Chem.* 164:63–79

93. Lamanna, C., McElroy, O. E., Eklund, H. W. 1946. *Science* 103:613–14
94. DasGupta, B. R., Boroff, D. A., Rothstein, E. 1966. *Biochem. Biophys. Res. Commun.* 22:750–56
95. DasGupta, B. R., Boroff, D. A. 1968. *J. Biol. Chem.* 243:1065–72
96. Gerwing, J., Dolman, C. E., Bains, H. S. 1965. *J. Bacteriol.* 89:1383–86
97. Boroff, D. A., DasGupta, B. R., Fleck, U. S. 1968. *J. Bacteriol.* 95:1738–44
98. Hauschild, A. H. W., Hilsheimer, R. 1968. *Can. J. Microbiol.* 14:805–7
99. Knox, J. N., Brown, W. P., Spero, L. 1970. *Infect. Immunol.* 1:205–6
100. Burgen, A. S. V., Dickens, F., Zatman, L. J. 1949. *J. Physiol.* 109:10–24
101. Brooks, V. B. 1956. *J. Physiol.* 134:264–77
102. Simpson, L. L., Tapp, J. T. 1967. *Neuropharmacol.* 6:485–92
103. Simpson, L. L. 1971. *Neuropharmacol.* 10:673–84
104. Simpson, L. L. 1973. *Neuropharmacol.* 12:165–76
105. Schantz, E. J., Spero, L. 1957. *J. Am. Chem. Soc.* 79:1623–25
106. Spero, L., Schantz, E. J. 1957. *J. Am. Chem. Soc.* 79:1625–28
107. Simpson, L. L., Rapport, M. M. 1971. *J. Neurochem.* 18:1341–43
108. Simpson, L. L., Rapport, M. M. 1971. *J. Neurochem.* 18:1751–59
109. Burton, M. R., Howard, R. E., Baer, S., Balfour, Y. M. 1964. *Biochim. Biophys. Acta* 84:441–47
110. Kuriyama, K., Roberts, E., Vos, J. 1968. *Brain Res.* 9:231–52
111. Fex, S., Sonesson, B., Thesleff, S., Zelena, J. 1966. *J. Physiol.* 184:872–82
112. Duchen, L. W., Strich, S. J. 1968. *Quart. J. Exp. Physiol.* 53:84–89
113. Duchen, L. W. 1970. *J. Neurol. Neurosurg. Psychiat.* 33:40–54
114. Duchen, L. W. 1971. *J. Neurol. Sci.* 14:47–60
115. Matsuda, T., Saito, K., Katsuki, S., Hata, F., Yoshida, H. 1971. *J. Neurochem.* 18:713–19
116. Musick, J., Hubbard, J. I. 1972. *Nature* 237:279–81
117. Ramwell, P. W., Shaw, J. E., Kucharski, J. 1965. *Science* 149:1390–91
118. Laity, J. L. H. 1969. *Brit. J. Pharmacol.* 37:698–704
119. Silinsky, E., Hubbard, J. I. 1973. *Nature* 243:404–5
120. Axelsson, J., Thesleff, S. 1959. *J. Physiol.* 147:178–93
121. Miledi, R. 1960. *J. Physiol.* 154:190–205
122. Thesleff, S. 1960. *J. Physiol.* 151:598–607

123. Birks, R., Katz, B., Miledi, R. 1960. *J. Physiol.* 150:145–68
124. Miledi, R. 1960. *J. Physiol.* 151:1–23
125. Drachman, D. B., Witzke, F. 1972. *Science* 176:514–16
126. Stromblad, B. C. R. 1960. *Experientia* 16:458–60
127. Jirmanova, I., Sobotkova, M., Thesleff, S., Zelena, J. 1964. *Physiol. Bohemoslov.* 13:467–72
128. Drachman, D. B. 1964. *Science* 145: 719–21
129. Drachman, D. B. 1967. *Arch. Neurol.* 17:206–18
130. Duchen, L. W. 1971. *J. Neurol. Sci.* 14:61–74
131. Drachman, D. B. 1971. *Neuropoisons: Their Pathophysiological Actions,* ed. L. L. Simpson, 325–48. New York-London: Plenum. 361 pp.

APPLICATION OF QUANTUM CHEMISTRY TO DRUGS AND THEIR INTERACTIONS

❖6596

Jack Peter Green, Carl L. Johnson, and Sungzong Kang
Department of Pharmacology, Mount Sinai School of Medicine, of the City University of New York, New York, NY

INTRODUCTION

Whether or not quantum mechanics is the supreme intellectual accomplishment of man—an allegation that appears less of a conceit as one reads its history (1–3)—it has certainly fostered philosophical speculation (1, 4–7) and a great deal of very practical achievements. It is reassuring to learn that quantum mechanics does not exclude life (8) and at the same time that it can account for laboratory observations that otherwise elude explanation. Molecular orbital (MO) methods, which have been more widely applied than the other method of quantum mechanics (the valence-bond or resonance method), have explained many of the physical and chemical properties of molecules of interest to the chemist (9–15). Evidence is accumulating that MO methods can also explain the physical and chemical properties of large biomolecules and, by inference, their biological activities (16–18). The relative ionization potentials and dipole moments of a series of purines (18, 19) were consistent with those predicted ten years earlier in the Pullmans' laboratory by MO theory. MO calculations on biomolecules have yielded information in agreement with that obtained by nuclear magnetic resonance spectroscopy (20–23), infrared spectroscopy (20), X-ray diffraction analysis (21, 24, 25) and, reasonably, with circular dichroic spectra (26). In most of this work, the results of the calculations have clear biological implications even to enzymatic mechanisms (16, 17, 27–32). Many of the inferences from MO calculations have been supported by subsequent experiment, a surprising number in consideration of the simple methods available when this work began and the inherent shortcomings of even modern MO techniques.

Despite these successes in accounting for the biological *properties* of molecules, there has been much less effort to use quantum-mechanical methods to account for the biological *effects* of molecules. This relative lack is strange, because the first application of quantum mechanics in biology was to analyze carcinogenic hydrocar-

319

bons. This work, begun by the Pullmans in the mid-forties (16, 33, 34), showed electronic correlates of carcinogenicity that have in large part been sustained (16, 35–42) even though the techniques they were obliged to use in this early work were primitive. It was in fact this success with the carcinogens that stimulated the use of quantum mechanics in biochemistry (16). Applications to pharmacology were sparse (43) even into the late fifties and early sixties. At a symposium in 1965, a review and some calculations of indoles were presented, but the paper was mainly a hortative plea that quantum mechanics be applied to pharmacology (44). Enough work has since been done to have impelled several reviews (45–50).

It has become clear that an understanding of the reactions of drugs with tissues or tissue components must rest on an understanding of the fundamental particles that control these events, the electrons and atomic nuclei that comprise the drug and its receptor. Such understanding requires information about the structural features of the molecules, the energies and distribution of the electrons, and the spatial arrangement of the atomic cores. Quantum mechanics provides such a description of matter, and molecular orbital theory is a quantum mechanical approach conveniently adapted to large molecules. It can yield quantitative information on electronic structure and on the geometry of molecules. Excellent texts and reviews of molecular orbital theory and methods are available at varying levels of formalism (9–13, 16, 20, 51–67). For the purposes of this article in this short space, it is sufficient to describe the information that these methods yield, particularly that which is germane to this article.

Theoretically, all the properties of the molecule are described in the wave equation. But existing techniques fall considerably short of that goal. Until recently, MO methods were confined to Hückel (H) method which considers only the π-electrons, i.e. the delocalized electrons that are usually pictured as contributing to double or triple bonds but that are extended over the whole conjugated part of the molecule. This highly approximative method has accounted for some of the chemical and biological behavior of aromatic compounds, probably because the π-electrons are the determinants of activity in many of these compounds. From the H method was developed the ω modification and then the Parr-Pariser-Pople (PPP) method which unlike the H procedure, includes an approximation to interelectron repulsion. The Del Re method was developed to include the localized σ electrons. A major step was taken with the simultaneous inclusion of both σ and π electrons: the extended Hückel (EH); CNDO (complete neglect of differential overlap) and modifications, e.g. CNDO/2; INDO (intermediate neglect of differential overlap); and the modified INDO (MINDO). Another approximate total valence technique is PCILO (Perturbative Configuration Interaction Using Localized Orbitals). Most recently various *ab initio* techniques have been applied to biologically interesting compounds (68–74). Not always do the all-valence and *ab initio* methods give a better account of aromatic properties than does the simple H (14, 60, 75–77), but the availability of these more sophisticated methods provides a means of studying saturated substances, saturated side-chains, conformation of molecules, and molecular interactions (73). The applications of these different methods to biomolecules has been reviewed (24, 73, 78), and their successes and failures in accounting for the properties of chemicals have been compared (14, 79–81). The enormous amount of work done with these methods on many different types of molecules vitiates any generality on their respective advantages. However, it is beginning to appear that the PCILO method gives a more realistic picture of molecular conformation than do other methods (21, 82). The CNDO/2 and INDO methods may best describe charge distributions, as they give dipole moments that most nearly correspond with measured ones, and the calculated electron densities correlate with the chemical shifts as measured by NMR spectroscopy (13).

In the development of these methods, the results of the calculations are compared with experimental facts; and in the semi-empirical methods, the method is adjusted to fit the laboratory results from, say, X-ray diffraction analysis, various spectroscopies, measurements of ionization potential, dipole moments, etc (14, 79–81). When results show agreement with laboratory findings in groups of molecules, the method is extended to other molecules. Although these methods evolve from abstract, inductive reasoning which historically was necessitated by anomalous laboratory findings that could not be explained by existing theories, they are rooted, as quantum mechanics has always been, in laboratory data. If the quantum chemical view of an electron is imaginary, then it is, like Marianne Moore's definition of a poem, "an imaginary garden with real toads in it."

As so much effort in quantum mechanics is directed to devise methods that reflect empirical laboratory findings, one may ask why not forego the computations and get on with the measurements. There are several practical reasons for using quantum mechanics. First, there is the hope, however wistful, that methodological advances will eventually provide a proper solution to the wave equation that will then yield all the properties of a molecule. Meantime the existing methods produce correct relative values of physicochemical measurements that can be determined by experiment either with great difficulty or not at all: resonance energies, dipole moments, ionization potentials, electron affinities, charges on atoms, transition states. And the studies can be carried out on molecules not yet available, the results of which can suggest what compounds to synthesize.

MO studies of molecular conformation proceed much more rapidly than by X-ray diffraction analysis and NMR spectroscopy. The conformation obtained by X-ray diffraction analysis is influenced by the free energy of crystal packing, which is not a consideration in a biological system. Crystal structure is influenced by intramolecular and intermolecular forces that may not occur in a biological system. Intramolecular forces, which are determinant of the conformation of large molecules like proteins, are less important in the conformation of molecules of pharmacological interest in a biological milieu; and intermolecular associations between two identical molecules are even less likely in a biological milieu. Also X-ray studies must often be done on salts of the compound of interest, e.g. acetylcholine chloride or bromide, which may not reflect the conformation of the free cation. Of great advantage in conformational studies is that MO calculations reveal the relative likelihood of occurrence of all possible conformers. At the very least, MO theory can account for the unmeasurable events that give rise to the observed ones, and in helping to interpret experiments it can suggest new ones. This assertion of the value and purpose of molecular orbital studies in no way denigrates the value of other methods. Information from all sources will have to be used to infer the conformation of molecules at a biological site and the forces controlling their biological activities.

Studies of molecular conformation or geometry are carried out by calculating the energies of a series of possible configurations of the rotatable bonds. For example, the atoms of the side-chain of an aromatic biogenic amine, $-CH_2-CH_2-NH_2$, are rotated with respect to each other and with respect to the aromatic ring (the geometries of all aromatic rings are virtually planar and fixed). For each rotamer, the energies are calculated to determine the relative likelihood of existence of the various conformations.

Electronic characteristics are expressed as reactivity indices. The energy of the highest occupied molecular orbital (E_H) correlates with ionization potential and indicates ability of a molecule to donate an electron. It contributes to charge transfer complexation. The energy of the lowest empty molecular orbital (E_L) correlates with electron affinities and polarigraphic reduction potentials and indicates ability of a molecule to accept an electron. Also it contributes to charge transfer complexes. The electron density of atom r, q_r, describes the electronic charge in the region of the atom; it can be used to calculate dipole moments. The net charge of atom r, q^n_r, is obtained by subtracting from q_r the number of electrons considered as contributed by that atom to the molecule. Frontier electron density in the case of an electron-donating reaction, f^e_r, is the electronic density in the E_H associated with atom r. For an electron-accepting reaction, f^n_r, is the electronic density in E_L associated with atom r.

Frontier density is associated with electron transfer rather than electrostatic interaction. Superdelocalizability (S_r) indicates the stabilization energy in the formation of a complex with another molecule; for an electron-donating reaction it is large when the electron density in the highest occupied orbital is large. The approximate superdelocalizability (S'_r) reflects the degree of contribution of the frontier orbitals to S: if the frontier electrons play a more significant role in the course of reaction than do the other π-electrons, the S'_r would be a better index of reactivity than is S_r, for the latter, by including the other electrons, can obscure the contribution of the frontier electrons. These indices are relatively simple to calculate and are formally similar to other indices that have been described: S_r to Wheland's localization energy, and S'_r to Dewar's approximate localization energy (57, 61, 62).

Static indices such as q_r have been surprisingly successful in correlating with chemical reactivity, probably because they mimic what is happening in the transition state: in the application of static indices, especially to a series of similar compounds, it is assumed that relative electronic structures are altered in a similar way or that the initial and transitional states are similar especially for very reactive molecules (83, 84). But it cannot be presumed that the electronic properties in the initial and transitional state are similar. Relative reactivity varies with the magnitude of the perturbation of the molecule by another (83, 84). S and localization energy (and the formally equivalent indices) are dynamic indices that reflect the transition state during a chemical reaction. Perturbation theory has been expanded

(83–85) and considered in drug-receptor interactions (46). In another method (86) a transition state for the enzymatic reduction of acetophenone was approximated by calculating the interaction energy as a hydride ion approached the carbonyl group of the acetophenone. In addition the energy difference between the ground state and the approach to a transition state was calculated. Others have calculated the electrostatic energy generated around the molecule by the approach of a charge and applied these methods to biomolecules (73, 87, 88) and to cholinergic agents (89, 90). It is likely that these approaches will have wide application in pharmacology.

SCOPE AND LIMITATIONS

Quantum mechanics is used as a tool to learn the molecular forces determining drug activity. This information can be used to infer the nature of the biological substances with which the drug reacts and hopefully as a guide to the synthesis of useful new agents. Like any other tool or any laboratory procedure, quantum mechanics can give rise to spurious or misleading information, and its use requires the same critical sense in resisting a too facile conclusion that one needs in evaluating data from ultraviolet spectroscopy, X-ray diffraction analysis, or from any other source.

MO theory has been used to study the conformation of drugs with the hypothesis that the results are applicable to the conformation of drugs at the receptor site and that the results can also help in the understanding of the structure of the active site of the receptor or enzyme reacting with the drug. In this work, the total energy of the molecule is calculated as a function of bond rotation with bond lengths and bond angles being held constant to avoid an impractical computing problem. It is clear, however, that the conformational energies are influenced by bond lengths and angles: the *ab initio* calculation (91) of acetylcholine (ACh) based on the bond lengths and angles from X-ray studies of ACh chloride showed the *gauche* form to be 3.2 kcal/mole more stable than the *trans,* whereas with the standard geometric input the *trans* form is 3.4 kcal/mole more stable than the *gauche* (91). Analogously, PCILO calculations based on geometric input from X-ray studies of ACh chloride or ACh bromide produced different preferred conformers of ACh (92). A similar ambiguity was found in studies of acetyl-α(R)-methylcholine (92), based on two geometric inputs derived from the same crystal. However, the differences are small (about 5 kcal/mole) and do not invalidate the conclusion that the most stable conformer is found in the vicinity of the theoretically calculated lowest conformation. Implicit in all this is the fact that X-ray studies present similar ambiguities, the salt form influencing conformation; and even in a single unit cell, one compound can have more than one conformation.

As it is unlikely that the conformation calculated to have the lowest energy is necessarily the conformer at the receptor, or the only important conformer, it is necessary to decide from the energy map what conformers are allowable. A consideration of 20 kcal/mole as an upper limit is high (93), for it often includes all possible conformers, i.e. the entire energy contour of mescaline is less than 10 kcal/mole (94). It is reasonable to suggest that all conformers within 6 kcal/mole of the conformer of lowest energy be considered allowable. Within this falls hydrogen bonding energy, electrostatic forces, van der Waals forces, and usually charge-transfer energy. This range of energy minima could encompass environmental effects. MO studies do not otherwise consider the environment, a fault shared by laboratory studies of conformation carried out on crystals or simple aqueous solutions. Also, the probability of finding conformers in various energy minima depends not only on the differences in energy but also on the width of the energy minima.

Some MO methods like X-ray studies suggest important conformers with intramolecular interactions that may not occur in a solvent. The CNDO and INDO methods especially overestimate nonbonded attractive forces; the EH method underestimate them. The PCILO method gives conformations of drugs (95) more nearly like those found in crystals than do the other methods. The relative energies of specific rotamers vary with different methods, as has been shown for ACh (91–93, 96–98), but in this example, all methods showed the *gauche* form to be more stable than the *trans,* in agreement with experiment (99–104). Whatever ambiguities evolve from MO studies on conformation can be reduced by studying series of similar compounds, as pharmacologists and medicinal chemists and crystallographers have always done.

The other objective in MO calculations on drugs is to account for the relationship between chemical structure and biological activity. In this work, studies are made on a series of structurally related substances differing in potency but appearing to act on the same receptor. Environmental effects are not considered, as it is assumed that they would alter the relative electronic structures of similar compounds in a consistent way. Attempts are made to find electronic indices of reactivity that correlate, preferably in a quantitative way, with potency. From the correlation, one attempts to deduce some information about the receptor. Implicit in the correlation are predictions of the activities of compounds not yet tested, the synthesis and examination of which not only tests the initial inference but could result in interesting and useful new compounds.

MO theory considers the molecule as a unit, not simply its specific atoms or groups. For example, putting a substituent on an aromatic ring, e.g. a hydroxyl group on the ring of tryptamine, influences the whole ring system. The π-electron cloud now has a different shape, and the distortion results in the alteration of the reactivity of other atoms in the ring. A hydroxyl group in different positions of the ring (e.g. 4-, 5-, or 6-hydroxytryptamine) alters the electronic characteristics in different ways in atoms far removed from the hydroxy group (44). Each molecule has properties different from its component system. In some instances, particularly for saturated portions of a molecule, substitution leads to only small changes in the electronic properties of atoms remote from the site of substitution. This circumstance raises a question about the significance of these indices in regressions analysis programs. Examination of this question in a series of molecules led to the conclusion (105) that both CNDO and *ab initio* methods are probably adequate for predicting qualitative charge variations in atoms separated from a molecular modification by as many as three saturated bonds. In general, EH charges correlated with CNDO charges but were exaggerated approximately threefold. For atoms far removed from the modification site, EHT predicted essentially random charge variations with respect to the CNDO results; therefore EH should be used with caution in structure-activity studies. This type of analysis indicates only that the CNDO and *ab initio* methods are reasonably self-consistent. The fact that these methods also yield quantitatively realistic estimates of certain experimentally measurable quantities, such as dipole moments, suggests that the calculated charge densities may be physically meaningful, although correlation of a charge term (or any other index) with biological activity does not imply a cause–effect relationship.

One of the hypotheses in this work is that the indices do in fact relate to chemical reactivity. Although many correlations between these indices and different types of chemical and biological activity have been found, there is no assurance that the indices describe reaction mechanisms. As noted above, the static properties of a molecule are probably different from those of the molecule when it is perturbed by a receptor or a chemical reagent, and the examples where MO theory correctly predicted chemical properties could be fortuitous, the ground state reflecting the perturbed state while still differing from it. Nevertheless, with the correlation is a testable prediction that depends on the assumption that the new compound(s) differ only quantitatively from the others. If it is found to differ qualitatively, the new finding may be more interesting than the correlation. If the quantitative activity is correctly predicted and with enough compounds, the inferences are supported, although it would be difficult to hold that the molecular mechanisms are truly understood (Ptolemaic astronomy accurately predicted eclipses) without independent chemical evidence.

Extrapolating from the electronic correlate of pharmacological activity to mechanism is less risky if the pharmacological activity is relatively free of competing reactions. A drug given to a whole animal is subject to many independent processes, all of which should have an independent correlate (44): absorption, distribution, binding to plasma proteins and other sites of loss ("silent receptors"), penetration through special membranes (e.g. the blood–brain barrier), enzymatic metabolism (sometimes to an active compound), and excretion. At the site of action, the compounds must have the same mechanism of action (drugs may cause the same gross effect by different mechanisms) and must act at the same site. At the site of action, potency is a function of both affinity for the receptor and intrinsic activity (106–108). The correlate is mechanistically more meaningful when the number of intervening biological steps are reduced to a minimum, e.g. intrinsic activity or K_I for an enzyme inhibitor. When the biological measurement requires many intervening steps, e.g. the potency of hallucinogens, the hope for a simple correlate diminishes. One becomes dependent on the assumption that all compounds are similarly susceptible to the intervening reactions, e.g. metabolic destruction; one can use multiple regression analysis to find the independent variables that account for activity. Work reviewed below shows that more than one variable is often needed to account for the relative potencies of similar compounds. For even in an isolated system, e.g. a muscle in a bath, the relative potency of congeners in causing contraction is influenced by the activity of the metabolizing enzyme (109) and ability to penetrate the tissue (110).

In most studies trying to relate chemical structure to biological activity, it is assumed that agonists and competitive antagonists act at the same receptor, the latter having affinity but no intrinsic activity. This assumption may not hold for all compounds. For example, it has been suggested that the receptors for agonist and antagonist opioids differ (111). The nonselectivity of many antagonists, their faint structural similarity to their agonists, and their large size suggest that antagonists may not neatly fit the receptor but react with sites adjoining the receptor (106). Other experiments have shown the exquisite selectivity of some receptors, e.g. the muscarinic and nicotinic receptors (106), even in particulate material (112).

In view of all these complexities it is appropriate that studies attempting to account for pharmacological activity not be confined to one approach. As noted below, MO methods can be fruitfully combined with empirical methods (113) that account for properties, e.g. lipid solubility, imperfectly handled by MO methods (114). This eclectic approach could yield inferences about receptor mechanisms complementing those obtained by isolation techniques (112, 115).

APPLICATIONS TO SPECIFIC SUBSTANCES

Cholinergic Substances

On the basis of EH calculations (96, 116) the nature of the cholinergic receptor was suggested, the difference between nicotinic and muscarinic activity being determined by the conformation of the $-C-O-C-CH_3$ portion of ACh, $120°$ for the nicotinic site and $180°$ for the muscarinic site (96, 117). The interatomic distances for muscarinic activity were suggested to be: $N-O_1 = 3.0–3.4$ Å, $N-O_2 = 5.4–5.8$ Å [or 4.4–5.6 Å in a later paper (118)], and $O_1-O_2 = 2.2–3.4$ Å. Neither X-ray studies (119) nor INDO (93) CNDO (120) PCILO calculations (92) support such flexibility of $-C-O-C-CH_3$; all show this angle to be $180°$. A similar model had been proposed (121, 122) without the aid of MO theory which also tried to explain the different activities of enantiomers: $L(+)$-muscarine is 700 times more potent than the $D(-)$-enantiomer, and $D(-)$-muscarone is three times more potent than the $L(+)$-enantiomer. The interheteroatomic distances of the enantiomers are the same. The deduction (96, 117) that the $N-O_1$ distance is 3.0–3.4 Å is not supported by the activities of rigid muscarinic compounds such as arecoline, pilocarpine, and others (123), in all of which the $N-O_1$ distance is 4.4 Å. Also, a model requiring three heteroatoms cannot account for the muscarinic activity of meprochol (123) which lacks a carbonyl oxygen or any analogous atom. Finally, the proposed model is a *gauche* form; the studies on three different types of rigid muscarinic agonists show that the *trans* form is active (124–126). It is interesting that preference of a *gauche* form is suggested by all MO calculations (although the *trans* form is not ruled out) and by X-ray (119) and NMR (99, 127–129) studies; yet work on rigid molecules show the *trans* form to be active at the muscarinic site.

All the MO calculations show that the positive charge of the onium head is spread out over the attached methyl groups, the nitrogen itself being electronegative as had been shown in another quaternary nitrogen compound (130).

The electronic structure of muscarine (131), nicotine (131), 3-acetoxyquinuclidine (132), and phencyclidines (89, 90) show clear analogies to that of ACh. Both the CNDO/2 and EH calculations (133) yield a relatively greater net negative charge on the carbonyl oxygen of carbamylcholine than that of ACh, a difference that fits with the suggestion (134) that the magnitude of this charge is a determinant of nicotinic activity.

The nicotinic activity of a series of nine compounds, mostly phenyl choline ethers, paralleled the H E_H (135). The search for an atom-localized correlate of the activities of phenyl choline ethers showed that $S\frac{E}{2}$ (135–138), $S\frac{E}{4}$ (135), and f^E of the ether oxygen (138) inexactly paralleled activity. These results could imply that these compounds may interact with the nicotinic receptor through a charge-transfer reaction involving electron donation from the phenyl ring or the ether oxygen or both. EH calculations of phenyl choline ether (139) showed that the distance separating the 2-position of the ring from the onium group is nearly the same as that between the carbonyl oxygen and the onium group in ACh.

All calculations on ACh show a positively charged carbon of the carbonyl group, which Wilson had suggested (140) reacts with a nucleophilic site on cholinesterase, and a positively charged onium head that reacts with the anionic site. All-valence electron calculations suggest that the enzymatic hydrolysis of acetylcholine is an exception to the postulate that hydrolysis usually occurs at a bond between atoms that both carry net positive charges (16). PCILO calculations showed that acetylthiocholine, which is a good substrate for acetylcholinesterase, is exclusively in the *trans* form (141) in agreement with X-ray (142) and NMR (127) studies.

The rate of hydrolysis of a series of nine phenyl acetates by butyrylcholinesterase, though not by acetylcholinesterase, correlated with $f\frac{E}{1}$ (136, 137), suggesting that the carbon at the 1-position of the phenyl ring is involved in binding to the active site of the enzyme through electron donation. The positive π-charge, derived from the H method, on the phosphorus atom of three organophosphate congeners paralleled their potencies as inhibitors of cholinesterase, a relationship that was also obtained with diisopropyl phosphofluoridate and mepafox (143), in agreement with the idea that inhibitory potency depends on the affinity of the phosphorus atom for an electron-rich site of the enzyme. The potency of four nicotinic acid derivatives in inhibiting acetylcholinesterase correlated with f^N of the carbonyl carbon (137), implying that this atom is the acceptor for electron transfer from a nucleophilic site in the enzyme, presumably the same site that attacks the carbonyl carbon of ACh. It was also suggested that the ring nitrogen binds to the anionic site of the esterase. One factor that tended to reflect cholinesterase inhibition in five carbamoylpiperidines was the net charge on the amide nitrogen, activity increasing as the nitrogen becomes more positive (144, 145). It was suggested that this circumstance increases the electrostatic attraction between the amide nitrogen and the serine hydroxyl group of the enzyme (146). The inference that a hydrogen bond is involved in the interaction of 3-hydroxyphenyltrimethylammonium derivatives with cholinesterase (147) was supported by σ-π calculations on six of these derivatives (148). An EH calculation on the cholinesterase reactivator, pralidoxime (i.e. 2-PAM), showed that the oxygen atom is strongly electronegative (130) which could account for its serving as a nucleophile in reactivating phosphorylated cholinesterase according to the mechanism proposed by Wilson (140).

Factors contributing to the potencies of 21 aryl-substituted styrylpyridines in inhibiting rat brain choline acetyltransferase correlated (149) with the sums of the S^E and the sums of the total charges of all atoms on the aryl portion of the molecule (H method). These sums had been shown to correlate with partition coefficient (150).

Other MO calculations have been done on cholinergic agonists and cholinesterase inhibitors (151–158).

Adrenergic Substances

Based on an EH study of ephedrine and ψ-ephedrine, a model for the alpha adrenergic receptor pharmacophore was proposed involving a *trans* arrangement of phenyl and amino groups and a β-OH to amino nitrogen distance of 2.9 Å (159). Favorable and unfavorable arrangements of the phenyl ring and α-methyl groups were proposed to explain the rank order of potency of the four ephedrine isomers. This model was supported by the X-ray crystallographic study of (–) norepinephrine (160) and a subsequent EH study of the same molecule (161). The distance of the β-OH to center of the ring was shown as 2.5 Å (158) and changed to 3.6 Å (162).

An INDO calculation on norepinephrine showed that the *gauche* arrangement of phenyl and amino groups was 2.5 kcal/mole more stable than the *trans* form, a difference that would not exclude either form as possible receptor pharmacophores (163). The O–N distance in either the *trans* or *gauche* conformations would be the same, 2.9 Å. PCILO calculations (164) on phenylethylamines as well as naphazoline, an α-adrenergic agent of significantly different structure, suggested a similar model for the α-receptor pharmacophore, a N to β-O distance of 2.8 Å, a N to ring center distance of 5.1 Å, and a N to ring plane distance of 1.3 Å. Some support for this model was provided by PCILO calculations (165) on α-sympatholytics having the molecular structure ϕ-O-C-C-N (e.g. piperoxan). The calculations showed preferred conformations for these antagonists that give interatomic distances like those noted above. It has been suggested that the selectivity for α- or β-receptors observed in norepinephrine or isoproterenol was due either to an effect of the N-alkyl group on *gauche/trans* conformational preference (166) or to changes in the charge of the onium group with substitution (167). Neither of these theories was verified by EH conformational studies or by CNDO and *ab initio* charge calculations (168). It was suggested that α-activity requires an unhindered onium hydrogen atom whereas β-activity depends on the presence of an alkyl substituent capable of dispersion interaction with the receptor, this interaction being optimal with the isopropyl group. Studies on rigid analogs of the phenylethanolamines (3-amino-2-phenyl-*trans* -2-decalols) cast considerable doubt on the significance of the MO preferred conformations: four isomers, one *trans* and three *gauche* arrangements of the β-OH and amino groups, were equipotent on α-receptors in the rat vas deferens (169).

CNDO calculations on norepinephrine and dopamine showed that the *gauche* forms were slightly more stable than the *trans*; it was suggested that an interatomic distance between two heteroatoms of about 6 Å was required for the uptake process at adrenergic nerve terminals (170). In a related CNDO study of polyhydroxy-phenylethylamines the following requirements for activity in long-term reduction of cardiac norepinephrine uptake were proposed: an interatomic distance between two heteroatoms of about 6 Å, ease of oxidation to 1,4-quinones by anion-radical mechanisms when a third hydroxyl group is present in the ring, and adequate uptake at the active site (171).

Other H calculations on adrenergic substances have been published (172, 173).

Dopaminergic Substances

EH calculations (174) suggested that dopamine, unlike norepinephrine and ephedrine, could exist only in a *gauche* conformation, results allegedly supported by NMR data. These observations were used as evidence for dissimilarity in the adrenergic and dopaminergic receptors. Other EH calculations (175, 176) as well as NMR (175) and X-ray studies (177) showed the *trans* form of dopamine to be only slightly more stable than the *gauche* forms. A PCILO calculation also indicated that the *trans* and *gauche* forms had about the same energy (164).

A comparison of the two N–O interatomic distances in one of the *gauche* conformations of dopamine and the N–N and N–O distances in the EH preferred conformation of oxotremorine (178) led to the proposal that tremorogenic compounds react with the same receptor. To test this idea, 18 drugs, as different as possible from dopamine and oxotremorine yet with the appropriate heteroatom distances fixed in a rigid molecule, were examined for dopaminergic properties. The results were negative (179).

Inhibition of synaptosomal dopamine uptake by six antihistaminic pheniramines was correlated with the E_H values from ω-Hückel calculations (180). It is confusing that this is an inverse correlation: the greater the electron-donating capacity of the molecule, the poorer the inhibitory activity. The significance of the E_H values in this study is not clear since both electron donating and withdrawing groups change E_H in the same direction, and the E_H orbital appears as an anti-bonding orbital, probably in artifact of the method of calculation.

Serotonergic Substances

Based on EH calculations of 5-hydroxytryptamine (5-HT), which showed only one preferred conformation (extended), a model was proposed (181) for the serotonergic pharmacophore consisting of three heteroatoms separated by specific distances: hydroxyl to alkylamine of 7.0 Å, hydroxyl to indole nitrogen of 5.7 Å, and indole nitrogen to alkylamine of 5.8 Å. There appears to be little justification for including the hydroxyl group as a part of the model pharmacophore, because other tryptamine derivatives without this function are active at 5-HT receptors. The prediction that only the extended conformation is energetically allowed was not confirmed by a more extensive EH calculation (182). The extended conformation was only slightly more stable then the folded conformations. INDO (183) and PCILO (184) calculations indicated that the folded forms were more stable than the extended. However, the few kcal/mole differences in the energies of the various low-energy conformers did not warrant exclusion of any of them as pharmacophore models (182, 185, 186).

Both extended and folded forms have been observed experimentally (187–189). The fact that the extended form of 5-HT and the rigid LSD molecule have a somewhat similar arrangement of heteroatoms and the fact that LSD acts on the 5-HT receptors in many pharmacological systems were offered (181) as support for the postulated pharmacophoric pattern (also see section on hallucinogens).

The potencies of 5-substituted tryptamines in contracting the rat fundus strip correlated with the resonance contribution of the substituents to the indole ring (190) as estimated by the empirical resonance parameters. This result suggested that the effect of the substituent group on potency was related to an effect on the π-electron density of the indole ring. INDO calculations on a larger number of derivatives supported this hypothesis and demonstrated several correlations of potency with charge densities and frontier electron densities at the C-4 and C-5 positions of the ring (191). It was suggested that the greater potency of 5-HT was mainly due to the influence of the hydroxy group on the electronic structure of the indole ring.

In an effort to explain the neuroleptic activities of chlorpromazine and haloperidol, the EH-preferred conformations (192) of these compounds were compared with those of dopamine and 5-HT obtained in previous EH studies. The pattern of heteroatom distances in the neuroleptics was not consistent with the predicted conformations of dopamine but was stated to be similar to the serotonergic pharmacophore. The amine to hydroxy distance in 5-HT was stated to be 5.6 Å in this paper, whereas in the original study (181) and subsequent reviews (117, 193) this distance was given as 6.96 Å.

Histaminergic Substances

Histamine has dual receptor activity: stimulation of H_1 receptors (e.g. guinea pig ileum) which is blocked by the conventional antihistamines, and stimulation of H_2 receptors (e.g. gastric secretion) which is blocked by burimamide (194). EH calculations on histamine showed two equally stable conformations with amino nitrogen – imino nitrogen interatomic distances of 4.55 and 3.60 Å (195). From molecular models of a potent H_1-antihistamine, triprolidine, an amino nitrogen-pyridyl nitrogen distance of 4.8 ± 0.2 Å was obtained, suggesting that the conformation of histamine relevant to H_1 receptor activity had a N–N distance of 4.55 Å; the second conformation with N–N of 3.6 Å was proposed as the H_2-receptor pharmacophore (195). NMR studies supported the EH conformations (196–198) but not those from other methods (199, 200). Only the extended form (equivalent to the postulated H_1 pharmacophore) was observed in crystals of histamine free base and histamine dication (201–203). Support for the extended form of histamine as the H_1 pharmacophore has also been provided by X-ray crystallography on the H_1-antihistamines, methapyrilene • HCl (204), and brompheniramine maleate (205). However, in the latter study the N–N distance was found to be 5.3 Å, considerably larger than the 4.6 Å predicted for the histamine pharmacophore. This comparison of histamine and antihistamine structures may be misleading because many of the latter do not have a nitrogen in a position analogous to the ring nitrogen of histamine. It is also questionable to assume that an aryl carbon atom could act as a ring nitrogen.

Comparison of EH calculations on histamine and molecular models of anti-ulcer compounds (which may not be appropriate) suggested a model for the H_2 pharmacophore involving two heteroatoms, 3.7 ± 0.2 Å apart, one with lone pair electrons in a σ-type hybrid orbital and the other involved in a π-electron system (206). It was stated that the model is supported by EH calculations of the preferred conformations of two anti-ulcer drugs, 2-phenyl-2-(2-pyridyl)thioacetamide (206) and prostaglandin E_1 (207). The rigid structures of two other anti-ulcer drugs give N–N or N–O distances of 3.8 Å in agreement with the model.

Several experimental studies argue against the proposed H_1 and H_2 pharmacophore models (195). N,N-dimethylhistamine, in which the *trans* isomer is preferred over *gauche* forms, is more active as a gastric stimulant than histamine and is less active than histamine on H_1 receptors (197). *trans*-2-(4-Imidazolyl)cyclopropylamine has weak but significant activity at H_2 receptors (208). EH calculated *trans/gauche* ratios for α- and β-methyl- and N,N-dimethylhistamines are quite different, yet none of these compounds shows selectivity for H_1 or H_2 receptors; 2- and 4-methylhistamines, on the other hand, have very similar conformer ratios but show a marked difference in receptor selectivity (198).

The relatively high activity of 4-methylhistamine on H_2 receptors and very weak activity on H_1 receptors and the observation that the 4-methyl group precludes a planar extended conformation has led to a new model for the H_1 pharmacophore in which the ethylamine side chain is coplanar with the imadazole ring in a *trans* conformation with N–N distance of 5.1 Å (209).

Hallucinogens

Early H calculations (210) on LSD suggested that its unusually high E_H might account for the activity of this drug. In a series of seven hallucinogens (including LSD, tryptamines, and methoxyamphetamines) a good correlation was found between activity and H E_H values (44, 211). These results were confirmed and extended by INDO calculations to 12 hallucinogenic methoxyamphetamines and to a series of N,N-dimethyltryptamines (212, 213). INDO calculations showed that E_H values do not correlate with potency among structurally different hallucinogens (213). It is also worth noting that since E_H values are sensitive to the conformation of aromatic ring substituents such as methoxy groups, care should be taken in interpretation of correlations based on calculations of molecules of uncertain geometry. E_H values do not adequately explain the presence of hallucinogenic activity in dialkyl-substituted tryptamines as opposed to the lack of activity in the nonalkylated analogs. Recent INDO calculation (186) and modified H calculations (214) on some LSD analogs failed to uncover any relationship between hallucinogenic potency and E_H. Thus, it is not clear that E_H is a realistic correlate of hallucinogen potency. This question can only be answered by testing the predictions stemming from apparent correlations with E_H (212, 213). One such prediction, that 7-hydroxy-2-aminotetralin would be mescaline-like (213) has been experimentally verified in animals (215).

The question of whether a charge-transfer reaction is involved in the mechanism of action of these psychotomimetics as implied by the E_H correlations has been approached experimentally by spectroscopic studies of donor-acceptor complexes.

Only moderate electron donating power among indoles and methylsergate was found, suggesting that LSD is not as good an electron donor as indicated by H calculations (216). A correlation was observed between hallucinogenic potency of eight methoxylated amphetamines and ability to form a molecular complex with the electron acceptor, 1,4-dinitrobenzene; three other amphetamines did not fit the correlation (217). It was suggested that the lack of correlation of E_H values among the different hallucinogens (LSD, tryptamines, and amphetamines) and the relatively low potency of the latter two groups of drugs may rest on the fact that only a small proportion of a dose of these hallucinogens exists in the correct conformation for binding to the LSD receptor (94, 186). It has also been emphasized (44) that such a molecularly gross characteristic as high E_H, possessed by many substances, cannot explain so specific a biological activity, and that E_H is probably correlated with a more subtle molecular characteristic.

It was suggested that the conformations of the hallucinogenic tryptamines (e.g. psilocin) and phenylalkylamines (e.g. methoxyamphetamines) at the receptor were such that their six-membered aromatic rings were congruent with the A ring of LSD, and their alkylamino nitrogens were congruent with the amino nitrogen of LSD (213). The stereochemical arguments upon which this model was based are supported by NMR studies (218) and biological experiments including the mescaline-like activity of rigid structures related to mescaline (215, 219). The proposed conformations of psilocin and mescaline are congruent with LSD within 3 kcal/mole of the global minimum (94). PCILO calculations on phenylethylamine (164) showed similar results. Thus only small energy barriers—less than the energy of a hydrogen bond—need to be overcome in order to attain close congruency. These energy barriers, however, could be sufficient to result in a relatively small amount of the appropriate conformer being available to the receptor, a circumstance that could partly account for the relatively low potencies of these compounds compared with LSD.

If LSD interacts with 5-HT receptors it is possible that a close congruence of the amines and aromatic rings is required for binding to the receptor. INDO calculations showed that the conformation of 5-HT having *closest* congruence to LSD was about 10 kcal/mole above the global minimum and 4 kcal/mole above a nearby local minimum (182, 183). A point should be made concerning this comparison of the energy of a particular conformation to an energy minimum. It is obvious that an energy minimum occurs due to specific stabilizing effects. In some cases, the stabilizing effects may be observed in the isolated molecule, but their presence in solution may be unlikely because of solvent effects. This may well be the situation for the global minimum in the 5-HT map because this conformation appears to be stabilized by N–H—π-electron hydrogen bonding (83). It is probably more reasonable in this case to compare the congruent conformation to the nearby local minimum.

EH calculations have also been made on cannabinoids (220).

Neuroleptics

The phenothiazines have been a subject of interest since H calculations suggested (16, 210) that they could function as electron donors, which was supported by other calculations (221–225) and, importantly, by measurements of ionization potentials (see 16, 223) and charge-transfer complexation (226, 227). There was no correlation between potency of neuroleptics (phenothiazines, butyrophenones, and others) and stabilization energies of their complexes with chloranil (227).

PCILO calculations (228) on promazine showed that it is folded along the N–S axis, the angle between the two planes being 140°. X-ray studies (229, 230) showed that chlorpromazine and two other phenothiazine tranquilizers are folded to the same degree. The degree of folding influenced the conformation of the side-chain, a finding supported by the PCILO calculations (228). EH calculations (192) on chlorpromazine and haloperidol showed similar distances between two heteroatoms, a conclusion not supported by the PCILO and crystallographic studies.

Other Neurally Active Substances

PCILO calculations (231) indicated that three local anesthetics, with side-chains of different lengths, have allowable conformers in which the distance between the carbonyl oxygen and amino groups is about 4.1 Å. In other local anesthetics this distance was significantly less than 4.1 Å, and in cocaine the distance between these groups is large, about 5.7 Å. In cocaine the distance between the ester oxygen near the phenyl ring and the carbonyl oxygen of the other ester group is about 4.1 Å (231), and the possibility was raised that the cabonyl oxygen of cocaine is positioned similarly to the amino group of the other local anesthetics (231). The functional implication of this positioning is not clear. It is unlikely that an oxygen in cocaine functions as the amino group in other local anesthetics through their lone pair electrons. Quaternary amines, which lack a lone pair, are effective local anesthetics, and further, an amino group is not required for activity, e.g. benzocaine (232, 233). In the PCILO calculations (231) it was assumed that a *trans* relationship exists between the carbonyl oxygen and the amino group in both ethanolamino and propanolamino local anesthetics; studies on cyclic analogs suggest that a *trans* configuration is important in the ethanolamine derivative, whereas a *gauche* configuration is important in the propanolamine (234). Dreiding models of these cyclic compounds show that despite these different configurations, the distance between the ester oxygen and nitrogen atoms is 3.6–3.7 Å; in two other cyclic derivatives with activity this distance was 4.2 and 2.9 Å (234).

In one attempt to account for the relative potency of eight anilide local anesthetics, the interaction between each compound and the electron-acceptor thiamine was considered (235) because spectroscopic observations showed that local anesthetics form complexes with thiamine. Each compound was sterically oriented to the pyrimidine ring of thiamine to maximize the electrostatic attactions. Stabilization energy, calculated by the H method, tended to correlate with local anesthetic potency (235).

In a large and heterogeneous group of substances, ranging from methyl alcohol to tricyclic compounds, the ability to block excitation of a frog nerve was a function of the polarizability and the H E_H (236). Examination of the data suggests that polarizability is a sufficient correlate of potency, the introduction of E_H not significantly improving the correlation.

The conformations of five barbiturates obtained by the PCILO method agreed well with available crystallographic studies. Noncyclic aliphatic substituents tend to fold toward the barbiturate ring, whereas cyclohexanyl and phenyl substituents eclipse the bonds attached to C-5 of the barbiturate ring. The substituents had little effect on the atomic charges of the ring (237). EH and CNDO/2 calculations of 19 compounds, barbiturates, and related anticonvulsants, failed to reveal any electronic correlate with biological activity (105).

A correlation between the analgesic activity of six aryl ethers of imidazolinyl methanol, substituted on the benzene ring, could be accounted for by a combination of E_H (Huckel) and the lipophilic substituent (238), suggesting that both charge-transfer and hydrophobic bonding are important in determining activity.

Other calculations of local anesthetics have appeared (239, 240). Morphine has been calculated by two methods (225, 241) and acetanilide (242) and salicylic acid (243) by the CNDO/2 method. Iproniazid was calculated by the PCILO method (244) and α-aminobutyric acid by the EH method (245).

Metabolism

MO calculations have been applied to the oxidation, reduction, and conjugation of pharmacological substances. Correlations with MO indices have sometimes been obtained.

The results of MO calculations on hydroxylation and oxidation allow no generality on mechanisms to emerge, and the conclusion of ten years ago, that metabolic hydroxylation is difficult to explain on the basis of the electronic properties of the ground state, appears valid today (246). Enzymatic hydroxylation of aromatic heterocycles occurs on electronegative sites, implicating electrophilic species like OH^+. No evidence for the occurrence of a hydroxyl cation has been found (247). It has been postulated that in some enzymatic oxygenations the attack is made by an oxygen with an oxenoid structure, defined as an electrophilic particle with six valence electrons (247), but it is not known how this could be formed from molecular oxygen. Hydroxylation of proline and lysine in collagen synthesis occurs on the carbons with the most negative EH charge, also suggesting an electrophilic mechanism (248). The rate of oxidative N-demethylation of six derivatives of 4-dimethylaminoazobenzenes, some of which are carcinogens, correlated with the H π-electron density on the amino nitrogen (249). The rate of O-demethylation seemed to depend on the net positive charge of the oxygen (250). The site of oxidation of purines by xanthine oxidase was suggested to be nucleophilic with OH^- serving as a nucleophilic agent (251, cf 252). For oxidation by ceruloplasmin, amines seemed to require a high E_H, as deduced from the H method (253).

Four possible mechanisms were considered for dechlorination of chlorethanes by the microsomal oxidase system (254): (a) radical or anionic displacement of a H by an OH group; (b) insertion of an O between a C–H bond; (c) radical cleavage of either a C–H or C–Cl bond; (d) anionic displacement of a Cl by an OH group. Nine compounds were calculated by the iterative EH method. The rate of dechlorination did not correlate with the C–Cl bond order, the carbon charge, or the Cl charge, suggesting that C–Cl bond cleavage was not the initial rate-determining step. Similarly, dechlorination did not correlate with C–H bond order, the carbon charge, or the H charge, suggesting that C–H bond cleavage, including insertion of an O in the C–H bond, was not the initial reaction. However, dechlorination did correlate rather well with the degree of electron deficiency in the most electron-deficient carbon valence orbital (the orbital involved exclusively in bonding to the Cl atom), which indicates that anionic attack by an OH⁻ group might occur at this orbital. A fair correlation was noted between dechlorination and the number of nonbonding electrons on the Cl atom, suggesting that C–Cl cleavage may be by C–Cl—H–R bond formation with a proton of the enzyme. Preliminary results with OH⁻ approach and Cl⁻ loss indicate that initial bonding overlap of the approaching OH⁻ group is indeed with the electron-deficient carbon orbital noted above and that C–Cl bond order (a measure of the strength of the bond) rapidly and preferentially drops as the OH⁻ group approaches.

Among antimetabolites that inhibit dihydrofolate reductase studied by the H method, both the 2-amino group and N–1 in the antimetabolites were, by these calculations, shown to be more basic than the corresponding groups in folic acid (255, 256). Basicity was calculated by a method (257) that has been criticized (258) but which gave values that correlated with measured pK_a's (259) and with potency in inhibiting the enzyme (260, 261). It was also suggested that for compounds to be active as substrates, the 4-substituent must have a positive charge greater than 0.1, which is reduced to a lower value by the enzyme, and are thereby displaced easily from the enzyme by other substrate molecules. In a challenge of these inferences, it was observed (262) that the p-aminobenzoylglutamic acid portion of the molecules was ignored in the calculations, that alkylation of the 2,4-diamino groups results in inhibitors with low activity, that insertion of phenyl groups in the pyrazine ring increases activity, and that the atom deduced to be most basic from calculations is not the one that is alkylated. It should be noted that ignoring the p-aminobenzoylglutamic does not imply that it is inconsequential; it is a necessary portion of the molecules, but, as it occurs in all analogs its contribution to the varied potencies of the molecules is constant and it would have a slight and consistent effect on the electronic characteristics of the pyrimidine portion of the ring. The fall in activity with alkylation could be attributable to a steric effect. Increased activity of phenyl derivatives could be accounted for by increased van der Waals or hydrophobic binding. The fact that the apparently most basic atom is not alkylated could be explained by factors other than basicity determining alkylation; also, the electronic correlate that seems to imply basicity may in fact indicate a more subtle kind of reactivity.

Inhibition of enzymatic conversion of orotic acid into uridine monophosphate by five orotic acid analogs correlated with f_i^r by the H method (263).

Both the EH and CNDO/2 methods were applied to the analysis of ten acetophenones that are substrates for a reductase (86). In this work, attempts were made to mimic the reduction of the compounds by studying the effect on the carbonyl carbon of an approaching hydride ion and to calculate the energy differences between the approach to a transition state with the hydride ion and the ground state of the molecules. Although the correlations of substrate reactivity with the MO indices were not quite as good as those obtained with the empirical constants, i.e. Hammett and Hansch, a significant correlation was found between charge density near the carbonyl carbon atom and V_{max}. Similar results were obtained with E_L or incipient-transition state energy difference, which is the difference between the ground state energy and the energy in the presence of a hydride ion near the carbonyl carbon. The meaning of the correlation with the transition state energy difference is hard to understand, because the energy difference is greater with a greater V_{max}. The values for the electron density for the carbonyl group (0.3 Å above the carbon) do not vary much with substitution: less than 0.002 electron by CNDO. A further confusion is that the EH and CNDO/2 values are quite different in magnitude and sign.

With the PPP method, the rate of phosphorylation of 15 adenosine analogs tended to correlate with f^e of N–3 (264). It was suggested that a magnesium chelate may form among this nitrogen, the 5'-hydroxyl group, and adenosine kinase. No evidence for such a chelate has appeared.

Data are not strong in supporting the idea that the rate of enzymatic acetylation of amines is reflected in π-electronic charge of the nitrogen atom (265). It was suggested that the rate of deacetylation reflected the dispositivity of the dissociable bond (265), but the data supporting this idea are also inconclusive. A dipositive bond is not required for deacetylation of acetylcholine (see above).

The H electronic charge on the hydroxyl oxygen of a series of coumarins seemed to reflect the extent to which they are conjugated in vivo (43), and H E_H reflected the inhibition of histamine methyltransferase (222). The potency of ten coumarins in inducing hepatic drug-metabolizing enzymes could be accounted for by several regression equations (266): in one equation, the lipophilic component, E_H, and the net charges on the carbonyl carbon and oxygen while in another, the lipophilic component, E_H, and the net charges on the ring oxygen and the carbonyl carbon. The third and best correlation was the electronic transition energy (the difference between E_H and E_L) and the net charges at the ring oxygen and carbonyl carbon. These and the other correlations, all obtained with the EH method, implicate in enzyme induction the –O–C–O portion of the molecule, perhaps as a site of electron transfer or of H-bonding. It was suggested that the electronic transition, indicating the excitation energy of the molecule, may reflect the free energy of reaction or activation. It may be interesting that inclusion of the electronic transition term made inclusion of the lipophilic term gratuitous.

ACKNOWLEDGMENTS

This work was supported by a grant (MH 17489–04) from the National Institute of Mental Health. We thank Dr. K. P. Dressler for suggestions, Mr. Michael Bergamini for a stimulating conversation, and Miss Doris Jaeger for help in the library.

Literature Cited

1. Heisenberg, W. 1971. *Physics and Beyond. Encounters and Conversations.* New York: Harper and Row. 247 pp.
2. Mulliken, R. S. 1967. *Science* 157: 13–24
3. Mulliken, R. S. 1970. *Pure Appl. Chem.* 24:203–15
4. Reichenbach, H. 1965. *Philosophic Foundations of Quantum Mechanics.* Berkeley: Univ. Calif. Press. 182 pp.
5. Petersen, A. 1968. *Quantum Physics and The Philosophical Tradition.* Cambridge: MIT. 200 pp.
6. Andrade e Silva, J., Lochak, G. 1969. *Quanta.* New York: McGraw. 255 pp.
7. Hoffmann, B. 1959. *The Strange Story of the Quantum.* New York: Dover. 285 pp.
8. Landsberg, P. T. 1964. *Nature* 203: 928–30
9. Daudel, R., Lefebvre, R., Moser, C. 1959. *Quantum Chemistry.* New York: Interscience. 572 pp.
10. Salem, L. 1966. *The Molecular Orbital Theory of Conjugated Systems.* New York: Benjamin. 567 pp.
11. Streitwieser, A. Jr. 1966. *Molecular Orbital Theory for Organic Chemists.* New York: Wiley. 489 pp.
12. Dewar, M. J. S. 1969. *The Molecular Orbital Theory of Organic Chemistry.* New York: McGraw. 484 pp.
13. Pople, J. A., Beveridge, D. L., Ostlund, N. S. 1967. *Int. J. Quantum Chem.* 1s:293–305
14. Dewar, M. J. S. 1971. *Fortschr. Chem. Forsch.* 23:1–30
15. Trinajstić, N. 1971. *Rec. Chem. Prog.* 32:85–97
16. Pullman, B., Pullman, A. 1963. *Quantum Biochemistry.* New York: Interscience. 867 pp.
17. Pullman, B. 1969. *Ann. NY Acad. Sci.* 158:1–19
18. Pullman, A., Pullman, B. 1972. *Jerusalem Symp. Quantum Chem. Biochem. Pt. 4, The Purines—Theory and Experiment,* ed. E. D. Bergmann, B. Pullman, 1–20. Jerusalem: Israel Acad. Sci. 61 pp.
19. Bergmann, E. D., Weiler-Feilchenfeld, H., Lifshitz, C. 1969. *Jerusalem Symp. Quantum Chem. Biochem. Pt. 1, Physico-Chemical Mechanisms of Carcinagenesis,* ed. E. D. Bergmann, B. Pullman, 72–77. Jerusalem: Israel Acad. Sci. Humanities. 338 pp.
20. Náray-Szabo, G. 1971. *Kémiai Közlemények* 36:293–310
21. Saran, A., Pullman, B., Perahia, D. 1972. *Biochim. Biophys. Acta* 287: 211–31
22. Günther, H. 1972. *Angew. Chem. Int. Ed. Engl.* 11:861–74
23. Blagdon, E. D., Rivier, J., Goodman, B. 1973. *Proc. Nat. Acad. Sci. USA* 70: 1166–68
24. Pullman, B. 1971. *Aspects De La Chimie Quantique Contemporaine,* ed. R. Daudel, A. Pullman, 261–301. Paris: Centre Nat. Rech. Sci. 339 pp.
25. Long, K. R., Goldstein, J. H. 1972. *Theor. Chim. Acta* 27:75–79
26. Bailey, M. L. 1972. *Biopolymers* 11: 1091–1102
27. Fischer-Hjalmars, I. 1969. *Quart. Rev. Biophys.* 1:311–45
28. Rein, R., Renugopalakrishnan, V., Bernard, E. A. 1971. *Proc. Eur. Congr. Biophys., 1st,* 6:35–41
29. Comorosan, S., Murgoci, P. 1971. *Bull. Math. Biophys.* 33:373–86
30. Alving, R. E., Laki, K. 1972. *J. Theor. Biol.* 34:199–214
31. Gasper, R. 1972. *Acta Biochim. Biophys.* 7:275–84
32. Davydov, A. S. 1973. *J. Theor. Biol.* 38:559–69
33. Coulson, C. A. 1953. *Advan. Cancer Res.* 1:1–56
34. Pullman, A., Pullman, B. 1955. *Advan. Cancer Res.* 3:117–69
35. Daudel, P., Daudel R. 1966. *Chemical Carcinogenesis and Molecular Biology.* New York: Interscience. 158 pp.
36. Chalvet, O., Daudel, P., Daudel, R., Moser, C., Prodi, J. 1966. *Wave Mechanics and Molecular Biology,* ed. L. de Broglie, 106–30. Reading, Mass.: Addison-Wesley. 186 pp.
37. Dipple, A., Lawley, P. D., Brookes, P. 1968. *Eur. J. Cancer* 4:493–506
38. Pullman, A., Pullman, B. See Ref. 19, pp. 9–24
39. Meyer, A. V., Bergmann, E. D. See Ref. 19, pp. 78–84
40. Hoffmann, F. 1969. *Theor. Chim. Acta* 15:393–412
41. Popp, F. A. 1972. *Z. Naturforsch. B* 27:850–63
42. Grover, P. L., Hewer, A., Sims, P. 1972. *Biochem. Pharmacol.* 21:2713–26
43. Pullman, B. 1964. *Electronic Aspects of Biochemistry,* ed. B. Pullman, 559–78. New York: Academic. 582 pp.

44. Green, J. P. 1967. *Molecular Basis of Some Aspects of Mental Activity,* ed. O. Walaas, 2:96–111. New York: Academic. 515 pp.
45. Schnaare, R. L., Martin, A. N. 1965. *J. Pharm. Sci.* 54:1707–13
46. Cammarata, A. 1968. *J. Med. Chem.* 11:1111–15
47. Kier, L. B. 1971. *Molecular Orbital Theory in Drug Research.* New York: Academic. 258 pp.
48. Purcell, W. P., Clayton, J. B. 1971 *Advan. Chem. Ser.* 108:123–40
49. Schnaare, R. L. 1971 *Drug Design,* ed. E. J. Ariens, 1:405–49. New York: Academic. 581 pp.
50. Kier, L. B. 1972. *Advan. Chem. Ser.* 114:278–97
51. Liberles, A. 1966. *Introduction to Molecular-Orbital Theory,* New York: Holt, Rinehart and Winston. 198 pp.
52. Arcos, J. C., Argus, M. F., Wolf, G. 1968. *Chemical Induction of Cancer.* 1:88–224. New York: Academic. 491 pp.
53. Jaffé, H. H. 1962. *Comprehensive Biochemistry. Vol. I, Atomic and Molecular Structure,* ed. M. Florkin, E. H. Statz, 34–112. New York: Elsevier. 253 pp.
54. Sebera, D. K. 1964. *Electronic Structure and Chemical Bonding.* New York: Blaisdell. 298 pp.
55. Fernández-Alonso, J. I. 1964. *Advan. Chem. Phys.* 7:3–84
56. de Broglie, L., Ed. 1966. *Wave Mechanics and Molecular Biology.* Reading, Mass.: Addison-Wesley. 186 pp.
57. Fukui, K. 1964. *Molecular Orbitals in Chemistry, Physics and Biology,* ed. P. O. Lowdin, B. Pullman, 513–38. New York: Academic. 578 pp.
58. Pullman, A. 1964. *Molecular Biophysics,* ed. B. Pullman, M. Weissbluth, 81–115. New York: Academic. 452 pp.
59. Ladik, J. 1972. *Quantenbiochemie für Chemiker und Biologen.* Stuttgart: Ferdinand Enke. 252 pp.
60. Löwdin, P. O. 1968. *Molecular Associations in Biology,* ed. B. Pullman, 539–49. New York: Academic. 571 pp.
61. Greenwood, H. H. 1972. *Computing Methods in Quantum Organic Chemistry.* New York: Wiley—Interscience. 213 pp.
62. Fukui, K. 1970. *Fortschr. Chem. Forsch.* 15:1–85
63. von Bunau, G. 1972. *Angew. Chem. Int. Ed. Engl.* 11:393–404
64. Pauling, L. E. 1960. *The Nature of the Chemical Bond.* Ithaca, NY: Cornell Univ. 644 pp.
65. Murrell, J. N., Harget, A. J. 1972. *Semi-Empirical Self-Consistent-Field Molecular Orbital Theory of Molecules.* New York: Wiley-Interscience. 180 pp.
66. Eyring, H., Ed. 1970. *Physical Chemistry. An Advanced Treatise. Vol. V, Valency.* New York: Academic. 732 pp.
67. McWeeny, R. 1972. *Quantum Mechanics: Principles and Formalism.* New York: Pergamon. 155 pp.
68. Ryan, J. A., Whitten, J. L. 1972. *J. Am. Chem. Soc.* 94:2396–2400
69. Jansen, H. B., Ros, P. 1972. *Theor. Chim. Acta* 27:95–107
70. Del Bene, J. E., Pople, J. A. 1973. *J. Chem. Phys.* 58:3605–8
71. Newton, M. D. 1973. *J. Am. Chem. Soc.* 95:256–8
72. Shipman, L. L., Christoffersen, R. E. 1973. *J. Am. Chem. Soc.* 95:4733–44
73. Pullman, A. 1972. *Forschr. Chem. Forsch.* 31:45–103
74. Perricaudet, M., Pullman, A. 1973. *Int. J. Peptide Protein Res.* 5:99–108
75. Pullman, B. 1969. *Int. J. Quantum Chem.* 3s:83–102
76. Castro, E. A., Sorarrain, O. M. 1972. *J. Chim. Phys. Physiochim. Biol.* 69:513–55
77. Murrell, J. N., Schmidt, W., Taylor, R. 1973. *J. Chem. Soc. Perkin Trans. 2,* 179–81
78. Bergmann, E. D., Pullman, B. 1973. See Ref. 19, Pt. 5. *Conformation of Biological Molecules and Polymers.* 831 pp.
79. Jaffé, H. H. 1969. *Accounts Chem. Res.* 2:136–43
80. Klopman, G., O'Leary, B. 1970. *Fortschr. Chem. Forsch.* 15:445–534
81. Pople, J. A. See Ref. 24, pp. 17–33
82. Perahia, D., Pullman, A. 1973. *Chem. Phys. Lett.* 19:73–75
83. Klopman, G., Hudson, R. F. 1967. *Theor. Chim. Acta* 8:165–74
84. Klopman, G. 1968. *J. Am. Chem. Soc.* 90:223–34
85. Yanez, M., Macias, A., Fernandez-Alonso, J. I. 1972. *Chem. Phys. Lett.* 17:63–65
86. Hermann, R. B., Culp, H. W., McMahon, R. E., Marsh, M. M. 1969. *J. Med. Chem.* 12:749–54
87. Bonaccorsi, R., Pullman, A., Scrocco, E., Tomasi, J. 1972. *Theor. Chim. Acta* 24:51–60
88. Giessner-Prettre, C., Pullman, A. 1972. *Theor. Chim. Acta* 25:83–88
89. Strebrenik, S., Weinstein, H., Pauncz, R. 1973. In preparation

90. Weinstein, H., Maayani, S., Srebrenik, S., Cohen, S., Sokolorsky, M. 1973. In preparation
91. Pont, G. N. J., Pullman, A. 1973. *J. Am. Chem. Soc.* 95:4059–60
92. Pullman, B. Courrière, P. 1972. *Mol. Pharmacol.* 8:612–22
93. Radna, R. J., Beveridge, D. L., Bender, A. L. 1973. *J. Am. Chem. Soc.* 95: 3831–42
94. Kang, S., Johnson, C. L., Green, J. P. 1973. *Mol. Pharmacol.* 9:640–48
95. Pullman, B., Courrière, P. 1973. See Ref. 19, *Pt. 5. Conformation of Biological Molecules and Polymers,* 547–68
96. Kier, L. B. 1967. *Mol. Pharmacol.* 3: 487–94
97. Beveridge, D. L., Radna, R. J. 1971. *J. Am. Chem. Soc.* 93:3759–64
98. Genson, D. W., Christoffersen, R. E. 1973. *J. Am. Chem. Soc.* 95:362–68
99. Culvernor, C. C. J., Ham, N. S. 1966. *Chem. Commun.* 15:537–39
100. Canepa, F. G., Pauling, P., Sörum, H. 1966. *Nature* 210:907–9
101. Martin-Smith, M., Smail, G. A., Stenlake, J. B. 1967. *J. Pharm. Pharmacol.* 19:649–59
102. Shefter, E., Mautner, H. G. 1969. *Proc. Nat. Acad. Sci. USA* 63:1253–60
103. Brennan, T. F., Ross, F. K., Hamilton, W. C., Shefter, E. 1970. *J. Pharm. Pharmacol.* 22:724–25
104. Herdklotz, J. K., Sass, R. L. 1970. *Biochem. Biophys. Res. Commun.* 40: 583–88
105. Andrews, P. R. 1969. *J. Med. Chem.* 12:761–64
106. Ariëns, E. J. 1971. See Ref. 49, pp. 1–270
107. Blank, M. 1972. *J. Colloid Interface Sci.* 38:470–76
108. Rang, H. P. 1973. *Neurosci. Res. Program Bull.* 11:220–24
109. Vane, J. R. 1959. *Brit. J. Pharmacol.* 14:87–98
110. Handschumacher, R. E., Vane, J. R. 1967. *Brit. J. Pharmacol.* 29:105–18
111. Collier, H. O. J. 1969 *Scientific Basis of Drug Dependence,* ed. H. Steinberg, 49–65. London: Churchill. 429 pp.
112. O'Brien, R. D. 1973. *Neurosci. Res. Program Bull.* 11:242–46
113. Hansch, C. 1971. See Ref. 49, pp. 271–342
114. Cammarata, A., Rogers, K. S. 1971. *J. Med. Chem.* 14:269–74
115. Cuatrecasas, P. 1973. *Neurosci. Res. Program Bull.* 11:215–19

116. Kier, L. B. 1968. *Mol. Pharmacol.* 4: 70–76
117. Kier, L. B. 1970. *Fundamental Concepts in Drug-Receptor Interactions,* Ed. J. F. Canielli, J. F. Moran, D. J. Triggle, 15–45. New York: Academic. 261 pp.
118. Jhon, M. S., Cho, U. I., Chae, Y. B., Kier, L. B. 1972. *Daehan Hwahak Hwoejee* 16:70–73
119. Baker, R., Chothia, C., Pauling, P., Weber, H. 1973. *Mol. Pharmacol.* 9:23–32
120. Saran, A., Govil, G. 1972. *J. Theor. Biol.* 37:181–85
121. Beckett, A. H., Harper, N. J., Clitherow, J. W., Lesser, E. 1961. *Nature* 189:671–73
122. Beckett, A. H. 1967. *Ann. NY Acad. Sci.* 144:675–88
123. Beers, W. H., Reich, E. 1970. *Nature* 228:917–22
124. Smissman, E. E., Nelson, W. L., LaPidus, J. B., Day, J. L. 1966. *J. Med. Chem.* 9:458–65
125. Chiou, C. Y., Long, J. P., Cannon, J. G., Armstrong, P. D. 1969. *J. Pharmacol. Exp. Ther.* 166:243–48
126. Robinson, J. B., Belleau, B., Cox, B. 1969. *J. Med. Chem.* 12:848–51
127. Cushley, R. J., Mautner, H. G. 1970. *Tetrahedron* 26:2151–59
128. Behr, J. P., Lehn, J. M. 1972. *Biochem. Biophys. Res. Commun.* 49:1573–79
129. Chynoweth, K. R., Ternai, B., Simeral, L. S., Maciel, G. E. 1973. *Mol. Pharmacol.* 9:144–51
130. Giordano, W., Hamann, J. R., Harkins, J. J., Kaufman, J. J. 1968. *Proc. Int. Pharmacol. Congr., 3rd, 1966* 7:327–54
131. Pullman, B., Courrière, P., Coubeils, J. L. 1971. *Mol. Pharmacol.* 7:397–405
132. Weinstein, H., Apfelderfer, B. Z., Cohen, S., Maayani, S., Sokolovsky, M. 1973. See Ref. 19, *pt. 5. Conformation of Biological Molecules and Polymers.* 531–46
133. Ajo, D. et al 1972. *J. Theor. Biol.* 34: 15–20
134. Sekul, A. A., Holland, W. C. 1963. *Arch. Int. Pharmacodyn.* 146:93–98
135. Crow, J., Wassermann, O., Holland, W. C. 1969. *J. Med. Chem.* 12:764–66
136. Inouye, A., Shinagawa, Y. 1962. *Bull. Chem. Soc. Jap.* 35:701–6
137. Inouye, A., Shinagawa, Y., Takaishi, Y. 1963. *Arch. Int. Pharmacodyn.* 144: 319–36
138. Fukui, K., Nagata, C., Imamura, A. 1960. *Science* 132:87–89
139. Kier, L. B., George, J. M. 1971. *J. Med. Chem.* 14:80–81

140. Wilson, I. B. 1959. *Fed. Proc.* 18: 752–58
141. Pullman, B., Courrière, P. 1972. *Mol. Pharmacol.* 8:371–73
142. Chothia, C., Pauling, P. 1969. *Nature* 223:919–21
143. Pullman, B., Valdemoro, C. 1960. *Biochim. Biophys. Acta* 43:548–50
144. Purcell, W. P. 1966. *J. Med. Chem.* 9: 294–97
145. Millner, O. E., Purcell, W. P. 1971. *J. Med. Chem.* 14:1134–36
146. Purcell, W. P., Beasley, J. G., Quintana, R. P., Singer, J. A. 1966. *J. Med. Chem.* 9:297–303
147. Wilson, I. B., Quan, C. 1958. *Arch Biochem. Biophys.* 73:131–38
148. Cammarata, A., Stein, R. L. 1968. *J. Med. Chem.* 11:829–33
149. Allen, R. C., Carlson, G. L., Cavallito, C. J. 1970. *J. Med. Chem.* 13:909–12
150. Rogers, K. S., Cammarata, A. 1969. *J. Med. Chem.* 12:692–97
151. Fukui, K., Morokuma, K., Nagata, C., Imamura, A. 1961. *Bull. Chem. Soc. Jap.* 34:1224–27
152. Neely, W. B. 1965. *Mol. Pharmacol.* 1:137–44
153. Ban, T., Nagata, C. 1966. *Jap. J. Pharmacol.* 16:32–38
154. Mutschler, E., Scherf, H., Wassermann, O. 1967. *Arzeim. Forsch.* 17:833–37
155. Mutschler, E., Wassermann, O., Woog, H. 1967. *Arzneim. Forsch.* 17:837–41
156. Crow, J. W., Holland, W. C. 1972. *J. Med. Chem.* 15:429
157. Crow, J. W. *J. Med. Chem.* In press
158. Farkas, M., Kruglyak, J. A. 1969. *Nature* 223:523–24
159. Kier, L. B. 1968. *J. Pharmacol. Exp. Ther.* 164:75–81
160. Carlstrom, D., Bergin, R. 1967. *Acta Crystallogr. B* 23:313–19
161. Kier, L. B. 1969. *J. Pharm. Pharmacol.* 21:93–96
162. Kier, L. B. See Ref. 47, p. 187
163. Pedersen, L., Hoskins, R. E., Cable, H. 1971. *J. Pharm. Pharmacol.* 23:217–19
164. Pullman, B., Coubeils, J. L., Courrière, P., Gervais, J.-P. 1972. *J. Med. Chem.* 15:17–23
165. Coubeils, J. L., Courrière, P., Pullman, B. 1972. *J. Med. Chem.* 15:453–55
166. Larsen, A. A. 1969. *Nature* 224:25–26
167. Pratesi, P., Grava, E. 1965. *Advan. Drug Res.* 2:127–42
168. George, J. M., Kier, L. B., Hoyland, J. R. 1971. *Mol. Pharmacol.* 7:328–36
169. Smissman, E. E., Gastrock, W. H. 1968. *J. Med. Chem.* 11:860–64

170. Katz, R., Heller, S. R., Jacobson, A. E. 1973. *Mol. Pharmacol.* 9:486–94
171. Katz, R., Jacobson, A. E. 1973. *Mol. Pharmacol.* 9:495–504
172. Mutschler, E., Scherf, H., Voss, P., Wassermann, O. 1967. *Naunyn Schmiedebergs Arch. Pharmakol. Exp. Pathol.* 256:367–82
173. Nagy, M., Nador, K. 1967. *Arzeim. Forsch.* 17:1228–31
174. Kier, L. B., Truitt, E. B. 1970. *J. Pharmacol. Exp. Ther.* 174:94–98
175. Bustard, T. M., Egan, R. S. 1971. *Tetrahedron* 27:4457–69
176. Rekker, R. F., Engel, D. J. C., Nys, G. G. 1972. *J. Pharm. Pharmacol.* 24: 589–91
177. Bergin, R., Carlstrom, D. 1968. *Acta Crystallogr. B* 24:1506–10
178. Kier, L. B. 1970. *J. Pharm. Sci.* 59: 112–14
179. Martin, Y. C. et al 1973. *J. Med. Chem.* 16:147–50
180. Kumbar, M., Sankar, D. V. S. 1972. *Res. Commun. Chem. Pathol. Pharmacol.* 4:707–22
181. Kier, L. B. 1968. *J. Pharm. Sci.* 57: 1188–91
182. Kang, S., Johnson, C. L., Green, J. P. 1973. *J. Mol. Struct.* 15:453–57
183. Kang, S., Cho, M-H. 1971. *Theor. Chim. Acta* 22:176–83
184. Courrière, P., Coubeils, J.-L., Pullman, B. 1971. *C.R. Acad. Sci.* 272:1697–1700
185. Johnson, C. L., Kang, S., Green, J. P. 1973. See Ref. 19, *Pt. 5. Conformation of Biological Molecules and Polymers.* 517–28
186. Johnson, C. L., Kang, S., Green, J. P. 1974. *LSD-A Total Study,* ed. D. V. S. Sankar. Hicksville, NY: PJD Publ. In press
187. Karle, I. L., Dragonette, K. S., Brenner, S. A. 1965. *Acta Crystallogr. B* 19: 713–16
188. Bugg, C. E., Thewalt, U. 1970. *Science* 170:852–54
189. Ison, R. R., Partington, P., Roberts, G. C. K. 1972. *J. Pharm. Pharmacol.* 24: 82–85
190. Kang, S., Green, J. P. 1969. *Nature* 222:794–95
191. Green, J. P., Kang, S. 1970. *Molecular Orbital Studies in Chemical Pharmacology,* ed. L. B. Kier, 105–20. New York:Springer. 290 pp.
192. Kier, L. B. 1973. *J. Theor. Biol.* 40:211–17
193. Kier, L. B. 1971. See Ref. 24, pp. 303–20

194. Wyllie, J. H., Hesselbo, T., Black, J. W. 1972. *Lancet* 2:1117–20
195. Kier, L. B. 1968. *J. Med. Chem.* 11: 441–45
196. Casy, A. F., Ison, R. R., Ham, N. S. 1970. *J. Chem. Soc.* 20:1343–44
197. Ham, N. S., Casy, A. F., Ison, R. R. 1973. *J. Med. Chem.* 16:470–75
198. Ganellin, C. R., Pepper, E. S., Prot, G. N. J., Richards, W. G. 1973. *J. Med. Chem.* 16:610–16
199. Margolis, S., Kang, S., Green, J. P. 1971. *Int. J. Clin. Pharmacol. Ther. Toxicol.* 5:279–83
200. Coubeils, J.-L., Courrière, P., Pullman, B. 1971. *C. R. Acad. Sci. D* 272: 1813–16
201. Veidis, M. V., Palenik, G. J., Schaffrin, R., Trotter, J. 1969. *J. Chem. Soc. A* 17:2659–66
202. Thewalt, U., Bugg, C. E. 1972. *Acta Crystallogr. B* 28:1767–73
203. Bonnet, J. J., Ibers, J. A. 1973. *J. Am. Chem. Soc.* 95:4829–33
204. Clark, G. R., Palenik, G. J. 1970. *J. Am. Chem. Soc.* 92:1777–78
205. James, M. N. G., Williams, G. J. B. 1971. *J. Med. Chem.* 14:670–75
206. Bustard, T. M., Martin, Y. C. 1972. *J. Med. Chem.* 15:1101–5
207. Hoyland, J. R., Kier, L. B. 1972. *J. Med. Chem.* 15:84–86
208. Burger, A., Bernabe, M., Collins, P. W. 1970. *J. Med. Chem.* 13:33–35
209. Ganellin, C. R. 1973. *J. Med. Chem.* 16:620–23
210. Karreman, G., Isenberg, I., Szent-Gyorgyi, A. 1959. *Science* 130:1191–92
211. Snyder, S., Merrill, C. 1965. *Proc. Nat. Acad. Sci. USA* 54:258–66
212. Kang, S., Green, J. P. 1970. *Nature* 226:645
213. Kang, S., Green, J. P. 1970. *Proc. Nat. Acad. Sci. USA* 67:62–67
214. Kumbar, M., Sankar, D. V. S. 1973. *Res. Commun. Chem. Pathol. Pharmacol.* 6:65–100
215. Green, J. P., Dressler, K. P., Khazan, N. 1973. *Life Sci. Pt. I* 12:475–79
216. Millie, P., Malrieu, J. P., Benaim, J., Lallemand, J. Y., Julia, M. 1968. *J. Med. Chem.* 11:207–11
217. Sung, M.-T., Parker, J. A. 1972. *Proc. Nat. Acad. Sci. USA* 69:1346–47
218. Bailey, K., Grey, A. A. 1972. *Can. J. Chem.* 50:3876–85
219. Cooper, P. D., Walters, G. C. 1972. *Nature* 238:96–98
220. Archer, R. A., Boyd, D. B., Demarco, P. V., Tyminski, I. J., Allinger, N. L. 1970. *J. Am. Chem. Soc.* 92:5200–6

221. Orloff, M. K., Fitts, D. D. 1961. *Biochim. Biophys. Acta* 47:596–99
222. Merrill, C. R., Snyder, S. H., Bradley, D. F. 1966. *Biochim. Biophys. Acta* 118:316–24
223. Malrieu, J. P. 1967. *Molecular Basis of Some Aspects of Mental Activity,* ed. O. Walaas, 2:83–93. New York: Academic. 515 pp.
224. Bloor, J. E., Gilson, B. R., Haas, R. J., Zirkle, C. L. 1970. *J. Med. Chem.* 13: 922–25
225. Kaufman, J. J., Kerman, E. 1972. *Int. J. Quantum Chem.* 6:319–35
226. Mercier, M. J., Dumont, P. A. 1972. *J. Pharm. Pharmacol.* 24:706–12
227. Saucin, M., van de Vorst, A. 1972. *Biochem. Pharmacol.* 21:2673–80
228. Coubeils, J. L., Pullman, B. 1972. *Theor. Chim. Acta* 24:35–41
229. McDowell, J. J. H. 1969. *Acta Crystallogr. B* 25:2175–81
230. McDowell, J. J. H. 1970. *Acta Crystallogr. B* 26:954–64
231. Coubeils, J. L., Pullman, B. 1973. *Mol. Pharmacol* 8:278–84
232. Ritchie, J. M. 1972. *Int. Encyclo. Pharmacol. Ther.* 1:131–46
233. Büchi, J., Perlia, X. 1972. *Int. Encycl. Pharmacol. Ther.* 1:39–130
234. Borne, R. F., Clark, C. R., Holbrook, J. M. 1973. *J. Med. Chem.* 16:853–56
235. Yoneda, F., Nitta, Y. 1965. *Chem. Pharm. Bull.* 13:574–79
236. Agin, D., Hersh, L., Holtzman, D. 1965. *Proc. Nat. Acad. Sci. USA* 53: 952–58
237. Pullman, B., Coubeils, J. L., Courrière, P. 1972. *J. Theor. Biol.* 35:375–85
238. Neely, W. B., White, H. C., Rudzik, A. 1968. *J. Pharm. Sci.* 57:1176–80
239. Lakik, J., Kobor, G. 1971. *Acta Biochim. Biophys. Acad. Sci. Hung.* 6: 449–52
240. Yoneda, F., Nitta, Y. 1964. *Chem. Pharm. Bull.* 12:1264–68
241. Dinya, Z., Makleit, S., Bognár, R., Jekel, P. 1972. *Acta Chim. Acad. Sci. Hung.* 71:125–26
242. Olsen, J. F., Kang, S. 1970. *Theor. Chim. Acta* 17:329–33
243. Catalan, J., Fernandez-Alonso, J. I. 1973. *Chem. Phys. Lett.* 18:37–40
244. Coubeils, J. L., Courrière, Ph., Pullman, B. 1971. *C.R. Acad. Sci.* 273: 1164–66
245. Kier, L. B., Truitt, E. B. 1970. *Experientia* 26:988–89

246. Diner, S. 1964. *Electronic Aspects of Biochemistry,* ed. B. Pullman, 237–81. New York: Academic. 582 pp.
247. Ullrich, V. 1972. *Angew. Chem. Int. Ed. Eng.* 11:701–12
248. Zahradnik, R., Hobza, P., Hurych, J. 1971. *Biochim. Biophys. Acta* 251:314–19
249. Ishidate, M., Hanaki, A. 1961. *Nature* 191:1198–99
250. Perault, A. M., Pullman, B. 1963. *Biochim. Biophys. Acta* 75:1–11
251. Perault, A. M., Valdemoro, C., Pullman, B. 1961. *J. Theor. Biol.* 2:180–87
252. Song, P.-S., Moore, T. A. 1967. *Int. J. Quantum Chem.* 1:699–719
253. Pettersson, G. 1970. *Acta Chem. Scand.* 24:1838–39
254. Loew, G., Trudell, J., Motulsky, H. 1973. *Mol. Pharmacol.* 9:152–62
255. Perault, A. M., Pullman, B. 1961. *Biochim. Biophys. Acta* 52:266–80
256. Collin, R., Pullman, B. 1964. *Biochim. Biophys. Acta* 89:232–41
257. Nakajima, T., Pullman, A. 1958. *J. Chim. Phys.* 55:793–97
258. Brown, R. D. 1964. *Proc. Roy. Aust. Chem. Inst.* 31:1–14
259. Pullman, A., Pullman, B. 1962. *Horizons in Biochemistry,* ed. M. Kasha, B. Pullman, 553–82. New York: Academic. 604 pp.
260. Neely, W. B. 1967. *Mol. Pharm.* 3:108–12
261. Neely, W. B., 1967. *Ann NY Acad. Sci.* 186:248–55
262. McCormack, J. J. 1967. *Ann NY Acad. Sci.* 186:256–57
263. Kaneti, J. J., Golovinsky, E. V. 1971. *Chem. Biol. Interact.* 3:421–28
264. Kaneti, J. 1973. *J. Theor. Biol.* 38:169–79
265. Perault, A. M., Pullman, B. 1963. *Biochim. Biophys. Acta* 66:86–92
266. Wald, R. W., Feuer, G. 1971. *J. Med. Chem.* 14:1081–84

CELLULAR PHARMACOLOGY OF LANTHANUM

❖6597

George B. Weiss

Department of Pharmacology, University of Texas Southwestern Medical School, Dallas, Texas

The general chemical characteristics of the rare earth or lanthanide series of elements resemble those of the alkaline earth elements in many respects (1). Of the lanthanides, lanthanum has long been considered to have chemical properties most similar to the alkaline earths (2). Recent interest in the biological actions of lanthanum ion (La^{3+}) is almost entirely based upon use of this rare earth ion as a substitute or antagonist for Ca^{2+} in a variety of cellular and subcellular reactions. The rapid and widespread employment of La^{3+} in the last few years is a measure of the complex and varied functions of Ca^{2+} in membrane and coupling reactions. In this review article, I attempt to concentrate upon the cellular actions of La^{3+} in muscle, nerve, and related tissues. A considerable literature has also accumulated concerning use of La^{3+} to discern the presence or absence of anatomical barriers and to delineate the molecular nature and specificity of subcellular Ca^{2+} transport systems and membrane structure. References to these areas of research (as well as to the general pharmacology of La^{3+}) will be limited to those studies most relevant to a consideration of the cellular basis of the actions of La^{3+}.

As long ago as 1910, Mines (3) examined the inhibitory effects of La^{3+} upon contractile function in frog heart. However, the recent proliferation of La^{3+}-related studies can quite clearly be traced to a prediction in 1964 by Lettvin and co-workers (4) that La^{3+}, by virtue of an ionic radius similar to Ca^{2+} and a higher valence than Ca^{2+}, will bind at superficially located Ca^{2+} sites in a less reversible manner than does Ca^{2+}. The subsequent testing of this prediction (5) demonstrated that La^{3+} did indeed exert a blocking action in lobster axons and that it acted in a manner equivalent to an extremely high Ca^{2+} concentration.

The high affinity of La^{3+} for membrane binding sites was of particular interest when related to evidence that the distribution of La^{3+} in many different preparations was confined to membrane areas contiguous with the extracellular space (6–12). Thus, use of La^{3+} as a relatively specific Ca^{2+} substitute or antagonist at well-defined

343

cellular locations appeared justified by both electrophysiological and anatomical criteria.

NERVE AND SKELETAL MUSCLE

Demonstration of blockade of Ca^{2+} fluxes by La^{3+} can be accomplished with least ambiguity in artificial membranes and in nerve cells. In a porous phospholipid-cholesterol artificial membrane, addition of 1 mM La^{3+} changed the membrane from a cation exchanger to an anion exchanger (13). This effect was interpreted as being due to the ability of La^{3+} to associate with fixed negative groups in a more pronounced manner than Ca^{2+}. More directly relevant for biological membranes is the demonstration by van Breemen & de Weer (14) that La^{3+} decreases the ^{45}Ca efflux rate by 87% when added to the solution bathing a squid giant axon previously injected with ^{45}Ca. The ^{45}Ca uptake in rabbit vagus nerve was also reduced by La^{3+} and the decrease was maintained (15). Thus, this effect of La^{3+} on Ca^{2+} uptake in vagus nerve can be interpreted as a blockade of at least a fraction of Ca^{2+} uptake rather than a decreased rate of uptake. In the same manner, La^{3+} irreversibly inhibited a lithium-sensitive Na^+ efflux component which was also abolished by removal of external Ca^{2+} (16). Again, the specific action of La^{3+} could be a Ca^{2+}-antagonistic action affecting the Ca^{2+} uptake component of a Na^+-Ca^{2+} exchange system.

Frog sartorius muscle is a tissue in which Ca^{2+} movements, contractile responses, and mechanisms of drug actions can be considered in terms of extensively character-ized cellular structures (see 17, 18). The alteration by La^{3+} of specific ^{45}Ca move-ments in this muscle also can be readily described. In sartorius muscle, La^{3+} decreased ^{45}Ca uptake, transiently increased ^{45}Ca release, and blocked the increased ^{45}Ca uptake and tension response usually obtained with 80 mM K^+ but not with caffeine (19). Potassium ions act at least partially at sites in the transverse tubules (17, 20), whereas the effects of caffeine on sartorius contracture and ^{45}Ca efflux appear to be independent of the extracellular Ca^{2+} concentration (21, 22). Thus, in frog sartorius muscle, La^{3+} acts specifically at superficial sites (at cellular and transverse tubule membranes) to displace Ca^{2+} and to prevent tension responses and ionic movements associated with these sites (19). However, La^{3+} did not inhibit the caffeine-induced increase in ^{45}Ca uptake, an uptake which has been attributed to an increased cellular permeability to Ca^{2+} in both polarized and depolarized muscles (23). On this basis, it appears that not all Ca^{2+} uptake mechanisms in frog sartorius muscle are blocked by La^{3+}.

In frog sartorius muscle even contractile responses to high K^+ are not quantita-tively related to the magnitude of the Ca^{2+} influx (24, 25) but, instead, the Ca^{2+} influx may act as a trigger for subsequent release of cellular Ca^{2+} (24). However, in some other muscle systems, Ca^{2+} entry is quantitatively important for both contractile responses and at least part of the depolarizing current.

Under these circumstances, the effects of La^{3+} on Ca^{2+} entry and subsequent events are quite pronounced. Of a number of divalent and trivalent ions tested, Hagiwara & Takahashi (26) found that La^{3+} was most potent in suppressing the

Ca-spike potential of the barnacle muscle fiber membrane. Binding of La^{3+} at the membrane surface appeared to be irreversible. In amphioxus muscle, La^{3+} also blocked the Ca^{2+}-dependent membrane conductance increases—presumably by occupying Ca^{2+} sites near or at the membrane (27).

In some situations involving either Ca^{2+}-dependent transmitter release mechanisms at the neuromuscular junction or slow twitch fibers (as in frog rectus abdominis muscle), La^{3+}-Ca^{2+} relationships appear more complex. In frog rectus abdominis muscle, La^{3+} inhibited ^{45}Ca uptake and the increase in residual ^{45}Ca content induced by high K^+ or acetylcholine (but not by nicotine); however, La^{3+} had only weak inhibitory effects on tension responses to high K^+, acetylcholine, or nicotine (28). Because removal of Ca^{2+} readily abolishes tension responses in rectus abdominis muscle, it is likely that responses dependent in some manner upon relatively superficial Ca^{2+} are resistant to inhibition by La^{3+}. Thus, even though La^{3+} is a relatively specific Ca^{2+} antagonist, it cannot be assumed that all responses dependent upon Ca^{2+} uptake or superficial binding of Ca^{2+} are susceptible to La^{3+} or even accessible to La^{3+}. More than one type of effect of La^{3+} on junctional transmission also has been described. A number of reports show that La^{3+} effectively increased spontaneous miniature endplate potential (MEPP) frequency (29–34) even in the absence of extracellular Ca^{2+} (31). At the same time, La^{3+} inhibited both the endplate (EP) potential (31) and the inward movement of Ca^{2+} necessary for normal transmitter release (35), whereas La^{3+} increased the rate of carbamylcholine-induced desensitization (36). Explanations offered for the potentiating effect of La^{3+} on spontaneous transmitter release (seen as an increase in MEPP frequency) include (a) accumulation of La^{3+} inside the nerve terminals and subsequent release of sequestered Ca^{2+} by this intracellular La^{3+} (31), and (b) an action of La^{3+} at superficial membrane sites to initiate release of Ca^{2+} from less superficial cellular stores (31, 33). Even though Heuser & Miledi (32) reported that La^{3+} causes structural changes in nerve terminals after longer incubation intervals (more than 1 hr), these changes paralleled a decline in spontaneous MEPP frequency and were not seen at shorter exposure intervals when increased spontaneous MEPP frequencies were observed. In the absence of evidence that significant amounts of La^{3+} enter the nerve terminal at a rapid rate, it seems more consistent with the actions of La^{3+} in other tissues to attribute the stimulatory action of La^{3+} to a postulated coupling between the binding of La^{3+} at external membrane sites and the release of sequestered Ca^{2+}.

CARDIAC MUSCLE

In cardiac muscle, the relationship between the development of contractile force and the level of extracellular calcium is a much more direct and obvious one than exists in fast twitch skeletal muscle. A recent review by Langer (37) provides a summary of heart muscle excitation-contraction coupling material and includes reference to some La^{3+} experiments in this area (38–40). Initial studies by Sanborn & Langer (38) on rabbit heart muscle demonstrated quite clearly that low concentrations of La^{3+} (5–40 μM) elicited both a transient increase in ^{45}Ca efflux and a decreased tension response without significant alteration of the action potential. The La^{3+}-induced inhibition of tension was generally reversible if the exposure to La^{3+} was brief, and increased extracellular Ca^{2+} yielded a small and transient increase in the efflux of ^{140}La. The primary and specific action of La^{3+} in mammalian heart tissue thus appears to be an inhibition of Ca^{2+} uptake (and subsequent release) at superficial membrane sites (38, 41) from which Ca^{2+} release may not be directly related to induction of contraction but, rather, essential for the release of relevant Ca^{2+} from less superficial sites (41). The superficially located Ca^{2+} binding sites in cardiac muscle appear to be affected by both lack of oxygen and exposure to drugs. Naylor and co-workers have reported that the amount of Ca^{2+} displaced by La^{3+} from superficially located membrane sites is reduced in ischemic or hypoxic muscle (42) and by pentobarbital (43), whereas ouabain, in concentrations sufficient to give a positive inotropic response without contracture, increased the amount of Ca^{2+} displaced by La^{3+} (40). Thus, the superficial Ca^{2+} fraction affected by La^{3+} appears to be important for induced alterations in cardiac function.

Extrapolations of data obtained from hearts of only one mammalian species may not result in an accurate general picture. Dietrich & Diacono (44) employed La^{3+} in perfused hearts from rats and guinea pigs and found that ouabain-induced contractions were more directly dependent on Ca^{2+} influx in rat hearts, whereas in guinea pig hearts the amplitude and duration of depolarization (and, presumably, subsequent release of Ca^{2+} from membrane stores) was relatively more important. Cellular parameters affected by La^{3+} in heart cells can be described with more precision in heart cell cultures or embryonic heart cells. In chick embryonic hearts, the Ca^{2+} channels present during early development are blocked by La^{3+} (45). In cultured rat heart cells, La^{3+} prevents Ca^{2+} uptake, greatly reduces Ca^{2+} efflux, abolishes contractile tension but not the action potential, displaces Ca^{2+} at superficial membrane sites, and binds specifically to the basement membrane without penetrating beyond this region (39). Though cultured cells may differ in structural detail from intact adult heart cells, similarities in effects of La^{3+} indicate that contractile responses in most cardiac muscle systems are regulated by a superficially located and rapidly exchangeable Ca^{2+} component. The high degree of specificity with which La^{3+} interacts with these Ca^{2+} sites facilitates a dissociation of at least two functional Ca^{2+} compartments in cardiac muscle.

SMOOTH MUSCLE

Use of La^{3+} as a tool to block some but not all Ca^{2+} movements in various isolated smooth muscle preparations is particularly valuable because the morphological basis for storage and release of Ca^{2+} in this type of muscle cannot be described as clearly as has been done for other muscle systems. Attempts to obtain specific physiological and pharmacological alterations in Ca^{2+} movements and distribution in terms of ^{45}Ca fluxes in a variety of preparations including guinea pig ileal longitudinal smooth muscle (46, 47) and taenia coli (48–50), rat uterine smooth muscle (51–54), and rabbit aortic smooth muscle (55–57) have been hampered by the presence of quantitatively large and apparently unrelated ^{45}Ca movements. There appear to be distinct differences between the manner in which contractile responses depend upon extracellular Ca^{2+} when responses to high K^+ are compared with those obtained with norepinephrine and histamine in rabbit aorta (56), norepinephrine in the rabbit ear vascular bed (58), epinephrine in rat ventral tail artery (59) and rat aorta (60, 61), and acetylcholine in rat uterus (62) and guinea pig taenia coli (63). In all of these preparations, removal of extracellular Ca^{2+} inhibits K^+-induced contractions more readily than contractile responses elicited with various stimulatory agents. Generally, this has led to a further inference concerning the nature of the Ca^{2+} important for contractile responses to K^+ and to other agents. Briefly, this hypothesis states that most of the Ca^{2+} important for K^+-induced smooth muscle contractions originates in the extracellular fluid or at superifical cellular sites or stores, whereas the major portion of the Ca^{2+} utilized by other stimulatory agents is located at less superficial or more sequestered sites or stores.

The presumption that smooth muscle contraction is linked to either depolarization by high K^+ or drug-receptor interactions by a number of intermediary steps that include Ca^{2+} movements or Ca^{2+}-mediated reactions has resulted in many investigations designed to elucidate the nature of these Ca^{2+}-dependent effects. This has been most conveniently accomplished by use of different types of inhibitory agents. Initial use of the local anesthetic cocaine in this manner led to the report by Hurwitz (64) that cocaine and Ca^{2+} exerted antagonistic actions on tension in K^+-depolarized longitudinal smooth muscle from guinea pig ileum. In polarized longitudinal smooth muscle, tone is inhibited by either high Ca^{2+} or cocaine (65). This indicates that interactions in depolarized smooth muscle are not the consequences of repolarization but, rather, are more closely related to events leading directly to smooth muscle contraction. The competitive nature of the inhibitory effects of local anesthetics upon Ca^{2+}-induced contractions in depolarized rat uterus has been described by Feinstein (66). Other inhibitory agents and the depolarized smooth muscle systems in which they exert a Ca^{2+}-antagonistic effect on contractile tone include ethanol in guinea pig ileal longitudinal smooth muscle (65), papaverine in guinea pig taenia coli (67), and phenoxybenzamine (68), desipramine (69), caffeine (70), cinnarizine, and chlorpromazine (71) in vascular smooth muscle preparations. However, K^+-depolarized preparations represent systems in which the patterns of Ca^{2+} binding and flux are substantially altered from the polarized state (72). Thus, effects of pharmacological agents on Ca^{2+} movements and contractile tone may also be qualitatively different in polarized and K^+-depolarized smooth muscles.

The effect of La^{3+} on membrane potential has not been measured directly in smooth muscle, though Anderson et al (73) found inhibition of both peak transient and steady-state currents in rat myometrical strips. However, if the role of La^{3+} is similar to that in nerve (5), a stabilizing or even hyperpolarizing action is likely. On this basis, Weiss & Goodman (74) predicted that La^{3+} would directly exert a stabilizing action at superficial Ca^{2+} sites but would only indirectly affect those Ca^{2+} sites or stores inaccessible to the extracellular bathing solution. The use of La^{3+} is then of particular value as a potential and specific antagonist of only a portion of total cellular Ca^{2+}. The idea that La^{3+} would, in essence, help dissociate Ca^{2+}-dependent actions has been successful in a number of important respects and has increased understanding of drug-Ca^{2+} interactions in several different types of smooth muscle. Not surprisingly, the degree of dissociation between responses to high K^+ and other types of Ca^{2+}-dependent responses varies with the manner in which Ca^{2+} is taken up, stored, and utilized.

In ileal longitudinal smooth muscle, comparisons between effects of acetylcholine and those of high K^+ indicate that Ca^{2+} acting at superficial sites decreases membrane permeability to inorganic ions (65, 75). Depletion of Ca^{2+} (by washing out muscles in a calcium-free medium) rapidly abolishes responses to both high K^+ and acetylcholine (76). Furthermore, either high K^+ (77, 78) or acetylcholine (79) will increase smooth muscle tone in ileal longitudinal smooth muscles after incubation in a high Ca^{2+} solution and subsequent washout in a calcium-free medium. Under these conditions, Ca^{2+} mobilization from less superficial sites or stores may occur. The relationship between superficial Ca^{2+} and Ca^{2+} located at less superficial sites or stores in guinea pig ileal longitudinal smooth muscle has been studied in some detail by Hurwitz and co-workers (77–79). It appears that removal of superficial or stabilizing Ca^{2+} is linked to cellular Ca^{2+} release so that agents may initiate inward Ca^{2+} movements by removal of superficial Ca^{2+}. Conversely, inhibitory agents can prevent contractile responses in ileal longitudinal smooth muscle either by blocking loss of stabilizing Ca^{2+} or by displacing and replacing this Ca^{2+}. Thus, Weiss & Goodman (74) explained the effects of La^{3+} in this muscle by postulating that La^{3+} displaces Ca^{2+} from surface sites, binds well at these sites, and exerts a stabilizing action that prevents inward release of Ca^{2+} from less accessible membrane sites. Uptake of ^{45}Ca is also inhibited, and contractile responses to both acetylcholine and high K^+ are blocked. Further investigation by Goodman & Weiss (80) of the effects of lower La^{3+} concentrations on ileal longitudinal smooth muscle contractions elicited with high K^+ or acetylcholine indicates that no differential inhibitory effects were observed. Contractions in both cases were inhibited about 50% by a concentration of 0.9 μM La^{3+}. Thus, La^{3+} could not dissociate actions of agents affecting Ca^{2+} uptake from effects resulting from translocation of cellular Ca^{2+} in this smooth muscle system.

Use of La^{3+} to dissociate different cellular actions of stimulatory agents in other types of smooth muscle systems has been more successful. In rat uterine strips Goodman & Weiss (80) found that high K^+-induced contractions were inhibited by a 100-fold lower concentration of La^{3+} than were acetylcholine-induced contractions, and responsiveness to acetylcholine returned much more rapidly after exposure to La^{3+} than did that to high K^+. Similarly, in rabbit aortic smooth muscle, La^{3+} had a greater inhibitory effect on high K^+-induced contractions than on responses elicited with norepinephrine (81, 82). In aortic smooth muscle, La^{3+} inhibited the contractions obtained with histamine to a lesser degree than those by norepinephrine (82), whereas Ca^{2+} depletion (56) had the reverse effect (inhibition of histamine-induced contractions was greater than those elicited with norepinephrine). Lanthanum ion also irreversibly inhibited contractile responses to a number of agonists in the rabbit anterior mesenteric-portal vein (83) and blocked the tonic (high K^+-induced) response in guinea pig vas deferens (84). A recent postulation by van Breemen and co-workers (85) that histamine, norepinephrine, and angiotensin II may affect the same limited intracellular Ca^{2+} fraction in rabbit aorta was based upon the observation that, after La^{3+}, only one drug-induced contraction can be obtained with histamine, norepinephrine, or angiotensin II. These important drug interactions are complicated by the increased inhibitory activity of La^{3+} on smooth muscle contractile responses as the exposure interval is lengthened (G. B. Weiss and F. R. Goodman, unpublished observations). Further documentation of the time-dependent drug relationships involved would help clarify the manner in which these different agents may utilize similar Ca^{2+} stores. The uptake of ^{45}Ca is also blocked by La^{3+} in intestinal (74, 86), uterine (80), and vascular (82) smooth muscle under appropriate conditions.

An indirect approach to measurement of changes in cellular Ca^{2+} in smooth muscle has been proposed by van Breemen and co-workers (85, 87). Their idea, which they have termed "the Lanthanum method," is based upon the assumptions that a sufficiently high concentration of extracellular La^{3+} will *(a)* displace and replace extracellular Ca^{2+}, *(b)* block both Ca^{2+} uptake and efflux, and *(c)* not enter the cell in appreciable quantities to displace or alter cellular Ca^{2+} distribution. On this basis, tissues could be exposed to a variety of stimulatory agents or conditions in the presence of ^{45}Ca and subsequently placed into washout solutions containing a concentration of La^{3+} high enough to replace all extracellular or superficial Ca^{2+} and to prevent any further uptake or efflux of cellular ^{45}Ca. In this manner, effects on cellular ^{45}Ca uptake that have been obscured by much larger quantities of extracellular ^{45}Ca and by nonspecific ^{45}Ca movements can be detected. However, the method, as it has been used, is subject to some serious criticisms. First, Hodgson, Kidwai & Daniel (88) reported that ^{140}La entered the rat myometrial cell in significant quantities. Their evidence for this is based primarily on binding of La^{3+} to isolated subcellular components. There is no direct demonstration in any smooth muscle system that La^{3+} either enters or is excluded from the intracellular compartment of stimulated as well as nonstimulated cells. The most convincing experimental approach would employ autoradiographic or electron microscopic techniques. In the absence of this, the possibility cannot be excluded that La^{3+} may enter the cell in differing quantities (which may even relate to the prior treatment regime) and alter the pattern of ^{45}Ca washout in a differential manner.

Determination of the actual rate of ^{45}Ca washout during the period of exposure to La^{3+} is also essential. Van Breemen et al stated (89) that efflux of ^{45}Ca is blocked by La^{3+} in smooth muscle, but they demonstrated this only for smooth muscle treated with monoidoacetic acid and 2,4-dinitrophenol (89) and for other systems such as squid axon (85) and artificial phospholipid membranes (81). Actually, it is not essential that La^{3+} totally block ^{45}Ca efflux, but only that ^{45}Ca emerge at similar and constant rates from control and treated tissues during washout in the presence of La^{3+}. This should be ascertained for each type of preparation by measuring the rate of loss of ^{45}Ca during the period of exposure to La^{3+}. In the absence of evidence that desaturation-type washout curves are parallel, the possibility exists that small but significant variations in the rate of loss of ^{45}Ca during the period of exposure to La^{3+} may be in large part responsible for the differences observed in residual ^{45}Ca content. The concentration of La^{3+} also appears rather critical. Earlier experiments of this type were performed with 2 mM La^{3+} (85, 87), but later work indicated that 10 mM La^{3+} might be a more satisfactory concentration (86, 89). In guinea pig ileal longitudinal muscle, Burton & Godfraind (90) reported that this La^{3+} concentration is sufficient to block all ^{45}Ca uptake and binding, because the resultant ^{45}Ca space of 0.35 ml/g equals the ^{14}C-inulin space. The use of such a high concentration of La^{3+} (10 mM) raises the possibility that nonspecific membrane stabilizing actions of La^{3+} may now be more prominent than specific Ca^{2+}-antagonistic actions. This high concentration of La^{3+} appears to inhibit the uptake of ^{14}C-sorbitol in this manner in metabolically depleted taenia coli (91). Hyperpolarization with La^{3+} in lobster axon membrane was reported by Takata and co-workers (5) to be about 20 times as effective as with equivalent concentrations of Ca^{2+}. If similar actions occur in smooth muscle, it is possible that polarization-induced changes with 10 mM La^{3+} could alter the binding and mobility of cellular Ca^{2+}. Thus, increased cellular residual ^{45}Ca levels might be more a function of nonspecific stabilizing actions of La^{3+} rather than of specific Ca^{2+}-antagonistic effects.

OTHER SYSTEMS

The relationship between Ca^{2+} and many secretory processes has been extensively studied, and this area is summarized in a recent review by Rubin (92). The analogy between excitation-contraction coupling in muscle and stimulus-secretion coupling is firmly based upon the necessity for Ca^{2+} as a coupling agent in both types of processes. Thus, in view of the successful use of La^{3+} as a specific Ca^{2+} antagonist in muscle and nerve, it is not surprising that similar approaches with La^{3+} would be attempted in various secretory systems.

It might be expected that physiological similarities between hormonal release mechanisms and myoneural junction transmission would result in analogous stimulatory and inhibitory effects of La^{3+}. The Ca^{2+}-dependent secretory actions that La^{3+} has been reported to alter include catecholamine release from adrenal medulla (93) and histamine release from mast cells (94). In isolated bovine adrenals, Borowicz (93) found that only the first exposure to La^{3+} stimulated release of a large quantity of catecholamine and, conversely, La^{3+} inhibited the increased catecholamine release obtained with acetylcholine or high K$^+$. In a similar approach, Foreman & Mongar (94) report that La^{3+} can increase the spontaneous release of histamine but is a potent inhibitor of the calcium-dependent component of antigen-stimulated histamine release. The stimulatory actions of La^{3+} on spontaneous release of stimulatory agents, and the inhibitory actions of La^{3+} on induced release of stimulatory agents obviously parallel similar actions of La^{3+} (29–35) on spontaneous MEPP frequency and on end plate potential and Ca^{2+} uptake in junctional transmission. In neither of these two studies (93, 94) involving secretory actions was ^{45}Ca movement examined, but in both cases the La^{3+}-induced inhibition of Ca^{2+}-dependent stimulated release was attributed to a specific block by La^{3+} of Ca^{2+} uptake. Perhaps the stimulatory action of La^{3+} is also similar in mechanism to that observed in junctional transmission and may result from a coupling action between the binding of La^{3+} at superficial membrane sites and the release of sequestered Ca^{2+}. Another study involving effects of La^{3+} on a secretory system (rat mammary tissue) was performed by Lawson & Schmidt (95). The oxytocin-induced milk ejection response of the tissue was markedly reduced by La^{3+}, and this action was attributed to a displacement by La^{3+} of superficial Ca^{2+} important for contraction of the myoepithelial cell. Unfortunately, as the authors noted, examination for possible displacement of superficially bound ^{45}Ca by La^{3+} was not undertaken in the absence of prior exposure to extracellular Ca^{2+}, and the resultant lack of effect is not conclusive. Similarly, failure to observe an oxytocin-induced increase in ^{45}Ca influx might be due to use of too low a concentration of La^{3+} (1 mM) to achieve substantial inhibition of ^{45}Ca efflux during the subsequent washout.

Employment of La^{3+} as a tool to examine Ca^{2+}-dependent actions has been attempted in numerous biological systems under various conditions. Though it is not feasible to discuss all of these studies at this time, some of the more interesting ones include (a) a reduction by La^{3+} in the increased frequency of ciliary beating, which results from mechanical stimulation and is related to the extracellular Ca^{2+} concentration and, presumably, to the Ca^{2+} influx which follows (96), (b) a removal by La^{3+} of large quantities of extracellular ^{45}Ca during washout of rat cerebral cortex slices (97), (c) an increase in membrane potential stability of Ehrlich ascites tumor cells in La^{3+}-containing solutions (98), (d) an enhancement by La^{3+} of in vitro calcification of the excised tibial epiphyses of Ca^{2+}-deficient (rachitic) rats (99), and (e) substitution of La^{3+} for Ca^{2+} essential for the postulated formation of an amiloride-receptor complex that blocks access of Na^+ to frog skin transport channels (100).

The effects of La^{3+} on Ca^{2+} uptake important for the binding and transport of Ca^{2+} in various subcellular structures and proteins has been the focal point for a number of studies concerned with the relevant biochemical and molecular mechanisms. Though a detailed discussion of these reports is outside the scope of this review, a summary of some basic views and concepts about binding of Ca^{2+} and La^{3+} is of considerable value. There is no doubt that La^{3+}, in extremely low concentrations, inhibits the uptake or binding of Ca^{2+} in rat liver mitochondria (101, 102) and in cardiac muscle sarcoplasmic reticulum (103, 104), but apparently not in dog cardiac microsomes (105). Of particular interest is the finding that specific high and low affinity sites for the binding of Ca^{2+} may exist in a protein fraction solubilized from rat skeletal muscle sarcoplasmic reticulum (106) and in rabbit skeletal muscle sarcoplasmic reticulum (103). Furthermore, La^{3+} is a relatively poor inhibitor of Ca^{2+} binding at specific Ca^{2+} sites in rabbit sarcoplasmic reticulum (103), and La^{3+} can also bind, in large amounts, to sites that differ from those normally occupied by Ca^{2+} (102). Thus, the suggestion emerges from these studies that the affinities of La^{3+} and Ca^{2+} for different membrane sites may be quite variable. The basis for differing affinities may be a function of access to sites, steric configurations in the vicinity of the sites, or other factors. Regardless of the molecular basis for these variations, the implication to be derived for isolated tissue studies is that, in a given cellular system, it cannot be assumed that La^{3+} has a greater affinity than Ca^{2+} for all relevant binding sites. The existence of specific La^{3+}-insensitive Ca^{2+} binding sites or uptake mechanisms may account for lack of inhibition by La^{3+} of the increased ^{45}Ca uptake elicited by caffeine in frog sartorius muscle (19) or by nicotine in frog rectus abdominis muscle (28).

GENERAL CONSIDERATIONS

The major point which emerges from consideration of the cellular pharmacology of La^{3+} is that this ion is a specific antagonist of Ca^{2+} in biological systems. It is possible to explain all of the effects of reasonable concentrations of La^{3+} by postulating that La^{3+} can replace Ca^{2+} at well-defined tissue loci or sites and, in this manner, either impede or augment Ca^{2+}-dependent movements or reactions. Use of La^{3+} to elucidate Ca^{2+}-dependent mechanisms of action appears to provide a more precise approach than use of a procedure such as Ca^{2+} depletion, whether accomplished by ionic variation or by addition of Ca^{2+}-chelating agents. Thus, the experimental value of La^{3+} has received rapid recognition, and La^{3+} has been used in a variety of investigations of Ca^{2+}-dependent processes over the last few years. Even with the increased current knowledge of La^{3+}-Ca^{2+} interactions, a number of significant problems remain. In each isolated system employed, dose-response relationships for La^{3+} as well as for Ca^{2+} should be ascertained routinely to prevent erroneous comparisons and extrapolations. This is particularly true if conclusions are to be based upon assumptions that La^{3+} blocks all Ca^{2+} movements or displaces virtually all Ca^{2+} from particular binding sites. It is clear that different types of preparations vary considerably in their sensitivity to inhibitory effects of La^{3+}. It is also possible that the relative affinities of Ca^{2+} and La^{3+} for different membrane binding sites may not be the same. Furthermore, high concentrations of La^{3+} may well exert non-specific (e.g. stabilizing) effects or even actions that are deleterious to cellular integrity. More complete understanding of these potentially toxic actions of La^{3+} would be valuable. Related to this is the question of possible cellular penetration of La^{3+} under physiological conditions. Resolution of this problem, preferably by use of established electron microscopic techniques in each type of isolated tissue system, is essential for validation of much of the work based on use of La^{3+} to dissociate different cellular Ca^{2+} sites or stores.

Finally, it should be recognized that even though use of techniques involving La^{3+} will contribute greatly to resolution of Ca^{2+}-dependent actions, development of other tools and approaches also will be necessary. For example, an agent or agents that would specifically displace Ca^{2+} from sequestered cellular stores (particularly in smooth muscle systems) would be of value in correlating pharmacological effects with actions of Ca^{2+} at clearly defined cellular sites. In this manner, employment of La^{3+} as a partial and specific Ca^{2+} antagonist may well serve as a model for eventual use of additional agents in similarly defined roles in the elucidation of other Ca^{2+}-dependent biological actions.

ACKNOWLEDGMENTS

Experimental work from this laboratory was supported in part by USPHS Grant HL 14775 and by the American Medical Association Education and Research Foundation.

Literature Cited

1. Moeller, T. 1963. *The Chemistry of the Lanthanides.* New York: Reinhold. 117 pp.
2. Levy, S. I. 1915. *The Rare Earths,* 171. New York: Longmans, Green
3. Mines, G. P. 1910. *J. Physiol. London* 40:327–46
4. Lettvin, J. Y., Pickard, W. F., McCulloch, W. S., Pitts, W. 1964. *Nature* 202:1338–39
5. Takata, M., Pickard, W. F., Lettvin, J. Y., Moore, J. W. 1966. *J. Gen. Physiol.* 50:461–71
6. Laszlo, D., Ekstein, D. M., Lewin, R., Stern, K. G. 1952. *J. Nat. Cancer Inst.* 13:559–71
7. Revel, J. P., Karnovsky, M. J. 1967. *J. Cell. Biol.* 33:C7–12
8. Brightman, M. W., Reese, T. S. 1969. *J. Cell. Biol.* 40:648–77
9. Payton, B. W., Bennett, M. V. L., Pappas, G. D. 1969. *Science* 166:1641–43
10. Zacks, S. I. 1970. *J. Histochem. Cytochem.* 18:302–4
11. Garant, P. R. 1972. *J. Ultrastruct. Res.* 40:333–48
12. Lane, N. J., Treherne, J. E. 1972. *Tissue Cell* 4:427–36
13. van Breemen, C. 1968. *Biochem. Biophys. Res. Commun.* 32:977–83
14. van Breemen, C., de Weer, P. 1970. *Nature* 226:760–61
15. Kalix, P. 1971. *Pfluegers Arch.* 326:1–14
16. Baker, P. F., Blaustein, M. P., Hodgkin, A. L., Steinhardt, R. A. 1969. *J. Physiol. London* 200:431–58
17. Sandow, A. 1965. *Pharmacol. Rev.* 17:265–320
18. Bianchi, C. P. 1968. *Cell Calcium.* London: Butterworth
19. Weiss, G. B. 1970. *J. Pharmacol. Exp. Ther.* 174:517–26
20. Hodgkin, A. L., Horowicz, P. 1960. *J. Physiol. London* 153:370–85
21. Bianchi, C. P. 1961. *Biophysics of Physiological and Pharmacological Actions,* ed. A. M. Shanes, 281–92. Washington: AAAS
22. Isaacson, A., Sandow, A. 1967. *J. Gen. Physiol.* 50:2109–28
23. Bianchi, C. P. 1961. *J. Gen. Physiol.* 44:845–58
24. Weiss, G. B., Bianchi, C. P. 1965. *J. Cell. Comp. Physiol.* 65:385–92
25. Bianchi, C. P., Bolton, T. C. 1966. *J. Pharmacol. Exp. Ther.* 151:456–63
26. Hagiwara, S., Takahashi, K. 1967. *J. Gen. Physiol.* 50:583–601
27. Hagiwara, S., Kidokoro, Y. 1971. *J. Physiol. London* 219:217–32
28. Weiss, G. B. 1973. *J. Pharmacol. Exp. Ther.* 185:551–59
29. Blioch, Z. L., Glagoleva, I. M., Liberman, E. A., Nenashev, V. A. 1968. *J. Physiol. London* 199:11–35
30. Lambert, D. H., Parsons, R. L. 1970. *J. Gen. Physiol.* 56:309–21
31. DeBassio, W. A., Schnitzler, R. M., Parsons, R. L. 1971. *J. Neurobiol.* 2:263–78
32. Heuser, J., Miledi, R. 1971. *Proc. Roy. Soc. London B* 179:247–60
33. Bowen, J. M. 1972. *Can. J. Physiol. Pharmacol.* 50:603–11
34. Kajimoto, N., Kirpekar, S. M. 1972. *Nature* 235:29–30
35. Miledi, R. 1971. *Nature* 229:410–11
36. Parsons, R. L., Johnson, E. W., Lambert, D. H. 1971. *Am. J. Physiol.* 220:401–5
37. Langer, G. A. 1973. *Ann. Rev. Physiol.* 35:55–86
38. Sanborn, W. G., Langer, G. A. 1970. *J. Gen. Physiol.* 56:191–217
39. Langer, G. A., Frank, J. S. 1972. *J. Cell. Biol.* 54:441–55
40. Naylor, W. G. 1973. *J. Mol. Cell. Cardiol.* 5:101–10
41. Ong, S. D., Bailey, L. E. 1972. *Experientia* 28:1446–47
42. Naylor, W. G., Stone, J., Carson, V., Chipperfield, D. 1971. *J. Mol. Cell. Cardiol.* 2:125–43
43. Naylor, W. G., Szeto, J. 1972. *Am. J. Physiol.* 222:339–44
44. Dietrich, J., Diacono, J. 1972. *Thérapie* 27:861–71
45. Shigenobu, K., Sperelakis, N. 1972. *Circ. Res.* 31:932–52
46. Lüllmann, H., Siegfriedt, A. 1968. *Pfluegers Arch.* 300:108–19
47. Weiss, G. B. 1972. *Agents Actions* 2:246–56
48. Urakawa, N., Holland, W. C. 1964. *Am. J. Physiol.* 207:873–76
49. Bauer, H., Goodford, P. J., Hüter, J. 1965. *J. Physiol. London* 176:163–79
50. Goodford, P. J. 1965. *J. Physiol. London* 176:180–90
51. van Breemen, C., Daniel, E. E., van Breemen, D. 1966. *J. Gen. Physiol.* 49:1265–97
52. van Breemen, C., Daniel, E. E. 1966. *J. Gen. Physiol.* 49:1299–1317

53. Krejci, I., Daniel, E. E. 1970. *Am. J. Physiol.* 219:256–62
54. Krejci, I., Daniel, E. E. 1970. *Am. J. Physiol.* 219:263–69
55. Briggs, A. H. 1962. *Am. J. Physiol.* 203:849–52
56. Hudgins, P. M., Weiss, G. B. 1968. *J. Pharmacol. Exp. Ther.* 159:91–97
57. Hudgins, P. M., Weiss, G. B. 1969. *Am. J. Physiol.* 217:1310–15
58. Hiraoka, M., Yamagishi, S., Sano, T. 1968. *Am. J. Physiol.* 214:1084–89
59. Hinke, J. A. M. 1965. *Muscle,* ed. W. M. Paul, E. E. Daniel, C. M. Kay, G. Monckton, 269–84. London: Pergamon
60. Peiper, U., Griebel, L., Wende, W. 1971. *Pfluegers Arch.* 324:67–78
61. Peiper, U., Griebel, L., Wende, W. 1971. *Pfluegers Arch.* 330:74–89
62. Edman, K. A. P., Schild, H. O. 1962. *J. Physiol. London* 161:424–41
63. Durbin, R. P., Jenkinson, D. H. 1961. *J. Physiol. London* 157:90–96
64. Hurwitz, L. 1961. *Biophysics of Physiological and Pharmacological Actions,* ed. A. M. Shanes, 563–77. Washington: AAAS.
65. Hurwitz, L., Battle, F., Weiss, G. B. 1962. *J. Gen. Physiol.* 46:315–32
66. Feinstein, M. B. 1966. *J. Pharmacol. Exp. Ther.* 152:516–24
67. Kadlec, O., Bauer, V. 1971. *Experientia* 27:815–16
68. Bevan, J. A., Osher, J. V., Su, C. 1963. *J. Pharmacol. Exp. Ther.* 139:216–21
69. Hrdina, P., Garattini, S. 1967. *J. Pharm. Pharmacol.* 19:667–73
70. Somlyo, A. V., Somlyo, A. P. 1968. *J. Pharmacol. Exp. Ther.* 159:129–45
71. Godfraind, T., Kaba, A. 1969. *Brit. J. Pharmacol.* 36:549–60
72. Weiss, G. B. 1974. *Methods in Pharmacology. Vol. III, Smooth Muscle,* ed. E. E. Daniel, D. Paton. In press
73. Anderson, N. C., Ramon, F., Snyder, A. 1971. *J. Gen. Physiol.* 58:322–39
74. Weiss, G. B., Goodman, F. R. 1969. *J. Pharmacol. Exp. Ther.* 169:46–55
75. von Hagen, S., Hurwitz, L. 1967. *Am. J. Physiol.* 213:579–86
76. Weiss, G. B., Hurwitz, L. 1963. *J. Gen. Physiol.* 47:173–87
77. Hurwitz, L., Joiner, P. D., von Hagen, S. 1967. *Proc. Soc. Exp. Biol. Med.* 125:518–22
78. Hurwitz, L., Joiner, P. D., von Hagen, S. 1967. *Am. J. Physiol.* 213:1299–1304
79. Hurwitz, L., von Hagen, S., Joiner, P. D. 1967. *J. Gen. Physiol.* 50:1157–72
80. Goodman, F. R., Weiss, G. B. 1971. *Am. J. Physiol.* 220:759–66
81. van Breemen, C. 1969. *Arch. Int. Physiol. Biochem.* 77:710–16
82. Goodman, F. R., Weiss, G. B. 1971. *J. Pharmacol. Exp. Ther.* 177:415–25
83. Collins, G. A., Sutter, M. C., Teiser, J. C. 1972. *Can. J. Physiol. Pharmacol.* 50:300–9
84. Magaribuchi, T., Ito, Y., Kuriyama, H. 1971. *Jap. J. Physiol.* 21:691–708
85. van Breemen, C., Farinas, B. R., Gerba, P., McNaughton, E. D. 1972. *Circ. Res.* 30:44–54
86. Mayer, C. J., van Breemen, C., Casteels, R. 1972. *Pfluegers Arch.* 337:333–50
87. van Breemen, C., McNaughton, E. 1970. *Biochem. Biophys. Res. Commun.* 39:567–74
88. Hodgson, B. J., Kidwai, A. M., Daniel, E. E. 1972. *Can. J. Physiol. Pharmacol.* 50:730–33
89. van Breemen, C. et al 1973. *Phil. Trans. Roy. Soc. London B* 265:57–71
90. Burton, J., Godfraind, T. 1973. *Arch. Int. Pharmacodyn. Ther.* 204:181–83
91. Casteels, R., van Breemen, C., Wuytack, F. 1972. *Nature* 239:249–51
92. Rubin, R. P. 1970. *Pharmacol. Rev.* 22:389–428
93. Borowicz, J. L. 1972. *Life Sci.* 11:959–64
94. Foreman, J. C., Mongar, J. L. 1972. *Nature New Biol.* 240:255–56
95. Lawson, D. M., Schmidt, G. H. 1972. *Proc. Soc. Exp. Biol. Med.* 140:481–84
96. Murakami, A., Eckert, R. 1972. *Science* 175:1375–77
97. Bull, R. J., Trevor, A. J. 1972. *J. Neurochem.* 19:999–1009
98. Smith, T. C., Mikiten, T. M., Levinson, C. 1972. *J. Cell. Physiol.* 79:117–25
99. Harris, A. F., Cotty, V. F. 1970. *Arch. Int. Pharmacodyn. Ther.* 186:269–78
100. Cuthbert, A. W., Wong, P. Y. D. 1972. *Mol. Pharmacol.* 8:222–29
101. Mela, L. 1968. *Arch. Biochem. Biophys.* 123:286–93
102. Lehninger, A. L., Carafoli, E. 1971. *Arch. Biochem. Biophys.* 143:506–15
103. Chevallier, J., Butow, R. A. 1971. *Biochemistry* 10:2733–37
104. Krasnow, N. 1972. *Biochim. Biophys. Acta* 282:187–94
105. Entman, M. L., Hansen, J. L., Cook, J. W. Jr. 1969. *Biochem. Biophys. Res. Commun.* 35:258–64
106. Ohnishi, T., Masoro, E., Bertrand, H. A., Yu, B. P. 1972. *Biophys. J.* 12:1251–65

URIC ACID IN NONHUMAN PRIMATES WITH SPECIAL REFERENCE TO ITS RENAL TRANSPORT

❖6598

George M. Fanelli Jr. and Karl H. Beyer Jr.
Merck Institute for Therapeutic Research, West Point, Pennsylvania

INTRODUCTION

This review is limited to renal uric acid transport and to any ancillary data on plasma or urinary urate concentrations and uricase in nonhuman primates only. Recently a very comprehensive review on renal mechanisms for the regulation of uric acid excretion in man and numerous other species has been published (1); this excellent review should be consulted by all individuals interested in uric acid. Older reviews that briefly touch upon urate metabolism in nonhuman primates have also appeared (2, 3).

There has been considerable confusion in the literature in which nonhuman primates have been utilized as experimental subjects because the word monkey was usually used in the materials section without regard to genus, species, or sex. However, this unfortunate situation is improving. All primates are mammals but not all mammals are primates. Man is the highest primate; the nonhuman primates comprise the Old and New World monkeys, the anthropoids or great apes (chimpanzee, orangutan, gorilla), and the lesser apes (gibbon and siamang). It is to be stressed that an ape is not a monkey. Excellent volumes on the classification of living primates are available (4, 4a).

In previous years the increased demand for nonhuman primates in biomedical research has precipitated a dangerous and alarming depletion of these animals in their natural habitat to the point that some are now classified as endangered and vanishing species. Therefore, the use of nonhuman primates must not be indiscriminate; wherever possible, they should not be used for terminal studies. In the interests of conservation, there should be a provision for propagation of the species. The Regional Primate Research Centers in the United States and several other institutions are actively engaged in breeding programs.

355

Because there is a paucity of renal urate studies in nonhuman primates recorded in the literature, we have attempted to be as complete as possible and have included all known references, even those remotely concerning urate. A comprehensive tabulation of uric acid values in plasma and urine has been made available by the Primate Information Center of the Regional Primate Research Center at the University of Washington (5).

ENDOGENOUS PLASMA OR SERUM URATE IN NONHUMAN PRIMATES

Old World Species

All Old World (Africa, Asia, Far East) monkeys have extremely low circulating serum urates. An early report of blood uric acid in a "monkey" (presumably a rhesus) was 0.4 mg/100 ml (6).

Macacca mulatta, the well-known rhesus, possess endogenous urate levels in males and females of 0.28–0.65 mg/100 ml (7), and the following mean values: 0.35 mg/100 ml (8), 0.88 mg/100 ml (9), 0.3 mg/100 ml (10, 11). Doloway et al (12) reported a plasma urate range of 0.9–1.4 mg/100 ml in female rhesus monkeys. Species other than the rhesus such as the stump-tailed macaque (*M. arctoides*) have a plasma urate less than 0.5 mg/100 ml (13) and 0.3 mg/100 ml (10, 11); the crab-eating monkey (*M. fasicularis*) was 0.5 mg/100 ml (10, 11). Recently Tisher, Schrier & McNeil (11a) listed values for mean serum uric acids of 0.5, 0.7, and 0.7 mg/100 ml for the rhesus, crab-eating macaque, and stump-tailed macaque, respectively. Similarly another species of macaque, the male Celebes black ape (*Cynopithecus niger*), had a plasma urate less than 0.5 mg/100 ml (13). A group of monkeys closely related to the macaques, i.e. the baboons of Africa, have been reported to possess no detectable serum uric acid by the uricase method (14). Using a colorimetric method, de la Pena, Matthijssen & Goldzieher (15) presented plasma urate values from *Papio* sp. with a mean of 0.7 and a range of 0.1–1.6 mg/100 ml; the male olive baboon (*P. anubis*) has a plasma urate less than 0.5 mg/100 ml (13). Weber et al (16) found mean plasma urates of 0.4 mg/100 ml in the chacma baboon of South Africa (*P. ursinus*) whereas Murphy et al (17) gave a mean figure of 0.21 for this species. Mean values for the yellow baboon *(P. cynocephalus)* of 0.4 mg/100 ml have been recorded (10, 11). One study in the Guinea baboon (*Papio papio*) (18) reported much higher values of 3.35 (range 2.13–5.43) mg/100 ml for randomly sexed mature animals. This large difference from other reported values for the baboon remains unexplained. Serum uric acid values for the Gelada baboon (*Theropithecus gelada*) were 1.2 mg/100 ml (K. F. Burns, personal communication). In the male Mandrill (*Mandrillus sphinx*) and the male African green monkey (*Cercopithecus aethiops*), endogenous plasma urate was less than 0.5 mg/100 ml (13); the patas monkey (*Erythrocebus patas*) has a plasma urate of about 0.2 mg/100 ml (unpublished observations). A prosimian, the male thick-tailed bushbaby (*Galago crassicaudatus*), possessed a mean plasma urate concentration of 0.5 mg/100 ml (13). In another primitive prosimian, the tree shrew (*Tupaia glis*), a serum urate concentration of 0.5 mg/100 ml was reported (10, 11); unpublished observations from our laboratory for endogenous plasma urate in this species were less than 0.5 mg/100 ml.

New World Species

New World (South America) monkeys with the exception of the *Cebus* (10, 11, 13, 19–25) and spider (13) and woolly monkeys (D. E. Duggan and R. M. Noll, personal communication) have vanishing low endogenous plasma urates. Endogenous plasma urate in the spider monkey (*Ateles* sp.) was reported to range from 3.3–6.3 mg/100 ml (13), whereas the woolly monkey (*Lagothrix lagothricha*) had a mean plasma urate of 3.2 mg/100 ml (unpublished observation). In another study, mean serum urate in the latter species was 3.1 mg/100 ml (10, 11). *C. capucinus* (males and females) maintain plasma levels within a range of 1.5–6.0 mg/100 ml, whereas *C. albifrons* and *C. apella* have plasma urate of 0.8–6.0 (13, 25) and 1.5–6.0 mg/100 ml (13), respectively. The common squirrel monkey (*Saimiri sciureus*) possesses endogenous urate concentrations of 0.5 mg/100 ml (10, 11) or less (13). Other studies in this species reported plasma urates with a mean of 1.0 mg/100 ml (26) and 1.0 with a range of 0.2–2.1 mg/l00 ml (27). In the authors' laboratory, it was found that plasma urate in the howler monkey was 0.3 mg/100 ml (unpublished observations). For the night monkey (*Aotus trivirgatus*), Wellde et al (28) tabulated a mean plasma uric acid level of 0.5 mg/100 ml. In the marmoset family, mean serum urates of 2.7 mg/100 ml (range 0–7.7) for the cottontop pinché (*Saguinus oedipus*) have been reported (29); these same authors also report mean values of 1.8 (range 0.6–3.1 mg/100 ml) for the moustached tamarin (*S. mystax*). These values seem rather high for this primitive family but Christen et al (10, 11) reported serum urates of 2.1 mg/100 ml for *S. oedipus*.

Great Apes

In a study by the United States Air Force (30), serum uric acid in male and female chimpanzees aged 1.5–16 years ranged from 2.7 to 5.8 mg/100 ml with the mean being 4.1. This report represented the first published data of its kind. Subsequently, mean serum urate figures for juvenile and mature chimpanzees of 3.57 and 4.68 mg/100 ml, respectively, appeared (18). The authors' laboratory (13) tabulated plasma urates of 2–5 mg/100 ml in male chimpanzees, but we have since noted endogenous levels of 6 mg/100 ml and higher. Clevenger, Marsh & Perry (31) noted serum urates of 2.2–2.7, 3.0, and 1.9–2.8 mg/100 ml for the gorilla, chimpanzee, and orang, respectively. Mean serum urates of 2.4 mg/100 ml (range 1.6–3.4) have been published for the gorilla (32); the same authors (33) reported mean figures for serum urates of 4.4, 2.8, and 2.7 mg/100 ml for infant, juvenile, and adult orangs, respectively. McClure, Keeling & Guilloud (33a) also recently found a mean serum uric acid value of 3.6 mg/100 ml (range 1.7–9.8) for the chimpanzee.

Lesser Apes

Mean plasma urate from the white-handed gibbon (*Hylobates lar*) was ascertained to range from 2–5 mg/100 ml (13), and in a more extensive study the mean value was 3.0 mg/100 ml (5). Also, a plasma urate of 2.6 mg/100 ml (5) was recorded for a female siamang (*H. syndactylus*).

URICASE: PRESENCE OR ABSENCE AND URIC ACID AND ALLANTOIN EXCRETION

The oxidative enzyme uricase catalyzes the aerobic oxidation of uric acid to the more soluble and readily excretable allantoin (for review see reference 3). The presence of uricase is responsible for the relatively low concentrations of circulating serum urate in most monkeys when compared with man and the great apes who maintain serum levels at much higher concentrations because of the mutational loss of this enzyme during the course of evolution (1). The first report that liver uricase was present in any nonhuman primate came from Wells (34) who confirmed its presence in the rhesus monkey. Subsequently, Wells & Caldwell (35, 36) showed that, like man, the chimpanzee and orang liver was devoid of uricase. They also agreed with the earlier important finding of Wiechowski (37) that the chimpanzee, also like man, excretes uric acid but no allantoin in the urine, whereas monkeys excrete chiefly allantoin. Hunter & Givens (38) showed that allantoin was a true urinary end product in the guenon [classified then as *Cercopithecus callitrichus,* while this species name is not mentioned by Napier & Napier (4) but is noted by Chiarelli (4a) to be *C. aethiops* or the green monkey]; only traces of uric acid were excreted. In a subsequent study by the same authors (39) using the same monkey in which they fed purine bases, allantoin was again confirmed to be the chief urinary end product with the appearance of only small amounts of uric acid. Hunter & Ward (40) put man and the chimpanzee in a class by themselves, characterized by the loss of uricolytic power and the consequent replacement of allantoin by uric acid as an end product of purine metabolism. From the historical point of view the papers by Wells, Hunter, and especially Wiechowski are of much interest. Friedemann (41) found that the orang, like the chimpanzee and man, excreted purines mainly as uric acid.

In an extensive study, Rheinberger (42) found that the orang and especially the chimpanzee excreted more uric acid as a percentage of total nitrogen than for the Old World monkeys studied. She also noted that the capuchin or *Cebus* and spider monkeys eliminated more urinary uric acid, thus presaging more definitive studies to be recounted later in this review. Although it was assumed that *C. albifrons* lacked liver uricase because of the rather high circulating uric acid (21), we found that *C. capucinus, C. albifrons,* and *C. apella* did in fact possess liver uricase but that the activity of the oxidative enzyme was present at a very low level (13). Subsequently Simkin (24, 25) and Simkin, Healey & Smuckler (43) demonstrated that even though uricase activity was present in the liver of *C. albifrons,* the relatively high circulating urate was the result of far higher rates of urate synthesis and destruction (formation of allantoin) than in man. Essentially the same results have been found by Duggan and Noll of these laboratories (unpublished observations). Urate pool sizes, turnover times, and biosynthetic rates have been determined by in vivo kinetic studies in the spider monkey, gibbon, and chimpanzee (44).

Hexose infusions in *C. albifrons* led to a rapid increase in plasma and urinary uric acid (45, 46). Data from these studies indicated a prompt increase in urate pool size and were consistent with an accelerated catabolism of a limited pool of preformed purines.

An editorial on the evolutionary aspects of the loss of uricase and nonhuman primate uricase has also appeared (47).

Uricase Demonstration by Histochemical and Electron Microscopic Techniques

Using morphologic techniques alone, Hruban & Swift (48) showed that there was a resemblance between the crystalloid of hepatic microbodies and uricase crystals. Histochemically, de la Iglesia, Porta & Hartroft (49) demonstrated uricase activity in hepatic microbodies of squirrel monkeys (*S. sciureus*). Shnitka (50), although presenting no direct evidence of uricase in hepatic microbodies in nonhuman primates, has presented an interesting account of interspecies differences in these subcellular structures. An excellent review by de la Iglesia (51) on comparative analysis of these hepatic microbodies has appeared in which he showed that *Cebus* and squirrel monkey possess uricase. Tisher et al (52) found that renal microbodies in the rhesus monkey did not contain detectable uricase activity, thus confirming earlier work (34) in which no uricase activity was detected in the kidney. Nakajima & Bourne (53) demonstrated hepatic uricase activity histochemically in various nonhuman primates; they also found no uricase in the kidneys of the chimpanzee, orang, rhesus, and Java monkey (*M. irus*). Hruban & Rechcigl (54, 55) have presented extensive evidence for uricase in monkeys and its absence in the great apes; included is an extensive bibliography on microbodies.

RENAL URATE TRANSPORT

Old World Monkeys

The only study on renal clearances of urate in relation to inulin clearance (C_{ur}/C_{In}) showed that in the species examined, uric acid was avidly secreted by the renal tubules (13) i.e. ($C_{ur}/C_{In} > 1.0$, or urate clearance was greater than the simultaneous inulin clearance (a measure of glomerular filtration rate or GFR). The only exception was that of the thick-tailed bushbaby in which there was limited evidence for net tubular reabsorption of urate ($C_{ur}/C_{In} < 1.0$). In the olive baboon, apparent net urate secretion can be readily inhibited by high doses of *p*-aminohippurate (PAH), probenecid and pyrazinoic acid (unpublished observations). In fact high doses of PAH and probenecid can convert net secretion to net reabsorption giving clearance ratios as low as 0.78 from initial values as high as 2.0 and thus furnishing evidence for bidirectional renal tubular transport of urate. These monkeys were urate loaded by constant intravenous infusion, for they all possess abundant liver uricase and consequently maintain low levels of endogenous urate, the accurate determination of which presents numerous technical difficulties (13). Bidirectional transport of urate is not unique, as it has been demonstrated in various other species (1), but the baboon studies represent the first observance of this general phenomenon in any nonhuman primate.

In slices of kidney cortex in a monkey (presumably a rhesus), Platts & Mudge (56) found that there was no accumulation of uric acid. Cannon, Symchych & DeMartini (57) showed that in antidiuretic *M. mulatta* infused with sodium urate, there was an increasing urate gradient from renal cortex to medulla with the highest concentration in the papillary tip, whereas in hydrated monkeys, similar infusions were not associated with a urate concentration gradient.

New World Monkeys

In a variety of monkeys, net reabsorption of varying degree was shown (13); C_{ur}/C_{In} from certain members of the family Cebidae varied from about 0.03 representing extensive urate reabsorption to 0.93 (approximately the level of glomerular filtration). The only exception was the red howler monkey in which net secretion was seen ($C_{ur}/C_{In} = 1.8$). The reason for this exception remains unexplained. Unpublished values from this laboratory of C_{ur}/C_{In} for the woolly monkey averaged about 0.13.

In the *Cebus* monkey, Skeith & Healey (21) showed that infusions of probenecid, sulfinpyrazone, and chlorothiazide increased urate clearance whereas β-hydroxybutyrate, lactate, and pyrazinoic acid produced a fall in this parameter. These observations were confirmed and extended to show an apparent tubular maximum (*Tm*) for urate in the *Cebus* that was enhanced by pyrazinoic acid (PZ) and reduced by probenecid (22). Also in this work, it was postulated that high loads of PAH inhibited the secretory moiety for urate by depressing the clearance ratio although not to the degree produced by PZ. Even though net urate secretion could not be demonstrated, the above results strongly suggested that it does exist. Urate was not bound to serum proteins in the *Cebus* (22, 58). May & Weiner (59) reported that *m*-hydroxybenzoic acid (*m*-HBA) was both secreted and reabsorbed by the kidney of *C. albifrons,* both of which processes were "carrier mediated." Also *m*-HBA was a powerful inhibitor of uric acid secretion and a weak inhibitor of PAH secretion; it behaved very much like PZ. Their data suggested that there may be one or more organic anion secretory mechanisms with overlapping specificities. Blanchard et al (60) examined the uricosuric potency of 2-substituted analogs of probenecid in the same species of monkey and found that they were about 10 times as potent as probenecid. Each analog was actively secreted albeit at different rates, and their enhanced uricosuric activity was due to the fact that they are all stronger acids than probenecid. Weiner & Tinker (61) in an extensive study of pyrazinamide and its principal metabolite, the free acid (PZ), conclusively indicated that PZ was bidirectionally transported by active mechanisms in *C. albifrons* in that its clearance was subject to competitive inhibition and insensitive to other manipulations characteristic of passive processes.

In *C. albifrons,* Vinay et al (62–64) ascribed the potent uricosuric action of benziodarone to a stimulation of urate secretion. Recently, Lemieux et al (65), extending their studies with benziodarone in *C. albifrons,* have apparently relinquished their earlier untenable assumption that benziodarone stimulated urate secretion. The marked uricosuric action of benziodarone results from inhibition of urate reabsorption in the proximal tubule in the *Cebus* (66).

Roch-Ramel & Weiner (67, 68), in the only free flow micropuncture studies to date in *C. albifrons,* found that at least 70–80% of urate was reabsorbed in the proximal tubule with no reabsorption of urate detectable in Henle's loop or distal tubules of surface nephrons. 2-Nitroprobenecid, a uricosuric agent, inhibited net urate reabsorption from the proximal tubule (68).

Known uricosuric drugs in man, with the exception of the potent zoxazolamine, were uricosuric in the *Cebus* (69). Also in the *Cebus,* mercurial diuretics in the absence of PAH loading were only slightly uricosuric; Tm for PAH was variably reduced (70).

Great Apes

It has been long recognized that the animals closest to man are the great apes. The chimpanzee (*Pan troglodytes*), however, is most closely related to man both serologically and immunologically (71). Because of wide species differences in the renal handling of urate (1, 72), we undertood a project to study renal urate transport in the chimpanzee systematically. Our very first experiments were carried out through the generous cooperation of the United States Air Force at Holloman AFB, New Mexico. Thereafter, through acquired knowledge and experience, our own small chimpanzee colony was established.

The first published work employing conventional renal clearance techniques in the chimpanzee was that of Smith & Clarke (73), although they did not measure urate clearance. Similarly, Gagnon & Clarke (74) enlarged on these earlier studies (73), but no urate data were presented. In another baseline study (75) of renal function in immature chimpanzees, urate clearances were not performed.

Elmadjian (76) reported that young chimpanzees (18.2 kg) excreted an average of 348 mg of uric acid/day or 0.267 mg/min, but no plasma urate values were given. Gagnon (77), assuming a plasma level of urate of 2 mg/100 ml, calculated that uric acid clearance would be about 13 ml/min or 0.73 ml/kg/min; this value was much greater than was found in an extensive study of urate clearances in adult chimpanzees (78) in which C_{ur}/GFR based on 417 observations was 0.104±0.008. The corresponding figure for C_{ur} was 0.215 ± 0.022 ml/min/kg. Pyrazinoic acid greatly diminished C_{ur}/GFR, the effect of which was not overcome by probenecid (78). Also in this study, the increased urate clearance brought about by probenecid was promptly nullified by pyrazinoic acid. It is also true that all known uricosuric drugs in man are effective in the chimpanzee (79).

The mercurial diuretics mersalyl (Salyrgan) and chlormerodrin (Neohydrin) markedly reduced Tm_{PAH} (80). Conclusive proof was presented that intravenous mersalyl, in the absence of PAH loading, readily converted net urate reabsorption to unequivocal net secretion; the highest C_{ur}/GFR noted was 1.98 (81). Also in the latter study, certain inhibitors of organic anion secretory transport prevented the appearance of net urate secretion; the magnitude of the uricosuric response correlated fairly closely with the excretion of mercury (81). Pyrazinoate (PZ) was apparently secreted and reabsorbed by active transport processes for the clearance ratio (C_{PZ}/GFR), normally greater than 1.0 was reduced to values well below control by probenecid, PAH, Diodrast, mersalyl, sulfinpyrazone, etc (82); PZ had a dual effect on urate excretion, for at a concentration in plasma of less than 10 μg/ml, there was a concentration related fall in C_{ur}/GFR. This ratio was maximally depressed at plasma PZ concentrations of 10–100 μ/ml. At PZ concentrations greater than

600 μg/ml, a definite uricosuric response was seen. These results were consistent with a model of urate transport in the chimpanzee involving high rates of bidirectional transtubular fluxes (82).

A new hypolipidemic-uricosuric agent, halofenate, was found to be uricosuric in the chimpanzee; halofenate free acid was actively secreted and passively reabsorbed (83) and was thought to act like other uricosuric drugs by partially inhibiting renal tubular reabsorption of urate at the luminal membrane.

A review on the morphology and anatomy of the urinary system in nonhuman primates has also appeared (84).

In summary, we have tried to show that, even among the nonhuman primates, marked species differences do exist regarding plasma urate concentrations, presence or absence of uricase, and the net renal clearance of uric acid. The complexities of urate transport are great, and this is eminently apparent in this specialized animal order. Even the superficial resemblance of the renal handling of urate between the chimpanzee and man can be misleading whenever one endeavors to extrapolate results to man. It is the relationship of the relative affinities (differing susceptibilities) of the urate transport mechanisms to various drugs, including the important area of drug interactions, which contributes to these highly complex renal mechanisms. There is also evidence that the chimpanzee urate transport system is more sensitive to the action of various drugs than is the case for man (Weiner and Fanelli, unpublished observations).[1]

Literature Cited

1. Gutman, A. B., Yü, T. F. 1972. *Sem. Arthritis Rheum.* 2:1–46
2. Folin, O., Berglund, H., Derick, C. 1924. *J. Biol. Chem.* 60:361–471
3. Keilin, J. 1959. *Biol. Rev. Cambridge Phil. Soc.* 34:265–96
4. Napier, J. R., Napier, P. H. 1967. *A Handbook of Living Primates.* London: Academic. 456 pp.
4a. Chiarelli, A. B. 1972. *Taxonomic Atlas of Living Primates.* London: Academic. 363 pp.
5. Morrow, A. C., Terry, M. W. 1972. *Urea nitrogen, uric acid and creatinine in the blood of nonhuman primates.* Seattle: Primate Info. Ctr., Regional Primate Res. Ctr. Univ. Washington. 30 pp.
6. Maddock, S., Svedburg, A. 1938. *Am. J. Physiol.* 121:203–8
7. Asatiani, V. S., Pichkhaya, T. P., Agieva, A. K. 1959. *Bull. Exp. Biol. Med.* 47:203–6 (in Russian)
8. Annenkov, G. A. 1965. *Inst. Exp. Path. Therap. Akad. Med. Nauk SSSR,* 99–103 (in Russian)
9. Petery, J. J. 1967. *Lab. Anim. Care* 17:342–44
10. Christen, P., Peacock, W. C., Christen, A. E., Wacker, W. E. C. 1970. *Eur. J. Pharmacol.* 12:3–5
11. Christen, P., Peacock, W. C. Christen, A. E., Wacker, W. E. C. 1970. *Folia Primatol.* 13:35–9
11a. Tisher, C. C., Schrier, R. W., McNeil, J. S. 1972. *Am. J. Physiol.* 223:1128–37
12. Dolowy, W. C., Henson, D., Cornet, J., Sellin, H. 1966. *Cancer* 19:1813–19
13. Fanelli, G. M., Bohn, D. L., Russo, H. F. 1970. *Comp. Biochem. Physiol.* 33:459–64
14. Vagtborg, H. 1967. *The Baboon in Medical Research,* ed. H. Vagtborg, III. Austin, Texas: Univ. Texas Press. 908 pp.
15. de la Pena, A., Matthijssen, C., Goldzieher, J. W. 1970. *Lab. Anim. Care* 20:251–61
16. Weber, H. W., Brede, H. D., Retief, C. P., Retief, F. P., Melby, E. C. Jr. 1971. *The Baboon in Medical Research: Base-*

[1]Since submission of this review, values for serum uric acid from the rhesus monkey of 1.0–1.4 mg/100 ml have been noted (85).

line Studies in Fourteen Hundred Baboons and Pathological Observations. In *Defining the Laboratory Animal,* 528–49. Washington DC: Nat. Acad. Sci. 628 pp.

17. Murphy, G. P. et al 1968. *S. Afr. Med. J.* 42:26–37

18. Burns, K. F., Ferguson, F. G., Hampton, S. H. 1967. *Am. J. Clin. Pathol.* 48:484–94

19. Healey, L. A., Skeith, M. D. 1966. *Arthritis Rheum.* 9:510

20. Skeith, M. D., Healey, L. A. 1967. *Clin. Res. 15:114*

21. Skeith, M. D., Healey, L. A. 1968. *Am. J. Physiol.* 214:582–84

22. Fanelli, G. M. Jr., Bohn, D., Stafford, S. 1970. *Am. J. Physiol.* 218:627–36

23. Simkin, P., Fortune, K. M., Healey, L. A. 1969. *Arthritis Rheum.* 12:697

24. Simkin, P. 1971. *Clin. Res.* 19:142

25. Simkin, P. 1971. *Am. J. Physiol.* 221:1105–9

26. Manning, P. J., Lehner, N. D. M., Feldner, M. A., Bullock, B. C. 1969. *Lab. Anim. Care* 19:831–37

27. New, A. E. 1968. *Baseline Blood Determinations of the Squirrel Monkey.* In *Squirrel Monkey* eds. L. A. Rosenblum, R. W. Cooper, 416–19. New York: Academic. 451 pp.

28. Wellde, B. T., Johnson, A. J., Williams, J. S., Langbehn, H. R., Sadun, E. H. 1971. *Lab. Anim. Sci.* 21:575–80

29. Holmes, A. W., Passovoy, M., Caps, R. B. 1967. *Lab. Anim. Care* 17:41–47

30. Staten, F. W. et al 1961. *Air Force Missile Develop. Ctr. Tech. Rep. 61–21. 15 pp.*

31. Clevenger, A. B., Marsh, W. L., Perry, T. M. 1971. *Am. J. Clin. Pathol.* 55:479–88

32. McClure, H. M., Keeling, M. E., Guilloud, N. B. 1972. *Folia Primatol.* 18:300–16

33. McClure, H. M., Keeling, M. E., Guilloud, N. B. 1972. *Folia Primatol.* 18:284–99

33a. McClure, H. M., Keeling, M. E., Guilloud, N. B. 1972. *Folia Primatol.* 18:444–62

34. Wells, H. G. 1910. *J. Biol. Chem.* 7:171–83

35. Wells, H. G., Caldwell G. T. 1914. *J. Biol. Chem.* 18:157–65

36. Wells, H. G., Caldwell, G. T. 1914. *Proc. Soc. Exp. Biol. Med.* 11:153–54

37. Wieckowski, W. 1912. *Prager Med. Wochenschr.* 37:275–76

38. Hunter, A., Givens, M. H. 1912. *J. Biol. Chem.* 13:371–88

39. Hunter, A., Givens, M. H. 1914. *J. Biol. Chem.* 17:37–53

40. Hunter, A., Ward, F. W. 1919. *Trans. Roy. Soc. Can.* Sec. 5:13:7–11

41. Friedemann, T. E. 1934. *J. Biol. Chem.* 105:335–41

42. Rheinberger, M. B. 1936. *J. Biol. Chem.* 115:343–60

43. Simkin, P. A., Healey, L. A. Jr., Smuckler, E. 1970. *N. Engl. J. Med.* 283:823–24

44. Noll, R. M., Duggan, D. E. 1971. *Pharmacologist* 13:208

45. Simkin, P. A. 1969. *Clin. Res.* 12:332

46. Simkin, P. A. 1972. *Metab. Clin. Exp.* 21:1029–36

47. Wacker, W. E. C. 1970. *N. Engl. J. Med.* 283:151–52

48. Hruban, Z., Swift, H. 1964. *Science* 146:1316–18

49. de la Iglesia, F. A., Porta, E. A., Hartroft, W. S. 1966. *J. Histochem. Cytochem.* 14:685–87

50. Shnitka, T. K. 1966. *J. Ultrastruct. Res.* 16:598–625

51. de la Iglesia, F. A. 1969. *Acta Hepato Splenol.* 16:141–60

52. Tisher, C. C., Finkel, R. M., Rosen, S., Kendig, E. M. 1968. *Lab. Invest.* 19:1–6

53. Nakajima, Y., Bourne, G. H. 1970. *Histochemie* 22:20–24

54. Hruban, Z., Rechcigl, M. Jr. 1967. *Fed. Proc.* 26:513

55. Hruban, Z., Rechcigl, M. Jr. 1969. *Intern. Rev. Cytol. Suppl. I.* 296 pp.

56. Platts, M. M., Mudge, G. H. 1961. *Am. J. Physiol.* 200:387–92

57. Cannon, P. J., Symchych, P. S., De martini, F. E. 1968. *Proc. Soc. Exp. Biol. Med.* 129:278–84

58. Simkin, P. A. 1972. *Proc. Soc. Exp. Biol. Med.* 139:604–6

59. May, D. G., Weiner, I. M. 1971. *J. Pharmacol. Exp. Ther.* 176:407–17

60. Blanchard, K. C., Maroske, D., May, D. G., Weiner, I. M. 1972. *J. Pharmacol. Exp. Ther.* 180:397–410

61. Weiner, I. M., Tinker, J. P. 1972. *J. Pharmacol. Exp. Ther.* 180:411–34

62. Vinay, P., Gougoux, A., Michaud, G., Lemieux, G. 1971. *Am. Soc. Nephrol. Meet.* 85

63. Vinay, P., Gougoux, A., Michaud, G., Lemieux, G. 1971. *Clin. Res.* 19:812

64. Vinay, P., Gougoux, A., Michaud, G., Lemieux, G. 1972. *Clin. Res.* 20:614

65. Lemieux, G., Gougoux, A., Vinay, P., Michaud, G. 1973. *Am. J. Physiol.* 224:1431–39

66. Lemieux, G., Vinay, P., Gougoux, A., Michaud, G. 1973. *Am. J. Physiol.* 224:1440–49
67. Roch-Ramel, F., Weiner, I. M. 1973. *Kidney Int.* 3:275
68. Roch-Ramel, F., Weiner, I. M. 1973. *Am. J. Physiol.* 224:1369–74
69. Fanelli, G. M. Jr., Bohn, D. L., Reilly, S. S. 1970. *J. Pharmacol. Exp. Ther.* 175:259–66
70. Fanelli, G. M. Jr., Bohn, D. L., Reilly, S. S. 1973. *Am. J. Physiol.* 224:993–96
71. Kratochvil, C. H. 1969. *Ann. N.Y. Acad. Sci.* 162:301–10
72. Weiner, I. M., Mudge, G. H. 1964. *Am. J. Med.* 36:743–62
73. Smith, H. W., Clarke, R. W. 1938. *Am. J. Physiol.* 122:132–39
74. Gagnon, J. A., Clarke, R. W. 1957. *Am. J. Physiol.* 190:117–20
75. Hamlin, R. L., Smith, C. R., Carter, W. T. 1964. *Aeromed. Res. Lab. Tech. Document. Rept.,* 64–18. 22 pp.
76. Elmadjian, F. 1963. *Aeromed. Res. Lab. Tech. Document. Rept.,* 63–18. 10 pp.
77. Gagnon, J. A. 1970. *Renal Function in the Chimpanzee.* ed. G. H. Bourne, 69–99. In *The Chimpanzee,* Vol. 2. Baltimore: Univ. Park Press. 417 pp.
78. Fanelli, G. M. Jr., Bohn, D. L., Reilly, S. S. 1971. *Am. J. Physiol.* 220:613–20
79. Fanelli, G. M. Jr., Bohn, D. L., Reilly, S. S. 1971. *J. Pharmacol. Exp. Ther.* 177:591–99
80. Fanelli, G. M. Jr., Bohn, D. L., Reilly, S. S. 1972. *J. Pharmacol. Exp. Ther.* 180:759–66
81. Fanelli, G. M. Jr., Bohn, D. L., Reilly, S. S., Weiner, I. M. 1973. *Am. J. Physiol.* 224:985–92
82. Fanelli, G. M. Jr., Weiner, I. M. 1973. *J. Clin. Invest.* 52:1946–57
83. Fanelli, G. M. Jr., Bohn, D. L., Reilly, S. S., Baer, J. E. 1972. *J. Pharmacol. Exp. Therap.* 180:377–96
84. Straus, W. L., Arcadi, J. A. 1958. *Primatologia* 3:507–41
85. Bourne, G. H., de Bourne, N. G., Keeling, M. E. 1973. *AGARD Conf. Proc.* 110:C6–1–6

MECHANISM OF ACTION OF INSULIN

❖6599

S. J. Pilkis and C. R. Park
Department of Physiology, Vanderbilt University, School of Medicine,
Nashville, Tennessee

INTRODUCTION

The literature on the mechanism of action of insulin on cells lacks a unifying concept despite the welter of experimental data. References to the classic experiments on insulin action and to recent reviews on various aspects of insulin action are found at the end of this article (1–10). Though insulin action has not been previously reviewed in this series, we restrict ourselves to work done over the last four to five years. This review reports in biochemical terms the effects of insulin on carbohydrate, fat, protein, and nucleic acid metabolism in the principal insulin sensitive tissues. After noting the individual effects of the hormone, we attempt to delineate possible mechanisms of action that account for these separate effects. This review emphasizes the effects of insulin action on carbohydrate metabolism, protein, and nucleic acid synthesis, and on the level of cyclic adenylate in cells.

EVIDENCE THAT THE ACTION OF INSULIN RESULTS FROM INITIAL INTERACTION WITH THE PLASMA MEMBRANE

Narahara (260) has reviewed past work on binding of insulin to tissues in relation to biological activity. The binding of insulin to tissue was first reported by Stadie et al (25) twenty years ago. This work was carried out using the isolated rat diaphragm exposed to iodoinsulin in vitro. The results were difficult to interpret, however, because of uncertainties as to whether the modified insulin had full biological potency (250, 251) and whether the hormone was actually bound or simply trapped in the interstices of the tissue. Antoniades & Gershoff (261) and later Crofford (22) showed that isolated fat cells could take up native insulin in a reaction that was so rapid that the uptake could be ascribed with reasonable certainty to binding to the plasma membrane. Since the insulin-membrane complex is stable in the cold (23, 251), these cells could be washed extensively at 0° to remove all

365

hormone not actually bound. Crofford (22), and subsequently Kono in detailed studies (43, 45), and others (23, 40, 54, 270, 271) have shown that the binding constant (K_c) for the hormone is much higher (3–7 nmol) than the concentration that gives half maximal activation of glucose utilization ($K_e = 50$ pmol). Cuatrecasas (27), and others (271, 272) have reported the existence of binding proteins of much higher affinity than the above. Kono (43, 45) and others (22, 23, 251) have proposed that only a small fraction of insulin receptors needs to interact with the hormone to generate a sufficient signal to induce metabolic changes. Kono (53) emphasizes that some processes (e.g. protein synthesis or lipolytic activation by insulin; see later), require much stronger signals than others (e.g. antilipolysis or glucose transport). The presence of many receptors allows strong signals to be developed, if necessary, and establishes sensitivity of the cell to low concentrations of hormone at all times. Sensitivity is promoted because the presence of receptors in large numbers, by mass action, increases the probability of hormone-receptor collision. Others (23, 27, 262) have suggested that cells have a small number of high affinity "specific" receptor sites and a large number of nonspecific sites. Kono & Colowick (263), Wohltmann & Narahara, (23) and Crofford (22) found that adipocytes washed at room temperature quickly lose insulin. Crofford (22) reported that insulin could not be found in the wash medium in an immunologically or biologically active form. This observation, along with his subsequent study (252, 253) with adipocyte plasma membranes, suggests that binding to the receptor may be followed by inactivation of the hormone. This is in line with the thought that any rapidly acting regulatory system must have very effective mechanisms to turn signals off as well as on. Others (27, 40, 264) using higher concentrations of insulin or unphysiological methods of dissociating the insulin receptor complex have found some of the hormone to be released in an active form. Recent work (264) suggests that the insulin receptor and an insulin degrading system in liver cell membranes are different.

Freychet et al (26) showed that lightly iodinated, fully biologically active insulin is bound to purified plasma membranes of rat liver. A number of investigators have extended this work and shown that plasma membranes from liver and fat cells (27–31), fibroblasts (32), lymphocytes (32), and the central nervous system (33) contain insulin-binding protein. The insulin-binding protein has been successfully dispersed from plasma membranes from fat cells and liver membranes (34, 35) using detergents. The binding protein of liver cells and adipocytes appears to be an asymmetrical protein, molecular weight about 300,000 with a frictional ratio of 1.7 and a Stokes radius of 71 Å (34). Cuatrecasas (35) has used affinity chromatography to isolate and purify an insulin-binding protein. It is not known, however, whether this is the physiological receptor, because no biological tests have been applied to it. Furthermore, it has been observed that membrane fractions exposed to phospholipase (C or A) show a great increase in insulin binding (27), whose significance is unknown.

It has been postulated that the binding of insulin to the membranes involves formation of disulfide bonds between the hormone and receptor (24, 36–38). Wohltmann & Narahara (23), however, were unable to relate the quantity of radioactive insulin that is covalently bound through disulfide bridges with the effect of the hormone on transport. Recently, Cuatrecasas (27, 39) and Pilkis et al (40) showed that insulin binding to fat cell membranes or purified liver plasma membranes is not affected by sulfhydryl-blocking agents.

Exposure of muscle (254) or fat cells (41–43) to proteases in low concentrations can induce insulin-like effects. Kono first noted that treatment of fat cells with trypsin or other proteases in very high concentrations results in a loss of insulin binding (42–43) and of biological effects. Cuatrecasas (44) reported that the affinity of the binding protein for insulin is diminished by such treatment, whereas Kono & Barham (45) found a decreased number of binding sites with no change in affinity. The insulin "receptors" regenerate upon further incubation of the cells in the presence of soybean trypsin inhibitor at a rate of about 3% of the total number per hour (42, 44, 45). Prior addition of insulin protects the "receptor" from proteolytic attack (30). Cuatrecasas found that exposure of fat cells to neuraminidase reduces the basal rate of glucose uptake and prevents the action of insulin (49). Neuraminidase digestion, however, does not affect insulin binding to fat cells (49) or to purified liver plasma membranes (50).

Reduced binding of insulin has been found in liver membranes of obese-hyperglycemic mice (51) suggesting that a deficiency of receptor may be an important component of some insulin-resistant states. No alteration in the binding of insulin to fat cells of rats treated with steroid or streptozotocin has been found (52).

Cuatrecasas (11) has reported that insulin bound covalently to sepharose beads will increase glucose oxidation and inhibit lipolysis in isolated fat cells. He claimed that the insulin sepharose complex is stable during incubation with tissue and that the sepharose bead is not taken up by cells. Cuatrecasas concludes, therefore, that insulin does not need to enter the cell to exert an effect. Others have shown that insulin-Sepharose or insulin-Dextran has insulin-like effects in various cell types and in the intact animal in these ways: it stimulates incorporation of precursors into RNA in mammary cells (12), accumulation of amino isobutyric acid in isolated mammary cells (13), glycogen synthesis in tadpole liver (14), glucose oxidation and glycogen synthesis in diaphragm muscle (15), and causes hypoglycemia in the rat (265).

These data must still be accepted only with reservations. Davidson (16) & Fritz (17) have presented evidence that insulin begins to leak off the Sepharose bead, commencing shortly after washing and continuing progressively. Davidson et al (16, 21) have concluded that insulin-Sepharose may be useful for isolating detergent-dispersed insulin-binding protein but it is not a suitable model for studying the biological effects of bound insulin. Katzen & Vlahakes (18) have recalculated the data of Cuatrecasas (11) on insulin-Sepharose and question the validity of his results. For example, only a few beads, and in some cases, only a fraction of a bead per milliliter would have been present in an incubation flask in his experiments, although the biological effects obtained were purportedly equal to those given by the same amount of unbound insulin (19, 20). It is important to clarify these Sepharose-insulin experiments because they constitute potentially an ingenious and useful tool for determining that a hormone need not enter a cell to exert a biological effect.

Much data already suggest that this is true for insulin, in particular the studies (42, 43, 46–48) with trypsin in which the evidence seems good that the enzyme attacks only structures on the surface of the plasma membrane.

The insulin-receptor complex formation can be postulated to induce a conformational change in the receptor that leads to generation of a signal. Light exposure to trypsin (41–43) or to p-chloromercuribenzoate (273) apparently also triggers effectively the generation of this or a similar signal which activates glucose utilization, inhibits lipolysis, and lowers the level of cAMP. Heavy exposure to trypsin or other proteases destroys the capacity of the receptor to bind hormone or to generate a signal. A very light exposure to N-ethylmaleimide blocks the insulin stimulation of transport without affecting the basal rate of transport or other metabolic parameters (266, 268). Binding of insulin is not blocked under these conditions but is apparently blocked by substantially heavier exposure to maleimide (22). These results suggest that the receptor is in part, at least, a peptide or protein. Kono & Barham (43, 45) estimate that a fat cell possesses about 160,000 receptors and that glucose utilization is maximally stimulated when 4000 of these sites are occupied. Crofford (22) reported that binding of 3000 molecules of insulin would stimulate glucose utilization maximally and that complexing of about 100 insulin molecules can generate a detectable metabolic response.

What is the nature of the signal generated by insulin-receptor interaction? This is the central, unanswered question with regard to the mechanism of insulin action. Some speculations are considered later.

EFFECTS OF INSULIN ON MUSCLE

Protein Metabolism

The molecular mechanism whereby insulin controls protein metabolism has been most extensively studied in muscle (55). So far as presently known, insulin appears to stimulate synthesis of all proteins in muscle, whereas in some other tissues, synthesis of specific enzymes is involved. Wool & Krahl (56) first demonstrated that the effect of insulin on incorporation of amino acids into diaphragm muscle protein was independent of the action of the hormone on glucose transport. This is also true of the perfused rat heart (55).

A number of observations regarding insulin effects on protein synthesis have been made using ribosome preparations. It has been shown that ribosomes from heart and skeletal muscle of diabetic animals do not synthesize protein as well as do preparations from normal animals (55, 57). Furthermore, insulin treatment of the diabetic animal increases the assembly of polysomes and the synthesis of protein by ribosomes by a mechanism that does not require RNA synthesis (58). That is, the effect of insulin is on translation of mRNA, not its synthesis. Martin & Wool (59) showed a defect in the 60S ribosomal subunit of diabetic muscle as regards its ability to carry on poly(U)-stimulated protein synthesis and to bind phenylalanine tRNA. This defect probably derives from the fact that ribosomes from normal liver retain greater amounts of bound peptidyl-tRNA when dissociated than do ribosomes isolated from the diabetic tissue (60, 61). Apparently peptidyl-tRNA bound to the ribosome acts as an initiator of peptide bond formation and aminoacyl-tRNA binding. Since some peptidyl-tRNA remains bound to the 60S ribosomal subunit when ribosomes are dissociated (60), the differing amounts of peptidyl-tRNA bound to muscle ribosomes from normal and diabetic animals would appear to be a plausible explanation for the difference in activity between the two preparations.

The reduction in peptidyl-tRNA bound to ribosomes from diabetic animals is probably explained by decreased initiation of endogenous protein synthesis. Rannels et al (62) have shown that levels of ribosomal subunits are increased in skeletal muscle but not in hearts from diabetic animals. Moreover, when protein synthesis of normal hearts perfused with glucose and amino acid is stimulated by addition of insulin, levels of subunits decrease and levels of polysomes rise, indicating that insulin has stimulated the initiation of peptide chains (63). Jefferson et al (64), employing an isolated perfused preparation of rat hemicorpus, have also shown that insulin decreases the levels of ribosomal subunits in this tissue.

In an attempt to study the initiation process itself, Wool et al (61) have studied the translation of polyuridylic acid and a viral mRNA by ribosomes from normal and diabetic animals. Ribosomes from diabetic animals were less efficient than ribosomes from normal animals. However, the difference tended to disappear after ribosomes were dissociated to subunits and then reconstituted (61). Wool et al (61) have also reported that ribosomal subunits isolated from muscle of diabetic animals reassociate less readily than normal in the presence of an initiation factor from rat liver.

Chain & Sender (65) report that protein synthesis by the perfused heart as well as the polysome profiles and amino acid incorporation by ribosomal preparations of these hearts are unaltered by streptozotocin-induced diabetes. These findings agree with those of Rannels et al (62) but are at variance with those of Wool et al (55).

It has been suggested that in heart, but not in skeletal muscle (65), elevated plasma concentrations of free fatty acids may be important in maintaining normal rates of protein synthesis (64).

Sender & Garlick (66) report that insulin stimulates labeling of all proteins separated by disc gel electrophoresis from extracts of the heart perfused with radioactive amino acid. They could detect no selective effect of the hormone on synthesis of specific proteins. Wool et al (55) earlier presented evidence that insulin stimulates the synthesis of a specific protein in diaphragm muscle, but this observation has not been confirmed.

The question of whether insulin may affect protein metabolism, and ultimately even ribosomal activity, by an effect on transport of amino acids across the cell membrane is still unanswered. It has been shown, in this connection, that raising the concentration of amino acids perfusing a rat heart (63) or liver preparation (274) will promote ribosome aggregation and increase incorporation into protein, thus duplicating effects of the hormone. Insulin in vitro stimulates the transport of some amino acids and not of others (67) whereas it stimulates incorporation of all naturally occurring amino acids, including those formed intracellularly into protein (68).

This would suggest that increased incorporation is not due entirely to increased uptake. This conclusion remains uncertain, however, because it is unclear whether amino acids entering the cell are incorporated preferentially into protein or mix with the pool of free amino acids within the tissue (67, 69). Manchester (69) has reviewed the effects of insulin on uptake of amino acids into muscle and the relation of this accumulation to the stimulation of amino acid incorporation into protein. In general, enhancement of amino acid transport in muscle by insulin does not appear to be a sufficient explanation for the hormone effect on protein synthesis (69).

Pozefsky et al (70) have shown recently that insulin reduces the plasma content of amino acids, in part at least, through suppression of release from msucle. All amino acids are affected, though quantitatively to different degrees.

Carbohydrate Metabolism in Muscle

The effects of insulin on carbohydrate metabolism have been well reviewed (5, 17, 88).

Glucose transport is the principal rate-limiting step for use of glucose in muscle under physiological conditions. The conclusion that insulin accelerates glucose transport has been confirmed by many investigators. Effects of insulin on kinetic parameters of transport have been investigated in perfused heart where the hormone increases the maximal rate of transport and appears to decrease the affinity somewhat (71–74). An increase in the maximal rate is also observed in skeletal muscle (75). The biochemical mechanism accounting for these changes is unknown (78), except that the movement of the carrier across the membrane is presumably increased. The rapidity of insulin action suggests that synthesis of new carrier is not involved. Weis & Narahara (254), using the frog sartorius preparation, have shown that trypsin stimulates glucose transport in a manner similar to insulin. This has also been observed in adipose cells (see later).

Gould & Chaudry (76) have studied the effect of cations on the action of insulin on glucose uptake by isolated rat soleus muscle. They found that stimulation of glucose uptake by insulin does not depend on monovalent cations in the incubation medium. Muscle depleted of Ca^{2+} and Mg^{2+} by EDTA treatment has a depressed glucose uptake which is not stimulated by insulin. Replacement of Mg^{2+} and Ca^{2+} restores the basal uptake to normal. However, Mg^{2+}, and not Ca^{2+}, is required for the stimulation by insulin. It is postulated that Mg^{2+} participates in the mechanism whereby insulin promotes the binding of glucose to the transport carrier. In our opinion, however, these studies do not distinguish between effects on transport and intracellular events. Gould & Chaudry also report (77) that anoxia does not stimulate glucose uptake in EDTA-treated muscle but does so in the presence of a low concentration of insulin, which by itself has no effect.

Tarui et al (15) have shown that insulin bound to dextran (molwt 40,000) stimulates glycogen formation in parallel with the facilitation of glucose transport in a manner similar to that of native insulin. This suggests that insulin exerts its effects in muscle on glycogen synthesis as well as glucose transport without entering the cell. Under certain conditions, an effect of insulin to control transport is seen without an effect on glycogen synthesis, while insulin can, under other conditions, affect glycogen synthesis without influencing glucose transport (89). Chain et al (90) have studied the effect of insulin on the pattern of glucose metabolism in the isolated perfused rat heart. In agreement with many previous studies, insulin stimulates glucose oxidation to CO_2, glycogen synthesis, and formation of phosphorylated sugar and lactate. Increasing the concentration of glucose in the perfusion medium leads to changes in the pattern of glucose metabolism that are quite different from those brought about by insulin. The effect of a work load on the pattern of glucose metabolism is also different from that of insulin. Beitner & Kalant (91), using rat hemidiaphragms, and Ozand & Narahara (92), using frog sartorius muscle, have shown that insulin stimulates the rate of glycolysis in muscle independently of its effect on glucose transport. Both groups conclude that insulin stimulates the phosphofructokinase reaction.

The Adenylate Cyclase System and Insulin Effects in Muscle

Wool et al (55) have reported that cAMP and caffeine inhibit amino acid incorporation in the isolated rat diaphragm. However, protein synthesis by ribosomes isolated from normal and diabetic rats is not influenced by addition of cAMP and caffeine to the cell-free systems (55).

Walaas et al (79) and Craig et al (80) have found no effect of insulin on cAMP content in the rat diaphragm. Insulin can increase the level of glycogen synthetase I without influencing that of cAMP (81), although, under certain conditions, a decreased cAMP concentration may be seen. Insulin injection into rats causes a slight increase in skeletal muscle cAMP content (82). Insulin does not alter the level of cAMP in perfused rat heart under conditions in which glucose transport is strongly stimulated (275). Goldberg et al (82) have reported that insulin in the presence of epinephrine elevates cAMP slightly in the isolated diaphragm. Although incubation of diaphragm with insulin augmented the rise in cAMP induced by epinephrine, glycogen phosphorylase activation was unaffected. Keely et al (83) have found that insulin in combination with epinephrine elevates cAMP in heart as in diaphragm.

Drummond et al (86) have reported that insulin in vitro does not affect the adenylate cyclase of purified plasma membranes of skeletal muscle in the presence or absence of epinephrine. Das & Chain (87) have reported a stimulating effect on cAMP phosphodiesterase in extracts of the isolated rat heart perfused with insulin. At present, it seems unlikely that cAMP is directly involved as a mediator of insulin action in muscle.

Larner (84) has postulated that insulin leads to formation of a nucleotide intermediate (in analogy to Murad et al, 85) that is in chemical equilibrium with cAMP. This "second messenger" would mediate the effects of insulin. The idea of a second messenger for insulin is an old one (269) but continues to be the leading theory of insulin action in many laboratories. There is, however, no experimental evidence whatsoever for the existence of such a compound.

EFFECTS OF INSULIN ON MAMMARY GLAND

Study of the effect of insulin and other hormones on cell proliferation in organ culture of mammary gland has yielded much information concerning the control of DNA, RNA, and protein synthesis. It is clear that this regulation in many types of cells is dependent upon exposure to several hormones in a well-defined sequence.

In explants of mammary glands cultured on chemically defined medium, 70% or more of the epithelial cells can be induced by insulin to proliferate (93, 94). Insulin stimulates incorporation of precursors into RNA and protein during the first 8–12 hr of culture, and shortly thereafter an increase in DNA synthesis is observed (94). Turkington and co-workers (95, 96) have also observed increased precursor incorporation into ribosomal RNA and rapidly labeled RNA after addition of insulin to intact cells. Addition of insulin to cells also results in an increased RNA polymerase activity measured in isolated nuclei (95, 96). Associated with these changes are increased rates of phosphorylation of histones and nonhistone proteins (97). Insulin induces initiation of DNA replication in the epithelial cells (93, 98) and, subsequent to this, cell division occurs. Both growth hormone and epithelial growth factor have similar effects on these cells (93, 99, 100).

Alevolar cell differentiation is dependent on the interaction of many hormones (94). Insulin, hydrocortisone, and prolactin increase the number of functionally differentiated cells (101, 102). The addition of all three hormones is necessary for a maximal response, but insulin or epithelial growth factor alone is adequate to stimulate cell division and differentiation in the proliferative stage (103). However, the effects of prolactin seen in the postmitotic period require insulin (103).

Stimulation of precursor incorporation into rapidly labeled RNA of isolated mammary cells has been reported using insulin covalently bound to Sepharose (12). Insulin did not change the specific activity of the intracellular precursor pool (12). These observations suggest action of the hormone at the cell membrane to stimulate an intracellular process. The reliability of insulin-sepharose as a tool is questionable, however, in view of the reservations already discussed.

Majumder & Turkington (104) have provided evidence that the level of cAMP is not rate limiting in the developing mammary gland. In organ cultures of mouse mammary tissue and in isolated epithelial cells, prolactin induces the synthesis of protein kinases in cells formed in vitro by insulin-mediated cell division (104). Insulin acts synergistically with prolactin for induction of the catalytic subunit of protein kinase, but induction of the cAMP-binding protein requires prolactin only. Neither hormone affects the activity of mammary cell plasma membrane adenylate cyclase. Addition of cAMP, dibutyryl cAMP, or theophylline to the incubation medium does not substitute for insulin, hydrocortisone, or prolactin. The regulatory polypeptide hormones in this system interact initially with the cell membrane (12, 104), but they do not affect adenylate cyclase activity. These data on the lack of role of cAMP in regulation of metabolism in developing mammary gland have not yet been confirmed by other workers.

INSULIN EFFECTS ON LIVER METABOLISM

Effects of Insulin on Liver Protein and Nucleic Acid Metabolism

As in muscle, insulin appears to have a general anabolic (or anticatabolic) effect in liver, but, in addition, insulin influences the levels of a number of specific proteins. Miller and co-workers have emphasized the essential nature of insulin in promoting positive nitrogen balance in the perfused liver (105). Mortimore & Mondon (106) have reported that insulin diminishes the release of $1\text{-}C^{14}$-valine from prelabeled proteins in the perfused liver. They have evidence that this is an effect of the hormone on lysosomal-induced proteolysis. It has also been postulated that insulin may stabilize hepatic lysosomes (107). Vavrinkova & Mosinger (177) reported that insulin administration decreases rat hepatic acid phosphatase, while glucagon elevates this activity. These authors conclude that the release of lysosomal enzymes in liver is hormonally sensitive and suggest that this process may well be under control of cAMP.

Microsomal and purified ribosomal preparations from livers of diabetic animals incorporate amino acids less efficiently than do such preparations from normal animals (108–111). Pilkis & Korner (110) find that this defect is most prominent in the free polysome fraction which has a lower than normal proportion of large polysomal aggregates. Insulin administration for 4 hr in vivo completely restores the activity and profile of the free polysome fraction to normal. As in diabetic muscle, ribosomes from diabetic liver have less bound peptidyl-tRNA, which may account for their reduced ability to incorporate amino acids into protein. Wittman et al have reported detectable effects of insulin injection within 5 min on rat liver polysome profiles (112).

The effect of insulin on the biosynthesis of hepatic enzymes has been well reviewed by Steiner (116). Insulin administration to diabetic rats over a period of days decreases the levels of gluconeogenic enzymes (pyruvate carboxylase, phosphoenolpyruvate carboxykinase, fructose-1,6-diphosphatase, and glucose-6-phosphatase), and increases the levels of the glycolytic enzymes (glucokinase, phosphofructokinase, and pyruvate kinase) (113). Protein and RNA synthesis are required for these hormone effects, but there is no evidence that insulin acts directly as an inducer or repressor of enzyme synthesis (116). In general, it seems likely that these slow changes in enzyme levels in liver of diabetic rats are a result of altered levels of substrates which protect the enzymes against degradation or promote their induction.

Surprisingly, there have been few detailed studies on insulin's effect on liver RNA synthesis despite the above data on hepatic enzyme synthesis (116). Steiner and associates have reported that insulin administration to diabetic rats stimulates incorporation of precursors into rapidly labeled total RNA and increases total RNA content in the liver (117). It has subsequently been shown that insulin administered to diabetic animals stimulates incorporation of labeled precursors into total nuclear RNA (118). Both nucleolar and extranucleolar labeling is stimulated, although the effect is first seen in the extranucleolar fraction (119). Insulin administration stimulates both the nucleolar and extranucleolar RNA polymerase activities. It seems likely that the effect of the hormone on incorporation of precursors into RNA is on the activity or quantity of the synthetic enzymes involved rather than on the pool size of precursor (118).

Relation between Insulin Action in the Liver and Hepatic cAMP Level

Exton and associates (reviewed by Park, 120) have presented evidence that many of the hepatic actions of insulin can be accounted for by a fall in intracellular levels of cAMP (121, 122). It should be pointed out, however, that these investigators do not believe that this phenomenon can account for all the effects of insulin in this or other tissues (120). Hepatic cAMP is elevated by both glucagon and catecholamines in the isolated perfused rat liver (122, 123). Many if not all the effects of these hormones on metabolic parameters can be mimicked by the addition of exogenous cAMP. If insulin action were due, even in part, to the lowering of cAMP levels, the hormone should counteract these effects. Park et al (120) have summarized the effects of cAMP (or glucagon or catecholamines) on the isolated rat liver and the antagonistic action of insulin. Insulin opposed the effects of glucagon (and epinephrine and exogenous cAMP where tested) on glycogenolysis (122, 124), gluconeogenesis (122), ureogenesis (122, 124), K^+ loss (122, 125), and proteolysis (107). Mackrell & Sokal (124) have also found that insulin generally antagonizes the metabolic effects of glucagon in the perfused liver. However, these authors showed that low doses of insulin also block urea production from endogenous substrate in the absence of glucagon. Williams et al (126) have shown that insulin antagonizes the glucagon stimulation of K^+ loss from the liver, and that the hormone also suppresses basal K^+ loss under conditions where there is no detectable alteration in cAMP levels.

In general, an effect of insulin on cAMP-mediated processes is most clearly seen when the level of cAMP is elevated submaximally by another hormone (123). A doubling of the basal level of cAMP is sufficient to stimulate maximally the rate of glucose output (glycogenolysis plus gluconeogenesis) in the perfused liver. A stimulation of this high degree can be understood if one postulates that most of the basal cAMP is bound or inactive. Thus, under basal condtions, the "free" cAMP level is near to zero as also suggested by the extremely low leakage (presumably by a transport system) of the nucleotide from the liver (122, 123). Upon addition of glucagon, relatively large amounts of cAMP appear in the perfusate, suggesting formation of another pool of cAMP that has better access to the plasma membrane (122, 123). In line with this idea, insulin is without detectable effect on the basal level of cAMP but does suppress the hormone-induced rise in tissue as well as movement of the nucleotide into the perfusate (122, 123). This effect is seen clearly with epinephrine or with low, physiological doses of glucagon but becomes undetectable at a high concentration of the latter hormone, for reasons that may be technical in nature (122, 123). Insulin also lowers glucagon-stimulated cAMP levels in isolated liver cells (127) and in organ culture of mature rat liver (128).

Mackrell & Sokal (124) reported that insulin inhibits urea formation but not phosphorylase activation in perfused livers in the presence of glucagon. An explanation for this selectivity of insulin action might be the presence of multiple adenylate cyclase systems controlling the concentrations of different intracellular cAMP pools. Some evidence has been presented for separate adenylate cyclase systems for glucagon and epinephrine (129), but this point is not firmly established. Another explanation for the finding of Mackrell & Sokal is based on the much greater sensitivity of phosphorylase to activation by cAMP than urea formation. Thus a reduction in cAMP sufficient to block stimulation of ureogenesis might be insufficient to inactivate phosphorylase (123).

Epinephrine is a much weaker stimulus than glucagon to cAMP formation in the perfused liver (123) and isolated liver cells (132). For example, epinephrine does not stimulate urea formation, although it does activate glycogenolysis and gluconeogenesis fully. In line with this relatively weak effect of the catecholamine on cAMP, its effect is very readily suppressed by insulin (123).

The mechanism by which insulin lowers cAMP in liver is controversial. Hepp & Renner (130) and Illiano & Cuatrecasas (131) have reported that insulin in vitro inhibits glucagon-stimulated adenylate cyclase in particulate preparations of mouse and rat liver. Neither of these preparations can be designated plasma membranes but rather are microsomal membranes contaminated with small amounts of plasma membranes. Both preparations have adenylate cyclase specific activities that are 1/8 to 1/10 that of purified plasma membrane preparations (132). The inhibitory effect of insulin on liver adenylate cyclase activity has not been seen in other laboratories (Thompson et al 133, Pilkis et al 127, and Pohl et al 144) in studies of similar crude or purified plasma membrane preparations. Failure to show in vitro effects of insulin on adenylate cyclase have been attributed to excessively high insulin concentrations (134–139). Illiano & Cuatrecasas (131) reported maximal inhibition of the cyclase at a concentration of 50 μU/ml ($3 \times 10^{-11} M$) whereas higher concentrations were stimulatory. However, the insulin concentration in portal venous blood of fasting humans is 40–50 μU/ml and levels as high as 1000 μU/ml have been observed in fed individuals (140). Very high concentrations of insulin suppress cAMP levels in the perfused rat liver (123).

It is possible that insulin could affect cyclic AMP production by an effect on membrane ATPase. Hepp & Renner (130) employed low ATP concentrations and an ATP-regenerating system in their assay. A direct action of insulin on plasma membrane ATPase activity in human lymphocytes has been reported (141),whereas the hormone did not affect the activity of adenylate cyclase. Krahl (142) has also suggested that insulin may alter membrane ATPase in cultured rat uteri. Luly et al (143) report that epinephrine, glucagon, cAMP, and insulin affect rat liver plasma membrane ($Na^+ + K^+$)-ATPase. In both the reports of Illiano & Cuatrecasas and Hepp & Renner (130, 131), a radioactive assay of adenylate cyclase employing ^{32}P-ATP was used. The specificity of this assay for cAMP is uncertain when used with crude enzyme preparations. Pohl et al (144), using this radioactive assay, have not detected an effect of insulin on adenylate cyclase in partially purified rat liver plasma membranes. Rosselin et al (145), using a radioimmunoassay to assay adenylate cyclase, were also unable to observe an insulin effect on the enzyme. In considering all the above reports, it would appear that an effect of insulin has not been demonstrated in a way that can be generally reproduced. This is reminiscent of many claims of insulin action on broken cell preparations in the past, virtually all of which have proved not to be reproducible.

Senft et al (146) first reported that insulin treatment increases the activity of phosphodiesterase in liver and adipose tissue, but others could not confirm their findings (147–151) until recently (153, 154). House & Weidemann (152) reported that insulin in vitro activates a liver plasma membrane-bound phosphodiesterase, but this has not been confirmed (153, 154). Thompson et al (153) and Pilkis et al

(154) have found that the rat liver plasma membrane, low K_m phosphodiesterase activity is decreased in liver of diabetic rats and increased after insulin treatment of the animal. These effects on phosphodiesterase in liver of diabetic animals are probably secondary to effects on protein synthesis (146).

Carbohydrate Metabolism

Mondon & Burton (155) have shown that when livers from fed animals are perfused with a glucose concentration of 240 mg% in 90% rat blood, glucose uptake is equal to glucose release, and insulin does not affect the net carbohydrate balance. When glucose release is increased by perfusion with 45% blood, which limits O_2 utilization in the liver, insulin decreases glucose output. Glycogen synthesis in the liver in vitro is slower than in vivo and is increased by raising the perfusate glucose concentration but not by addition of insulin or acetylcholine. However, insulin plus acetylcholine markedly increase glucose uptake and glycogen synthesis. The authors conclude that insulin affects hepatic carbohydrate metabolism by inhibiting catabolic processes and enhances glycogen synthesis when combined with cholinergic stimulation. Kotoulas et al (156) have presented morphological evidence to suggest that insulin and glucose may delay formation of lysosomes and thereby delay mobilization of glycogen in the postnatal period. Seglen (157) and Johnson et al (158) have shown that insulin stimulates glycogen synthesis in isolated liver cells, but only if the cell donors are starved.

Blatt et al (161) have reported that activation of hepatic glycogen synthetase and glycogen deposition in tadpoles are dependent on insulin. They have also shown that insulin in vitro promotes conversion of glycogen synthetase to the I form in minced tadpole liver preparations (162). Addition of ouabain prevents this effect of insulin (163), suggesting involvement of $Na^+ + K^+$ ATPase. Nichols & Goldberg (160) report that the activity of glycogen synthetase D-phosphatase activity is decreased in the alloxan diabetic rat. Insulin administration has been reported to raise this activity to normal (164, 165), and similar observations have been made using leukocytes of diabetic humans (166). Gold (164) reports a stimulation by insulin of glycogen synthetase activity within 15 min but no alteration in phosphatase activity until 1 hr. The control of liver glycogen synthetase D-phosphatase has recently been linked to changes in levels of active phosphorylase (167).

Bishop (179) has reported a rapid increase in liver glycogen synthetase D-phosphatase after insulin infusion into dogs. Activity is reduced by subsequent infusion of glucagon. This rapid activation-inactivation suggests that there are interconvertible forms of the phosphatase. In diabetic animals, however, insulin is unable to elevate phosphatase activity (179). Hornbrook (159) and Nichols & Goldberg (160) have shown that cortisol administration to alloxan diabetic animals fails to promote the activation of glycogen synthetase.

It would seem highly probable that one mechanism by which insulin activates hepatic glycogen synthetase involves a decrease in cellular cAMP. Jefferson et al (121) and Nichols & Goldberg (160) have shown that the elevated levels of hepatic cAMP found in the liver of alloxan diabetic animals are returned to normal within 75 min by injection of insulin into the animal. Insulin also decreases hepatic cAMP in perfused liver within 20 min when the level has been raised by continuous infusion of a low concentration of glucagon (123). An effect of insulin on glycogen synthetase or phosphorylase in perfused liver was not shown by Glinsmann et al (168) but has recently been obtained by Miller & Larner (180). Nichols & Goldberg (160), Miller & Larner (180), and Curnow et al (181) have reported a stimulatory effect of insulin on glycogen synthetase I formation without any significant change in cAMP levels under appropriate conditions. As mentioned earlier, insulin may lower cAMP in a small free (active) pool of cAMP, a change which may be undetectable in the presence of a large pool of bound cAMP. It is possible, as suggested for muscle by Villar-Palasi & Wenger (169) and others in this group (170–172), that the sensitivity of glycogen synthetase kinase (i.e. protein kinase) to cAMP is altered by insulin. There are, of course, other possible mechanisms not involving cAMP.

An insulin effect to suppress gluconeogenesis in the perfused rat liver has been obtained by Jefferson et al (21). The findings of Friedmann et al (173) and others (174–176) also support the view that insulin can suppress gluconeogenesis and enhance glycogenesis by moderating the level of cAMP. This effect of insulin is rapid and is not likely to be due to enzyme synthesis.

Inhibitory effects of cAMP on insulin-stimulated enzyme activities in liver have been reported. Pilkis (114) and Ureta et al (115) have shown that in vivo administration of cAMP can prevent the insulin mediated induction of rat liver glucokinase. Lakshmanan et al (178) have shown that the in vivo synthesis of rat liver fatty acid synthetase was stimulated by insulin administration and inhibited by glucagon and cAMP.

Wieland et al (182) have reported that administration of insulin to normal rats causes an increase in the active form of pyruvate dehydrogenase in rat liver (182). They (182) suggest that plasma free fatty acids play an important role in control of pyruvate dehydrogenase interconversion. They find no effect of insulin in vitro on this process in the perfused liver. The control of pyruvate dehydrogenase will be more fully discussed in the next section.

EFFECTS OF INSULIN ON ADIPOSE TISSUE

Carbohydrate, Protein, and Lipid Metabolism in Relation to the Adenylate Cyclase System

Insulin effects on isolated adipose tissue have been extensively reviewed (183–187). Some of the important actions of the hormone in vitro on adipose tissues are as follows: (*a*) enhancement of the transport of sugars that employ the glucose carrier system (glucose, galactose, and 3-O-methyl glucose; 188); (*b*) increased conversion of glucose intracellularly to CO_2, glyceride glycerol, fatty acids, and glycogen (186, 187); (*c*) stimulation of transport of amino acids, such as α-amino isobutyric acid and methionine, independent of the presence of glucose in the medium (189); (*d*) increased incorporation of amino acids into protein (5); (*e*) inhibition of lipolysis induced by epinephrine or other agents which enhance lipolysis, independent of the presence of glucose in the medium (187).

In intact fat cells, Sneyd et al (267) have shown that insulin stimulates sugar transport apparently independently of the level of cAMP, and Rodbell (186) has shown that various lipolytic hormones, which elevate cyclic AMP in fat cell ghosts, do not block insulin-stimulated glucose utilization (glucose transport). The possibility cannot be excluded, although it seems highly unlikely, that insulin affects transport through changes in cAMP level in a small compartment of the cell.

Avruch et al (190) have reported that a sonicated plasma membrane preparation from insulin-treated adipocytes of the rat epididymal fat pad shows an accelerated uptake and/or release of D-glucose. Addition of insulin directly to the plasma membranes was without effect (190). The hormone effect is presumably on glucose transport in vesicles formed in processing the preparation. No changes in the physical properties and protein composition of the plasma membrane were observed (190).

Soifer et al (192) report that insulin promotes microtubule assembly in fat cells. Colchicine inhibits this effect and also the stimulation of lipid and glycogen synthesis but does not affect acceleration of glucose oxidation (presumably glucose transport). Colchicine did not block the insulin-like, metabolic effects of high cocentrations of glucose (192). Murthy & Steiner (193) have shown that insulin increases lipogenesis from acetate in brown adipose tissue through an effect that is independent of any action on glucose transport or metabolism. Jungas (194) and Halperin & Robinson (195) reported that insulin augments the rate of fatty acid synthesis in white adipose tissue by a mechanism distinct from the stimulation of glucose transport. The insulin effect on fatty acid synthesis does not appear to involve changes in the level of cAMP.

Jungas and others have shown that insulin treatment of adipose tissue stimulates pyruvate dehydrogenase activity. This regulation may explain, in part, how insulin promotes fatty acid synthesis from lactate, pyruvate, or endogenous sources (see 196–198 for review). This effect of insulin appears also to be independent of any effect on glucose transport (197). Coore et al (199) have shown that the effect of insulin on pyruvate dehydrogenase activity is inhibited by adrenaline, ACTH, or dibutyryl cAMP. The adipose tissue enzyme is similar to the pyruvate dehydrogenase in heart, kidney, and liver where evidence has been given that activation and inactivation were catalyzed by an ATP-dependent kinase and Mg^{2+}-dependent phosphatase (200). Insulin has been postulated to act by increasing the proportion of active (dephosphorylated) pyruvate dehydrogenase (199, 201). It seems unlikely that insulin activation of the enzyme is mediated by cAMP directly. Taylor et al (202) found no effect of cAMP on the protein kinase or phosphatase for pyruvate dehydrogenase (198). Furthermore, they were unable to demonstrate any effect of cAMP or cGMP on the pyruvate dehydrogenase complex in adipose tissue. Coore et al (199) have obtained similar negative results. Martin et al (259) have very interesting evidence to suggest that the insulin effect on this enzyme system is mediated by a change in the cellular distribution of Ca^{2+}. This ion is an activator of the pyruvate dehydrogenase phosphatase.

Sica & Cuatrecasas (203) report that insulin stimulates the total activity of adipose tissue pyruvate dehydrogenase by a process that is inhibited by high concentrations of puromycin and cycloheximide but not by actinomycin.

Addition of insulin in vitro to adipose tissue stimulates the incorporation of labeled amino acids into protein (5). It does so in isolated fat cells, in the absence or presence of glucose in the medium. Minemura et al (204) have reported that insulin affects peptide bond synthesis rather than amino acid transport. These workers also find that insulin counteracts the inhibition of protein synthesis caused by ACTH, suggesting involvement under these conditions of cAMP. However, insulin added by itself to adipose tissue stimulates protein synthesis with no detectable alteration in cAMP levels (205). Under conditions in which protein synthesis is inhibited by cycloheximide, insulin has an inhibitory effect on proteolysis. This hormone effect is too small, however, to account for the increased net incorporation of amino acids into protein noted above. Little or no work on subcellular systems has been attempted in adipose tissue, probably because of technical difficulties. Insulin stimulates uridine incorporation into adipose tissue RNA (206).

Insulin inhibits lipolysis in isolated fat cells (207, 208) in the absence of glucose. This effect can be accounted for under certain conditions by a lowering of cellular cAMP. Under physiological conditions, however, where glucose is always present, the antilipolytic effect of insulin may for the most part be due to the stimulation of fatty acid reesterification consequent to increased glucose uptake (187). The effect of insulin to lower cAMP is seen most readily if the nucleotide level has been elevated by low (215–217) or moderate (210, 211) concentrations of epinephrine, caffeine, or both. A small lowering of the basal level has been reported recently (210). Insulin counteracts the lipolytic effect of exogenous cAMP (210, 211, 218), which must be added in very high concentrations because of poor penetration, and counteracts low but not high concentrations of exogenous dibutyryl cAMP (148, 150, 218, 255–257). Insulin is strongly antilipolytic in fat cells stimulated by ACTH. The level of cAMP may be reduced only slightly under these conditions and to an insufficient degree to account for the antilipolysis unless compartmentation of cAMP is invoked (210). Kuo et al (212) have presented evidence for separate pools of cAMP in adipose tissue. Jarett et al (205) and Khoo et al (220) suggest that insulin does not lower cAMP levels sufficiently to account for antilipolysis in adipose tissue exposed to catecholamine under certain conditions. There have been reports that insulin inhibits adipose tissue adenylate cyclase (130, 131) and other reports that it has no effect (134–139). Loten & Sneyd (214) and Vaughan (213) have found a small, activating effect of insulin on phosphodiesterase activity in homogenates of adipose tissue pretreated briefly with insulin. The effect is greatest on the membrane-bound enzyme (213). It has been reported (146) and denied (147) that phosphodiesterase is reduced in adipose tissue of diabetic rats. It is not stimulated by injection of insulin into diabetic or normal animals (148–151). Crofford and co-workers (219) have postulated that the ability of lipolytic agents to inhibit the stimulation by insulin of glucose oxidation and protein synthesis is a consequence of their ability to elevate cAMP levels. Fain (216) has suggested that this inhibition of insulin action by lipolytic agents is due to an accumulation of intracellular fatty acids which, in turn, could be the consequence of lipolytic activation by cAMP.

Khoo et al (220) have studied the effects of epinephrine and insulin on the control of lipase, phosphorylase kinase, phosphorylase, and glycogen synthetase in adipose cells. They suggest that the antagonistic effects of insulin and epinephrine on the activation of these enzymes cannot be fully accounted for by changes in the level of cAMP.

Lavis et al (257) and Kono (210, 211) showed that insulin in a concentration of 150 μU/ml or higher enhances the lipolytic activity of epinephrine or ACTH but not of caffeine. Increased lipolysis is associated with a rise in the level of cAMP. Insulin by itself does not have this effect. Hepp & Renner (130) and Illiano & Cuatrecasas (131) report that low but not high concentrations of insulin inhibit hormone-stimulated adipose tissue adenylate cyclase.

Effects of Insulin on Adipose Tissue; Relationship to Ions

Taubai & Jeanrenaud (221) have reported that insulin counteracts concomitantly the lipolysis and decreased K^+ uptake induced by lipolytic hormones in fat tissue. These authors suggest that insulin prevents a fall in phosphate bond energy level by reducing reesterification. In this connection, Bihler & Jeanrenaud (222) have shown that insulin partly prevents the depression of ATP levels induced by lipolytic agents in the absence of glucose.

Rodbell (223) reported a potassium requirement for the insulin stimulation of glucose transport in isolated fat cells of the rat. Letarte & Renold (224) and Letarte et al (225), however, found no consistent effect of potassium deficiency on the hormone effect in mouse adipocytes. In contrast to muscle, adipose tissue does not require magnesium for an insulin effect on transport (224).

A number of investigators have found that insulin effects on glucose oxidation and lipogenesis are inhibited in a medium low in sodium. Clausen (226) concluded that sodium was not required for transport stimulation but that it may effect oxidation and lipogenesis. However, Letarte & Renold (224) concluded that insulin-enhanced glucose transport was sodium dependent. In their experiments sodium lack did not completely prevent the effect of insulin, and there is no conclusive evidence that insulin action on transport in adipose tissue has an absolute requirement for this ion.

Krishna et al (227) have shown that norepinephrine causes a depolarization of the cell membrane of brown fat. Insulin counteracts the depolarization caused by norepinephrine but does not by itself alter the membrane potential. Propranolol also blocks the depolarization. These authors suggested that norepinephrine and insulin modify membrane potential by modifying the entry of K^+ into the cell. Dibutyryl cAMP did not alter the membrane potential of the fat cell (225). The resting membrane potential of adipose tissue cells of young rats is increased by insulin in the absence of glucose (228).

As already noted, Martin et al (259) suggest that activation of pyruvate dehydrogenase in adipose tissue by insulin is associated with an intracellular flux of Ca^{2+}.

EFFECTS OF INSULIN ON CELLS IN CULTURE

Addition of insulin to serum starved 3T3 cells results in what has been referred to as a positive pleiotypic response (229). This is characterized by increased uridine uptake, RNA synthesis, polysome aggregation, protein synthesis, increased glucose utilization, and decreased protein degradation.

A number of investigators have studied the effect of insulin on tyrosine transaminase activity in hepatoma cell cultures. In general, insulin increases the activity of this enzyme (230–233) and also of pyruvate kinase in a rat liver cell line. Insulin completely supresses the stimulatory effects of dexamethasone and dibutyryl cAMP on phosphoenolpyruvate carboxykinase in Reuber H35 cells. Immunochemical-isotope data indicate that insulin specifically stimulates the synthesis of tyrosine transaminase at the post-transcriptional or -translational level (232, 233). The effect of insulin on pyruvate kinase requires de novo RNA synthesis (235). Insulin increases the uptake of α-aminoisobutyrate in hepatoma cell cultures (234).

In BHK-21 cells insulin stimulates glucose uptake and protein synthesis (236). Jimenez de Asua et al (237) have reported that insulin has a dramatic stimulatory effect on the growth of fibroblasts in culture. Insulin inhibits adenylate cyclase in crude homogenates of these cells (237) and also in homogenates of neurospora (276).

Gerschenson et al (238) have shown that insulin stimulates growth and formation of polyribosomes in cultured rat liver cells. Insulin causes morphologic changes in explanted chicken embryos (239).

EFFECTS OF INSULIN ON OTHER TISSUES

Goldfine and associates (240, 241) have shown that insulin stimulation of α-aminoisobutyric acid transport in rat thymocytes correlates with ^{125}I-insulin binding and that the change in α-aminoisobutyric acid influx is blocked by inhibitors of protein synthesis. cAMP does not appear to be involved (241).

Peck and co-workers (242, 243) have reported that insulin enhances the incorporation of labeled uridine into the free uridine pool and into RNA in isolated bone cells. These workers suggest that insulin acts by stimulating uridine uptake and phosphorylation. Dithiothreitol has an effect similar to insulin. Hahn et al (244) have shown that insulin stimulates amino acid transport in fetal rat calvaria by a process that is blocked by inhibitors of protein synthesis and by ouabain.

The human red blood cell is generally thought to be an insulin insensitive tissue. In line with this is the fact that insulin does not bind appreciably to red blood cells. However, Zipper & Mawe (245) report that insulin elevates the maximal net flux of glucose across the cell membrane.

RELATION OF INSULIN STRUCTURE TO FUNCTION

The three-dimensional structure of the insulin molecule has been determined by single crystal X-ray analysis by Hodgkin and associates (246). They have shown that the B chain has a rigid central helical region extending between residues B9 and B19. This central structure holds the cysteines B7 and B19 a definite distance apart. The terminal residues on both sides of the helix extend as arms to form a pocket for the A chain. The A chain conformation is compact and is confined by the interchain disulfide bonds connecting to A7 and A20 and by the interchain bond connecting A6 and A11.

In the crystals, the monomers of insulin align in pairs in such a way as to bury the hydrophobic residues that make up the helices of the B chains. In the presence of zinc, there is aggregation of these dimers to form hexamers. This aggregation occurs not only in the crystals used for X-ray analysis but also in the pancreas (258). Hydrophobic residues are very evident in intermolecular contacts, but only two hydrophobic groups, A10 isoleucine and B25 phenylalanine, are exposed to the surface. On the other hand, certain hydrophilic residues of the A chain, A1 glycine, A5 glutamine, A19 tyrosine, and A21 asparagine are on the surface of the molecule and are not involved in aggregation. Their deletion affects activity and function. Arquilla and associates (247), using immunological data, have been able to construct a three dimensional model of insulin that is amazingly similar to the model constructed by X-ray analysis.

The question of whether the physiologically active form of insulin is monomeric or dimeric is as yet unanswered. Evidence for an active monomer is the retention of biological activity of insulin after covalent linkage to sepharose beads where dimer interaction is unlikely.

Frazier et al (248) have summarized a large amount of data that points out that nerve growth factor and insulin (or proinsulin) are similar in structure, function, and origin. Both effectors stimulate many anabolic processes (248).

Somatomedin competes with insulin for binding sites on liver plasma membranes (249) suggesting that insulin and somatomedin also are related structurally and functionally.

CONCLUSIONS

The plasma membrane of insulin sensitive cells contains specific receptors for the hormone. These receptors have peptide elements that face the external surface of the cell and are presumably the sites of insulin complex formation. It seems likely that there is a single class of specific receptors, on adipocytes at least, with an insulin-receptor dissociation constant of about 5×10^{-9} mol. An insulin binding protein, which may be the specific receptor, has been extensively purified. It has a molecular weight of about 300,000.

It seems likely that only a small fraction of the total number of receptors in a cell needs to complex with insulin in order to generate a signal of sufficient strength to modify cell function. It is speculated that the signal results from a conformational change in the receptor. Complexing with the receptor may be coupled to inactivation of the hormone.

As regards the nature of the signal, it is frequently theorized that an intracellular mediator substance, X, may be generated. The compound is postulated to affect transport systems in the membrane and intracellular enzymes to produce the changes characteristic of insulin action. Certain cyclic nucleotides (277), Ca^{2+}, and other ions have been suggested to fulfill the role of X, in part, at least. Another theory is that the signal consists of a modification of cell structure. As a consequence, transport systems and enzyme reactions would be affected. This theory would also account for the persistent problem of demonstrating a reproducible effect of insulin preparations. Neither theory has any firm experimental support. It is possible that more than one type of signal is generated.

Some of the consequences of signal generation are rapid. These include effects on transport of sugars, amino acids, some inorganic ions, and probably many other compounds. Other consequences are relatively slow and include acceleration of growth and the synthesis of specific proteins. The signal affects protein turnover in several ways. It may modify the levels of substrates that protect or "induce" various enzymes; it may affect the level of cAMP or act by other as yet unknown mechanisms. The signal, probably through many steps, stimulates RNA polymerase activity, the initiation of peptide chains, and ribosomal aggregation, It also probably reduces protein catabolism by stabilization of lysosomes.

The signal can lead to a reduction in the level of cAMP in adipocytes, hepatocytes, and probably certain other cells, but not detectably in skeletal muscle or cardiac cells. The reduction is prominent if the level of cAMP has first been elevated slightly or moderately by other hormones, notably catecholamines (β activity) and glucagon. In this way, insulin action is antagonistic to these hormones in all of their cAMP-mediated effects. From a physiological point of view, the effect on the level of cAMP would seem particularly important in hepatic metabolism (glycogenolysis, gluconeogenesis, ion fluxes, protein turnover), and it probably contributes to antilipolysis in the adipocyte.

Literature Cited

1. Banting, F. G., Best, C. H. 1922. *J. Lab. Clin. Med.* 7:251
2. Cori, C. F. 1931. *Physiol. Rev.* 11:234
3. Steiner, D. F., Freinkel, N., Eds. 1971. *Handb. of Physiol. Sect. 7: Endocrinol.* Vol. I
4. Houssay, B. A. 1947. *Le Prix Nobel,* p. 129
5. Krahl, M. E. 1961. *Action of Insulin on Cells.* New York: Academic
6. Krahl, M. E. 1957. *Perspect. Biol. Med.* 1:69
7. Lukens, F. C. 1944. *J. Clin. Invest.* 23:233
8. Mirsky, I. A. 1956. *Metab. Clin. Exp.* 5:138
9. Randle, P. J. 1957. *Ciba Found. Colloq. Endrocrinol.* 11:115
10. Soskin, S., Levine, R. 1962. *Carbohydrate Metabolism.* Chicago: Univ. Chicago Press. 2nd ed.
11. Cuatrecasas, P. 1969. *Proc. Nat. Acad. Sci. USA* 63:450
12. Turkington, R. W. 1970. *Biochem. Biophys. Res. Commun.* 41:1362
13. Oka, T., Topper, Y. 1971. *Proc. Nat. Acad. Sci. USA* 68:2066
14. Blatt, L. M., Kim, K. H. 1971. *J. Biol. Chem.* 246:4897
15. Tarui, S., Saito, Y., Suzuki, F., Takeda, Y. 1972. *Endocrinology,* p. 1442

16. Davidson, M. B., Gerschenson, L. E., Van Herle, A. J. 1972. *Diabetes* 21: Suppl. 1, 335
17. Fritz, I. 1972. In *Biochemical Actions of Hormones,* ed. G. Litwack, II:165–214. New York: Academic
18. Katzen, H. M., Vlahakes, G. J. 1973. *Science* 179:1142–43
19. Cuatrecasas, P. 1973. *Science* 179: 1143–44
20. Katzen, H. M., Soderman, D. D. 1972. In *Membranes in Metabolic Regulation,* ed. M. A. Mehlman, R. W. Hanson, p. 212. New York: Academic
21. Davidson, M. B., Gerschenson, L. E., Van Herle, A. J. 1972. *Diabetes* 21: Suppl. 1, 335
22. Crofford, O. B. 1968. *J. Biol. Chem.* 243:362
23. Wohltmann, H. J., Narahara, H. T. 1966. *J. Biol. Chem.* 241:4931
24. Cadenas, E., Kaji, H., Park, C. R., Rasmussen, H. 1961. *J. Biol. Chem.* 236:PC63
25. Stadie, W. C., Haugaard, N., Vaughan, M. 1953. *J. Biol. Chem.* 199: 729
26. Freychet, P., Roth, J., Neville, D. M. Jr. 1971. *Biochem. Biophys. Res. Commun.* 43:400

27. Cuatrecasas, P. 1972. In *Insulin Action,* ed. I. Fritz, 137–66. New York: Academic
28. Freychet, P., Kahn, R., Roth, J., Neville, D. M. 1972. *J. Biol. Chem.* 247:3953
29. Freychet, P., Roth, J., Neville, D. M. 1971. *Proc. Nat. Acad. Sci.* 68:1833
30. Cuatrecasas, P., Desbuquois, B., Krug, F. 1971. *Biochem. Biophys. Res. Commun.* 44:333
31. Cuatrecasas, P. 1971. *Proc. Nat. Acad. Sci. USA* 68:1264
32. Gavin, J. R. III, Roth, J., Jen, P., Freychet, P. 1972. *Proc. Nat. Acad. Sci. USA* 69:747–51
33. Szabo, O., Szabo, A. J. 1972. *Diabetes* 21:Suppl. 1, 337
34. Cuatrecasas, P. 1972. *J. Biol. Chem.* 247:1980–91
35. Cuatrecasas, P. 1972. *Proc. Nat. Acad. Sci. USA* 69:318–22
36. Fong, C. T. O., Silver, L., Popenoe, E. A., DeBons, A. F. 1962. *Biochim. Biophys. Acta* 56:190
37. Edelman, P. M., Rosenthal, S. L., Schwartz, F. E. 1963. *Nature* 197:878
38. Whitney, J. E., Cutlar, O. E., Wright, F. E. 1963. *Metabolism* 12:352
39. Cuatrecasas, P. 1971. *J. Biol. Chem.* 246:7265
40. Pilkis, S. J., Johnson, R. A., Park, C. R. 1972. *Diabetes* 21:Suppl. 1, 335
41. Kuo, J. F., Dill, I. K., Holmlund, C. E. 1967. *J. Biol. Chem.* 242:3659
42. Kono, T. 1969. *J. Biol. Chem* 244:5777
43. Kono, T., Barham, F. W. 1971. *J. Biol. Chem.* 246:6204–9
44. Cuatrecasas, P. 1971. *J. Biol. Chem.* 246:6522–31
45. Kono, T., Barham, F. W. 1971. *J. Biol. Chem.* 246:6210
46. Kono, T. 1969. *J. Biol. Chem.* 244:1772
47. Fain, J. N., Loken, S. C. 1969. *J. Biol. Chem.* 244:3500
48. Czech, M. P., Fain, J. N. 1970. *Endocrinology* 87:191–93
49. Cuatrecasas, P., Illiano, G. 1971. *J. Biol. Chem.* 246:4938
50. Cuatrecasas, P. 1971. *J. Biol. Chem.* 246:6532
51. Kahn, C. R., Neville, D. M., Gorden, P., Freychet, P., Roth, J. 1972. *Biochem. Biophys. Res. Commun.* 48:135
52. Bennett, G. V., Cuatrecasas, P. 1972. *Science* 176:805
53. Kono, T. See Ref. 27, pp. 171–78
54. House, P. D. R. 1971. *FEBS Lett.* 16:339
55. Wool, I. G. et al 1968. *Recent Progr. Horm. Res.* 24:139
56. Wool, I. G., Krahl, M. E. 1959. *Am. J. Physiol.* 196:961–64
57. Wool, I., Cavicchi, P. 1967. *Biochemistry* 6:1231
58. Wool, I. G., Cavicchi, P. 1966. *Proc. Nat. Acad. Sci. USA* 56:991
59. Martin, T. E., Wool, I. G. 1968. *Proc. Nat. Acad. Sci. USA* 60:569–74
60. Stirewalt, W. S., Castles, J. J., Wool, I. G. 1971. *Biochemistry* 10:1594
61. Wool, I. G., Wettenhall, R. E. H., Kleen-Bremhaar, H., Abayang, N. 1972. In *Action of Insulin,* ed. I. Fritz, 415–25. New York: Academic
62. Rannels, D. E., Jefferson, L. S., Hjalmairson, A. C., Wolpert, E. B., Morgan, H. E. 1970. *Biochem. Biophys. Res. Commun.* 40:1110
63. Morgan, H. E., Jefferson, L. S., Wolpert, E. B., Rannels, D. E. 1971. *J. Biol. Chem.* 246:2163–70
64. Jefferson, L. S., Koehler, J. O., Morgan, H. E. 1972. *Proc. Nat. Acad. Sci. USA* 69:816–20
65. Chain, E. B., Sender, P. M. 1973. *Biochem. J.* 132:593–601
66. Sender, P. M., Garlick, P. J. 1973. *Biochem. J.* 132:603–8
67. Manchester, K. L. 1970. *Biochem. J.* 117:457–65
68. Manchester, K. L., Krahl, M. E. 1959. *J. Biol. Chem.* 234:2938–42
69. Manchester, K. L. 1972. *Diabetes* 21: Suppl. 2, 447–51
70. Pozefsky, T., Felig, P., Tobin, J. D., Soeldner, J. S., Cahill, G. F. 1969. *J. Clin. Invest.* 48:2273–82
71. Post, R. L., Morgan, H. E., Park, C. R. 1961. *J. Biol. Chem.* 236:269
72. Morgan, H. E., Regen, D. M., Park, C. R. 1964. *J. Biol. Chem.* 239:369
73. Bihler, I., Cavert, H. M., Fisher, R. B. 1965. *J. Physiol.* 180:157
74. Fisher, R. B., Gilbert, J. C. 1970. *J. Physiol.* 210:297
75. Narahara, H. T., Ozand, P. 1963. *J. Biol. Chem.* 238:40
76. Gould, M. K., Chaudry, H. 1970. *Biochim. Biophys. Acta* 215:249
77. Gould, M. K., Chaudry, H. 1970. *Biochim. Biophys. Acta* 215:258
78. Zierler, K. L. 1958. *Am. J. Physiol.* 192:283
79. Walaas, O., Walaas, E., Wick, A. 1969. *Diabetologia* 5:79–87
80. Craig, J. W., Rall, T. W., Larner, J. 1969. *Biochim. Biophys. Acta* 177:586–90
81. Larner, J. et al 1968. *Advan. Enzyme Regul.* 6:409

82. Goldberg, N. D., Villar-Palasi, C., Sasko, H., Larner, J. 1967. *Biochim. Biophys. Acta* 148:665–72
83. Keely, S., Corbin, J., Park, C. R. 1973. *Fed. Proc.* 32:643
84. Larner, J. 1972. *Diabetes* 21: Suppl. 2, 428–38
85. Murad, F., Rall, T., Vaughan, M. 1969. *Biochim. Biophys. Acta* 192:430–45
86. Drummond, G. I., Severson, D. L., Sulahke, P. V. See Ref. 27, pp. 277–95
87. Das, I., Chain, E. B. 1972. *Biochem. J.* 128:95P–96P
88. Randle, P. J. et al 1966. *Recent Progr. Horm. Res.* 22:1
89. Larner, J., Villar-Palasi, C. 1972. In *Current Topics in Cellular Regulation,* ed. B. Horecker, E. W. Stadtman, 3: 195–236
90. Chain, E. B., Mansford, K. R. L., Opre, L. H. 1969. *Biochem. J.* 115:537
91. Beitner, R., Kalant, N. 1971. *J. Biol. Chem.* 246:500–3
92. Ozand, P., Narahara, H. T. 1964. *J. Biol. Chem.* 239:3146
93. Turkington, R. W. 1968. *Endocrinology* 82:540
94. Turkington, R. W. See Ref. 17, pp. 55–80
95. Turkington, R. W., Riddle, M. 1970. *J. Biol. Chem.* 245:5145–52
96. Turkington, R. W. 1970. *J. Biol Chem.* 245:6690–97
97. Turkington, R. W., Riddle, M. 1969. *J. Biol. Chem.* 244:6040
98. Stockdale, F. E., Topper, Y. J. 1966. *Proc. Nat. Acad. Sci. USA* 56:1283–89
99. Turkington, R. W. 1969. *Exp. Cell Res.* 57:79
100. Turkington, R. W. 1969. *Cancer Res.* 30:104
101. Rivera, E. M., Bern, R. A. 1961. *Endocrinology* 69:340–53
102. Stockdale, F. E., Juergens, W. G., Topper, Y. J. 1966. *Develop. Biol.* 13: 266–81
103. Turkington, R. W. 1971. In *Developmental Aspects of the Cell Cycle,* ed. I. L. Cameron, G. M. Padilla, A. M. Zimmerman, 315–55 New York: Academic
104. Majumder, G. C., Turkington, R. W. 1971. *J. Biol. Chem.* 246:5545–54
105. Miller, L. L., Griffin, E. E. See Ref. 27, pp. 487–507
106. Mortimore, G. E., Mondon, C. E. 1970. *J. Biol. Chem* 245:2375
107. Neely, A. N., Mortimore, G. E. 1973. *Fed. Proc.* 32:299
108. Robinson, W. S. 1961. *Proc. Soc. Exp. Biol. Med.* 106:115–16

109. Korner, A. 1960. *J. Endocrinol.* 20: 256–60
110. Pilkis, S. J., Korner, A. 1971. *Biochim. Biophys. Acta* 247:597–608
111. Tragl, K. H., Reaven, G. M. 1971. *Diabetes* 20:27–32
112. Wittman, J. S., Miller, O. N. 1971. *Am. J. Clin. Nutr.* 24:770–76
113. Weber, G., Singhal, R. L., Srivastava, S. K. 1965. *Advan. Enzyme Regul.* 3:43
114. Pilkis, S. J. 1970. *Biochim. Biophys. Acta* 215:461–76
115. Ureta, T., Radojkovic, J., Niemeyer, H. 1970. *J. Biol. Chem.* 245:4819
116. Steiner, D. F. 1966. In *Vitamins and Hormones,* ed. R. S. Harris, I. G. Wool, J. A. Lorame, p. 1. New York: Academic
117. Steiner, D. F., King, J. 1966. *Biochim. Biophys. Acta* 119:517
118. Pilkis, S. J., Salaman, D. F. 1972. *Biochim. Biophys. Acta* 272:327–39
119. Pilkis, S. J., Oravec, M., Salaman, D. F., Korner, A. 1971. *Fed. Proc.* 30: 1317
120. Park, C. R., Lewis, S. B., Exton, J. H., 1972. *Diabetes* 21: Suppl. 2: 439–46
121. Jefferson, L. S., Exton, J. H., Butcher, R. W., Sutherland, E. W., Park, C. R. 1968. *J. Biol. Chem.* 243:1031
122. Exton, J. H., Park, C. R. 1972. In *Handb. Physiol. Sect. 7: Endocrinol.* I:437–55
123. Exton, J. H., Lewis, S. B., Ho, R. J., Robison, G. A., Park, C. R. 1971. *Ann. NY Acad. Sci.* 185:85
124. Mackrell, D., Sokal, J. 1969. *Diabetes* 18:724
125. Glinsmann, W. H., Mortimore, G. E. 1968. *Am. J. Physiol.* 215:553–59
126. Williams, T. F., Exton, J. H., Friedmann, N., Park, C. R. 1971. *Am. J. Physiol.* 221:1645–51
127. Pilkis, S. J., Claus, T. H., Johnson, R. A., Wasner, H., Park, C. R. 1973. *Congr. Int. Diabetes Congr., 8th,* p. 80
128. Siddle, K., Kane-Maguire, B., Campbell, A. K. 1973. *Biochem. J.* 132: 765–73
129. Bitensky, M. W., Russell, V., Robertson, W. 1968. *Biochem. Biophys. Res. Commun.* 31:706
130. Hepp, K. D, Renner, R. 1972. *FEBS Lett.* 20:191
131. Illiano, G., Cuatrecasas, P. 1972. *Science* 175:906
132. Pilkis, S. J., Johnson, R. A. Unpublished observations
133. Thompson, W. J., Williams, R. H., Little, S. A. 1973. *Biochim. Biophys. Acta* 302:329–37

134. Manganiello, V. C., Murad, F., Vaughan, M. 1971. *J. Biol. Chem.* 246: 2195

135. Vaughan, M., Murad, F. 1969. *Biochemistry* 8:3092

136. Cryer, P. E., Tarret, L., Kipnis, D. M. 1969. *Biochim. Biophys. Acta* 177:586

137. Butcher, R. W., Baird, C. E., Sutherland, E. W. 1968. *J. Biol. Chem.* 243: 1705

138. Butcher, R. W., Sneyd, J. G. T., Park, C. R., Sutherland, E. W. 1966. *J. Biol. Chem.* 241:1651

139. Jungas, R. L. 1966. *Proc. Nat. Acad. Sci. USA* 56:757

140. Blackard, N. G., Nelson, N. C. 1970. *Diabetes* 19:302–6

141. Hadden, J. W., Hadden, F. M., Wilson, E. E., Good, R. A., Coffey, R. G. 1972. *Nature New Biol.* 235:174

142. Krahl, M. E. 1972. *Diabetes* 21: Suppl. 2, 695–702

143. Luly, P., Barnabei, O., Tria, E. 1972. *Biochim. Biophys. Acta* 282:447–52

144. Pohl, S. L., Birnbaumer, L., Rodbell, M. 1971. *J. Biol. Chem.* 246:1849

145. Rosselin, G., Freychet, P. 1973. *Biochim. Biophys. Acta* 304:541–51

146. Senft, G., Schultz, G., Munske, K., Hoffmann, M. 1968. *Diabetologia* 4: 322

147. Mueller-Oerlinghausen, B., Schwabe, U., Hasselblatt, A., Schmidt, F. H. 1968. *Life Sci.* 7:593

148. Blecher, M., Merlino, N. S., Roane, J. T. 1968. *J. Biol. Chem.* 243:3973

149. Hepp, K. D., Menahan, L. A., Wieland, O., Williams, R. H. 1969. *Biochim. Biophys. Acta* 184:554

150. Hepp, K. D., Menahan, A., Wieland, O., Williams, R. H. 1969. *Biochim. Biophys. Acta* 184:554

151. Menahan, A., Hepp, K. D., Wieland, O. 1969. *Eur. J. Biochem.* 8:435

152. House, P. D. R., Poulis, P., Weidemann, M. J. 1971. *Eur. J. Biochem.* 24: 429

153. Thompson, W. J., Little, S. A., Williams, R. H. 1973. *Biochemistry* 12: 1889–94

154. Pilkis, S. J., Exton, J. H., Johnson, R. A., Park, C. R. 1973. *Fed. Proc.* 32:299

155. Mondon, C. E., Burton, S. 1971. *Am. J. Physiol.* 220:724

156. Kotoulas, O. B., Ho, J., Adachi, F., Weigensberg, B. I., Phillips, M. J. 1971. *Am. J. Pathol.* 63:23–36

157. Seglen, P. O. 1973. *FEBS Lett.* 30: 25–28

158. Johnson, M. E., Das, N. M., Butcher, F., Fain, J. 1972. *J. Biol. Chem.* 247: 3229–35

159. Hornbrook, K. R. 1970. *Diabetes* 19: 916

160. Nichols, W. K., Goldberg, N. 1972. *Biochim. Biophys. Acta* 279:245–59

161. Blatt, L. M., Sevall, J. S., Kim, K. H. 1971. *J. Biol. Chem.* 246:873

162. Blatt, L. M., Kim, K. H. 1971. *J. Biol. Chem.* 246:7256–61

163. Blatt, L. M., McVerry, P. H., Kim, K. 1972. *J. Biol. Chem.* 247:6551–54

164. Gold, A. H. 1970. *J. Biol. Chem.* 245: 903

165. Bishop, L., Larner, J. 1970. *Biochim. Biophys. Acta* 208:208

166. Esmann, V., Hedeskou, C. J., Rosell-Perez, M. 1968. *Diabetologia* 4:1968

167. Stalmans, W., DeWulf, H., Hers, H. G. 1971. *Eur. J. Biochem.* 18:582

168. Glinsmann, W., Pauk, G., Hern, E. 1970. *Biochem. Biophys. Res. Commun.* 39:774

169. Villar-Palasi, C., Wenger, J. 1967. *Fed. Proc.* 26:563

170. Shen, L. C., Villar-Palasi, C., Larner, J. 1970. *Phys. Chem. Physics* 2:536

171. Nuttal, F. Q., Larner, J. 1970. *Biochim. Biophys. Acta* 230:560

172. Villar-Palasi, C., Shen, L. C. 1971. *Fed. Proc.* 30:219

173. Friedmann, B., Goodman, E. H., Weinhouse, S. 1970. *Endocrinology* 86: 1264–71

174. Mondon, C. E., Mortimore, G. E. 1967. *Am. J. Physiol.* 212:173

175. Mortimore, G. E., King, E., Mondon, C. E., Glinsmann, W. H. 1967. *Am. J. Physiol.* 212:179

176. Glinsmann, W. H., Mortimore, G. E. 1968. *Am. J. Physiol.* 215:553

177. Vavrinkova, H., Mosinger, B. 1971. *Biochim. Biophys. Acta* 231:320–26

178. Lakshmanan, M. R., Nepokroeff, C. M., Porter, J. W. 1972. *Proc. Nat. Acad. Sci. USA* 69:3516–19

179. Bishop, J. S. 1970. *Biochim. Biophys. Acta* 208:208–18

180. Miller, T., Larner, J. 1973. *J. Biol. Chem.* 248:3483–88

181. Curnow, R. T., Rayfield, E. J., Derubertes, F. R., Zenser, T. V. 1973. *Diabetes* 22: Suppl. I, 309

182. Wieland, O., Patzelt, C., Löffler, G. 1972. *Eur. J. Biochem.* 26:426–33

183. Rodbell, M. 1965. *Handb. Physiol., Adipose Tissue,* pp. 471–83

184. Vaughan, M., Steinberg, D. 1963. *J. Lipid Res.* 4:1973

185. Ball, E., Jungas, R. L. 1964. *Recent Progr. Horm. Res.* 20:183

186. Rodbell, M., Jones, A. B., Chiappe de Cingolani, G. E., Birnbaumer, L. 1968.

Recent Progr. Horm. Res. 24: 215
187. Jeanrenaud, B., Renold, A. E. 1969. In *Physiopathology of Adipose Tissue,* ed. J. Vague, p. 20. Amsterdam: Excerpta Med.
188. Crofford, O. B., Renold, A. E. 1965. *J. Biol. Chem.* 240:3237
189. Riggs, T. R. 1970. In *Biochemical Actions of Hormones,* ed. G. Litwack, I:157–208. New York: Academic
190. Avruch, J., Carter, J. R., Martin, D. B. 1972. *Biochim. Biophys. Acta* 288: 27–42
191. Martin, D. B., Carter, J. R. 1970. *Science* 167:873–74
192. Soifer, D., Braun, T., Hechter, O. 1971. *Science* 172:269–71
193. Murthy, V. K., Steiner, G. 1972. *Am. J. Physiol.* 222:983
194. Jungas, R. L. 1970. *Endocrinology* 86: 1368
195. Halperin, M. L., Robinson, B. H. 1971. *Metabolism* 20:78
196. Denton, R. M., Halperin, M. L., Randle, P. J. See Ref. 187, p. 31
197. Jungas, R. L. 1971. *Metabolism* 20:43
198. Jungas, R. L., Taylor, S. I. See Ref. 27, p. 369
199. Coore, H. G., Denton, R. M., Martin, B. R., Randle, P. J. 1971. *Biochem. J.* 125:115–27
200. Reed, L. J. 1971. In *Proc. Symp. Metab. Regul.,* ed. M. A. Mehlman, R. A. Hanson. New York: Academic
201. Denton, R. M., Coore, H. G., Martin, B. R., Randle, P. J. 1971. *Nature New Biol.* 231:115
202. Taylor, S. I., Mukherjee, C., Jungas, R. 1973. *J. Biol. Chem.* 248:73–81
203. Sica, V., Cuatrecasas, P. 1973. *Biochemistry* 12:2282–91
204. Minemura, T., Lacy, W., Crofford, O. 1970. *J. Biol. Chem.* 245:3872–81
205. Jarett, L., Steiner, A. L., Smith, R. M., Kipnis, D. M. 1972. *Endocrinology* 90: 1277–84
206. Gellhorn, A., Benjamin, W. 1966. *Advan. Enzyme Regul.* 4:19
207. Mahler, R., Stafford, W. S., Tarrant, M. E., Ashmore, J. 1964. *Diabetes* 13:297–302
208. Jungas, R. L., Ball, E. G. 1963. *Biochemistry* 2:383–88
209. Butcher, R. W., Baird, C. E., Sutherland, E. W. 1968. *J. Biol. Chem.* 243: 1705–12
210. Kono, T. 1973. *Fed. Proc.* 32:581
211. Kono, T. 1972. *Fed. Proc.* 31:243
212. Kuo, J. F., DeRenzo, E. C. 1969. *J. Biol. Chem.* 244:2252–60

213. Vaughan, M. See Ref. 27, pp. 297–304
214. Loten, E. G., Sneyd, J. G. T. 1970. *Biochem. J.* 120:187
215. Fain, J. N., Kovacev, V. P., Scow, R. O. 1966. *Endocrinology* 78:773–78
216. Fain, J. N. 1971. *Mol. Pharmacol.* 7: 465–79
217. Fain, J. N., Rosenberg, L. 1972. *Diabetes* 21: Suppl. 2, 414–25
218. Goodman, H. M. 1968. *Proc. Soc. Exp. Biol. Med.* 130:97–100
219. Crofford, O. B., Minemura, T., Kono, T. 1970. *Advan. Enzyme Regul.* 8: 219–38
220. Khoo, J. C., Steinberg, D., Thompson, B., Mayer, S. E. 1973. *J. Biol. Chem.* 248:3823–30
221. Taubai, M., Jeanrenaud, B. 1970. *Biochim. Biophys. Acta* 202:486–95
222. Bihler, I., Jeanrenaud, B. 1970. *Biochim. Biophys. Acta* 202:496–506
223. Rodbell, M. 1967. *J. Biol. Chem.* 242: 5751
224. Letarte, J., Renold, A. E. 1969. *Biochim. Biophys. Acta* 183:350
225. Letarte, J., Jeanrenaud, B., Renold, A. E. 1969. *Biochim. Biophys. Acta* 183: 357
226. Clausen, T. 1970. In *Adipose Tissue Regulation and Metabolic Functions,* ed. B. Jeanrenaud, D. Hepp, p. 66. New York: Academic
227. Krishna, G., Moskowitz, J., Dempsey, P., Brodie, B. B. 1970. *Life Sci.* 9: 1353–61
228. Biegelman, P. M., Hollander, P. B. 1962. *Proc. Soc. Exp. Biol. Med.* 110: 590
229. Hershko, A., Mamont, P., Shields, R., Tomkins, G. M. 1971. *Nature* 232: 206–11
230. Gelehrter, T. D., Tomkins, G. M. 1970. *Proc. Nat. Acad. Sci. USA* 66:390–97
231. Barnett, C., Wicks, W. 1971. *J. Biol. Chem.* 246:7201–6
232. Lee, K. L., Reel, J. R., Kenney, F. T. 1970. *J. Biol. Chem.* 245:5806–12
233. Reel, J. R., Lee, K. L., Kenney, F. 1970. *J. Biol. Chem.* 245:5800–5
234. Krawitt, E. L., Baril, E., Becker, J. E., Potter, V. R. 1970. *Science* 169:294–96
235. Gerschenson, L. E., Andersson, M. 1971. *Biochem. Biophys. Res. Commun.* 43:1211
236. Ussery, M. A., Sagik, B. P. 1973. *Fed. Proc.* 32:489
237. Jimenez de Asua, L., Surian, E., S., Flavia, M. M., Torres, H. N. 1973. *Proc. Nat. Acad. Sci. USA* 70:1388–92

238. Gerschenson, L. E., Okigaki, T., Andersson, M., Molson, J., Davidson, M. B. 1972. *Exp. Cell Res.* 71:49–58
239. Hickey, E. D., Klein, N. 1969. *Teratology* 4:453–60
240. Goldfine, I. D., Gardner, J. D., Neville, D. M. 1972. *J. Biol. Chem.* 247: 6919–26
241. Goldfine, I. D., Sherline, P. 1972. *J. Biol. Chem.* 247:6927–31
242. Peck, W. A., Messinger, K. 1970. *J. Biol. Chem.* 245:2722–29
243. Peck, W. A., Messinger, K., Carpenter, J. 1971. *J. Biol. Chem.* 246:4439–46
244. Hahn, T. J., Downing, S., Phang, J. M. 1971. *Am. J. Physiol.* 220:1717
245. Zipper, H., Mawe, R. 1972. *Biochim. Biophys. Acta* 282:311–25
246. Blundell, T. L. et al 1971. *Nature* 231:506–11
247. Arquilla, E. R., Stanford, E. J. See Ref. 27, pp. 29–62
248. Frazier, W. A., Angeletti, R. H., Bradshaw, R. A. 1972. *Science* 176:482–88
249. Hintz, R. L., Clemmons, D. R., Underwood, L. E., Van Wyk, J. J., 1972. *Proc. Nat. Acad. Sci. USA* 69:2351–53
250. Izzo, J. L., Roncone, A., Izzo, M. T., Bale, W. F. 1964. *J. Biol. Chem.* 239: 3749–54
251. Garratt, C. J. 1964. *Nature* 201: 1324–28
252. Crofford, O. B., Okayama, T. 1970. *Diabetes* 19:369
253. Crofford, O. B., Rogers N. L., Russell, W. G. 1972. *Diabetes* 21: Suppl. 2, 403–13
254. Weis, L. S., Narahara, H. T. 1969. *J. Biol. Chem.* 244:3084–91
255. Solomon, S. S., Brush, J. S., Kitabchi, A. 1970. *Biochim. Biophys. Acta* 218: 167–69
256. Kono, T. Unpublished data
257. Lavis, V. R., Hepp, D., Williams, R. H. 1971. *Diabetes* 19:371
258. Grieder, M. H., Howell, S. L., Lacy, P. E. 1969. *J. Cell Biol.* 41:162

259. Martin, B. R., Clausen, T., Gliemann, J. 1973. *International Congress of Biochemistry, 9th* Stockholm, p. 376
260. Narahara, H. T. 1972. In *Handb. Physiol. Sect. 7: Endocrinol.* Vol. I
261. Antoniades, H. N., Gershoff, S. N. 1966. *Diabetes* 15:655–62
262. Garratt, C. J., Cameron, J. S., Menzinger, G. 1966. *Biochim. Biophys. Acta* 115:176–86
263. Kono, T., Colowick, S. P. 1961. *Arch. Biochem. Biophys.* 93:520–33
264. Freychet, P., Kahn, R., Roth, J., Neville, D. M. 1972. *J. Biol. Chem.* 247: 3953–61
265. Armstrong, K. J., Noall, M. W., Stouffer, J. E. 1972. *Biochim. Biophys. Res. Commun.* 47:354–60
266. Crofford, O. B., Minemura, T., Kono, T. 1970. *Advan. Enzyme Regul.* 8: 219–38
267. Sneyd, J. G. T., Corbin, J. D., Park, C. R. 1968. *Int. Symp. Pharmacol. Horm. Polypeptides Proteins, Milan,* p. 367
268. Crofford, O., Unpublished
269. Park, C. R. 1965. *Excerpta Med. Found. Int. Congr., Ser. n* 84, p. 564
270. El-Allowy, R. M. M., Gliemann, J. 1972. *Biochim. Biophys. Acta* 273:97–109
271. Hammond, J. H., Jarett, L., Mariz, I. K., Daughaday, W. H. 1972. *Biochim. Biophys. Acta* 49:1122–28
272. Robinson, C. A., Bashell, B. R., Reddy, W. J. 1972. *Biochim. Biophys. Acta* 290:84–91
273. Minemura, T., Crofford, O. B. 1969. *J. Biol. Chem.* 244:5181–88
274. Jefferson, L. S., Korner, A. 1969. *Biochem. J.* 111:703–12
275. Morgan, H. E., Unpublished results
276. Flawia, M. M., Torres, H. N. 1973. *FEBS Lett.* 30:74078
277. Illiano, G., Tell, G. P. E., Siegel, M. I., Cuatrecasas, P. 1973. *Proc. Nat. Acad. Sci. USA* 70:2443–47

DRUG EFFECTS AND HYPOTHALAMIC-ANTERIOR PITUITARY FUNCTION

❖6600

David de Wied and Wybren de Jong
Rudolf Magnus Institute for Pharmacology, University of Utrecht,
Utrecht, The Netherlands

This review is restricted to a discussion of recent data concerning the neuroendocrine control of anterior pituitary function, which has been studied with the use of drugs that affect the release of hypothalamic hypophysiotropic factors through their action on brain neurotransmitters. Our knowledge of the polypeptide hypophysiotropic factors, including releasing as well as inhibiting factors of hormones, has rapidly expanded in the past decade and has been competently reviewed elsewhere (1–3). The hypothalamic control of the secretion of the hypophysiotropic principles is not precisely known and is subject to multiple systems which govern their discharge into the hypophyseal portal blood supply. Negative and positive feedback mechanisms have been implicated (4), comprising negative feedback action of target gland hormones and of pituitary hormones on the respective hypophysiotropic factors. In addition, a negative feedback action of the hypophysiotropic factors themselves has been indicated (2, 5).

Part of the regulatory mechanism in the secretion of hypophysiotropic factors is of neural origin. Dopamine (DA) and norepinephrine (NE) containing hypothalamic pathways have been observed. An intrahypothalamic tubero-infundibular DA system with cell bodies in the arcuate nucleus ends in the external layers of the median eminence close to the capillary loops of the portal vessels (6, 7). In the hypothalamus, fibers containing NE and serotonin (5-hydroxytryptamine, 5-HT) are found. These are primarily axons of neurons whose cell bodies are located in the mesencephalon and lower brain stem (6, 8, 9). Cholinergic hypothalamic pathways also exist (10). During the past five years a great many studies were performed to elucidate the role of brain transmitter activity in the modulation of pituitary function. A number of symposia and conferences reflect the remarkable interest in this area. Part of the data and inspiration for writing this review originated from the satellite symposium of the Fifth International Congress on Pharmacology: "Drug

389

Effects on Neuroendocrine Regulation," held at Aspen, Colorado on July 17–19, 1972.

PITUITARY ADRENOCORTICOTROPIN (ACTH) RELEASE

Introduction

Variation in pituitary-adrenocortical activity and stress may affect the turnover rate of catecholamines (CA) in the brain. Hypophysectomy decreases the turnover of DA and NE, while adrenalectomy slightly increases NE turnover in the CNS (9, 11). This increased NE turnover in adrenalectomized rats is normalized by administration of glucocorticoids (9, 12). Adrenalectomy and administration of metyrapone increase hypothalamic monoamine oxidase (MAO) and catechol-O-methyltransferase (COMT) activity (13). ACTH has no significant effect on brain NE turnover in hypophysectomized rats (12), but ACTH and the ACTH analog $ACTH_{4-10}$ increase brain NE turnover of intact rats (9, 14). Immobilization stress increases the turnover of CA in the brain and the spinal cord (15), and this occurs in hypophysectomized rats as well (12). Increased central NE turnover has also been found during exercise and exposure to cold (16) and after electric shock (17, 18). Surgical stress produces a rapid fall in hypothalamic NE (19). The increase in the turnover of NE following restraint is blocked by the tranquilizer chlordiazepoxide but not by high doses of dexamethasone (12).

Catecholaminergic Input in ACTH Release

In a recent review, Ganong (2) marshalled evidence, obtained in rats and dogs, indicating that the release of ACTH is under the inhibitory control of central NE containing neurons. Tullner & Hertz (20) and Ganong and associates (21) found that α-ethyltryptamine, an antidepressant with MAO inhibiting activity, blocks the release of ACTH in surgically stressed dogs. This inhibition is probably exerted at the hypothalamic level and correlates with the sympathomimetic activity of α-ethyltryptamine (21, 22). Systemic administration of L-dihydroxyphenylalanine (L-Dopa) and of several sympathicomimetic compounds (amphetamine, methamphetamine, α-methyltryptamine, tyramine, clopane, 2-aminoheptane) inhibits stress-induced ACTH release (2, 21, 23). Administration of L-Dopa, DA, NE, tyramine, α-ethyltryptamine, isoproterenol, and 5-hydroxytryptophan (5-HTP) into the third ventricle has a similar effect (2, 21, 24). Although these data support the thesis of a central noradrenergic inhibitory system for ACTH release, they do not necessarily indicate a specific receptor, and unfortunately large doses of amines have been employed to demonstrate inhibition of ACTH release.

Inhibition of tyrosine hydroxylase by α-methyl-p-tyrosine (α-MT) and of dopamine β-hydroxylase by bis-(1-methyl-4-homopiperazinylthiocarbonyl)-disulfide (FLA-63) causes an increase in plasma corticosterone and a decrease in hypothalamic NE content. α-MT induces a decrease in brain DA content as well (21, 25–27). These data suggest a primary role of NE and not of DA in the regulation of ACTH release. An inverse relation has been found between hypothalamic NE and DA content and plasma corticosterone (25, 26). In rats treated with α-MT both the decrease of hypothalamic NE and the increase in plasma corticosterone are partially prevented by dihydroxyphenylserine (DOPS) (25). DOPS is directly decarboxylated into NE bypassing DA. Partial repletion of CA by administration of L-Dopa also reduces the effect of α-MT on plasma corticosterone (21, 26). Thus, making NE available in the hypothalamus counteracts ACTH release as a result of NE removal. Intraventricular guanethidine in rats increases plasma corticosterone and decreases hypothalamic NE. Guanethidine crosses the blood brain barrier poorly (28), and systemic injection of a dose 30 times the amount administered intraventricularly fails to affect plasma corticosterone (25). Systemically ineffective doses of α-MT given intraventricularly also cause a rise in plasma corticosterone (26).

The majority of available data that point to inhibition of ACTH release by NE containing brain neurons has been obtained in acute experiments. Chronic administration of α-MT fails to cause an increase in rat adrenal weight (2). Immediately after the intraventricular administration of 6-hydroxydopamine (6-OHDA), which acutely causes gross NE release, stress-induced ACTH release is blocked. One day after administration, an elevation of circulating corticosterone is associated with approximately 90% depletion of brain NE. However, no increase in plasma corticosterone is found 15 days after injection of 6-OHDA, although NE depletion is similar to that of day 1 (2, 29). Others reported 70–80% brain NE depletion one week after intraventricular 6-OHDA with normal or slightly elevated plasma corticosterone (30, 31). Provoost & De Jong (unpublished data) found a similar degree of brain NE depletion and failed to observe an increase in circulating corticosterone in rats 3 months after neonatal intraventricular 6-OHDA administration. This suggests that NE neurons are not necessarily involved in corticotropin releasing factor (CRF) or ACTH release. However, this treatment does not completely deplete hypothalamic NE (31), and supersensitivity to NE may occur under these conditions, resulting in a normal function at the receptor sites. Deafferentation of the hypothalamus may be a better means of removing the NE input to the hypothalamus, while the DA system from the arcuate nucleus remains more or less unaffected. Rats with a deafferented hypothalamus, or rats that have had section of the fornix, have chronically elevated resting corticosteroid levels (2, 32, 33). Deafferentation completely depletes NE but does not affect DA content of the hypothalamic island (34). This again points to NE as an inhibitory transmitter in the mechanism of ACTH release.

Only limited data are available concerning the type of receptor involved in the inhibitory central action of NE on ACTH release. The α-adrenergic blocking agent phentolamine, after systemic administration markedly increases plasma corticosterone in rats, while the β-adrenergic blocker propranolol was ineffective in this respect (25, 35). A systemic ineffective dose of phentolamine causes a similar rise in plasma corticosterone upon intraventricular administration (25). Inhibition of ACTH release by L-Dopa in dogs can be blocked by intraventricular administration of phenoxybenzamine, while phentolamine and also propranolol are ineffective (2). MAO inhibition prevents reserpine- and stress-induced ACTH release (36). De Schaepdryver et al (37), however, were unable to block the increase in plasma corticosterone as a result of restraint by the administration of nialamide. Laparotomy stress can be blocked by prior iproniazid and dexamethasone, but neither drug alone was effective under the conditions used. Phentolamine reduces the blockade of adrenocortical activation by iproniazid plus dexamethasone, while propranolol is without effect (25). It is possible therefore that the inhibitory central noradrenergic effect on ACTH release is mediated by an α-adrenergic receptor.

Iproniazid potentiates dexamethasone in blocking ACTH release following stress in rats (38). This may be due to an increase in NE levels in the hypothalamus which may enhance the inhibitory effect of dexamethasone on CRF-ACTH secretion (21). Other amines may also be involved (39). MAO inhibitors also prevent reserpine-induced ACTH release in rats (21) and potentiate dexamethasone blockade of ACTH secretion in Cushing's disease as well (40). These data suggest that the negative feedback action of corticosteroids may be mediated at least in part via noradrenergic control of ACTH release. Several investigators (37, 41, 42) reported that depletion of monoamines by α-MT or reserpine does not affect the ability of the pituitary to release ACTH in response to stress. Interestingly, rats treated with drugs that deplete brain NE exhibit a disturbance in circadian variation in ACTH secretion, an increased adrenocortical response to ACTH and to metyrapone, and a decreased suppressibility of ACTH secretion by glucocorticoids. These disturbances can be overcome by brain NE repletion after L-Dopa administration (21). Similar disturbances are found in patients with Cushing's syndrome. However, Krieger (43) failed to find an alteration in plasma cortisol levels in patients with ACTH dependent Cushing's disease following acute or chronic L-Dopa administration. In addition, adrenocortical function in L-Dopa treated patients seems to be normal (44). A single oral dose of L-Dopa, which increases circulating growth hormone (GH), does not affect cortisol levels (45). The same has been found in children (46). Thus, in man, clear evidence for an aminergic inhibitory control of ACTH release so far is lacking.

Marks and associates have contributed considerably to our knowledge on the mode of action of centrally acting drugs on pituitary-ACTH release (36, 47, 48). Treatment of rats with chlorpromazine (CPZ) or reserpine produces a marked and long lasting depletion of CRF activity in the hypothalamus. This indicates removal of a central inhibitory control by these neuroleptics. In fact, pretreatment with a MAO inhibitor (pargyline) prevents reserpine-induced ACTH release and the decrease in hypothalamic CRF activity. Pargyline also reduces ACTH release in response to ether and laparotomy stress (36, 48). Intraventricular carbachol, NE, and DA in rats stimulate ACTH release, but the amounts required are greater than the transmitter content in the brain (48). However, reserpine-induced ACTH release is terminated following a lower dose of intraventricular NE, while DA is less effective and carbachol further stimulates ACTH release (48). The doses employed have little effect on ACTH release and on blood pressure in nonreserpinized rats. However, reserpine implants in the median eminence fail to alter ACTH secretion (49). This may indicate that noradrenergic inhibition is outside the CRF producing region, that the brain area involved is too extensive to be completely effective, or that NE depletion had not been complete. Bhattacharya & Marks (47) proposed that CA and 5-HT are important as inhibitory neurotransmitters for the steady state secretion of CRF.

Serotonergic Input in ACTH Release

Immobilization stress causes depletion of brain 5-HT which has been observed to disappear 16 hr after the stress (15). This may be due to an increased corticosterone secretion, since cortisol can produce a short lasting depletion of 5-HT (50). However, De Schaepdryver et al (37) observed a slight increase in brain 5-HT of rats after 6 hr restraint associated with elevated plasma corticosterone. Other types of stress such as electric shock have also been found to increase 5-HT levels slightly in the brain (51) and to increase 5-HT turnover (17, 18, 52). These discrepancies may in part be explained by the different time intervals used. Marked changes in 5-HT levels caused by MAO and tryptophan hydroxylase inhibitors, tryptophan deficiency, and 4-chloramphetamine do not affect stress-induced ACTH release (37, 53).

Daily injections of corticosteroids do not change brain 5-HT levels (54), but a reduced 5-HT turnover has been found in adrenalectomized rats. This is restored to normal by cortisol or dexamethasone (12). Adrenalectomy decreases brain tryptophan hydroxylase activity, and administration of corticosterone and also of ACTH restores this activity (55, 56). Naumenko (57) reported that injection of 5-HT in the hypothalamus of intact and midbrain sectioned guinea pigs causes ACTH release. In unanesthetized cats, 5-HT implantation into the median eminence and septal area also causes an acute rise in circulating 17-hydroxycorticosteroids (17-OHCS) (58). 5-HTP produces adrenocortical activation in rats with complete deafferentation of the hypothalamus (59). The intraventricular injection of 5-HT, however, neither stimulates nor inhibits ACTH release in normal or reserpinized rats (48).

Scapagnini et al (60) have shown that the circadian variation of limbic 5-HT parallels changes in plasma corticosterone and that treatment with *p*-chlorophenylalanine (pCPA) abolishes the normal diurnal variation of plasma corticosterone (60, 61). Drugs that affect the level or action of 5-HT also abolish the daily rise in plasma 17-OHCS in cats but not the response to stress (62). These different treatments did not affect, or slightly decreased, the adrenocortical response to ACTH. Krieger & Rizzo (62) suggested a role of 5-HT in the nervous pathways mediating circadian periodicity of ACTH release. From these findings Scapagnini et al (60) suggested that the frontal cortex, hippocampus, and amygdala, which are rich in 5-HT fibers (63), are part of a serotonergic functional unit that plays a modulating role in the regulation of ACTH secretion. Vernikos-Danellis et al (39) studied the diurnal variation of plasma corticosterone in rats treated with pCPA for 2 or 4 days. These authors also found a disappearance of the diurnal rhythm in plasma corticosterone, but an enhancement of the circulating ACTH and corticosterone response to electric shock or ether stress and an increase in pituitary ACTH levels. They further showed that pCPA reduces the feedback action of prednisolone in stressed animals. Iproniazid potentiates dexamethasone in blocking ACTH release following stress (38). From these studies the hypothesis was proposed (39) that 5-HT mediates the corticosteroid negative feedback action. In this view, the absence of corticosterone due to adrenalectomy results in a decreased brain 5-HT turnover, thus allowing greater ACTH synthesis and release and an increased sensitivity to stress. In contrast, increased levels of corticosteroids stimulate 5-HT synthesis through which the hypothalamic-pituitary adrenal axis is suppressed. This is in accord with the reported potentiation of stress-induced ACTH release in 5-HT depleted rats. Conversely, treatment with 5-HTP to increase brain 5-HT level raises circulating corticosterone slightly and somewhat suppresses the response to the stress of ether and laparotomy. However, tryptophan administration to adrenalecto-mized rats abolishes stress-induced release of ACTH. In addition, oral administra-tion of the peripheral decarboxylase inhibitor L-α-hydrazinomethyldihydroxy-phenylalanine (MK–486) and 5-HTP for several days produced a marked drop in 17-OHCS excretion in urine in four normal human volunteers (39). These studies suggest that 5-HT is involved in the circadian variation of pituitary-adrenal activity, in stress-induced ACTH release, and in the negative feedback action of glucocorticos-teroids.

Cholinergic Input in ACTH Release

Krieger & Krieger (58) have investigated the chemical sensitivity of neurons in brain areas known to be associated with ACTH secretion in unanesthetized cats. They found that carbachol injections into the basal hypothalamus provoke ACTH release. This can be blocked by prior administration of atropine. In rats, in which ACTH release is blocked by pentobarbital even in the presence of morphine or CPZ, systemic carbachol is a powerful stimulus for the release of ACTH (64). Evidence for the existence of a cholinergic mechanism in the release of ACTH comes from studies by Hedge & Smelik (65) who showed that implantation of atropine in the anterior hypothalamus markedly inhibits stress-induced ACTH release. Interest-ingly, atropine in the same area does not block release of antidiuretic hormone activity which can under certain conditions be reduced by systemic atropine (66). In the dog, intraventricular atropine does not affect stress-induced ACTH release (2), and systemic administration of atropine fails to inhibit stress-induced ACTH release in dogs and cats (67, 68). In contrast, the circadian rhythm of circulating 17-OHCS in cats can be prevented by systemic administration of atropine just prior to the time of the expected circadian rise (68). Thus, a central cholinergic mecha-nism may be involved in the release of ACTH, but the significance of this mechanism is not well understood.

PITUITARY GONADOTROPIN AND PROLACTIN RELEASE

Introduction

Alterations in hypothalamic CA content, CA turnover, and MAO activity vary with the stage of the estrus cycle and the levels of circulating gonadal steroids (9, 69, 70). A steady increase in CA fluorescence from day one to estrus was found in the DA-containing nerve cells of the tuberal region, but not in the substantia nigra; ovariectomy prevents these changes (71, 72). Following removal of the inhibitory effects of gonadal steroids by castration, NE content and tyrosine hydroxylase activity increase and the rate of turnover of NE in the anterior hypothalamus is accelerated (73, 74), while DA turnover appears to decrease (9). No change in 5-HT synthesis was found in ovariectomized rats (74). The effect of castration disappears following hypophysectomy but can be reproduced in hypophysectomized-oophorectomized rats by treatment with follicle stimulating hormone (FSH) (75). Ovariectomy, but also FSH increases ^{3}H-CA accumulation in rat brain (73). In addition, ^{3}H-CA accumulation is almost four times as rapid during proestrus as during diestrus (75). Turnover of DA in the median eminence, on the other hand, decreases during proestrus and early estrus. This is associated with a drop in luteinizing hormone (LH) content in the pituitary (76). Nigro-neostriatal DA turnover does not change under these conditions. Moreover, DA turnover is high during low pituitary FSH secretion as occurs during pregnancy, lactation, and treatment with gonadal steroids (7).

PROLACTIN RELEASE

Catecholaminergic Input in Prolactin Release

Chronic deafferentation of the medial basal hypothalamus of rats induces a complete depletion of NE, leaving the DA content intact, while the 5-HT concentration of the deafferented island decreases to 30% (34, 77). In male deafferented rats, gonadal function remains relatively normal, while in females ovulation is blocked (78). Thus, cyclic release of gonadotropins depends on neural input to the medial basal hypothalamus. Others found that, following deafferentation, animals become diestrus and circulating levels of FSH and LH decrease, while serum prolactin levels remain normal (34, 79, 80). Administration of α-MT causes a rapid rise in circulating levels of prolactin in completely deafferented rats (34), suggesting that DA is involved in the secretion of prolactin. Donoso et al (81) found that α-MT also increases serum prolactin in castrated male and female rats. Diethyldithiocarbamate (DDC), which inhibits dopamine-β-hydroxylase, has no effect on circulating prolactin. L-Dopa lowers prolactin levels in nontreated and α-MT-treated castrated rats and blocks the prolactin response to suckling. The L-Dopa effect is maintained in the presence of DDC. Treatment with α-MT and DOPS results in a further rise in circulating prolactin (81, 82). It may be, therefore, that NE stimulates and DA inhibits prolactin secretion.

That DA exerts an inhibitory control on prolactin secretion has been suggested by Van Maanen & Smelik (83), who reported that implants of reserpine in the basal hypothalamus of rats induce pseudopregnancy. This local effect of reserpine is blocked by iproniazid. These authors suggested that DA is identical to prolactin inhibiting factor (PIF). This suggestion is supported by observations that not only DA but also NE and epinephrine (E) decrease prolactin secretion from incubated pituitaries in vitro without affecting GH release (84, 85). DA is most effective, and the effect is not due to destruction of prolactin (85) and can be abolished by α- and β-adrenergic blockers (84). However, the amounts of the various amines used in vitro are far greater than the physiological amounts that reach the pituitary from the median eminence (86). Koch et al (87) found that low concentrations of NE and E stimulate in vitro prolactin release while high doses of these amines reduce prolactin release from incubated rat pituitaries. In view of the stimulatory effects of low levels of NE and E on prolactin release in vitro (87), Nicoll (88) suggested that one of these catecholamines may function as the prolactin releasing factor

(PRF). However, intrapituitary infusion of DA, NE, E, or 5-HT has no effect on plasma prolactin, and injection of DA into the stalk median eminence complex via the peduncular artery fails to stimulate prolactin release (70). In contrast, intraventricular administration of 1.25 μg DA and of 100 μg NE or E in intact rats decreases circulating prolactin levels (70, 89), while intraventricular propranolol and phenoxybenzamine increase prolactin secretion (90). Systemically administered MAO inhibitors depress prolactin release, as does the COMT inhibitor pyrogallol in moderate amounts (81, 91). The precursor of DA and NE, L-Dopa, markedly affects prolactin release. L-Dopa decreases while methyldopa increases serum prolactin in young and aged male rats (92). L-Dopa in hypophysectomized rats with pituitary transplants decreases circulating prolactin and increases hypothalamic PIF (93). The same is found on hypothalamic PIF content in intact rats. Intravenous thyrotropin releasing factor (TRF) has been found to augment prolactin secretion in man (94, 95). Surprisingly, L-Dopa inhibits TRF-induced prolactin secretion (96). This would suggest a direct inhibitory action of L-Dopa on pituitary prolactin release if TRF acts on the pituitary directly in mediating prolactin secretion. L-Dopa reduces basal prolactin levels in normal individuals (96). Long-term treatment with L-Dopa decreases prolactin levels in patients with Forbes-Albright syndrome with galactorrhoea. Withdrawal of L-Dopa therapy is associated again with high prolactin levels and galactorrhoea (97).

Inhibition of prolactin secretion by ergot alkaloids has been extensively reviewed recently (98). Ergocornine and 2-Br-α-ergokryptine suppress prolactin secretion in rats (98, 99). These compounds seem to have DA receptor stimulatory effects (9) and reduce the increased turnover of DA in lactating rats with a high prolactin secretion. In rats with a pituitary tumor that secretes prolactin, treatment with ergocornine reduces circulating prolactin and the size of the tumor. The effect of ergocornine on PIF is believed to be of minor importance under these conditions (100). Various ergot alkaloids in lactating rats decrease circulating prolactin levels and lactation (98). The same is found in pituitary grafted hypophysectomized rats (101). Ergocornine also prevents the rise in circulating prolactin in rats bearing lesions in the median eminence (102). Thus, ergot alkaloids have a direct effect on the pituitary. Additional evidence for this has been obtained from in vitro studies (98). 2-Br-α-ergokryptine lowers circulating prolactin levels in normal subjects. Postpartum it causes a marked suppression of elevated serum prolactin and inhibits lactation. In patients with idiopathic galactorrhoea and amenorrhoea it leads to cessation of galactorrhoea and normal menstrual cycles (98, 103). L-Dopa has a similar effect, although it has a shorter duration of action and is more potent. 2-Br-α-ergokryptine decreases circulating prolactin in male and female patients with prolactin secreting tumors and in patients with Chiari-Frommel syndrome (104). The TRF effect on prolactin is inhibited by ergokryptine, suggesting a direct effect of the compound on prolactin secreting cells. Interestingly, during ergokryptine treatment, circulating FSH and LH levels rise considerably (104).

Psychotropic drugs markedly affect the release of prolactin (105). After a single injection, reserpine, CPZ, α-MT, and α-methyl-metatyrosine (α-MMT) elevate circulating prolactin in rats and decrease pituitary prolactin, except α-MMT which increases prolactin concentration in the pituitary (106). Reserpine and perphenazine increase prolactin secretion in rats without affecting GH release (85). Interestingly, the prolactin stimulatory effect of reserpine depends on the presence of estrogens, since it does not occur in ovariectomized rats (107). However, when the pituitary secretes high amounts of gonadotropins as in ovariectomy, the secretion of prolactin in response to perphenazine is markedly decreased (108). Reserpine and perphenazine also restore the reduced release of prolactin of incubated anterior pituitary tissue of rats bearing prolactin producing tumors (85). Perphenazine in rats increases plasma levels of prolactin by a factor of 10 in relatively low doses (109). Haloperidol, which is an antagonist of DA (110), also causes a marked increase in circulating prolactin in proestrus rats, while pituitary prolactin content decreases concomitantly with hypothalamic PIF. The same occurs in male rats although to a lesser extent (111). In vitro addition of perphenazine does not release prolactin from the pituitary, and this drug slightly affects the release of prolactin in vivo in rats with pituitary transplants in the kidney (109). Addition of low levels of haloperidol and perphenazine to incubated pituitary glands has no effect on prolactin release. However, in the presence of DA both drugs block the inhibitory effect of DA on prolactin release in vitro (112). The effect of apomorphine, a DA receptor stimulating agent (113), and ergokryptine on prolactin release from incubated pituitary glands is also blocked by haloperidol or perphenazine (114). The effect of the two neuroleptic drugs, therefore, may be partially explained by a direct action in the anterior pituitary.

Chronic treatment with CPZ, imipramine, amitriptyline, and haloperidol increases prolactin secretion in animal and man (96, 105, 115). CPZ in man markedly stimulates prolactin release which does not occur in patients with a disease of the hypothalamic-pituitary unit (116). These authors also found that L-Dopa inhibits CPZ-induced prolactin release in healthy volunteers. Apomorphine also blocks CPZ- and suckling-induced prolactin release in rats (117).

In conclusion, DA administration seems most effective in reducing prolactin secretion, and it follows that prolactin secretion may be under the inhibitory control of the tubero-infundibular DA neurons in the hypothalamus by affecting PIF release and/or by a direct action of DA on prolactin secreting cells in the anterior pituitary. Prolactin, but not FSH, LH, ACTH, or TSH, stimulates DA turnover in the median eminence of intact, castrated, and in particular of hypophysectomized rats, which also occurs following intraventricular administration of prolactin (9). This fact lends support to the existence of an intimate relation between this hormone and DA. However, central serotonergic stimulatory pathways may be involved in the release of prolactin as well.

Serotonergic and Cholinergic Input in Prolactin Release

Suckling-induced rise in prolactin secretion is inhibited when 5-HT synthesis is blocked 0–96 hr before the suckling stimulus (118). It reappears after 5 days when 5-HT stores are normal again or sooner if repleted by administration of 5-HTP. Kordon (118) suggests that increasing the 5-HT level in the hypothalamus facilitates prolactin release. Intraventricular administration of high doses (50 μg) of 5-HT and N-acetylserotonin in intact male and estrogen-treated female rats stimulates prolactin release. This, however, is not found in castrated rats (89). Intraventricular 5-HT and melatonin (1–50 μg) stimulate the release of prolactin in a dose-dependent fashion, as does systemic administration of 5-HTP (70). Electrical stimulation of the ventral medial hypothalamus augments prolactin secretion, which can be somewhat reduced by intraventricular atropine (90), and pilocarpine and physostigmine increase prolactin secretion in ovariectomized rats. This effect is blocked by atropine pretreatment (119). This may indicate the existence of cholinergic stimulatory influences on prolactin release.

FSH AND LH RELEASE

Catecholaminergic Input in FSH/LH Release

Many reports indicate that hypothalamic CA affect the release of gonadotropin hormones. Using an in vitro system, Schneider & McCann (120) found that DA releases LH releasing factor (LRF) from hypothalamic fragments, thus enhancing LH release from incubated pituitaries in vitro. DA had no direct effect on pituitary LH release and did not affect the pituitary response to LRF. In addition, DA injected via a hypophyseal portal vein did not affect FSH and LH release (121). DA injected intraventricularly stimulates LH release via release of LRF in intact rats and increases LRF in portal vessel and peripheral blood of hypophysectomized rats (121–123). Systemic administration of the α-blockers phentolamine and phenoxybenzamine, in contrast to β-blocking agents, prevents the release of hypophysiotropic factors from hypothalamic tissue in vitro by DA (70, 120, 124). The LH response to DA is blocked by prior intraventricular estradiol, while estradiol added in vitro also blocks the effect of DA (122, 124).

Discrepancies as to which of the catecholamines are involved in the release of gonadotropins still exist. Rubinstein & Sawyer (125) found that intraventricular E is more potent than other amines to trigger ovulation in proestrus pentobarbital blocked rats. L-Dopa stimulates LH- and FSH release in ovariectomized estrogen-progesterone primed rats (70). LH release by progesterone-induced stimulation of the preoptic area can be blocked by α-MT or a dopamine-β-hydroxylase inhibitor and is restored by DOPS, indicating NE as the mediator of LH release (123). A single intraventricular injection of 6-OHDA in male rats reduces LH secretion for approximately 8 hr only, while FSH release remains unaltered (126). Marked decrease of hypothalamic amine concentration as induced by reserpine, tetrabenazine, and α-methyldopa suppresses FSH and LH secretion in pregnant mare serum (PMS)-treated immature rats (127). When in PMS-treated immature rats, CA synthesis is blocked with α-MT prior to the "critical period," ovulation is reduced (reduced number of ova). α-MT reduces DA before NE levels in the hypothalamus are decreased (128). In fact, L-Dopa restores ovulation in α-MT-treated rats, while restoration of NE alone by DOPS is ineffective (82). Thus, DA may be involved in α-MT-induced blockade of ovulation. Conversely, α-methyldopa blocks ovulation only when applied to the region of the tubero-infundibular tract or the median eminence.

These data indicate that a stimulatory dopaminergic control is involved in PMS-induced ovulation. This is not in accord with data on DA turnover (76, 123), which appears low during the critical period in PMS-treated rats (9). The day after the critical period, DA turnover rates are high. Testosterone, in amounts that block ovulation and reduce LH release in PMS-treated immature rats, markedly increases DA turnover in the tubero-infundibular neurons during the critical period (9, 129, 130). These studies suggest that the tubero-infundibular DA neurons might act to inhibit LRF/LH release. Also, a mixture of DA and cholesterol implanted in the median eminence causes prolonged diestrus in normal, cycling rats (131). Although Cramer & Porter (89) failed to find an effect of DA on plasma LH in either intact or estrogen-treated animals, these authors found that DA is a potent inhibitor of LH release in the castrated male rat elicited by the intraventricular injection of 0.15 M NaCl via strain receptors in the vicinity of the ventricle. This measure does not release FSH. However, these authors used very high doses of DA. In this respect it is relevant to mention that intraventricular DA in relatively low doses and large amounts of NE and E stimulate LH and FSH release, while high amounts of DA appeared to decrease the discharge of the gonadotropins (70, 132). In man L-Dopa slightly decreases circulating LH (45), but in a study in children L-Dopa was unable to affect FSH or LH levels in blood (46), and L-Dopa in Parkinson patients does not alter the excretion of gonadotropins in urine (44). Chronic treatment with L-Dopa also fails to affect circulating LH and testosterone (133).

Castration hypersecretion of FSH and LH in rats is prevented by α-MT (134). This effect is counteracted by MAO inhibitors or CA precursors. Administration of L-Dopa or DOPS restores the post-castration rise of FSH but not of LH in orchidectomized α-MT-treated rats. L-Dopa shortly after α-MT treatment restores both FSH and LH secretion following castration (135). In contrast, α-methyldopa does not affect circulating LH levels in castrated female rats (118). Thus, the post-castration rise in gonadotropins, which occurs as a result of the removal of the negative feedback of gonadal steroids, may be due to increased NE or DA activity (135).

The positive feedback action of gonadal steroids also seems under CA influence. Using progesterone-induced release of FSH and estradiol-induced release of LH in spayed estrogen pretreated rats, Kalra & McCann (123) studied the interaction of catecholamines in the stimulatory effects of these steroids on the release of gonadotropins. Haloperidol and phenoxybenzamine block the surge of FSH and LH, following progesterone or estradiol respectively. The blockade by these drugs indicates the participation of an α-adrenergic component in the steroid-induced gonadotropin secretion. In fact, blockade of DA and/or NE synthesis with α-MT, DDC, or U 14,624 [1-phenyl-3-(2-thiazolyl)-2-thiourea] inhibits progesterone or estradiol-evoked stimulation of gonadotropin release. Whereas L-Dopa is effective in restoring steroid-induced release of gonadotropin secretion in α-MT-treated rats, it is ineffective when the conversion of DA to NE is blocked by DDC. Repletion of NE by

DOPS in the presence of a low DA concentration in the hypothalamus reverses the blockade (123). These studies suggest that NE plays a role in the regulation of the positive feedback action of estradiol and progesterone on the release of FSH and LH.

The phenothiazines have long been known to inhibit the release of FSH and LH and to block ovulation (for review see De Wied, 115). These drugs interfere with the release of FSH and LH and in particular in high doses, with the sensitivity of the gonads to gonadotropins. The same holds for reserpine. Barraclough & Sawyer (136) were among the first to show that reserpine and CPZ block ovulation when administered prior to the critical period of LH discharge at proestrus. This effect is counteracted by pretreatment with MAO inhibitors (137). PMS-induced ovulation in immature rats is also blocked by reserpine (138). Reserpine given after the critical period does not affect ovulation, suggesting that the effect of reserpine is mainly on LH release (137). PMS plus human chorionic gonadotropin (HCG)-induced ovulation in intact or hypophysectomized immature rats is also blocked by reserpine (139). This effect is not dose related and pargyline partially reverses the inhibitory action of reserpine. Thus, reserpine appears to act on both LH release and on the ovary. Treatment with reserpine on the morning of proestrus inhibits spontaneous ovulation and elevates the electrical threshold of the preoptic area to induce ovulation but not of the median eminence region (125). Reserpine 18–20 hr after treatment completely blocks ovulation evoked by electrical stimulation, and MAO inhibition in these rats restores electrically stimulated but not spontaneous ovulation. FSH release is also affected by reserpine. The depletion of FSH, which occurs in the pituitary of rats of 34–39 days of age, is reduced by reserpine (140). The foregoing discussion does not allow a conclusion as to which CA is involved in FSH/LH release. Presumably more than one transmitter participates in the cyclic and noncyclic secretion of these pituitary hormones.

Serotonergic Input in FSH/LH Release

The level of plasma testosterone in rats is reduced following treatment with α-MT or pCPA, indicating that both CA and serotonergic pathways are involved in the regulation of gonadotropic hormone release (141). Nialamide given during the critical period of PMS-treated immature rats (82) blocks ovulation. This blockade is prevented by prior treatment with pCPA but unaffected by α-MT. A tonically inhibitory effect of 5-HT neurons on copulation has been suggested (69), because pCPA can substitute for progesterone. In addition, progesterone is capable of reversing the antiovulatory effect of MAO inhibition (82). pCPA reduces ovarian weight increase in immature rats and prevents FSH depletion in rats of 34–39 days of age (140). A single injection of 5-HT or melatonin on the day of operation blocks compensatory ovarian hypertrophy and FSH release in a dose-related fashion. The blockade is most effective when substances are given on the day of diestrus. 5-HT is less effective than melatonin (142). Melatonin and 5-methoxytryptophol in the lateral ventricle of immature rats from the 25th day of birth delays vaginal opening, indicating blockade of gonadotropin release (143). Intraventricular 5-HT and melatonin in moderate amounts have been shown to suppress the release of FSH and LH. Systemic administration of 5-HTP in castrated male and female rats reduces LH and FSH release. The proestrus surge of FSH and LH can be inhibited by intraventricular administration of 5-HT and melatonin in rats (70).

5-HT administered systemically on the day before proestrus blocks spontaneous ovulation. This effect can be overcome by methysergide or LH (144). In addition, multiple intraventricular or intracardiac injections of 5-HTP or melatonin on the day of proestrus inhibit ovulation. 5-HT has the same effect upon central administration as 5-HTP after intracardiac injection. This blockade of ovulation is preceded by inhibition of gonadotropin release and is prevented by LH or hypothalamic extracts (70). Blockade of ovulation after the administration of MAO inhibitors has been specifically linked to increased brain 5-HT levels (82). Microinjection of a MAO inhibitor in the median eminence increases 5-HT levels and blocks ovulation (82). The same is found when the MAO inhibitor mebenazine is given in combination with 5-HTP. Mebenazine plus L-Dopa has no such effect (145). A single injection of α-MT, which inhibits DA and NE synthesis without affecting 5-HT synthesis, blocks ovulation, while α-MMT, which also decreases 5-HT, does not. Donoso et al (81) reported that α-MT does not affect FSH/LH release in castrated rats. The same was reported for pCPA. Kordon & Glowinski (82) found that pCPA facilitates ovulation only when administered just before the critical period. It has an opposite effect when given 20 hr before. This suggests that different 5-HT neurons are involved in cyclic and noncyclic LH release. This paradoxical effect of pCPA may partly explain existing controversies in the literature on the influence of 5-HT neurons on gonadotropin release.

In conclusion, the evidence summarized above indicates that serotonergic pathways exert an inhibitory control over the release of gonadotropins. These effects are exerted via FSH releasing factor (FRF) and LRF release, while the injection of 5-HT into the portal vessel system does not affect the release of gonadotropic hormones (70, 132).

Cholinergic Input in FSH/LH Release

Kato & Minaguchi (146) have reported changes in choline acetylase activity during cyclic changes of gonadotropin secretion. Atropine has been known for a long time to block ovulation (147), and atropine administered subcutaneously or intraventricularly suppresses FSH and LH release and blocks ovulation. This blockade can be reversed by LH or by a crude hypothalamic extract (70, 148). In the presence of hypothalamic fragments, acetylcholine stimulates the release of gonadotropins from anterior pituitary tissue in vitro (70, 148, 149), while atropine has the reverse effect. Atropine given intraventricularly on the day of proestrus suppresses FSH and LH surge and inhibits ovulation (149). Pilocarpine and physostigmine reduce plasma LH but not FSH levels. This reduction is followed by a sharp rise in LH 1.5–6 hr after injection. Atropine, which in itself does not affect FSH/LH release, partly prevented the effect of these cholinomimetics (119). Oxotremorine reduces LH secretion in ovariectomized rats. This effect is blocked by atropine but not by methylatropine. Thus, central muscarinic receptors are involved in the blocking effect of oxotremorine on LH secretion (150). Nicotine, when injected at half-hour intervals on the afternoon of proestrus, delays the ovulatory surge of LH and blocks spontaneous ovulation in rats, indicating an inhibitory effect of nicotine receptors in the neural mechanism of LH release (151).

PITUITARY GROWTH HORMONE (GH) RELEASE

Catecholaminergic Input in GH Release

Numerous reports have appeared indicating the existence of catecholaminergic regulation of GH secretion in man, monkey, sheep, and rat. However, contradictory data exists, and species differences in GH release complicate the picture. Man and rat respond differently to stress with respect to GH secretion. Stress stimulates the release of GH in man and monkey (152, 153), while it inhibits the discharge of GH in rats (154, 155). Administration of E to monkeys induces a significant rise in GH secretion (156). In baboons, intraventricular administration of DA inhibits GH secretion (157). The same is found after microinjection of DA in the ventromedial nucleus, while NE in the same structure stimulates GH release (158). In contrast, microinjection of 5-HT in the ventromedial nucleus does not affect GH release, while DA and NE in other hypothalamic areas do not change the secretion of GH in baboons. Phentolamine depresses, while β-adrenergic and ganglionic blockade increase GH levels in blood of baboons (159). The stimulatory action of β blockers and ganglionic blockade on GH release is prevented by phentolamine. Thus, in primates α-adrenergic activity stimulates, while DA- and β-adrenergic activity inhibit GH release. A recent study in rhesus monkeys points to a stimulatory influence of DA, NE, and 5-HT on GH release (160). In these monkeys, equipped with a chronic indwelling intraatrial cannula, L-Dopa infusion causes a GH peak, which is enhanced in animals pretreated with the dopamine-β-hydroxylase inhibitor disulfiram. DOPS also causes an increase in circulating GH, as does 5-HT infusion (160).

In sheep, infusion of E decreases circulating GH (161). In the same species, administration of E blocks the GH response to arginine (162). This effect of E is not blocked by phentolamine (163). Intracarotid injection of phenoxybenzamine or of arginine increases circulating GH in sheep, while L-Dopa blocks arginine-induced GH secretion (163). Because phenoxybenzamine does not block DA receptors (8), central NE activity may tonically inhibit GH release in sheep. Interestingly, Davis & Borger (163) found the same mechanism operating in the release of prolactin in sheep.

In rats, CPZ and reserpine, as well as α-methyldopa and α-MMT, block insulin-induced depletion of GH activity in the pituitary. This effect is prevented by prior administration of ipromiazid. Peripheral depletion of CA with guanethidine is ineffective (164, 165). Injection of low doses (0.1–0.5 μg) of NE and DA into the lateral cerebral ventricle of rats induces depletion of bioassayable GH activity in the pituitary. E is also active, but only at higher dose levels, and NE (5 ng) appeared to be the most active amine in this respect (166). Intraventricular injection of 5-HT, acetylcholine, histamine, vasopressin, or oxytocin is without effect (167). Intraventricular NE and DA in doses that cause depletion of pituitary GH activity, decrease GH releasing factor (GRF) activity in the hypothalamus of intact and hypophysectomized rats and increase circulating GRF activity (166). Rats with a transplanted pituitary tumor secreting high quantities of GH and prolactin have markedly lower circulating GH only if pretreated with L-Dopa (168). The authors suggest a direct effect of L-Dopa on GH secretion from the tumor. However, neither E, NE, nor DA affect the discharge of GH from rat pituitaries incubated in vitro (84).

Urethane anesthesia in rats induces constant and low circulating GH levels. Collu and associates (169), with the aid of a radioimmunoassay, explored the role of central CA on GH release in urethanized rats. It was found that intraventricular DA induces a decrease in GH level shortly after administration. NE has a similar effect. Propranolol had no effect in itself, but it prevented DA-induced suppression of GH release. Intraventricular administration of 5-HT was followed by a rapid rise in GH levels which was prevented by intraventricular phenoxybenzamine. Phenoxybenzamine elicited a prompt inhibition of GH release.

In view of this, Collu et al (170) proposed that in the rat, central DA tonically inhibits and 5-HT stimulates GH release. In fact, DA is found in the same band as GRF activity of fractionated nerve terminals of rat median eminence (171). However, Müller et al (172) were unable to affect GH release with 1 μg intraventricular 5-HT in urethane anesthetized rats. These authors found that central CA depletion by 6-OHDA or α-MT does not affect plasma GH level. L-Dopa in α-MT-treated rats, which is associated with high hypothalamic DA level, reduces GH secretion. FLA-63 plus L-Dopa had the same effect, while the DA receptor blocking agent pimozide had the reverse influence on GH release. Therefore DA may inhibit and NE may stimulate GH release in rats.

Evidence for an inhibitory DA control of GH secretion has also been obtained in deafferented rats. Ether stress and auditory stress reduce plasma GH levels in sham-operated rats, as well as in frontally and in incompletely deafferented rats. Auditory stress does not reduce GH release in totally deafferented rats but ether stress does (173). Treatment of totally deafferented rats with α-MT prevents GH reduction in response to ether stress. Because DA neurons are preserved in the totally deafferented rat hypothalamus, DA appears responsible for the inhibitory effect of stress on GH release in the rat. This is in accord with the fact that deafferented young rats grow fairly well (78).

A considerable number of reports has appeared on the influence of L-Dopa on GH release in humans. In contrast to rats, L-Dopa increases circulating GH levels of normal human subjects and of patients with Huntington's chorea (174). Chronic treatment of Parkinson patients with L-Dopa, however, is not associated with increased fasting levels of GH, although the GH response to insulin hypoglycemia is subnormal (175). In children, oral L-Dopa for several days increases GH levels within 0.5–2 hr. No such increase is found in children with idiopathic hypopituitarism (46). The same has been observed following a single oral dose of L-Dopa in normal subjects and in patients with Parkinson's disease (45, 175–177).

L-Dopa given orally induces a gradual rise in circulating GH. This effect is blocked by pretreatment with phentolamine (178). The effect on circulating GH after orally administered L-Dopa, is more consistent in young than in older subjects, and a high percentage of nonresponders is found in depressive illness (179). In acromegalic patients, however, L-Dopa suppresses GH release (180), while L-Dopa treatment in Cushing's disease fails to affect plasma GH levels (43). Phentolamine inhibits and propranolol enhances plasma GH response to insulin hypoglycemia in human subjects. Infusion of L-Dopa, and of E plus propranolol increases circulating GH and enhances insulin- and arginine-induced GH release (178, 181, 182). None of these treatments increases plasma GH levels in pituitary dwarfs (182). The increase in circulating GH following E and propranolol is blocked by phentolamine but not by glucose or aminophylline (178). In addition, exercise-induced GH release in normal and in nonobese juvenile diabetics is suppressed by phentolamine and enhanced by propranolol (183). Propranolol in a single oral dose augments glucagon-induced GH secretion in normal subjects. This does not occur in hypopituitarism (178). The poor GH response to glucagon in hypothyroid patients is converted to normal by propranolol treatment (184). Thus, α-adrenergic stimulation and possibly β-adrenergic inhibition in man are associated with GH release.

PITUITARY THYROTROPIN HORMONE (TSH) RELEASE

Catecholaminergic Input in TSH Release

It has been suggested that TSH release is also under the control of central CA activity (185). Martini (186) found that intraventricular administration of E in dogs increases plasma TSH. However, application of NE or E in the hypothalamus of rats failed to stimulate the release of TSH (187). In addition, propylthiouracil treatment has no effect on DA turnover in the median eminence of male rats (7). Deafferentation of the medial basal hypothalamus of rats slightly reduces TSH release as determined by ^{131}I uptake and biological half life of thyroidal ^{131}I (78). Thus, the absence of hypothalamic NE only slightly affects TSH release.

Direct stimulating effects of E added in vitro and of systemically administered CA and 5-HT on anterior pituitary and thyroid gland have been found (188, 189). Cervical sympathetic stimulation also increases thyroidal hormone release; this effect is blocked by phentolamine (190), but phenoxybenzamine and phentolamine reduce the thyroid response to TSH (191). Daily injection of propranolol for 21 days does not affect circulating TSH in intact rats. However, propranolol increases circulating thyroxin (T_4) levels in intact as well as in hypophysectomized rats (192), indicating a direct stimulatory effect of β-adrenergic receptor blockade on thyroid gland activity. Thus, a peripheral TSH-like effect of the biogenic amines and the β-blocking agents on thyroid hormone secretion is present. This is in accord with recent studies (193) in which the effect of various CA depleting agents on thyroid activity in rats was investigated. Thyroid activity was compared with NE depletion in hypothalamus and heart. Chronic treatment with reserpine, α-methyldopa, α-MT, and guanethidine reduces thyroid secretion rate. Tetrabenazine, which acts mainly centrally, did not affect thyroid secretion rate, while guanethidine, which acts mainly peripherally, decreased thyroid activity. Thus, peripheral NE depletion rather than depletion of central NE is correlated with a decrease in thyroid function (193). The effect of cold exposure, which causes an acute and marked increase in intrathyroidal colloid droplets, is blocked by phentolamine, reserpine, and atropine. These drugs do not interfere with the action of TSH releasing factor (TRF) on the pituitary-thyroid axis (194), suggesting that their effect on pituitary TSH release is centrally mediated.

The phenothiazines affect the pituitary-thyroid axis. Acute and chronic administration of CPZ and related phenothiazines depress thyroid activity. This probably is not only the result of inhibition of TSH release, but also of a direct effect on the thyroid gland and on the metabolism of T_4 in the body (for review see De Wied, 115). Onaya et al (195) found evidence for a direct inhibitory effect of CPZ on TSH-stimulated colloid droplet formation in dog thyroid slices. This is attributed to a stabilizing effect of CPZ on lysosomes. Reserpine given chronically to rats lowers circulating TSH and reduces TRF synthetase concentration in the hypothalamus (196). This was interpreted to indicate a central catecholaminergic input in pituitary TSH release. 5-HT, however, may be involved. Treatment of rats with pCPA for five days decreases circulating triiodothyronine (T_3) levels, without affecting T_4. However, a marked depression of serum TSH is associated with 5-HT depletion. The intrathyroidal 5-HT and 5-hydroxyindole acetic acid (5-HIAA) decrease induced by pCPA suggests a peripheral effect of pCPA, but the fall in TSH points to a central stimulatory influence of 5-HT neurons on TRF/TSH release (197).

Studies in man also fail to reveal a central aminergic control of TSH secretion. Eddy et al (177) found no change in circulating TSH following the acute administration of L-Dopa, and no alteration in various parameters of thyroid function was observed following two weeks of L-Dopa treatment in Parkinson's patients (44). In children, chronic L-Dopa does not affect plasma TSH levels (46). L-Dopa administration to normal human subjects and to patients with Parkinson's disease does not materially affect T_4 levels in blood. Chronic treatment increases circulating T_4 (175). This could be due to increased TSH levels, but also to alterations in distribution, binding, metabolism, and excretion of T_4, because infusion of E causes a decrease in fecal excretion of T_4, increased binding, and a shift of tissue T_4 stores to the vascular compartment (198). Ericson et al (199) obtained evidence for a direct stimulating effect of CA and 5-HT on thyroid hormone release in mice. Interestingly, chronic L-Dopa treatment in patients with Parkinson's disease results in inhibition of TSH secretion in response to TRF (200). Infusion of isoproterenol, NE, phentolamine, or propranolol does not alter TRF-induced TSH release nor do these agents affect circulating TSH levels (201). Neither α- nor β-adrenergic blockade has an effect on the serum TSH response to cooling in young adult human subjects (202).

GENERAL CONCLUSION

The evidence summarized in this review supports the hypothesis that monoamines and other transmitter substances participate in the control of hypophysiotropic hormones from the releasing factor cells in the median eminence of the hypothalamus. These cells can be regarded, as Wurtman (69) has put it, as neuroendocrine transducer cells that differ from neurons as well as from endocrine cells, in that they convert a neuronal input to a humoral output.

Variations in pituitary-adrenal activity and stress, and cyclic changes in pituitary gonadotropin release are associated with variations in neurotransmitter activity in the hypothalamus as determined by alteration in content, turnover, rate of synthesis from labeled precursors, enzyme activity, and histochemical fluorescence. The tubero-infundibular DA system, which is not affected following deafferentation of the hypothalamus, plays an important role in the release of various pituitary hormones. Conclusive evidence has been obtained that this system tonically inhibits the release of prolactin. This may be achieved by a stimulatory influence of DA on PIF, although a direct inhibitory effect of DA on pituitary prolactin release as demonstrated in in vitro studies cannot be excluded. These effects are brought about by amounts that probably never reach the pituitary under physiological conditions (86, 132). In addition, intrapituitary infusion and injection of these amines into the stalk median eminence complex via the local blood supply (70, 121) do not affect the release of prolactin. A number of studies point to a direct effect of L-Dopa on pituitary prolactin, TSH, and GH release, because TRF-induced release of prolactin and TSH in man is blocked by pretreatment with L-Dopa, and this amino acid in rats lowers circulating prolactin and GH from extrapituitary tumors.

The release of gonadotropins according to Fuxe et al (7) is also related to the tubero-infundibular DA neurons because DA turnover may be high when FSH/LH release is low and conversely low when FSH/LH release is high. This could be explained if the release of FSH/LH and prolactin would be inversely related as has been maintained for many years (203). In fact, when the pituitary secretes high amounts of gonadotropins as in ovariectomized animals, perphenazine has a much smaller effect on prolactin release as in intact rats (108). However, evidence has also been presented that NE is the transmitter involved in LH- and FSH release elicited by stimulation of the preoptic area (123), in PMS-induced ovulation in immature rats, and in the negative and positive feedback action of gonadal steroids on gonadotropin release. The issue, however, is not clear, and controversies as to which transmitter is involved exist.

An inhibitory noradrenergic control of ACTH release has been suggested (2), and available data support this hypothesis in acute preparations. In chronic situations a persistent depletion of brain NE as induced by α-MT and 6-OHDA is not associated with a rise in pituitary-adrenal activity and these observations suggest that either NE is not essentially involved in ACTH release or that the hypothalamus under these conditions is not completely devoid of this transmitter. A small active pool may be present (29), and supersensitivity to NE may exist. However, resting pituitary-adrenal activity is chronically increased in rats in which the medial basal hypothalamus is completely deafferented.

In various species, E, NE, and DA affect GH release. Phentolamine is capable of blocking the effect of these amines, suggesting that NE is the transmitter involved. α-Adrenergic blockade in various species has an effect on the release of GH opposite to β-adrenergic blockade. However, DA may also be the transmitter, since GH secretion is maintained in rats with a complete deafferentation of the medial basal hypothalamus (78), and GRF activity is found in the same band as DA in fractionated rat median eminence nerve terminals (171). Conclusions from the different studies on GH release are limited because of the existence of species differences and profound effects of stress and of anesthetics used.

Surprisingly, little is known of the neural input to the neuroendocrine TRF-producing transducer cell whose hormonal output was the first to be identified (3). Data on the neuroendocrine regulation of TSH release are scarce, but should be available soon, because the radioimmunoassay of TSH has come into operation. Studies on TSH release are obscured by a direct TSH-like effect on various amines on the thyroid gland.

Other transmitter systems seem to be involved in the input to the releasing factor cells as well. Atropine can block the diurnal variation in pituitary-adrenal activity and inhibits stress-induced ACTH release when implanted in the anterior hypothalamus but not when administered systemically. In addition, atropine is capable of blocking ovulation and reduces FSH/LH release. Depletion of brain 5-HT also abolishes the diurnal variation in plasma corticosterone (60, 62). Since there appears to be a correlation between the daily variation of 5-HT concentration in the limbic system and that of circulating corticosteroids (60), it is not surprising that circadian variation in pituitary-adrenal activity is disturbed when 5-HT levels in the brain are altered. The same may hold for other transmitters as well. A daily rhythm in anterior and posterior hypothalamic NE has been observed, the concentration being highest at the middle of the dark period (204), and drugs that deplete brain NE disturb the circadian variation in ACTH secretion (21). Depending on the time of the day the experiments were performed, depletion of amine stores, as has been used in many of the studies reported here, may interfere with cyclic phenomena and with pituitary hormone release. 5-HT is involved in other pituitary functions as well. It reduces the feedback action of adrenal steroids on pituitary ACTH release, and systemic administration of 5-HT blocks spontaneous ovulation. However, 5-HT also inhibits ovulation by local vasoconstriction in the ovary (205). Moreover, 5-HT may be a stimulatory transmitter in the release of GH. Thus, the input to the releasing factor cells is complex and of catecholaminergic, cholinergic, and serotonergic character.

Finally, the feedback action of target gland hormones on the release of anterior pituitary hormones may be mediated by brain neurotransmitter activity. Corticosteroid-sensitive neurons in the hypothalamus are inhibited by NE (206). Dexamethasone does not block the increased NE turnover following immobilization stress (12), but the corticosteroid negative feedback action on pituitary ACTH release is potentiated by MAO inhibition and reduced by pCPA (39). Testosterone in amounts that reduce LH release during the critical period increases DA turnover in the tuberoinfundibular DA system (129, 130), and estradiol blocks LH release as induced by intraventricular DA (122). pCPA can substitute for progesterone in copulatory behavior (69), and progesterone is as effective as pCPA in reversing the antiovulatory effect of MAO inhibitors (82). These are interesting observations that need additional experiments to explore the interaction of target gland and pituitary hormones with neurotransmitter activity in the hypothalamus.

ACKNOWLEDGMENTS

The authors wish to thank Miss Tine Baas and Mrs. Linda Philbert for typing the manuscript and assembling the references.

Literature Cited

1. Blackwell, R. E., Guillemin, R. 1973. *Ann. Rev. Physiol.* 35:357–90
2. Ganong, W. F. 1973. *The Neurosciences, Third Study Program,* ed. B. H. Ankeny. Cambridge: MIT Press
3. Schally, A. V., Arimura, A., Kastin, A. J. 1973. *Science* 179:341–50
4. Motta, M., Piva, F., Martini, L. 1970. *The Hypothalamus,* ed. L. Martini, M. Motta, F. Fraschini, 463–89. New York: Academic. 705 pp.
5. Motta, M., Fraschini, F., Martini, L. 1969. *Frontiers in Neuroendocrinology,* ed. W. F. Ganong, L. Martini, 211–53. New York: Oxford Univ. Press. 442 pp.
6. Ungerstedt, U. 1971. *Acta Physiol. Scand. Suppl.* 367:1–48
7. Fuxe, K., Hökfelt, T., Jonsson, G., Löfström, A. 1973. *Proc. Int. Catecholamine Symp., 3rd, 1973*
8. Fuxe, K., Hökfelt, T. See Ref. 4, 123–38
9. Hökfelt, T., Fuxe, K. 1972. *Brain-Endocrine Interaction: Structure and Function,* ed. K. M. Knigge, D. E. Scott, A. Weindl, 181–223. Basel: Karger. 368 pp.
10. Shute, C. C. D. See Ref. 4, 167–79
11. Javoy, F., Glowinski, J., Kordon, C. 1968. *Eur. J. Pharmacol.* 4:103–4
12. Fuxe, K., Corrodi, H., Hökfelt, T., Jonsson, G. 1970. *Progr. Brain Res.* 32: 42–56
13. Parvez, H., Parvez, S. 1973. *J. Neurochem.* 20:1011–20
14. Versteeg, D. H. G. 1973. *Brain Res.* 49:483–85
15. Corrodi, H., Fuxe, K., Hökfelt, T. 1968. *Life Sci. P. I.* 7:107–12
16. Gordon, R., Spector, S., Sjoerdsma, A., Udenfriend, S. 1966. *J. Pharmacol. Exp. Ther.* 153:440–47
17. Bliss, E. L., Ailion, J., Zwanziger, J. 1968. *J. Pharmacol. Exp. Ther.* 164: 122–34
18. Thierry, A. -M., Javoy, F., Glowinski, J., Kety, S. S. 1968. *J. Pharmacol. Exp. Ther.* 163:163–71
19. Stoner, H. B., Elson, P. M. 1971. *J. Neurochem.* 18:1837–46
20. Tullner, W. W., Hertz, R. 1964. *Proc. Soc. Exp. Biol. Med.* 116:837–40
21. Ganong, W. F. See Ref. 9, 254–66
22. Lorenzen, L. C., Ganong, W. F. 1967. *Endocrinology* 80:889–92
23. Van Loon, G. R., Hilger, L., King, A. B., Boryczka, A. T., Ganong, W. F. 1971. *Endocrinology* 88:1404–14
24. Van Loon, G. R., Scapagnini, U., Cohen, R., Ganong, W. F. 1971. *Neuroendocrinology* 8:257–72
25. Scapagnini, U., Preziosi, P. 1973. *Progr. Brain Res.* 39:172–84
26. Van Loon, G. R., Scapagnini, U., Moberg, G. P., Ganong, W. F. 1971. *Endocrinology* 89:1464–69
27. Kaplanski, J., Dorst, W., Smelik, P. G. 1972. *Eur. J. Pharmacol.* 20:238–40
28. Schanker, L. S., Morrison, A. S. 1965. *Int. J. Neuropharmacol.* 4:27–39
29. Scapagnini, U. See Ref. 2
30. Kaplanski, J., Smelik, P. G. 1973. *Res. Comm. Chem. Pathol. Pharmacol.* 5: 263–71
31. Ulrich, R. S., Yuwiler, A. 1973. *Endocrinology* 92:611–14
32. Halász, B. See Ref. 5, 307–42
33. Lau, C., Timiras, P. S. 1972. *Am. J. Physiol.* 222:1040–42
34. Weiner, R. I. 1973. *Progr. Brain Res.* 39:166–70
35. Govier, W. C., Lovenberg, W., Sjoerdsma, A. 1969. *Biochem. Pharmacol.* 18:2661–66
36. Bhattacharya, A. N., Marks, B. H. 1969. *Proc. Soc. Exp. Biol. Med.* 130: 1194–98
37. De Schaepdryver, A., Preziosi, P., Scapagnini, U. 1969. *Brit. J. Pharmacol.* 35:460–67
38. Dallman, M. F., Yates, F. E. 1967. *Memoirs of the Society for Endocrinology 17,* ed. V. H. T. James, J. Landon, 39–72. Cambridge: Cambridge Univ. Press. 311 pp.
39. Vernikos-Danellis, J., Berger, P., Barchas, J. D. 1973. *Progr. Brain Res.* 39: 301–10
40. Nicolescu-Catargi, A., Cristoveanu, A., Stan, M., Berceanu, A. 1970. *Abstr. Int. Congr. Hormonal Steroids, 3rd.* 210: 201–2. Amsterdam: Excerpta Med. Found. 248 pp.
41. Carr, L. A., Moore K. E. 1968. *Neuroendocrinology* 3:285–302
42. Preziosi, P., Scapagnini, U., Nisticó, G. 1968. *Biochem. Pharmacol.* 17: 1309–13
43. Krieger, D. T. 1973. *J. Clin. Endocrinol. Metab.* 36:277–84
44. Boyd, A. E. III, Lebovitz, H. E., Feldman, J. M. 1971. *J. Clin. Endocr. Metab.* 33:829–37
45. Boden, G., Lundy, L. E., Owen, O. E. 1972. *Neuroendocrinology* 10:309–15
46. Hayek, A., Crawford, J. D. 1972. *J. Clin. Endocr. Metab.* 34:764–66
47. Bhattacharya, A. N., Marks, B. H. 1969. *J. Pharmacol. Exp. Ther.* 165: 108–16

48. Marks, B. H., Hall, M. M., Bhatta-charya, A. N. 1970. *Progr. Brain Res.* 32:57–70
49. Smelik, P. G. 1967. *Neuroendocrinology* 2:247–54
50. Green, A. R., Curzon, G. 1968. *Nature* 220:1095–97
51. Thierry, A. -M., Fekete, M., Glowinski, J. 1968. *Eur. J. Pharmacol.* 4:384–89
52. Barchas, J. D. et al 1972. *Hormones and Behavior,* ed. S. Levine, 235–329. New York: Academic. 363 pp.
53. Dixit, B. N., Buckley, J. P. 1969. *Neuroendocrinology* 4:32–41
54. McKennee, C. T., Timiras, P. S., Quay, W. B. 1966. *Neuroendocrinology* 1: 251–56
55. Azmitia, E. C. Jr., McEwen, B. S. 1969. *Science* 166:1274–76
56. Millard, S. A., Costa, E., Gal, E. M. 1972. *Brain Res.* 40:545–51
57. Naumenko, E. V. 1968. *Brain Res.* 11: 1–10
58. Krieger, H. P., Krieger, D. T. 1970. *Am. J. Physiol.* 218:1632–41
59. Popova, N. K., Maslova, L. N., Naumenko, E. V. 1972. *Brain Res.* 47:61–67
60. Scapagnini, U., Moberg, G. P., Van Loon, G. R., De Groot, J., Ganong, W. F. 1971. *Neuroendocrinology* 7:90–96
61. Van Delft, A. M. L., Kaplanski, J., Smelik, P. G. 1973. *J. Endocrinol.* In press
62. Krieger, D. T., Rizzo, F. 1969. *Am. J. Physiol.* 217:1703–7
63. Fuxe, K., Hökfelt, T., Ungerstedt, U. 1968. *Advan. Pharmacol.* 6A:235–51
64. De Wied, D., Witter, A., Versteeg, D. H. G., Mulder, A. H. 1969. *Endocrinology* 85:561–69
65. Hedge, G. A., Smelik, P. G. 1968. *Science* 159:891–92
66. Hedge, G. A., De Wied, D. 1971. *Endocrinology* 88:1257–59
67. Guillemin, R. 1955. *Endocrinology* 56: 248–55
68. Krieger, D. T., Silverberg, A. I., Rizzo, F., Krieger, H. P. 1968. *Am. J. Physiol.* 215:959–67
69. Wurtman, R. J. 1971. *Neurosci. Res. Program Bull.* 9: No. 2
70. Kamberi, I. A. 1973. *Progr. Brain Res.* 39:261–80
71. Lichtensteiger, W., Korpela, K., Langemann, H., Keller, P. 1969. *Brain Res.* 16:199–214
72. Lichtensteiger, W. 1969. *J. Pharmacol. Exp. Ther.* 165:204–15
73. Anton-Tay, F., Anton, S. M., Wurtman, R. J. 1970. *Neuroendocrinology* 6:265–73
74. Bapna, J., Neff, N. H., Costa, E. 1971. *Endocrinology* 89:1345–49
75. Wurtman, R. J. 1973. *Proc. Int. Catecholamine Symp., 3rd, 1973*
76. Ahrén, K., Fuxe, K., Hamberger, L., Hökfelt, T. 1971. *Endocrinology* 88: 1415–24
77. Weiner, R. I., Shryne, J. E., Gorski, R. A., Sawyer, C. H. 1972. *Endocrinology* 90:867–73
78. Halász, B. 1972. *Progr. Brain Res.* 38: 97–122
79. Blake, C. A., Weiner, R. I., Gorski, R. A., Sawyer, C. H. 1972. *Endocrinology* 90:855–61
80. Blake, C. A., Weiner, R. I., Sawyer, C. H. 1972. *Endocrinology* 90:862–66
81. Donoso, A. O., Bishop, W., Fawcett, C. P., Krulich, L., McCann, S. M. 1971. *Endocrinology* 89:774–84
82. Kordon, C., Glowinski, J. 1972. *Neuropharmacology* 11:153–62
83. Van Maanen, J. H., Smelik, P. G. 1968. *Neuroendocrinology* 3:177–86
84. Birge, C. A., Jacobs, L. S., Hammer, C. T., Daughaday, W. H. 1970. *Endocrinology* 86:120–30
85. MacLeod, R. M., Fontham, E. H., Lehmeyer, J. E. 1970. *Neuroendocrinology* 6:283–94
86. Coppola, J. A. 1968. *J. Reprod. Fert. Suppl.* 4:35–45
87. Koch, Y., Lu, K.-H., Meites, J. 1970. *Endocrinology* 87:673–75
88. Nicoll, C. S. 1971. *Frontiers in Neuroendocrinology,* ed. L. Martini, W. F. Ganong, 291–330. New York: Oxford Univ. Press. 419 pp.
89. Cramer, O. M., Porter, J. C. 1973. *Progr. Brain Res.* 39:74–85
90. Gala, R. R., Janson, P. A., Kuo, E. Y. 1972. *Proc. Soc. Exp. Biol. Med.* 140: 569–72
91. Quadri, S. K., Knecht, E., Meites, J. 1973. *Fed. Proc.* 32:307 (Abstr.)
92. Euker, J. S., Shaar, C. J., Riegle, G. D. 1973. *Fed. Proc.* 32:307 (Abstr.)
93. Lu, K.-H., Meites, J. 1972. *Endocrinology* 91:868–72
94. Bowers, C. Y., Friesen, H. G., Hwang, P., Guyda, H. J., Folkers, K. 1971. *Biochem. Biophys. Res. Commun.* 45: 1033–41
95. Jacobs, L. S., Snyder, P. J., Wilber, J. F., Utiger, R. D., Daughaday, W. H. 1971. *J. Clin. Endocr. Metab.* 33: 996–98
96. Frantz, A. G. 1973. *Progr. Brain Res.* 39:311–22
97. Turkington, R. W. 1972. *J. Clin. Endocr. Metab.* 34:306–11

98. Floss, H. G., Cassady, J. M., Robbers, J. E. 1973. *J. Pharm. Sci.* 62:699–715
99. Wuttke, W., Cassell, E., Meites, J. 1971. *Endocrinology* 88:737–41
100. Quadri, S. K., Meites, J. 1973. *Proc. Soc. Exp. Biol. Med.* 142:837–41
101. Shaar, C. J., Clemens, J. A. 1972. *Endocrinology* 90:285–88
102. Welsch, C. W., Squiers, M. D., Cassell, E., Chen, C. L., Meites, J. 1971. *Am. J. Physiol.* 221:1714–17
103. del Pozo, E., Brun del Re, R., Varga, L., Friesen, H. 1972. *J. Clin. Endocrinol. Metab.* 35:768–71
104. Tolis, G., del Pozo, E., Goldstein, M. S. 1973. *Endocrinology Suppl.* 92:A–50
105. Sulman, F. G. 1970. *Hypothalamic Control of Lactation,* ed. F. G. Sulman, 1–235. Berlin: Springer-Verlag. 235 pp.
106. Lu, K.-H., Amenomori, Y., Chen, C.-L., Meites, J. 1970. *Endocrinology* 87:667–72
107. Van der Gugten, A. A., Verhofstad, F., Sala, M., Kwa, H. G. 1970. *Acta Endocrinol. Copenhagen* 65:309–15
108. Ben-David, M., Danon, A., Sulman, F. G. 1971. *J. Endocrinol.* 51:719–25
109. Blackwell, R., Vale, W., River, C., Guillemin, R. 1973. *Proc. Soc. Exp. Biol. Med.* 142:68–71
110. Janssen, P. A. J. 1967. *Int. J. Neuropsych.* 3:Suppl. 1,10–18
111. Dickerman, S., Clark, J., Dickerman, E., Meites, J. 1972. *Neuroendocrinology* 9:332–40
112. MacLeod, R. M., Lehmeyer, J. E. 1973. *Fed. Proc.* 32:307 (Abstr.)
113. Ernst, A. M. 1967. *Psychopharmacologia* 10:316–23
114. MacLeod, R. M., Lehmeyer, J. E. 1973. *Endocrinology Suppl.* 92:A–50
115. De Wied, D. 1967. *Pharmacol. Rev.* 19:251–88
116. Kleinberg, D. L., Noel, G. L., Frantz, A. G. 1971. *J. Clin. Endocrinol. Metab.* 33:873–76
117. Smalstig, E. B., Sawyer, B. D., Roush, M. E., Clemens, J. A. 1973. *Fed. Proc.* 32:308 (Abstr.)
118. Kordon, C. 1973. In *Excerpta Med. Found. Int. Congr. Ser. n 273,* 120–24
119. Libertun, C. 1973. *Endocrinology Suppl.* 92:A–240
120. Schneider, H. P. G., McCann, S. M. 1969. *Endocrinology* 85:121–32
121. Kamberi, I. A., Mical, R. S., Porter, J. C. 1970. *Endocrinology* 87:1–12
122. McCann, S. M. 1971. *Neurosci. Res. Program Bull.* 9 (2):218–26
123. Kalra, P. S., McCann, S. M. 1973. *Progr. Brain Res.* 39:185–98
124. McCann, S. M. et al. See Ref. 9, 224–35

125. Rubinstein, L., Sawyer, C. H. 1970. *Endocrinology* 86:988–95
126. Kitchen, J. H., Ruf, K. B., Younglai, E. V. 1973. *Endocrinology Suppl.* 92:A–234
127. Coppola, J. A. See Ref. 88, 129–43
128. Thierry, A. M., Blanc, G., Glowinski, J. 1971. *Eur. J. Pharmacol.* 14:303–7
129. Klawon, D. L., Sorrentino, S. Jr., Schalch, D. S. 1971. *Endocrinology* 88:1131–35
130. Fuxe, K., Hökfelt, T., Sundstedt, C.-D., Ahrén, K., Hamberger, L. 1972. *Neuroendocrinology* 10:282–300
131. Uemura, H., Kobayashi, H. 1971. *Endocrinol. Jap.* 18:91–100
132. Schwartz, N. B., McCormack, C. E. 1972. *Ann. Rev. Physiol.* 34:425–74
133. Sinhamahapatra, S. B., Kirschner, M. A. 1972. *J. Clin. Endocrinol. Metab.* 34:756–58
134. Donoso, A. O., Santolaya, R. C. 1969. *Experientia* 25:855–57
135. Ojeda, S., McCann, S. M. 1973. *Fed. Proc.* 32:227 (Abstr.)
136. Barraclough, C. A., Sawyer, C. H. 1957. *Endocrinology* 61:341–51
137. Meyerson, B. J., Sawyer, C. H. 1968. *Endocrinology* 83:170–76
138. Coppola, J. A., Leonardi, R. G., Lippman, W. 1966. *Endocrinology* 78:225–28
139. France, E. S. 1970. *Neuroendocrinology* 6:77–89
140. Brown, P. S. 1971. *Neuroendocrinology* 7:183–92
141. Bliss, E. L., Frischat, A., Samuels, L. 1972. *Life Sci.* 11:Pt. I, 231–38
142. Vaughan, M. K., Benson, B., Norris, J. T., Vaughan, G. M. 1971. *J. Endocrinol.* 50:171–75
143. Collu, R., Fraschini, F., Martini, L. 1971. *J. Endocrinol.* 50:679–83
144. Labhsetwar, A. P. 1971. *Acta Endocrinol.* 68:334–44
145. Labhsetwar, A. P. 1972. *J. Endocrinol.* 54:269–75
146. Kato, J., Minaguchi, H. 1964. *Neurosecretion and Neural Control of Internal Secretion,* ed. K. Kurosumi, 269–81. Maebashi, Japan: Gunma Univ. Press. 357 pp.
147. Everett, J. W., Sawyer, C. H., Markee, J. E. 1949. *Endocrinology* 44:234–50
148. Kamberi, I. A., Bacleon, E. S. 1973. *Fed. Proc.* 32:240 (Abstr.)
149. Kamberi, I. A., Bacleon, E. S. 1973. *Endocrinology Suppl.* 92:A–136
150. Marks, B. H. 1973. *Progr. Brain Res.* 39:331–38

151. Blake, C. A., Scaramuzzi, R. J., Norman, R. L., Kanematsu, S., Sawyer, C. H. 1972. *Endocrinology* 91:1253–58
152. Glick, S. M. 1968. *Ann. NY Acad. Sci.* 148:471–87
153. Knobil, E., Meyer, V. 1968. *Ann. NY Acad. Sci.* 148:459–70
154. Schalch, D. S., Reichlin, S. 1968. *Growth Hormone*, ed. A. Pecile, E. Müller, 211–25. Amsterdam: Excerpta Med. Found. 455 pp.
155. Takahashi, K., Daughaday, W. H., Kipnis, D. M. 1971. *Endocrinology* 88:909–17
156. Meyer, V., Knobil, E. 1967. *Endocrinology* 80:163–71
157. Toivola, P. T. K., Gale, C. C. 1970. *Neuroendocrinology* 6:210–19
158. Toivola, P. T. K., Gale, C. C. 1973. *Fed. Proc.* 32:265 (Abstr.)
159. Werrbach, J. H., Gale, C. C., Goodner, C. J., Conway, M. J. 1970. *Endocrinology* 86:77–82
160. Brown, G. M., Chambers, J. W., Feldmann, J. 1973. *Endocrinology Suppl.* 92:A–201
161. Wallace, A. L. C., Bassett, J. M. 1970. *J. Endocrinol.* 47:21–36
162. Hertelendy, F., Machlin, L., Kipnis, D. M. 1969. *Endocrinology* 84:192–99
163. Davis, S. L., Borger, M. L. 1973. *Endocrinology* 92:303–9
164. Müller, E. E., Saito, T., Arimura, A., Schally, A. V. 1967. *Endocrinology* 80:109–17
165. Müller, E. E., Sawano, S., Arimura, A., Schally, A. V. 1967. *Endocrinology* 80:471–76
166. Müller, E. E., Pecile, A., Felici, M., Cocchi, D. 1970. *Endocrinology* 86:1376–82
167. Müller, E. E., Dal Pra, P., Pecile, A. 1968. *Endocrinology* 83:893–96
168. Malarkey, W. B., Daughaday, W. H. 1972. *Endocrinology* 91:1314–17
169. Collu, R., Fraschini, F., Martini, L. 1973. *Progr. Brain Res.* 39:289–99
170. Collu, R., Fraschini, F., Visconti, P., Martini, L. 1972. *Endocrinology* 90:1231–37
171. Clementi, F. et al 1970. *J. Endocrinol.* 48:205–13
172. Müller, E. E., Cocchi, D., Jalanbo, H., Udeschini, G. 1973. *Endocrinology Suppl.* 92:A–248
173. Collu, R., Jéquier, J.-C., Letarte, J., Leboeuf, G., Ducharme, J. R. 1973. *Neuroendocrinology* 11:183–90
174. Podolsky, S., Leopold, N. A. 1973. *Progr. Brain Res.* 39:225–35

175. Kansal, P. C., Buse, J., Talbert, O. R., Buse, M. G. 1972. *J. Clin. Endocrinol. Metab.* 34:99–105
176. Boyd, A. E. III, Lebovitz, H. E., Pfeiffer, J. B. 1970. *N. Engl. J. Med.* 283:1425–29
177. Eddy, R. L., Jones, A. L., Chakmakjian, Z. H., Silverthorne, M. C. 1971. *J. Clin. Endocrinol. Metab.* 33:709–12
178. Massara, F., Camanni, F. 1972. *J. Endocrinol.* 54:195–206
179. Sachar, E. J. 1972. *Science* 178:1304–5
180. Liuzzi, A., Chiodine, P. G., Botalla, L., Cremascoli, G., Silvestrini, F. 1972. *J. Clin. Endocrinol. Metab.* 35:941–43
181. Cavagnini, F. et al 1972. *J. Endocrinol.* 54:425–33
182. Parra, A., Schultz, R. B., Foley, T. P. Jr., Blizzard, R. M. 1970. *J. Clin. Endocrinol. Metab.* 30:134–37
183. Hansen, A. P. 1971. *J. Clin. Endocrinol. Metab.* 33:807–12
184. Mitchell, M. L., Suvunrungsi, P., Sawin, C. T. 1971. *J. Clin. Endocrinol Metab.* 32:470–75
185. Ganong, W. F. 1972. *Progr. Brain Res.* 38:41–57
186. Martini, L. 1956. *Sui rapporti tra ipofisi e tiroide; l'ormone tireotropico.* Milano: Ganassini. 223 pp.
187. Greer, M. A., Yamada, T., Lino, S. 1960. *Ann. NY Acad. Sci.* 86:667–75
188. Wilber, J. F., Peake, G. T., Utiger, R. D. 1969. *Endocrinology* 84:758–60
189. Melander, A., Sundler, F. 1972. *Endocrinology* 90:188–93
190. Melander, A., Nilsson, E., Sundler, F. 1972. *Endocrinology* 90:194–99
191. Melander, A. 1971. *Acta Endocrinol.* 66:151–61
192. Tal, E., Biran, S., Sulman, F. G. 1972. *J. Endocrinol.* 53:503–4
193. Coleoni, A. H. 1972. *Pharmacology* 8:300–10
194. Kotani, M., Onaya, T., Yamada, T. 1973. *Endocrinology* 92:288–94
195. Onaya, T., Solomon, D. H., Davidson, W. D. 1969. *Endocrinology* 85:150–54
196. Reichlin, S. et al 1972. *Rec. Progr. Horm. Res.* 28:229–86
197. Shenkman, L. et al 1973. *Endocrinology Suppl.* 92:A–138
198. Hays, M. T., Solomon, D. H. 1969. *J. Clin. Invest.* 48:1114–23
199. Ericson, L. E., Melander, A., Owman, Ch., Sundler, F. 1970. *Endocrinology Suppl.* 92:A–138

200. Spaulding, S. W., Burrow, G. N. Donabedian, R., Van Woert, M. 1972. *J. Clin. Endocrinol. Metab.* 35:182–85
201. Woolf, P. D., Lee, L. A., Schalch, D. S. 1972. *J. Clin. Endocrinol. Metab.* 35:616–18
202. Fisher, D. A., Odell, W. D. 1971. *J. Clin. Endocrinol. Metab.* 33:859–62

203. Sawyer, C. H., Haun, C. K., Hilliard, J., Radford, H. M., Kanematsu, S. 1963. *Endocrinology* 73:338–44
204. Manshardt, J., Wurtman, R. J. 1968. *Nature* 217:574–75
205. Wilson, C., McDonald, P. G. 1973. *Acta Endocr. Suppl.* 177:138
206. Steiner, F. A., Ruf, K., Akert, K. 1969. *Brain Res.* 12:74–85

THE PHARMACOLOGY OF CONTRACEPTIVE AGENTS

❖6601

W. D. Odell and M. E. Molitch

Division of Endocrinology, Department of Medicine, Harbor General Hospital, UCLA School of Medicine, Torrance, California

INTRODUCTION

The number of publications on contraceptive and antifertility agents is increasing every year. We have attempted here to review some aspects of the pharmacology and physiology of the agents administered to women. We have avoided discussing minor modifications in dosage or techniques of administration, but instead have concentrated on classes of compounds and selected examples for illustration. We have eliminated discussion of prostaglandins used for abortion and the recent studies of testosterone or androgen treatment of males; the latter has had no clinical trials of contraceptive effectiveness or acceptance. We apologize for these large omissions and our selective view; our task was large and our space limited.

HORMONAL EVENTS DURING THE NORMAL MENSTRUAL CYCLE

A discussion of the mechanism of actions of contraceptive steroids administered to women is most easily understood in context of the physiology of the normal menstrual cycle. Figure 1 depicts the hormonal events occurring during a typical menstrual cycle. These events are centered around ovulation, which is arbitrarily drawn in this figure to occur on day 14 (day 1 is defined as the first day of menstrual flow). In the mature ovary, the primary follicle consists of an oogonium surrounded by a single layer of granulosa cells. Presumably, under the influence of follicle stimulating hormone (FSH), 10 to 15 of these primary follicles undergo development into secondary follicles; the granulosa cells proliferate to several layers thick and the oogonium increases in size during the first few days of the cycle. Through poorly understood local (ovarian) mechanisms, all but one of these secondary follicles undergo atresia and one (normally) is selected for further development. The granulosa cells of the selected follicle continue mitotic division under FSH stimulation, and fluid accumulates between the cells. At the preovulatory stage the follicle is large, and the ovum, called a secondary oocyte at this development stage, projects

413

into the large fluid-filled antral cavity (1). As this sequence of follicle growth occurs, estradiol concentrations increase in blood, reaching a maximum just prior to the LH-FSH surge (LH = luteinizing hormone). These changes in blood estradiol appear to be predominantly related to changing numbers of granulosa cells.

For a number of years after the development of the competitive binding assay for progesterone, using cortisol binding globulin (CBG) as a binding protein, it was believed that progesterone was secreted in low or undetectable and unchanging concentrations during the follicular phase of the cycle (2–4). CBG has a relatively low affinity for progesterone, and assays using CBG as the binding protein have inadequate sensitivity to quantify progesterone in the concentrations existing during the follicular phase. Many assumed that progesterone could not play any role in control of the process of ovulation. However, studies from our laboratory (5, 6) using more sensitive radioimmunoassays have revealed that progesterone concentrations fall during the first half of the follicular phase and rise again just prior to ovulation as shown in Figure 1. Once the preovulatory follicle has developed and these estradiol and progesterone changes have occurred, a surge of LH and FSH (ovulatory surge) can be detected, followed by ovulation and transformation of the follicle into the corpus luteum. During corpus luteum function, estradiol, progesterone, and other steroids are secreted in large amounts, and blood FSH and LH fall to low concentrations, lower than are observed during the follicular phase (7, 8).

Several facts have led to the conclusion [Odell & Swerdloff 1968 (9)] that timing of ovulation in women is related to an ovarian signal system and is not caused by an inherent central nervous system rhythmicity: (a) During carefully studied normal menstrual cycles one does not observe aberrantly timed LH-FSH ovulatory surges (ovulatory LH-FSH surges only occur when a preovulatory follicle is mature); (b) during estrogen suppression of castrated or postmenopausal women under defined conditions, rhythmic discharges of LH-FSH are not observed; (c) if one were to design a control system for ovulation, the ovarian signal-activated model would be the most efficient indicator, when a mature follicle is developed. To test this postulate, considering ovarian steroids to be the most likely hormonal signals, Odell & Swerdloff (9) administered sequential estrogens and progestogens to castrate and postmenopausal women. The estrogens suppressed elevated FSH and LH concentrations and maintained them at a low level until the progestogen was added. At this time an LH-FSH surge mimicking the ovulatory surge occurred. Subsequent studies by Yen (10) in postmenopausal women and by Weick et al in castrate monkeys (11) have shown that estrogens alone can induce ovulatory LH surges. Schwartz (12) has summarized evidence to indicate that the prime signal in rodents is related to changing estrogen concentrations. Ferin et al (13) have shown that antisera to estradiol, administered just prior to ovulation, blocked the ovulatory LH surge; antisera to progesterone did not block this surge. A review of all animal and human data is consistent with the concept that the changing estrogen concentration is the prime ovarian signal. Thus estrogens may act in two distinct ways upon the central nervous system: 1. in negative feedback to suppress LH and FSH secretion, and 2. in "positive feedback" to stimulate LH secretion. Whether the negative or the positive action is expressed appears to be dependent on change and dose of estrogen and the presence or absence of other hormones such as progestogens.

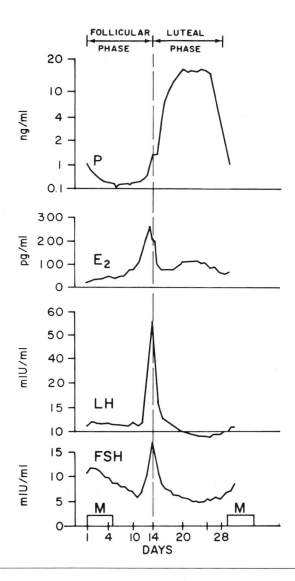

Figure 1 Schematized depiction of the fluctuations in progesterone (P), estradiol (E_2), luteinizing hormone (LH), and follicle stimulating hormone (FSH) during the normal menstrual cycle. Note that P in ng/ml (10^{-9} g/ml) is plotted on a log scale in order to show the small, but significant changes. Other abbreviations include pg/ml = picograms/ml (10^{-12} g/ml), mIU/ml = milliinternational units in terms of International Reference Preparation #2 of human menopausal gonadotropin. These data were modified from Abraham, Odell, Swerdloff & Hopper 1972 (6).

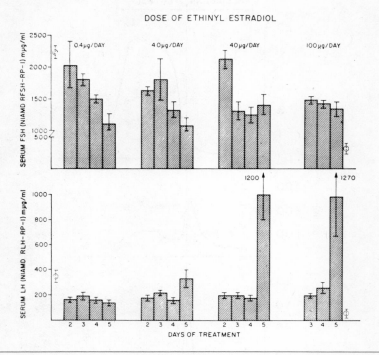

Figure 2a Serum FSH *(above)* and LH *(below)* in castrate female rats treated daily with ethinyl estradiol (EE) at various doses between 0.4 and 100 μg/day. LH and FSH fell with all doses of EE, but at the highest doses of EE a biphasic response in LH, but not FSH was noted.

C = castrate control, I = intact control. Reproduced from Swerdloff, Jacobs & Odell 1972 (14).

Swerdloff, Jacobs & Odell (14), performing studies in rodents, have assisted in clarifying the interplay of estrogens and progestogens. When ethinyl estradiol alone was administered in large doses (100 μg or 40 μg/day) to oophorectomized rats, the elevated LH concentrations fell progressively for 4 days until day 5 when a sharp surge in LH, but not FSH, occurred. This large dose of estradiol produced both negative and positive feedback. However, positive feedback was observed only for LH; no coincident FSH surge occurred. When lower doses of estradiol (4 μg or 0.4 μg/day) were administered, LH concentrations were suppressed, but no LH surge occurred on day 5 or any other day. Thus, under these conditions only negative feedback occurred. If, however, a single injection of progesterone or 20-hydroxy-pregnen-3-one[1] were given on day 5 in addition to the low dose of estradiol, a sharp

[1]This steroid is secreted in relatively large amounts by the rat. It does not appear to be of major importance in women. Conversely, 17-hydroxyprogesterone is secreted in large amounts in women, but did not increase LH or FSH in the studies in rats. Thus, different progestogens may be active in different species.

surge of LH and FSH occurred which exactly mimicked the ovulatory LH-FSH ovulatory surge in height and duration. These studies are illustrated in Figures 2a and 2b. One may thus hypothesize that estrogen secreted by the developing granulosal cells during the normal cycle is the prime ovarian signal determining the time of and triggering the LH ovulatory surge. Progesterone (or possibly other progestogens) appears to act as a fail-safe mechanism, lowering the threshold for estrogen stimulation of LH release. Progesterone (or another progestogen) appears to be necessary for the FSH surge that accompanies the LH ovulatory surge under normal circumstances.

Finally, the synergistic suppressive action of progestogens is important. Numerous studies show that estrogens alone in large doses suppress both FSH and LH but do not suppress them to undetectable concentrations (7–10). When FSH and LH are suppressed by estrogens to a maximal degree, the addition of large doses of a progestogen (if positive feedback does not occur) suppresses gonadotropins further. This phenomenon is observed during the normal menstrual cycle after the ovulatory surge; FSH and LH are lower during luteal phase than during follicular phase (4, 7, 8). FSH and LH concentrations rise toward the end of the luteal phase as estradiol and progesterone concentrations fall with functional corpus luteum death.

Therefore, like estrogens, progesterone (and in various species possibly other progestogens) acts in a complex way, both stimulating and inhibiting LH and FSH

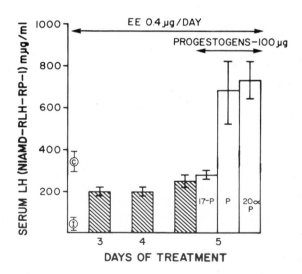

Figure 2b Serum LH after EE 0.4 μg/day plus either 17 ∝ hydroxyprogesterone (17 ∝ P), progesterone (P) or 20∝hydroxypregnen-3-one (20∝P). When a single dose of either P or 20∝P was added to the 0.4 μg of EE on morning of day #5, a surge of LH was observed; serum FSH was also increased.

From Swerdloff, Jacobs & Odell (14).

release. Sawyer & Everett (15) in 1959 first demonstrated this fact in rabbits. Because LH and FSH radioimmunoassays were not available, they used ovulation as an endpoint and demonstrated that ovulation in estrogen-primed rabbits was at first stimulated by progesterone and then inhibited. The explanation for this biphasic action of both progestogens and estrogens is unclear, but functionally it appears that once the positive stimulation or release of LH-FSH has occurred, then inhibition or negative feedback occurs and persists unless progestogens fall to low concentrations (or are discontinued).

In addition to their action as signals for the reproductive system, estrogens and progestogens of course have important other actions. Among their other effects are actions on the endometrium, cervix, and vagina in very specific ways to prepare for conception. Sperm entry through the cervical os is greatly affected by cervical mucous structure which is in turn modified by hormonal means (16). Once the sperm have entered the uterine cavity, migration to the fallopian tubes, the site of fertilization, is in major part hormonally controlled. After fertilization has occurred, the timing, migration of the fertilized ovum into the uterus, and implantation all require the orderly action of estrogens and progestogens. Contraceptive compounds, in addition to modifying the hormonal control of ovarian function, also may act on these later stages of fertility (i.e. sperm entry and postconception events up to and including implantation) (1).

CONTRACEPTIVE DRUGS FOR WOMEN

The contraceptive drugs in clinical use for women are all either combinations of or singly administered estrogens and/or progestogens. The estrogens used are usually potent synthetics, mestranol or some derivative of ethinyl estradiol. The progestogens are usually 19-nortestosterone or 17-hydroxyprogesterone derivatives. Most of the 19-nortestosterones (methyl group of carbon-19 absent) have androgenic effects in addition to their potent progestational effects. Figure 3 gives the structures of these families of steroids.

Combination Estrogen-Progestogen Contraceptives

The best understood contraceptives are the combined estrogen-progestogen preparations. These are generally administered daily for 20 days, then stopped for 5 days during which withdrawal bleeding occurs. Preparations that contain sufficiently large amounts of estrogens and progestogens act in continued negative feedback to suppress LH and FSH concentrations (7, 8, 17, 18) to normal luteal phase values. No LH-FSH ovulatory surge occurs to cause ovulation; no follicular phase rise in FSH exists to initiate follicle development. As a result of suppressed LH and FSH concentrations and the inhibition of follicle development, endogenous estradiol concentrations in blood also remain low (19). The early studies of Rock et al (20) and Garcia & Pincus (21), by directly observing the ovaries of women receiving these preparations, demonstrated that corpora lutea were absent and that developed

3A PHYSIOLOGIC HORMONES

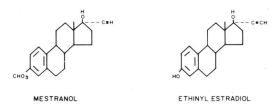

| ESTRADIOL-17β | PROGESTERONE | TESTOSTERONE |

3B ESTROGENS

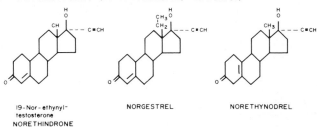

MESTRANOL   ETHINYL ESTRADIOL

3C PROGESTOGENS (19 Nortestosterone derivatives)

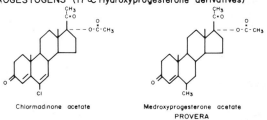

| 19-Nor-ethynyl-
testosterone
NORETHINDRONE | NORGESTREL | NORETHYNODREL |

3D PROGESTOGENS (17α Hydroxyprogesterone derivatives)

Chlormadinone acetate   Medroxyprogesterone acetate
PROVERA

Figure 3 Structures of some steroids involved in the normal menstrual cycle and used as contraceptive agents.

follicles were rare. In long term treatment the ovaries were reduced in size and presented an atrophic picture. In addition to exerting negative feedback, the contraceptive steroids act directly on the endometrium during the time of administration. When they are discontinued for 5 day periods, withdrawal bleeding occurs. Interestingly, during this 5 day withdrawal period, LH and FSH concentrations remain low when high dose estrogen-progestogen preparations are used. The mechanisms for this prolonged suppression are uncertain but could be sustained release of the steroids from fat stores, prolonged presence of steroids on hypothalamic or pituitary receptors even after blood concentrations fall, or prolonged changes in neuronal or pituitary cellular activity. When taken regularly, this form of contraceptive appears to be 100% effective. Adverse side effects are related to the estrogen component and, as discussed later, may be related to dosage. The original combined contraceptives contained relatively large doses of synthetic estrogens. In an attempt to reduce side effects, more recent forms containing less estrogens have been developed. Preston (22) reported a collaborative study of various oral contraceptive formulations containing 20, 40, and 60% reductions in both estrogen and progestogen components of combination contraceptives. Pregnancy rates were no different from the higher dose formulation. However, bleeding patterns showed alterations characterized by irregular bleeding episodes and occasional absence of withdrawal bleeding. Side effects reported such as headaches, nausea or vomiting, or weight gain were low. The lowest dose studied consisted of a combination of 20 μg of ethinyl estradiol and 1.0 mg norethindrone. The mechanism of action of these low dose combinations may be different and has not yet been studied in detail. (See following sections for the effects of low dose progestogens or estrogens alone as possible examples of alternate effects.)

Progestogens

While progestogens administered alone to castrate animals or humans are poorly effective in suppressing LH and FSH (14), they do suppress these hormones when administered in large doses to normal menstruating women, probably by acting synergistically with endogenous estrogen. Mishell & Odell (23) showed that very high doses of ethynodiol diacetate (1–2 mg/day) caused suppression of both LH and FSH while low doses (0.1–0.5 mg) were associated with irregular, high surges of LH (but not FSH) and an increase in average LH concentrations over normal values. Presumably this positive action is explained by lowering the threshold of endogenous estrogen stimulation with resulting positive feedback by endogenous estrogens. Other studies have confirmed these findings. Garmendia et al (24) in a well-controlled study showed that a single dose of 200 mg of norethindrone enanthate intramuscularly suppressed LH below control LH concentrations for 4 weeks after administration. Between 4 and 12 weeks after the injection, LH rose slowly and was above control concentrations by the 12th week. A second group of women received a low dose (0.03 mg orally/day) of d-norgestrel; irregular LH surges were observed and mean LH concentrations were higher than normal. Moghissi et al (25) showed that 359 μg/day of norethindrone inhibited both the FSH rise initiating follicle growth and the midcycle LH ovulatory surge. These changes alone would explain contraceptive actions. Foss et al (26) showed that the minimum contraceptive dose of *dl*-norgestrel was 50 μg/day. Rudel (27), quoting unpublished studies of Martinez-Manatou, stated that contraceptive effectiveness of chlormadinone acetate was directly related to the dosage between 0.1 and 0.5 mg/day, with megestrol between 0.25 and 5 mg/day and norethindrone between 0.05 and 0.5 mg/day. With sufficiently small doses of any of these progestogens, a normal secretory endometrium was observed. As the dosage was increased, there was progressive reduction in glandular secretion and tortuosity. Martinez-Manautou et al (28), Foss et al (26), and Wright et al (29) have shown that very low dose progestogen treatment is associated with ovulation in many cycles, indicating the hormonal mechanisms described for the normal cycle are still likely to be occurring in some cycles. If ovulation is common, mechanisms other than those discussed would appear to be of major importance, at least for some dosages of progestogen contraceptive. Moghissi et al (25) showed that properties of cervical mucous (spinnbarkeit and ferning) were altered with low dose progestogen. Probably as a result, sperm penetration into the uterine cavity was also abolished. Vaginal sperm number and motility were similar to nontreated controls postcoitally; uterine sperm were absent in the treated group and present in large numbers in the nontreated group. Roland (30) had shown previously that sperm migration into the uterine cavity was inhibited by microdose progestogens.

In summary, the mechanisms of action of progestogens administered alone are complex and relate to dosage. High doses suppress LH and FSH with inhibition of follicular development but also commonly inducing aberrant LH surges not timed to coincide with any follicular development. Still lower doses may be associated with normal follicular development and ovulation but also act as higher doses do by modifying cervical mucous composition and preventing sperm entry into the uterine cavity. Lastly, endometrial histology is altered which may interfere with implantation should fertilization occur.

Progesterone treatment, while effective as a contraceptive, is often not associated with regular menses; bleeding is irregular and unpredictable. High dose progestogen treatment is also associated with intermittent or unpredictable vaginal bleeding. In addition, high dose depo progestogen treatment may be associated with prolonged periods of amenorrhea. Because of these effects and the associated infertility, high dose depo injections of progestogens are not usually recommended for nulliparous women.

Estrogens

Low dose estrogens also decrease fertility when administered cyclically for 20 days, followed by discontinuation for 5 days. Estrogens administered alone to normal women act in positive feedback to stimulate LH surges in bizarre, unpredictable fashion, similar to the pattern observed following progestogens alone (18).

Recently, a once-a-month estrogen pill has received clinical trials and has been shown to be an effective contraceptive (31–36). Quinestrol (an estrogen) is stored in body fat and subsequently is released slowly and probably converted into ethinyl estradiol. Quingestanol acetate (a progestogen) is the 3-cyclopentylenol ether derivative of norethindrone acetate. Quingestanol is a short acting progestogen. Thus, when a combination pill of quinestrol and quingestanol is taken once each 4 weeks, menses usually occur 3–4 days after the pill because of the rapid falloff in progestational effects on the endometrium. The estrogen produces the contraceptive effect and is effective for prolonged periods due to its peculiar fat-soluble properties. Nudemberg et al (35) showed that this contraceptive abolished ovulation; FSH concentrations were quite constant during treatment and no follicular phase rise or midcycle FSH surges were observed. LH was variable, some patients were observed to have double surges to heights comparable to those causing ovulation in normal subjects. These actions, of course, are predictable from the effects of steroids discussed previously for control of the normal cycle. In animal and human studies, estrogens usually suppress FSH, and at times LH, but also may stimulate LH secretion due to positive feedback. As indicated, progesterone measurements were not consistent with ovulation. This contraceptive might also act by abolishing the FSH-induced follicular development.

Sequential Estrogen Plus Progestogen Preparations

These preparations consist of an estrogen administered alone for a number of days (usually 15) followed by estrogen plus progestogen for several days (usually 5). The drugs are discontinued for 5 days to permit withdrawal bleeding, and the sequence is repeated. The effects of these preparations, predictably, are suppression of FSH with a stimulation of erratic LH surges during the estrogen only phase, usually a stimulation of another LH surge at the onset of the progestogen, followed by a suppression of both LH and FSH as the combination is continued (18).

Postcoital Contraceptives

Estrogens administered in large doses are currently being used as postcoital contraceptives for large numbers of patients, particularly on college campuses. In large doses these substances greatly shorten transit time of the fertilized ova into the uterine cavity (36). In both the rat and mouse, the amount of estradiol required to prevent nidation is 50 to 100 times greater than that required to initiate nidation. Thus, the dose required for contraception postcoitally in humans is also large, usually 15 mg of diethylstilbestrol daily for several days (37, 38).

Recently, Kesseru et al (39) reported that a single dose of d-norgestrel (a progestogen) taken within 3 hr of sexual intercourse could prevent pregnancy. Doses of 150 to 400 μg were studied. The contraceptive action was poor with 150 and 200 μg doses but was excellent with the 400 μg dose. In 2801 patients receiving this dose for an average of 9.1 months and averaging 8 coital exposures per month, the corrected failure rate was 1.7. The only side effects noted were cycle disturbances, most often a shortening of cycles. One third had intervals between bleedings of less than 20 days. Fewer than 10% of the patients had any complaints other than cycle length disturbances. Discontinuation rate of the drug was lower than that observed for oral microdose or long acting parenteral methods.

Steroid Administration from Silastic Preparations

In 1964 Folkman & Long (40) demonstrated that physiologically active materials would diffuse through the wall of a silicone rubber capsule at a steady, sustained rate. Dziuk & Cook (41) reported that silicone implants into ewes would allow sustained and constant steroid administration. This technique has now been applied to administer progestogens at low constant doses to women. Segal & Croxatto (42) further documented the findings of Folkman & Long (40) and added that dosage of the steroid could be adjusted by varying the surface area and wall thickness of the capsule. Croxatto et al (43) implanted subcutaneous capsules in women and demonstrated effective contraception using low dose progestogens as the steroid. Tatum et al (44) also performed such a study. They showed that contraception effectiveness was directly related to the number of capsules implanted and thus to steroid dosage administered. These findings were similar to those reported by Martinez-Manautou (28) using oral progestogens. There were no local or systemic complications attributable to the implants in the 24 women studied by Tatum et al. Mishell et al (45) have recently reported the use of silicone rings (55 or 65 mm outside diameter) impregnated with progesterone which were inserted intravaginally on day 5 of the cycle in 24 women and left in place 3 weeks. Absorption was sufficient to inhibit ovulation. The only complication, observed in a few patients, was superficial vaginal ulceration which healed quickly and spontaneously. The smaller devices were not associated with such ulceration. There was less breakthrough bleeding than when such steroids were given orally. The concept of using silastic impregnated devices is attractive, since theoretically the steroids released could supply constant dosage for years. In addition, absorption through mucous and dermal membranes makes a variety of potential devices possible.

Intrauterine Devices

Intrauterine devices (IUDs) have been increasingly used as antifertility agents, especially in underdeveloped countries, because of low cost, high efficiency (96%), minimal side effects, and no necessity for daily pilltaking, physician attention, or laboratory follow-up. The IUDs are of three types: 1. the older, purely mechanical devices made of steel or polyethylene and barium sulfate mixtures, 2. The newer copper and zinc devices, and 3. the still experimental steroidal releasing IUDs.

The earlier mechanical devices consisted of various types of rings (Hall), bows (Birnberg), and loops (Margulies spiral, Lippes loop) which were associated with the side effects of abnormal uterine bleeding, cramping, and expulsion from forcing the uterine cavity to adjust to the size and shape of the IUD (46). Although the efficacy was 98–99%, the rate of discontinuance of these IUDs was 23% after 1 year and 35% after 2 years of use because of these side effects (46). More recent IUDs include a T-shaped device (in which the arms of the T extend into the cornua) with a low rate of side effects but an 18% pregancy rate, and the Dalkon shield, a small pear-shaped device covered with a plastic membrane, giving a large surface area. In two studies (47, 48) this latter device has been found to have a pregnancy rate of 1 and 2.4% and removal rate of 4.9 and 14.5% after 1 year of use, yielding a net retention rate of 94% at 1 year.

The mechanism of the antifertility action of these IUDs remains unclear. Normal ovulatory cycles do occur (49). The IUDs all induce a sterile inflammatory reaction in the endometrium with a polymorphonuclear outpouring into the intrauterine cavity. These leukocytes may contain a toxic substance that affects implantation of fertilized ova rather than sperm viability and motility. Other possible mechanisms include the acceleration of ova transport through the fallopian tube and the increase in endometrial development, causing an environment inhospitable to implantation (1, 49).

Copper wire-bearing IUDs have been in use since 1967 and the efficiency of pregnancy prevention is directly proportional to the surface area of the copper wire on the IUD (46). The pregnancy rate of the most current models (using approximately 200 mm^2 of surface area) is 0.8% using the T-shaped device (50) and 1.1% using a number 7-shaped device (51), with an overall IUD retention rate at one year of 79% for the T and 76.8% for the 7 (50,51). Other devices using zinc in addition to copper are also being tested, and preliminary reports show even greater effectiveness (52).

The copper in these IUDs causes an increased copper concentration in the secretory endometrium, in endometrial fluid, and in cervical mucous, but not in plasma. A gradual decrease of 7 to 26 mg of the copper content of the IUD occurs each year (46, 53, 54). A polymorphonuclear leukocyte outpouring similar to the inert IUDs is also seen (55). The presence of copper (and to a less extent, zinc and silver) in cervical mucous is inhibitory to sperm migration in humans and animals in vitro (56, 57). In addition, in vitro experiments have shown a toxic effect of cupric chloride on mouse blastocysts (58).

The most recent innovation in IUDs has been the steroidal releasing devices. Preliminary animal work has shown progestogens are slowly released locally from silicone elastomer IUDs, and significant contraceptive action was found (56). Clinical trials (59) using a T-shaped IUD that released 50 μg/day of progesterone showed a pregnancy rate of 1.4%, an overall expulsion rate of 2.3%, and a removal rate of 8.1%. The progesterone apparently induces the production of decidua that blocks implantation. It appears that this IUD will require periodic changing, however, to renew the hormone supply.

ORAL CONTRACEPTIVES—METABOLIC AND SYSTEMIC EFFECTS

The combination estrogen and progestogen and progestogen-only oral contraceptives (OC) currently available have been associated with many metabolic changes and adverse systemic effects, many of which have been reviewed elsewhere (60–64). In this next section we will attempt to review the most recent findings in this area (See Table 1).

Thromboembolic Phenomena

The retrospective studies of the British Research Council were the first to demonstrate an increased risk of thromoembolic phenomena in OC users; the risk was

Table 1 Systemic effects of combined estrogen-progestogen oral contraceptives

Venous thromboembolism	Depression
Cerebrovascular accidents	Nausea
Hypercoagulable state	Vomiting
Defective folate metabolism	Abdominal cramps
Altered hepatic protein synthesis	Dizziness
Abnormal glucose tolerance	Edema
Hyperlipidemia	Breast soreness
Hypertension	Backache
Defective lactation	Fatigue
Post-use amenorrhea	Increased appetite
Hepatic dysfunction	Weight gain
Melasma	Nervousness
Erythema nodosum	Leg cramps
Gall bladder disease	Photosensitivity

directly correlated with the dose of estrogen in the preparations (65–68). Similar findings have been reported in American (69, 70) and Swedish (71) studies. An association has also been described for intracranial venous thrombosis (72). Prospective studies, however, have not borne out the association between OC use and thromboembolism (73). Drill, in 1972, reviewed (74) several large-scale prospective studies and found an average figure of 0.92 cases per 1000 women per year of thromboembolic disease which he compared with a figure of 2.2 cases in women not on OC. However, this latter number was derived from several different studies and is thus also open to question. The conclusions reached in these analyses of prospective and retrospective studies are at marked variance and are difficult to explain. It would seem that an internally controlled, double-blind large prospective study of this problem is warranted.

Two mechanisms have been proposed for the controversial increased incidence of thromboembolism in women taking OC: 1. an increased tendency toward clotting (see below) and 2. venous stasis. A decrease in the elasticity and tone of the smooth muscle of the peripheral vascular system due to OC estrogens has been hypothesized as one of the causes of decreased flow and stasis (75).

Although the incidence of headache was not increased in women on OC, those reporting headaches often experienced significant relief when stopping OC (76). However, there is evidence for a definite association between cerebrovascular disease and OC use; about 25% of the patients having an occlusion suffered from an occlusion in the vertebrobasilar distribution (78). Recently, an extensive, collaborative, retrospective study was published (79) from 12 medical centers in the United States. Each subject with cerebrovascular disease had an age and race matched control from the hospital population and a second, healthy, similar control from the same neighborhood. This study showed that the risk of a thrombotic stroke was 9.5 times greater from combined OC users than for hospital controls and 8.8 times greater than for neighbor controls. The relative risk for hemorrhagic stroke was 2.0 for OC users vs hospital controls and 2.3 vs neighbor controls, with no increased risk for other types of stroke.

Other associations with vascular complications have been suggested but have been less well documented. For example, Inman and Vessey (77) found a slight increase in OC use in patients dying of coronary artery disease but this was not statistically significant. Mesenteric arterial insufficiency has also been reported in women on OC (80).

Progestogen-only OC have so far not been associated with increased risk of vascular disease (81–85). However, in the combined preparations, Inman et al (67) found that the progestogen (megestrol) was associated with venous thromboembolic disease but not cerebral or coronary disease.

Hematologic Changes

Combination OC have been reported to affect the coagulation process in several ways. Clotting factors II, VII, and X are elevated (86, 87) as is plasminogen (88), but fibrinogen has been reported as either elevated (88) or unchanged (87). Antithrombin III and antiplasmin have been found to be low (88, 89). Although there is a decrease in fibrinolytic inhibitor, there is normal fibrinolytic activity on combined OC (90). Clots formed in women on combined OC are also significantly more stable than in controls (91). The net effect of these changes is uncertain. Although some have suggested the existence of a "hypercoagulative state," present testing systems are inadequate to prove or disprove this. Progestogen-alone OC have been found to cause either no change in these parameters (88) or to decrease antithrombin III (92), increase factors VIII and IX and decrease V (93), and decrease fibrinolytic activity (90).

Platelet studies have yielded conflicting results. Although significant increases in platelet aggregation have been found (86, 94), no increases have been found in platelet adhesiveness (95). An increase in aggregation has also been found with progestogen-only OC, though not so marked as in the combined preparations (96).

Oski et al (97) have shown a decrease in RBC filterability within 3 days of onset of OC. These authors suggest a decrease in RBC deformability, with perhaps a tendency for these cells to be trapped in the microcirculation leading to stasis.

Although no changes in hemoglobin level (98) or platelet counts (95) have been found, women on combined OC have an absolute increase in neutrophil count and a smaller increase in lymphocyte count (99). Serum folic acid levels have been found to fall with time in women on OC in some studies (100) but not others (101) without a change in hemoglobin levels (100). The low folate has been attributed to defective absorption of dietary folate, the folate polyglutamates (102), or to an increased clearance of folate from plasma to tissues (101).

Combined OC have been found to increase serum transferrin, total iron binding capacity (TIBC), and iron (103–106) with the rise in TIBC and iron independent of each other (104). Increased synthesis by the liver is thought to cause the rise in transferrin, but the mechanism for the increased serum iron is unknown because iron absorption is normal (105). Progestogen-only OC have been reported to both increase (107) and not change (108) serum iron and TIBC levels.

Other hepatically synthesized proteins elevated by combined OC include α-1-globulins (109), α-2-macroglobulins, IgG (110), IgM, ceruloplasmin, α-1-antitrypsin (111), cryofibrinogens (112), tyrosine aminotransferase (113), α-amylase (114), Vitamin B_{12} binding capacity, thyroxine binding globulin (TBG), and cortisol binding globulin (CBG) (115). Albumin decreases in women on OC (111). Other circulating substances increased by OC include Vitamin A (116), copper (117, 118), phosphorus, and calcium (119), with no change in magnesium (119) and a decrease in zinc (117) and the amino acids proline, glycine, alanine, valine, leucine, tyrosine, glutamate, and isoleucine (120). Combined OC have induced positive lupus erythematosus cell preparations in some series but not in others (121).

The elevated TBG concentrations result in elevated total thyroxine and triiodothyronine concentrations, but the concentrations of the free hormones remain normal (122). In addition, increases in plasma cortisol result from the increased CBG and increased testosterone from the increased sex hormone binding globulin (124, 125). While the hypothalamic-pituitary axis has been reported to be normal (124), the single dose 1 mg dexamethasone suppression test is frequently abnormal because cortisol concentrations commonly remain above 1 $\mu g\%$ (due to increased CBG). Surprisingly, increased free cortisol in plasma and decreased urinary excretion in 17-hydroxy and 17-ketosteroids have been reported; these findings, if true, can not be explained by increases in cortisol binding globulin alone (124, 125). Contraceptives containing only progestogens do not increase TBG (123) or CBG and sex hormone binding globulin (125).

Glucose Tolerance

Combined OC have been found to induce a mild to moderate deterioration of glucose tolerance in many women (126–129). In addition, distinct worsening of the GTT (Glucose Tolerance Test) was correlated with previous gestationally abnormal GTT curves (130). Progestogen-only OC were not found to cause abnormal GTTs in most studies (131–135), but Vermeulen et al (135) found increased insulin values in some patients despite normal GTTs. This deterioration of glucose tolerance has also been found frequently in postmenopausal women treated with estrogens (136). Administering OC to panhypopituitary women in addition to their usual thyroid and cortisol replacement, Davidson & Holzman (137) found no evidence of insulin resistance on tolbutamide tolerance testing when compared to controls on OC, suggesting that growth hormone might be the cause of the deterioration of glucose tolerance in normal women on OC. The normals had exaggerated growth hormone responses to tolbutamide while the hypopituitary patients, of course, had no response.

Lipid Metabolism

Serum triglycerides have been found to be elevated in 60 to 96% of women taking combined OC (126, 138, 139), with an average rise of 33 mg/100 ml (139). These elevations are associated with increases in low density lipoproteins (LDL) and very low density lipoproteins (VLDL) (139). The elevations slowly return toward normal over several weeks when a progestogen-only OC is substituted for the combination (140), and a dose-response relationship between the dose of estrogen in the OC and the level of triglycerides has been found (141).

The mechanism for the rise in triglycerides is unclear. Post-heparin lipolytic activity (PHLA) is decreased in women on combined OC, but there is no actual defect in triglyceride removal from serum (142). Kekki & Nikkila (143) have demonstrated an increased triglyceride synthesis by the liver in women on OC.

Cholesterol has generally been found to be either unchanged or slightly elevated in women on combined OC (139, 144, 145). Occasionally very large increases in triglycerides and cholesterol have been found, usually in patients with an underlying hyperlipidemia (146–149). No changes in serum triglycerides or cholesterol have been demonstrated in patients on progestogen-only OC (132).

Hypertension

Both prospective (150–152) and retrospective (153–154) studies have generally agreed on a definite association between combined OC use and the development of hypertension in some women, although there are some dissenters (155, 156). The incidence figures range from 1% (151) to 15.41% (150); the former figure is in fact less than the 2% of the normal population expected to develop hypertension in the 25–34 year age group (157).

Studies of the renin-angiotensin-aldosterone system have shown increased renin substrate (158), plasma renin activity (158), angiotensin II (159), and aldosterone (160) in all women on combined OC. However, only some of these women develop hypertension, reflecting some additional genetic or environmental factor necessary to cause hypertension in certain individuals. Progestogen-only OC have as yet not been implicated in the development of hypertension.

Lactation

Reports of combined OC effects on postpartum lactation have been conflicting, with some investigators reporting increased milk production and baby weight (161) and others finding decreased milk production and baby weight gain (162–164) and decreased milk protein and fat content (165). In addition to the effects of OC on milk production, a significant correlation has been found between prior OC use and breast milk-related jaundice in the infant, due to estrogen interference with bilirubin conjugation by an unknown mechanism in the neonate (166).

Amenorrhea

A small percent of women taking combined OC develop prolonged amenorrhea upon discontinuation of medication. Although good incidence figures are lacking, Shearman (167) estimated that only 1% of women will develop amenorrhea persisting for more than 12 months. A few of the patients have elevated gonadotropin and premature menopause, but most have normal or low serum and urinary gonadotropins and urinary 17-ketosteroids when measured. In some series, over 50% of the women developing this syndrome had considerable menstrual irregularity before going on OC and a few of these proved to have the polycystic ovary syndrome. Clomiphene citrate with and without additional human chorionic gonadotropin (HCG) treatment has induced ovulatory cycles in 50–75% of these women with smaller proportions of these resuming normal ovulatory cycles or becoming pregnant. Interestingly 10–20% of women with this syndrome have galactorrhea with normal skull roentgenograms (167–171). As yet no studies have been done on large numbers of these patients utilizing daily serum LH, FSH, estrogen, and prolactin levels, although Frantz (190) has reported elevated prolactin levels in six of these patients. However, the data would seem to indicate that most of these patients have normal gonadotropins but probably fail to have an ovulatory surge of LH either because of a lack of the estrogen rise prior to the LH surge or because of a lack of response on the part of the hypothalamus to such a rise if it occurs. The significant percentage of such patients with galactorrhea and the response of many to clomiphene citrate implicate hypothalamic dysfunction as the possible etiology. Experience with low dose progestogen-only OC is too short to determine whether amenorrhea will be a problem with their use.

Depression

Anecdotal reports of depression associated with the use of combined OC, especially in women prone to premenstrual tension, have been found in the literature. However, large surveys (172, 173) and two double-blind studies using placebo controls (174, 175) have failed to confirm these reports. A preliminary report by Baumblatt & Winston (176) of 58 women with OC-related depression states that supplemental pyridoxine was able to reverse this depression in 44 (76%). Adams et al (191) have had similar results. The estrogenic component of OC increases pyridoxine utilization by inducing an increase in the enzyme tryptophan oxygenase and a general increase in tryptophan catabolism via pathways that use pyridoxine (177). This increased activity makes less pyridoxine available for the decarboxylation of 5-hydroxytryptophan to serotonin. Since low serotonin levels have been found in some depressed patients, according to these authors, supplemental pyridoxine would increase serotonin and reduce depression in some women on OC. Progestogen-only OC have not been associated with depression (84).

Hepatic Dysfunction

Combined OC have been associated with BSP retention in about 20% of patients, rises in alkaline phosphatase in 2%, and elevations of transaminases in up to 18%, but these elevations are usually transient and have not been regarded as necessitating discontinuance of the drug (62, 64). Cholestatic jaundice has also been reported in isolated cases (62). Recent investigations of giving OC to women with recently resolved viral hepatitis (178), obstructive jaundice (179), and previous jaundice of pregnancy (179) have not shown any deleterious effects, although serum transaminases did go up transiently after 3 weeks of use. Most authors would agree that liver function testing should be more frequent than usual in women with a prior history of liver disease. Although most investigators seem to accept slight elevations of BSP and continue with OC use (64), O'Malley et al (180) have shown impairment of antipyrine and phenylbutazone metabolism (the latter drug not statistically significant) in women on OC; both drugs are metabolized principally by the liver. More drugs should be studied with regard to this potentially widespread area of drug-drug interaction in which OC-induced liver changes might alter the metabolic degradation rates of various drugs.

Skin

Melasma is the most common skin complication and occurs in 5–8% of women on OC within 1–20 months of the start of therapy. Either component of the combined OC can cause an increase in pigmentation, but the combination brings it on more frequently. It appears that the estrogens stimulate melanocytes and the progestogens cause the pigmentation to spread. Sunlight worsens the condition. The pigmentation usually fades slowly after OC use is discontinued, but it may be permanent. Acne is usually improved due to the estrogenic component, although there may be a paradoxical worsening of the acne in the first few months of therapy. Vaginal moniliasis is more common in patients on OC as well as photosensitivity, erythema nodosum, telangiectasias, and spider nevi (181).

Miscellaneous Changes

OC use has not to date been associated with any breast disease. The incidence of OC use among patients with benign and malignant breast tumors was not increased in two separate studies (70, 182). Similarly, OC use has not been related to opthalmological abnormalities when compared to controls (183). On the other hand, surgically proven cholecystitis and cholelithiasis have been found slightly but significantly more frequently in OC users (70).

In cytogenetic studies some investigators have found significantly increased chromosome breakage and satellite association (184), but others have been unable to find such breaks or increases in mitotic indices (185, 186).

In addition to the above serious and sometimes irreversible side effects, there are many other symptomatic side effects of a more general nature that can be of such intensity and discomfort as to cause many patients to stop using OC. These effects include nausea, vomiting, abdominal cramps, dizziness, nervousness, edema, breast soreness, leg cramps, backache, fatigue, increased appetite, and weight gain. Many of these can be related on a dose basis to the estrogenic component of combined OC (22). Progestogen-only OC seem to be free of most of the above side effects, with most problems in patient acceptance being the abnormal bleeding (81, 82) and occasionally amenorrhea (187).

All of the above side effects condition the rate of patient acceptance and the reliability of use. In one 4 year prospective study of over 2000 women, the overall continuation rate for combined OC was 81% at 1 year and 50% at 4 years; the rates for sequential OC were 83% at 1 year and 36% at 1 year. The reasons for discontinuation included accidental pregnancy, planning future pregnancy, and personal reasons, with medical reasons being 13.1% of the total at 4 years with combined OC and 20.7% for sequential OC (188). A similar recent study by Hall (189) showed a 28% discontinuance of sequential OC at 2 years for medical reasons. With the progestogen-alone OC, abnormal bleeding caused most of the medical reasons for discontinuing the OC, with rates of 8% for continuous use (81) and 11.6% for cyclic use (30). Pregnancy rates for combined OC were 0.9% for 1 year and 2.1% cumulatively after 4 years (188), for sequential OC 2.0% at 1 year and 4.3% at 4 years cumulatively (188), and for continuous progestogen-only OC 4.5% per year (81).

Literature Cited

1. Odell, W. D., Moyer, D. L. 1971. *Physiology of Reproduction,* C. V. Mosby, St. Louis
2. Neill, J. D., Johansson, E. D. B., Datta, J. K., Knobil, E. 1967. *J. Clin. Endocrinol. Metab.* 27:1167–73
3. Yoshimi, T., Lipsett, M. B. 1968. *Steroids* 11:527–40
4. Ross, G. T., Cargille, C. M., Lipsett, M. B., Rayford, P. L., Marshall, J. R., Strott, C. A., Rodbard, D. 1970. *Rec. Prog. Horm. Res.* 26:1–62
5. Abraham, G. E., Swerdloff, R. S., Tulchinsky, D., Odell, W. D. 1971. *J. Clin. Endocrinol. Metab.* 32:619–24
6. Abraham, G. E., Odell, W. D., Swerdloff, R. S., Hopper, K. 1972. *J. Clin. Endocrinol. Metab.* 84:312–18
7. Odell, W. D., Ross, G. T., Rayford, P. L. 1967. *J. Clin. Invest.* 46:248–55
8. Odell, W. D., Parlow, A. F., Cargille, C. M., Ross, G. T. 1968. *J. Clin. Invest.* 47:2551–62
9. Odell, W. D., Swerdloff, R. S. 1968. *Proc. Nat. Acad. Sci. USA* 61:529–56
10. Yen, S. S. C., Tsai, C. C. 1971. *J. Clin. Endocrinol. Metab.* 33:882–87
11. Weick, R. F., Dierschke, D. J., Karsch, F. J., Yamaji, T., Knobil, E. 1972. *Endocrinology* 91:1528–30
12. Schwartz, N. B. 1969. *Rec. Prog. Horm. Res.* 25:1–55
13. Ferin, M., Tempone, A., Zimmering, P. E., Vande Wiele, R. L. 1969. *Endocrinology* 85: 1070–78
14. Swerdloff, R. S., Jacobs, H. S., Odell, W. D. 1972. *Endocrinology* 90:1529–36
15. Sawyer, C. H., Everett, J. W. 1959. *Endocrinology* 65:644
16. Davajan, V., Nakamura, R. M., Kharma, K. 1970. *Obstet. Gynecol. Survey* 25:1–43
17. Ross, G. T., Odell, W. D., Rayford, P. L. 1966. *Lancet* 2:1255–56
18. Swerdloff, R. S., Odell, W. D. 1969. *J. Clin. Endocrinol. Metab.* 29:157–63
19. Mishell, D., Thorneycroft, I. H., Nakamura, R. M., Nagata, Y., Stone, S. C. 1972. *Am. J. Obstet. Gynecol.* 114:923–28
20. Rock, J., Garcia, C. R., Pincus, G. 1957. *Rec. Prog. Horm. Res.* 13:323
21. Garcia, C. R., Pincus, G. 1964. *Int. J. Fert.* 9:95
22. Preston, S. N. 1973. *Contraception* 6: 17–35
23. Mishell, D. R., Odell, W. D. 1971. *Am. J. Obstet. Gynecol.* 109:140–49
24. Garmendia, F., Kesseru, E., Lierena, L. A. 1973. *Horm. Metab. Res.* 5: 134–38
25. Moghissi, K. S., Syner, F. N., McBride, L. C. 1973. *Obstet. Gynecol.* 41: 585–94
26. Foss, G. L., Svendsen, E. K., Fotherby, K., Richards, D. J. 1968. *Brit. Med. J.* 4:489–91
27. Rudel, H. W. 1970. *Fed. Proc.* 29: 1228–31
28. Martinez-Manautou, J. et al 1967. *Brit. Med. J.* 2:730–32
29. Wright, S. W., Fotherby, K., Fairweather, F. 1970. *J. Obstet. Gynaecol. Brit. Comm.* 77:65–68
30. Roland, M., Leisten, D., Caruso, L. J. 1973. *Obstet. Gynecol.* 41:595–601
31. Berman, E. 1970. *J. Reprod. Med.* 5: 196–201
32. Claman, A. D. 1970. *Am. J. Obstet. Gynecol.* 107:461–64
33. Guiloff, E., Berman, E., Montiglio, A., Osorio, R., Lloyd, C. W. 1970. *Fert. Steril.* 21:110–18
34. Larranaga, A., Berman, E. 1970. *Contraception* 1:137
35. Nudemberg, F., Kothari, M., Karam, K., Taymor, M. L. 1973. *Fert. Steril.* 24:185–90
36. Emmens, C. W. 1970. *Brit. Med. Bull.* 26:45–51
37. Morris, J. M., Van Wagenen, G. 1967. *Proc. 8th Int. Congr. Planned Parenthood,* Santiago de Chile, Ed. I. P. P. F.: London 1968 pp. 276–79
38. Haspels, A. A. 1972. *Bol. Med. I. P. P. F.* 6:2
39. Kesseru, E., Larranaga, A., Parada, J. 1973. *Contraception* 7:367–79
40. Folkman, J., Long, D. M. 1964. *J. Surg. Res.* 4:139–42

41. Dziuk, P. J., Cook, B. 1966. *Endocrinology* 78:208–11
42. Segal, S. J., Croxatto, H. 1967. *Meet. Am. Fert. Soc., 23rd* Wash., D.C.
43. Croxatto, H., Diaz, S., Vera, R., Etchart, M., Atria, P. 1969. *Am. J. Obstet. Gynecol.* 105:1135–38
44. Tatum, H. J., Coutinho, E. M., Filho, J. A., Santanna, A. R. 1969. *Am. J. Obstet. Gynecol.* 105:1139–43
45. Mishell, D. R., Lumkin, M., Stone, S. 1972. *Am. J. Obstet. Gynecol.* 113: 925–32
46. Tatum, H. J. 1972. *Am. J. Obstet. Gynecol.* 112:1000–23
47. Davis, H. J. 1970. *Am. J. Obstet. Gynecol.* 106:455–56
48. Horowitz, A. J. 1973. *Contraception* 7: 1–10
49. Corfman, P. A., Segal, S. J. 1968. *Am. J. Obstet. Gynecol.* 100:448–59
50. Tatum, H. J. 1972. *Contraception* 6: 179–89
51. Bernstein, G. S., Israel, R., Seward, P., Mishell, D. R. 1972. *Contraception* 6: 99–107
52. Zipper, J. A., Tatum, H. J., Medel, M., Pastene, L., Rivera, M. 1971. *Am. J. Obstet. Gynecol.* 109:771–74
53. Hagenfeldt, K. 1972. *Contraception* 6: 37–54
54. Hagenfeldt, K. 1972. *Contraception* 6: 219–30
55. Hagenfeldt, K., Johannisson, E., Brenner, P. 1972. *Contraception* 6:207–18
56. Kesseru, E., Camacho-Ortega, P. 1972. *Contraception* 6:231–40
57. Jecht, E. W., Bernstein, G. S. 1973. *Contraception* 7:381–401
58. Naeslund, G. 1972. *Contraception* 6: 281–85
59. Scommegna, A., Avila, T., Luna, M., Rao, R., Kulkarni, B., Dmowski, W. 1973. Presented at *Clinical Program, Am. Coll. Obstet. Gynecol.* Bal Harbour, Fla.
60. Council on Drugs. 1970. *J. Am. Med. Assoc.* 214:2316–21
61. Warren, M. P. 1973. *Am. J. Med. Sci.* 265:4–21
62. Doll, R., Vessey, M. P. 1970. *Brit. Med. Bull.* 26:33–38
63. Goldzieher, J. W. 1970. *Fed. Proc.* 29: 1220–27
64. Elgee, N. J. 1970. *Ann. Intern. Med.* 72:409–18
65. Medical Research Council. 1967. *Brit. Med. J.* 1:355–59
66. Vessey, M. P., Doll, R. 1968. *Brit. Med. J.* 2:199–205

67. Inman, W. H. W., Vessey, M. P., Westerholm, B., Engelund, A. 1970. *Brit. Med. J.* 2:203–09
68. Vessey, M. P., Doll, R., Fairbairn, A. S., Glober, G. 1970. *Brit. Med. J.* 3: 123–26
69. Sartwell, P. E., Masi, A. T., Arthes, F. G., Greene, G. R., Smith, H. E. 1969. *Am. J. Epidemiol.* 90:365–80
70. Boston Collaborative Drug Surveillance Program. 1973. *Lancet* 1:1399–1404
71. Bottiger, L. E., Westerholm, B. 1971. *Acta Med. Scand.* 190:455–63
72. Atkinson, E. A., Fairburn, B., Heathfield, K. W. G. 1970. *Lancet* 1:914–18
73. Wait, R. B., Sturtevant, F. M. 1970. *Contraception* 2:193–98
74. Drill, V. A. 1972. *J. Am. Med. Assoc.* 219:583–92
75. Wood, J. E. 1972. *Mod. Conc. Cardiovasc. Dis.* 41:37–40
76. Diddle, A. W., Gardner, W. H., Williamson, P. J. 1969. *Am. J. Obstet. Gynecol.* 105:507–11
77. Inman, W. H. W., Vessey, M. P. 1968. *Brit. Med. J.* 2:193–99
78. Masi, A. T., Dugdale, M. 1970. *Ann. Int. Med.* 72:111–21
79. Collaborative Group for the Study of Stroke in Young Women. 1973. *N. Engl. J. Med.* 288:871–78
80. Hurwitz, R. L., Martin, A. J., Grossman, B. E., Waddell, W. R. 1970. *Ann. Surg.* 172:892–96
81. Bernstein, G. S., Seward, P. 1972. *Contraception* 5:369–88
82. Jeppsson, S., Kullander, S. 1970. *Fert. Steril.* 32:307–13
83. Larsson-Cohn, U. 1970. *Acta. Endocrinol. (Kbh) Suppl.* 144:7–46
84. Editorial 1971. *Lancet* 1:25–26
85. Vessey, M. P., Mears, E., Andolset, L., Ogrinc-Oven, M. 1972. *Lancet* 1: 915–22
86. Poller, L., Thomson, J. M., Thomas, W. 1971. *Brit. Med. J.* 4:648–50
87. Lorrain, J., Harel, P. 1972. *Fert. Steril.* 23:422–27
88. Howie, P. W., Mallinson, A. C., Prentice, C. R. M., Horne, C. H. W., McNicol, G. P. 1970. *Lancet* 2:1329–32
89. Fagerhol, M. K., Abildgaard, U., Bergsjo, P., Jacobsen, J. H. 1970. *Lancet* 1:1175
90. Menon, I. S., Peberdy, M., Rannie, G. H., Weightman, D., Dewar, H. A. 1970. *J. Gynaecol. Brit. Comm.* 77:752–56
91. Shanberge, J. N., Tanaka, K., Gruhl, M. C., Ikemori, R., Inoshita, K. 1972. *Ann. NY Acad. Sci* 202:220–29

92. Bergsjo, P., Fagerhol, M. K., Abild-gaard, U. 1972. *Am. J. Obstet. Gynecol.* 112:938-40
93. Mink, J. B., Cowrey, N. G., Moore, R. H., Ambrus, C. M., Ambrus, J. L. 1972. *Am. J. Obstet. Gynecol.* 113:739-43
94. Adams, J. H., Mitchell, J. R. A., Soppitt, G. D. 1970. *Lancet* 2:333-35
95. Ham, J. M., Rose, R. 1969. *Am. J. Obstet. Gynecol.* 105:628-31
96. Poller, L., Thomson, J. M., Thomas, W., Wray, C. 1971. *Brit. Med. J.* 1: 705-07
97. Oski, F. A., Lubin, B., Buchert, E. D. 1972. *Ann. Intern. Med.* 77:417-19
98. Cruickshank, J. M. 1970. *Brit. J. Haematol.* 18:523-29
99. Cruickshank, J. M., Alexander, M. K. 1970. *Brit. J. Haematol.* 18:541-50
100. Shojania, A. M., Hornady, G. J., Barnes, P. H. 1971. *Am. J. Obstet. Gynecol.* 111:782-91
101. Stephens, M. Z. M., Craft, I., Peters, T. J., Hoffbrand, A. V. 1972. *Clin. Sci.* 42: 405-14
102. Necheles, T. F., Snyder, L. M. 1970. *N. Engl. J. Med.* 282:858-59
103. Jacobi, J. M., Powell, L. W., Gaffney, T. J. 1969. *Brit. J. Haematol.* 17:503-09
104. Mardell, M., Symmons, C., Zilva, J. F. 1969. *J. Clin. Endocrinol. Metab.* 29: 1489-95
105. Norby, A., Rybo, G., Solvell, L. 1972. *Scand. J. Haematol.* 9:43-51
106. Thein, M., Beaton, G. H., Milne, H., Veen, M. J. 1969. *Can. Med. Assoc. J.* 101:678-79
107. Briggs, M. H., Briggs, M. 1970. *Brit. Med. J.* 3:521
108. Powell, L. W., Jacobi, J. M., Gaffney, T. J., Adam, R. 1970. *Brit. Med. J.* 3: 194-95
109. Adlercreutz, H., Eisalo, A., Heino, A., Luukkainen, T., Penttila, I., Saukkonen, H. 1968. *Scand. J. Gastroenterol.* 3:273-84
110. Horne, C. H. W., Weir, R. J., Howie, P. W., Gondie, R. B. 1970. *Lancet* 1: 49-53
111. Mendenhall, H. W. 1970. *Am. J. Obstet. Gynecol.* 106:750-53
112. Chandra, R. K. 1972. *J. Reprod. Fert.* 28:463-64
113. Rose, D. P., Cramp, D. G. 1970. *Clin. Chim. Acta.* 29:49-53
114. Adlercreutz, H., Soininen, K., Harkonan, M. 1972. *Brit. Med. J.* 3:529
115. Barbos, J., Seal, U.S., Doe, R. P. 1973. *J. Clin. Endocrinol. Metab.* 36:706-14
116. Gal, I., Parkinson, C., Craft, I. 1971. *Brit. Med. J.* 2:436-38

117. Schenker, J. G., Hellerstein, S., Jungreis, E., Polishuk, W. Z. 1971. *Fert. Steril.* 22:229-34
118. O'Leary, J. A., Spellacy, W. N. 1969. *Am. J. Obstet. Gynecol.* 103:131-32
119. Simpson, G. R., Dale, E. 1972. *Fert. Steril.* 23:326-30
120. Craft, I. L., Peters, T. J. 1971. *Clin. Sci.* 41:301-07
121. Editorial. 1970. *Lancet* 1:72-73
122. Fisher, D. A. 1973. *J. Pediat.* 82:1-9
123. Goolden, A. W. G., Bateman, D. M., Pleehachinda, R., Sanderson, C. 1970. *Lancet* 1:624
124. Daly, J. R., Elstein, M. 1972. *J. Obstet, Gynaecol. Brit. Comm.* 79:544-49
125. Briggs, M. H., Briggs, M. 1972. *J. Obstet. Gynaecol. Brit. Comm.* 79:946-50
126. Beck, P. 1973. *Metabolism.* 22:841-55
127. Boshell, B. R., Roddam, R. F., McAdams, G. L., Fox, O. J. 1968. *J. Reprod. Fert., Suppl.* 5:77-88
128. Wynn, V., Doar, J. W. H. 1969. *Lancet* 2:761-66
129. Spellacy, W. N., Bendel, R. P., Buhi, W. C., Birk, S. A. 1969. *Fert. Steril.* 20: 892-902
130. Szabo, A. J., Cole, H. S., Grimaldi, R. D. 1970. *N. Engl. J. Med.* 282:646-50
131. Goldman, J. A., Ovadia, J. L., Eckerling, B. 1968. *Israel J. Med. Sci.* 4: 878-82
132. Beck, P. 1970. *J. Clin. Endocrinol.* 30: 785-91
133. Goldman, J., Eckerling, B., Zukerman, Z., Mannheimer, S. 1971. *J. Obstet. Gynaecol. Brit. Comm.* 78:255-60
134. Larrson-Cohn, U., Tengstrom, B., Wide, L. 1969. *Acta Endocrinol.* (Kbh) 62:242-50
135. Vermeulen, A., Daneels, R., Thiery, M. 1970. *Diabetalogia* 6:519-23
136. Ajabor, L. N., Tsai, C. C., Vela, P., Yen, S. S. C. 1972. *Am. J. Obstet. Gynecol.* 113:383-87
137. Davidson, M. B., Holzman, G. B. 1973. *J. Clin. Endocrinol. Metab.* 36:246-55
138. Gershberg, H., Hulse, M., Javier, Z. 1968. *Obstet. Gynecol.* 31:186-89
139. Wynn, V., Doar, J. W. H., Mills, G. L., Stokes, T. 1969. *Lancet* 2:756-60
140. Rossner, S., Larsson-Cohn, U., Carlson, L. A., Boberg, J. 1971. *Acta Med. Scand.* 190:301-05
141. Stokes, T., Wynn, V. 1971. *Lancet* 2: 677-81
142. Hazzard, W. R., Notter, D. T., Spiger, M. J., Bierman, E. L. 1972. *J. Clin. Endocrinol. Metab.* 35:425-37
143. Kekki, M., Nikkila, E. A. 1971. *Metabolism* 20:878-89

144. Aurell, M., Cramer, K., Rybo, A. 1966. *Lancet* 1:291–93
145. DeAlvarez, R. R., Jahed, F. M., Spitalny, K. J., Elkin, H., Jannakis, I. 1973. *Am. J. Obstet. Gynecol.* 116:727–49
146. Zorilla, E., Hulse, M., Hernandez, A., Gershberg, H. 1968. *J. Clin. Endocrinol.* 28:1793–96
147. Bank, S., Marks, I. N. 1960. *Postgrad. Med. J.* 46:576–88
148. Glueck, C. J., Scheel, D., Fishback, J., Steiner, P. 1972. *Metabolism* 21:657–66
149. Molitch, M. E., Oill, P., Odell, W. D. *J. Am. Med. Assoc.* In press
150. Spellacy, W. N., Birk, S. A. 1970. *Fert. Steril.* 21:301–06
151. Weir, R. J., Briggs, F., Mack, A., Taylor, L., Browning, J. Naismith, L., Witson, E. 1971. *Lancet* 1:467–71
152. Clezy, T. M., Foy, B. N., Hodge, R. L., Lumbers, E. R. 1972. *Brit. Heart. J.* 34:1238–43
153. Wallace, M. R. 1971. *Aust. N. Z. J. Med.* 1:49–52
154. Fisch, I. R., Freedman, S. H., Myatt, A. V. 1972. *J. Am. Med. Assoc.* 222:1507–10
155. Kunin, C. M., McCormack, R. G., Abernathy, J. R. 1969. *Arch. Intern. Med.* 123:362–65
156. Smith, R. W., 1972. *Am. J. Obstet. Gynecol.* 113:482–87
157. Wither, J. A., Barrow, J. G. 1972. *Am. J. Med.* 52:653–63
158. Saruta, T., Saade, G. A., Kaplan, N. M. 1970. *Arch. Intern. Med.* 1261:621–26
159. Cain, M. D., Walters, W. A., Catt, K. J. 1971. *J. Clin. Endocrinol.* 33:671–76
160. Crane, ., Harris, J. J., Winsor, W. III 1971. *Ann. Intern. Med.* 74:13–21
161. Kamal, I., Hefnawi, F., Ghoneim, M., Abdallah, M., Abdel Razek, S. 1970. *Am. J. Obstet. Gynecol.* 108:655–58
162. Miller, G. H., Hughes, L. R. 1970. *Obstet. Gynecol.* 35:44–50
163. Borglin, N. E., Sandholm, L. E. 1971. *Fert. Steril.* 22:39–41
164. Koetsawang, S., Bhiraleus, P., Chiemprajert, T. 1972. *Fert. Steril.* 23:24–28
165. Kader, M. M. A. et al 1969. *Am. J. Obstet. Gynecol.* 105:978–85
166. Wong, Y. K., Wood, B. S. B. 1971. *Brit. Med. J.* 4:403–04
167. Shearman, R. P. 1971. *Lancet* 2:64–66
168. Nillins, S. J., Gemzell, L. 1972. *Acta Endocrinol.* (Kbh) 69:445–58

169. Golditch, I. M., 1972. *Obstet. Gynecol.* 39:903–08
170. Rifkin, I., Nachtigall, L. E., Beckman, E. M. 1972. *Am. J. Obstet. Gynecol.* 113:420–32
171. Arrata, W. S. M., de Alvarez, R. R. 1972. *Am. J. Obstet. Gynecol.* 112:1025–30
172. Murawski, B. J., Sapir, P. E., Shulman, N., Ryan, G. M. Jr., Sturgis, S. H. 1968. *Fert. Steril.* 19:50–63
173. Herzberg, B. N., Draper, K. L., Johnson, A. L., Nicol, G. C. 1971. *Brit. Med. J.* 3:495–500
174. Marcotte, D. B., Kane, F. J., Obrist, P., Lipton, M. A. 1970. *Brit. J. Psychiat.* 116:165–67
175. Goldzieher, J. W., Moses, L. E., Averkin, E., Scheel, C., Taber, B. Z. 1971. *Fert. Steril.* 22:609–23
176. Baumblatt, M. J., Winston, F. 1970. *Lancet* 1:832–33
177. Rose, D. P., Braidman, I. P. 1971. *Am. J. Clin. Nutr.* 24:673–83
178. Eisalo, A., Konttinen, A., Hietala, O. 1971. *Brit. Med. J.* 3:561–62
179. Rannevik, G., Jeppsson, S., Kullander, S. 1972. *J. Obstet. Gynaecol. Brit. Comm.* 79:1128–36
180. O'Malley, K., Stevenson, I. H., Crooks, J. 1972. *Clin. Pharm. Ther.* 13:522–57
181. Jelinek, J. E. 1970. *Arch. Dermitol.* 101:181–86
182. Fechner, R. E. 1970. *Cancer* 25:1332–39
183. Connell, E. B., Kelman, C. D. 1969. *Fert. Steril.* 20:67–79
184. McQuarrie, H. G., Scott, C. D., Ellsworth, H. S., Harris, J. W., Stone, R. A. 1970. *Am. J. Obstet. Gynecol.* 108:659–65
185. Bishun, N. P., Mills, J., 1971. *Brit. Med. J.* 3:704
186. Shapiro, L. R., Graves, Z. R., Hirschhorn, K. 1972. *Obstet. Gynecol.* 39:190–92
187. Apelo, R., Veloso, I. 1973. *Fert. Steril.* 24:191–97
188. Feldman, J. G., Lippes, J. 1971. *Contraception* 3:93–104
189. Hall, L. 1973. *Am. J. Obstet. Gynecol.* 116:671–81
190. Frantz, A. G. 1973. In *Frontiers in Neuroendocrinology,* ed. W. F. Ganong, L. Martini, 337–74. New York: Oxford Univ. Press
191. Adams, P. W. et al 1973. *Lancet* 1: 897–904

NEWER CEPHALOSPORINS ❖6602
AND "EXPANDED-SPECTRUM"
PENICILLINS

Lauri D. Thrupp
University of California at Irvine, Irvine, California

The tremendous effort of the past two decades in developing semisynthetic modifications of existing antibiotics as well as in screening for new natural agents has produced a large number of new products, which suggested some time ago that a point of diminishing returns was being approached (1). In recent years the majority of new compounds reaching clinical investigation has resulted from evolution of the technology for semisynthetic modifications of either the 6-aminopenicillanic acid (6-APA) or the 7-aminocephalosporanic acid nucleus (2–6). Chemical alterations have been designed specifically to produce more desirable properties such as the following: (*a*) improved acid stability; (*b*) broadened microbiological spectrum; (*c*) improved activity against resistant organisms (by a variety of mechanisms such as improved resistance to enzymatic degradation, inhibition of degrading enzyme production, improved intrinsic activity through better steric fit, better cell penetration, etc); (*d*) improved metabolic or pharmacologic efficiency, such as better oral absorption, slower excretion, better tissue diffusion; and (*e*) decreased allergenecity (1). Significant advances have been made toward these goals.

Major among these advances has been enhanced resistance to degradation by staphylococcal β-lactamase, accomplished with the series of semisynthetic penicillins which have seen extensive clinical application begining with methicillin and subsequently including nafcillin and the isoxazolyl series (oxacillin, cloxacillin, dicloxacillin, and most recently under evaluation, flucloxacillin). The microbiology, pharmacology, and clinical applications of these drugs have been reviewed (7–12) and will not be included in this report because there are few new developments in the application of these agents.

In addition to high activity against Gram-positive cocci and bacilli, the action of penicillin G also includes moderately high activity against *Neisseria,* relatively modest activity against *Hemophilus,* and low-level activity against *Enterobacteriaceae* such as *Escherichia coli* and *Salmonella* (see Table 1). However, early

435

attempts at treatment of *Hemophilus* meningitis with penicillin G in moderate doses were not particularly successful, and primary treatment of serious *Hemophilus* infection with large doses has not been examined in recent years. Massive doses of penicillin have been used to treat Gram-negative septicemia (13); the results, though uncontrolled, were not conclusive and were complicated by penicillin neurotoxicity (14). Thus, except for Stamey's suggestion of penicillin G prophylaxis for recurrent cystitis (15), penicillin G treatment of infection due to Gram-negative bacilli is not widely recommended. Therefore, improved antimicrobial activity against Gram-negative bacilli (particularly *Hemophilus,* enterics, and *Pseudomonas*) and improved pharmacologic efficiency have been the other main objectives in developing semisynthetic penicillins and cephalosporins. This report reviews the present status of the "expanded-spectrum" penicillins and of newer cephalosporins. It has not been possible to include all compounds reported. [We have excluded, for example, two promising compounds, pivampicillin (16) and cephanone (16a, 16b), because development of these agents has apparently been delayed.]

NEWER "EXPANDED-SPECTRUM" PENICILLINS

Ampicillin, D-α-aminobenzyl penicillin, described in 1961, showed increased activity against enteric bacilli and *Hemophilus*. It was the first such agent to receive extensive clinical trial and has since achieved wide use and probable overuse. The microbiologic activity, pharmacology, and clinical applications have been reviewed (17–25) and will not be detailed here. For comparison, summaries of the antibacterial spectrum, relative activity, and clinical pharmacology of ampicillin are included in Tables 1–3, which summarize selected data for penicillins G and V and ampicillin for comparison with more recently developed compounds. Examples of drugs generally resembling ampicillin in spectrum, without clinically significant activity against penicillinase-producing staphylococci or against *Pseudomonas,* include hetacillin, amoxicillin, epicillin, azidocillin, and cyclacillin. Compounds with some activity against *Pseudomonas* include carbenicillin sodium, idanyl carbenicillin, and ticarcillin.

Hetacillin and Ampicillin

CLASSIFICATION   Hetacillin was produced by reacting ampicillin with acetone (22), producing a compound resembling ampicillin with the inclusion of a dimethylimidazolidinyl structure in the side chain (Figure 1). Hetacillin is rapidly and virtually quantitatively hydrolyzed both in vitro and in vivo so that the active agent remaining is apparently ampicillin.

ANTIMICROBIAL ACTIVITY   Because hetacillin is hydrolyzed to ampicillin the activity is that of ampicillin, including high activity against pneumococci, streptococci, and penicillin sensitive staphylococci, in the same range as penicillin G and V, but with significant activity also against *Hemophilus* and certain *Enterobacteriaceae* (See Table 1) but not against *Pseudomonas*.

CLINICAL PHARMACOLOGY   Conversion to ampicillin in the process of gastro-intestinal absorption or uptake from intramuscular sites takes place rapidly, with little

Table 1 Antibacterial activity of penicillin G and representative "expanded spectrum" staphylococcal β-lactamase-susceptible semisynthetic penicillins

Bacterial Species	Penicillin G MIC Mode (Range) (μg/ml)	Penicillin G Prop. "Resist."[a] (%)	Ampicillin MIC Mode (Range) (μg/ml)	Ampicillin Prop. "Resist."[a] (%)	Amoxicillin MIC Mode (Range) (μg/ml)	Amoxicillin Prop. "Resist."[a] (%)	Azidocillin MIC Mode (Range) (μg/ml)	Carbenicillin MIC Mode (Range) (μg/ml)	Carbenicillin Prop. "Resist."[a] (%)	Ticarcillin MIC Mode (Range) (μg/ml)	Ticarcillin Prop. "Resist."[a] (%)
Strep. pneumoniae	0.01(<0.01-0.02)	(0)	0.02(<0.01-0.1)	(0)	0.04(0.01-0.05)	(0)	<0.01	0.4(0.1-1)	(1)[b]	1(0.6-2.5)	(0)
Strep. pyogenes (A)	<0.01(<0.01-0.02)	(0)	0.01(<0.01-0.2)	(0)	0.01(<0.01-0.2)	(0)	<0.01	0.2(0.1-1)	(1)	0.8(0.3-2.5)	(0)
Staph. aureus (Non-Pase)	0.06(0.02-0.2)	(0)	0.1 (0.04-0.3)	(0)	0.1 (0.04-0.3)	(0)	0.06(0.01-0.5)	5(1-10)	(1)	2.5(1-10)	(1)
Enterococci	3(2-5)	(1)	1.25(0.5-5)	(1)	1.25(0.5-5)	(1)	(0.25-4)	50	(100)	25	(100)
N. gonorrhoeae	0.05(<0.01-2.5)	(v)[c]	0.02(0.01-1.0)	(v)	0.02(0.01-0.3)	(v)					
N. meningitidis	0.06	(0)	0.03	(0)	0.02			0.1			
H. influenzae	0.6 (0.1-3)	(1)	0.2 (0.05-1.0)	(5)	0.2 (0.02-1.0)	(5)	0.6 (0.1-3)	(0.5-125)[a]			
E. coli	(16->125)	(30)[a]	3(<1->125)	(20)[a]	3(<1->125)	(25)[a]	(32->125)	5(2->125)	(20)[a]	3(1->125)	(10)[a]
Salmonella	(2-64)		1(0.4->125)	(10)[a]	1(<0.5->125)	(10)[a]		(4-16)		(2-8)	
Proteus mirabilis	8(2->125)	(90)[a]	1(0.5->125)	(10)[a]	0.5(0.2->125)	(10)[a]	(16-128)	1(0.5->125)	(10)[a]	1(0.2->125)	(<10)[a]
Proteus (other)	(16->250)		125(32->125)	(90)[a]	125(50->125)	(90)[a]	125	2(0.5->125)	(15)[a]	2(0.2->125)	(10)[a]
K pneumoniae	>250		12(4->125)	(80)[a]	12(25->125)	(90)[a]	>125	>125(50->125)	(100)	>125(50->125)	(100)
Enterobacter	>250		50(25->125)	(85)[a]	>125		>125	32(6->125)	(25)[a]	6(3->125)	(25)[a]
Pseudomonas	>250		>250		>250		>125	32(8->250)	(20-[a])	16(2->250)	(15+[a])

[a] "Resistant" to serum concentrations of drug achieved with "normal" dosage. Proportion may vary markedly depending on strain selection, nosocomial origin, and testing methodology including inoculum size.

[b] 1 = Many strains intermediate in susceptibility.

[c] v = Variable proportion of strains (approximately 5-30%) with MICs at high end of range, depending on population studied.

Table 2 Clinical-pharmacologic characteristics of penicillin G, V and selected "expanded spectrum" semisynthetic penicillins

Drug	Proportion of Oral Dose Absorbed (%)	Protein-Bound (%)	Route of Admin.	Maximum Serum Level 0.5 g Dose Mode (Range) (μg/ml)	Serum Half-Life (hr.)	Recovery in Urine (% of Dose)
Penicillin G (benzyl)	20-30	20-60	oral	2.5 (2-6)	0.6	15-25
			im	4.5 (2-6)	0.5-1	90-100
			iv-inf.	10	0.4	90-100
Penicillin V (phenoxymethyl)	25-50	70-80	oral	2.5	0.5	35-50
Ampicillin	30-60	16-20	oral	3.5 (1.5-6)	1-2	35-45
			im	7.5 (6-9)	1.1	75
			iv-inf.	12	0.6-1.0	75
Amoxicillin	50-80	15-25	oral	8 (3-20)	1	60-90
Epicillin		10-30	oral	5 (2-9)	1	40
Azidocillin	75	85	oral	5-7	0.5	60-70
			im	6-9	1.0	85
Carbenicillin sodium	–	50	im	10-18	1.5	80-98
			iv-inf.	40 est.	1	
Carbenicillin indanyl	40	50	oral	5-7	1	50
Ticarcillin	–	45	im	22 (14-32)	2	85-98
			iv-inf.[a]	40 est.	1.1	

[a] 5 g given iv in 15-30 min will produce peak serum levels >300 μg/ml.

or no delay in absorption-excretion kinetics compared with administration of ampicillin. There are only minor variations in clinical pharmacology between ampicillin and hetacillin. One study showed slightly higher hetacillin serum levels following iv administration (23), while others (22) showed slightly lower levels compared with ampicillin following oral or intramuscular administration. Kirby & Kind noted slight delay in excretion and suggested that these resulted from greater acid stability of hetacillin together with a slight time lag for hydrolysis of hetacillin to ampicillin in vivo (25). Hetacillin was slightly more resistant than ampicillin to in vivo inactivation, presumably by the liver, and both ampicillin and hetacillin show lower renal clearance compared with penicillin G (23–25).

CLINICAL EFFECTIVENESS Treatment of a variety of infections with hetacillin has produced results which approximate those expected for ampicillin, including meningitis (26), respiratory infections (27), and typhoid fever (28–29). Hence, there is no

Table 3 Estimated minimum therapeutic ratio for penicillin G, V and selected "expanded spectrum" penicillins against common pathogens

Drug	Route of Admin. of 0.5 g Dose	Ratio (minimum peak serum level[a]/MIC[b])									
		Str. pn.	Str. A	St. aur. (N-Pase)	Enterococ.	H. infl.	E. coli	Klebs	Pr. mirab.	Prot. Other	Pseudo.
Penicillin G (benzyl)	oral	100	100	10-50	1	1	0.2	0	0.1	0	0
	im	100	100	10-50	1	1	0.2	0	0.1	0	0
	iv-inf.	1000	1000	50-100	3	3	1	0	0.5	0	0
Penicillin V (phenoxymethyl)	oral	75	75	10-25	1	1	0.02	0	0.2	0	0
Ampicillin	oral	20	10	10	0.5	2	1[c]	0.1[c]	1[c]	0	0
	im	30	20	30	1.5	6	2[c]	0.3[c]	3[c]	0	0
	iv-inf.	60	40	60	3	10-15	4[c]	1[c]	6[c]	0	0
Amoxicillin	oral	50	100	10	1	3	1[c]	0.1[c]	1[c]	0	0
Azidocillin	oral	500	500	10	1	1	0.2[c]	0	0.2[c]	0	0
	im										
Carbenicillin sodium	im	10	10	1	0.2		1[c]	0	5[c]	2[c]	0.2[c]
	iv-inf.[d]	40	40	4	1		4[c]	0	20[c]	10[c]	1[c]
Carbenicillin indanyl	oral	5	5	0.5	0.1		0.5[c]	0	2[c]	1[c]	0.1[c]
Ticarcillin	im	5	5	1.5	0.5		2[c]	0	6[c]	3[c]	0.5[c]
	iv-inf.[d]	50	50	5	1		10[c]	0	20[c]	10[c]	1[c]

[a]Minimum value from reported range of peak serum levels, unadjusted for duration of level, volume of distribution, etc.

[b]MIC = minimum inhibitory concentration (Maximum of range of MICs for species or strains considered "susceptible" to therapy, unadjusted for protein-binding, tissue diffusion, etc; used in deriving the ratio estimate.)

[c]Higher dosage would achieve higher ratios with some strains but a variable proportion are quite resistant and would not be amenable to any therapy. Others are inhibited at high levels such as achieved in urine.

[d]For treatment of *Pseudomonas septicemia* higher dosage necessary, e.g. 4-5 g infusions.

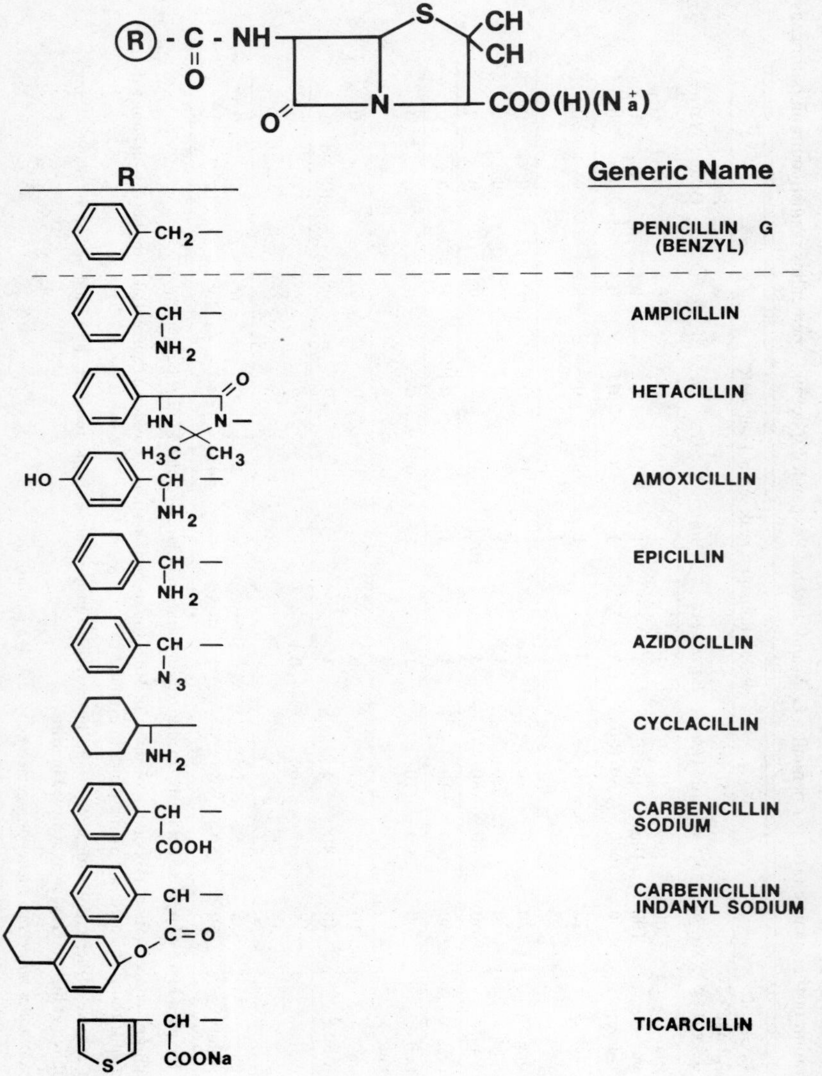

Figure 1 Structure of penicillin G, penicillin V, ampicillin, and representative newer, "expanded" spectrum, (penicillinase-susceptible), penicillins.

reason to suspect that hetacillin shows any advantage warranting its use instead of ampicillin.

TOXICITY AND HYPERSENSITIVITY   Direct pharmacologic toxicity should be almost nonexistent for hetacillin, as for ampicillin and penicillin, and would probably be limited to encephalopathy such as recorded with massive doses of penicillin (14) or ampicillin (30), particularly in the presence of renal failure.

The incidence of skin rashes, usually macular or maculopapular, and occasionally morbilliform, is clearly higher following ampicillin compared with the other penicillins (31) and is even higher in patients also receiving allopurinol (32), and in patients with infectious mononucleosis the incidence is so high as to be suggestively diagnostic (33). Bierman et al (34) studied hemagglutinating antibody and skin-test reactivity to benzyl penicillin, benzyl penicillaote, benzyl penicilloyl polylysine, ampicillin, and hetacillin in patients with a history of rashes induced by ampicillin or hetacillin. Their results indicated that few of the maculopapular type of eruptions were demonstrable as true immunologic allergy and seldom recurred on rechallenge, whereas urticarial reactions were much more likely to be immunologic in origin (34). The mechanism of these "toxic" rashes is not clear. Clinical data are not extensive enough to determine whether the other newer penicillin and ampicillin analogs will be associated with similar eruptions. Bierman's study (34) included hetacillin testing, and although details are not presented, it is likely that here again hetacillin is behaving essentially as ampicillin.

Amoxicillin

CLASSIFICATION   As indicated in Figure 1, the structure of amoxicillin, or α-amino-p-hydroxybenzyl-penicillin differs from ampicillin only in the addition of the parahydroxy group. Similar to ampicillin, amoxicillin is relatively insoluble in water but is soluble in pH8 phosphate buffer (35). It shows greater stability to gastric juice pH of 1.5 than ampicillin (half-lives of 17 hr for amoxicillin and 12 hr for ampicillin).

ANTIMICROBIAL ACTIVITY   In vitro activity of amoxicillin is virtually identical with that of ampicillin, both in its spectrum and relative activity (excellent activity against penicillin-sensitive Gram-positive pathogens and moderate activity against enterococci and certain Gram-negative bacilli). There is essentially complete cross-resistance between ampicillin and amoxicillin against a number of strains and species of Gram-negative enteric bacilli. Neither amoxicillin or ampicillin are active against *Pseudomonas* (35–37).

CLINICAL PHAMACOLOGY   Compared with ampicillin, amoxicillin shows remarkably improved absorption following oral administration (37–43). The pattern of renal excretion is similar to that of ampicillin, indicating that the higher serum levels and more complete recovery in the urine (70% in 6 hr for amoxicillin compared with 40–50% for ampicillin) are the result of more complete oral absorption rather than other basic differences in pharmacokinetics (Table 2, 40–42).

The effect of food on absorption of amoxicillin is not great, but peak serum levels are somewhat lower and the time of peak levels delayed in nonfasting subjects. Middleton et al (44) noted greater variability in serum levels in patients, compared with data from normal subjects (38–41), as might be anticipated because of difficulty controlling clinical variables such as food intake and gastrointestinal disorders in patient populations. Probenecid produced modest delay in urinary excretion and somewhat higher serum levels (37).

Because of the generally better absorption after oral dosing, with serum levels significantly higher compared with ampicillin, it is evident that amoxicillin theoretically should provide an improved "therapeutic ratio," as indicated in Table 3, which presents an arbitrary ratio between the lower end of the range of expected peak serum levels and the minimum inhibitory concentrations (MICs) of common pathogens. (No attempt has been made to adjust these ratios by taking into account additional, more complex factors, such as protein binding, tissue diffusion, lipid solubility, and membrane transport. Table 3 therefore provides only an arbitary reference ratio based on direct assays of serum levels and should not be taken to imply that such ratios can necessarily be translated into differences in clinical efficacy.)

Administration of amoxicillin and ampicillin to animals produced similar serum levels after parenteral administration but much higher levels following oral administration of amoxicillin (40), similar to the human phamacologic findings. In treatment of experimental infections, amoxicillin proved significantly superior to identical doses of ampicillin; however, the differences were evident not only after oral drug, which was expected, but also after parenteral administration, which was not anticipated in view of the similar serum levels and similar MICs of the infecting organism. It did not appear likely that differences in protein binding were responsible for the apparent paradox, and no other explanation was yet evident (40).

CLINICAL APPLICATION   No clinical evidence has appeared to prove that the pharmacologic advantage of improved absorption has necessarily resulted in better clinical response compared with ampicillin or with other drugs effective against similar pathogens. Satisfactory clinical and bacteriologic response has been recorded in uncontrolled studies of urinary tract infections (44) and in streptococcal infections of upper respiratory tract and skin (45). Additional clinical experience, including controlled trials, will be required to determine whether the pharmacologic advantage of improved absorption of amoxicillin can be fully used clinically by employing lower dosage or by substitution of oral instead of the parenteral dosage now required when high serum levels of ampicillin are needed.

Epicillin

CLASSIFICATION   Epicillin (amino-cydohexadienyl penicillin) is an acid-stable semisynthetic penicillin similar in structure to ampicillin (Figure 1). The low, reversible serum protein binding (46) and susceptibility to degradation by staphylococcal β-lactamase (47) are also similar to ampicillin.

ANTIMICROBIAL ACTIVITY   The antibacterial activity of epicillin is sufficiently close to that of ampicillin so that the characteristic MIC values are not listed separately in Table 1. In summary, epicillin shows high activity against Group A streptococci, pneumococci, non-penicillinase-producing staphylococci, and penicillin-sensitive anaerobes and *Neisseria,* and moderate activity against *Hemophilus* and against selected ampicillin-sensitive strains of enteric bacilli, notably *Proteus mirabilis* and *E. coli.* In addition, epicillin shows somewhat greater activity than ampicillin against certain strains of *Pseudomonas* and indol-positive *Proteus* (46), but this activity is less than that of carbenicillin against these strains and is not likely to be of clinical value. Otherwise, cross-resistance and spectrum seem virtually identical between epicillin and ampicillin.

CLINICAL PHARMACOLOGY   The clinical pharmacology of epicillin is similar to ampicillin (Table 2) with similar rates of oral absorption and a serum half-life of about 1 hr. Some 30% of the oral dose is recovered in the urine within 6 hr in full active form. Serum levels and total absorption following oral administration appear to be slightly less than for ampicillin, but it is unlikely that these differences would be significant clinically.

CLINICAL APPLICATION   A variety of infections in adults and children have been treated with parenteral and oral epicillin. These largely uncontrolled trials have included patients with infections of the upper and lower respiratory tact, *Salmonella* and *Shigella* infections, soft-tissue infections, and urinary tract infections (48–50). Clinical results appear as good as could have been anticipated. However, in the absence of detailed analyses of clinical pharmacologic and microbiologic data in individual patients or of controlled trials, further conclusions cannot be drawn beyond the apparent similarity to ampicillin.

Azidocillin

CLASSIFICATION   Azidocillin (α-azidobenzyl-penicillin) is also similar generally to ampicillin in structure (Figure 1), activity (Table 1), and pharmacology (Table 2). Its acid stability is similar to penicillin V, better than penicillin G, but somewhat less than ampicillin (51). It differs from ampicillin in the much greater protein binding (80–85%), compared with 15–20% for ampicillin (51).

ANTIMICROBIAL ACTIVITY   Against Gram-positive cocci the antibacterial activity of azidocillin is also generally similar to ampicillin and penicillin. Minor differences are as follows: against *Streptococcus pneumoniae, Strep. viridans,* and *Strep. pyogenes* it is slightly more active than ampicillin or penicillin G; against penicillin sensitive *Staphylococcus aureus* it is slightly less active than penicillin or ampicillin; and against *Haemophilus influenzae* and *H. parainfluenzae* it is similar to penicillun G but shows slightly higher MICs than ampicillin. It is susceptible to staphylococcal penicillinase and therefore is inactive against penicillin-resistant *Staph. aureus.* The activity against enterococci is similar to ampicillin but apparently fourfold better than penicillin G (52,53).

Azidocillin is not significantly active against Gram-negative enteric bacilli, showing similar or less activity against *E. coli* and *Proteus* than penicillin G or V, and is clearly less active than ampicillin against enteric bacilli (52, 53).

CLINICAL PHARMACOLOGY Azidocillin (Table 2) shows good (about 75%) oral absorption, more complete than ampicillin or penicillin G or V. Peak serum levels, reached within 1 hr after oral doses, are somewhat higher than either penicillin G, V, or ampicillin, and appear equally rapidly after oral or im administration. Some 70% appears in the urine after oral administration compared with 85% after im doses (54, 55). Peak serum levels are slightly higher than penicillin G, V, or ampicillin following oral doses; however, this combination of slightly higher peak serum levels, together with MICs, which are only slightly lower against streptococci and pneumococci, produces theoretical therapeutic ratios against these pathogens which exceed those of any of the other penicillins (Table 3). This greater therapeutic margin would be offset in theory by the somewhat greater protein-binding of azidopenicillin, and it is unlikely that the theoretical ratio difference would prove clinically significant.

In studying experimental *H. influenzae* meningitis, Lithander found azidocillin and benzyl-penicillin levels in cerebrospinal fluid (CSF) slightly lower than ampicillin (56) and confirmed earlier studies in meningitis patients that suggested that ampicillin reaches slightly higher levels in CSF than does penicillin (24).

CLINICAL APPLICATION Azidopenicillin is under clinical trial for respiratory infections (57) with the objective of determining the clinical efficacy of this active penicillin which shows good pharmacologic characteristics together with high activity against respiratory pathogens, but like penicillin G or V, remains narrow spectrum in its limited activity against facultative enteric bacilli. Indeed, should azidopenicillin produce fewer reactions, or because of its lower activity against enterics and more complete upper GI absorption produce less change in lower intestinal flora than ampicillin, then such decreased side effects might represent a potential therapeutic advantage. Unfortunately, this expectation was not realized in one 6-month placebo-controlled trial of ampicillin and azidocillin for continuous prophylaxis in 40 children with severe chronic bronchitis and bronchiectasis (57). One third of the patients carried ampicillin- and cephaloridine-resistant *E. coli* at the beginning of the trial; this proportion did not change in the placebo group (who reported somewhat more respiratory symptoms), but the number with resistant coliforms doubled in both the ampicillin and azidocillin-treated groups. Kerrebigin's findings suggested that exposure to the 6-APA nucleus was sufficient stimulus to induce and/or select penicillinase producing strains of *E. coli* (57).

Cyclacillin

CLASSIFICATION AND ANTIMICROBIAL ACTIVITY Cyclacillin (amino-cyclohexane penicillin) is an acid-stable penicillin that shows moderate activity in vitro against a spectrum of organisms similar to penicillin and ampicillin. It is somewhat more resistant to degradation by staphylococcal penicillinase, but despite partial effectiveness in experimental infections, it is not likely that the drug warrants clinical application in treatment of infections due to penicillinase-producing staphylococci. The activity against pneumococci, Group A streptococci, and nonpenicillinase-producing *Staph. aureus* is clearly less than ampicillin or penicillin G or V but is similar to that observed for cephalexin (58,59). Activity in vitro against selected Gram-negative bacilli is manyfold less than that of ampicillin, and from limited published data appears in the range expected for penicillin G or V (58, 59).

PHARMACOLOGY AND EXPERIMENTAL INFECTION From limited published data, cyclacillin appears to be reasonably well absorbed (60, 61), producing serum levels similar to penicillin V, but not as high as cephalexin (60, 61). Protein binding is a low 20%, similar to ampicillin, and produces a similarly small effect on MIC endpoints (58, 60).

The notable feature of cyclacillin is the marked discrepancy between its modest in vitro activity and its striking in vivo effectiveness in experimental infections particularly with Gram-positive pathogens. Not only were highly significantly lower ED_{50} values recorded for treatment of a variety of infections in mice, but the duration of effectiveness of single doses far exceeded that of ampicillin or penicillin (61). It seemed unlikely that low protein binding and good tissue diffusion were sufficient explanation for the differences between in vitro and experimental in vivo activity (61). This prolonged activity in vivo suggested the possibility that a metabolic product with residual antibacterial activity might be excreted slowly, such as the slow excretion of aminocyclopentane carboxylic acid found by Christensen in man and rat (62). Prolonged retention of such a metabolite would, if confirmed, also suggest careful study to rule out any unexpected tissue toxicity, for example, in the kidney which showed high levels of cyclacillin in animal tissue assays (58).

CLINICAL APPLICATIONS Clinical applications of cyclacillin are not well defined, and caution is indicated in view of the modest in vitro activity. Nevertheless, one controlled study of Group A streptococcal pharyngitis demonstrated equivalent effectiveness for cephalixin, penicillin V, and cyclacillin (63).

Carbenicillin Sodium

Disodium carbenicillin has been marketed extensively and has been the subject of recent reviews and symposia (64–67); the following summarizes the current status of parenteral carbenicillin.

CLASSIFICATION AND ANTIMICROBIAL ACTIVITY Carbenicillin (disodium α-carboxybenzyl-pencillin) is the first semisynthetic penicillin to reach extensive clinical application specifically because of its enhanced activity against selected Gram-negative bacilli, primarily *Pseudomonas* and indol-positive *Proteus*. It shows relatively modest activity against other Gram-positive and Gram-negative pathogens comprising an overall spectrum similar to that of ampicillin (68–72).

RESISTANCE OF PSEUDOMONAS AND ENTEROBACTERIACEAE TO CARBENICILLIN While most investigators have found that three fourths or more of *Pseudomonas* strains are inhibited by $100\mu g/ml$ or less, a part of the variability in various studies results from differences in methodology. Variation in endpoints results from differences in inocula, media, and test systems. On the other hand, the emergence of increasing proportions of resistant strains was predicted from early in vitro studies (71, 72). One common pattern of resistance observed in many strains seems to be a stable heterotypic manifestation not associated with production of specific inactivating enzymes, but manifest for example in discrepancies between inhibitory and bactericidal endpoints. A second mechanism for resistance has also been demonstrated. Episomal R-factors mediating linked resistance to carbenicillin, probably via carbenicillin β-lactamase, and to other antibiotics, have been transferred between *Pseudomonas* and other *Enterobacteriaceae* in vitro (73, 74), in vivo, and in burn wound infections with *Pseudomonas* and *Klebsiella* in mice (73), and such strains have emerged as major clinical problems (67, 73).

SYNERGISM BETWEEN CARBENICILLIN AND GENTAMICIN   Carbenicillin and gentamicin show apparent synergism against many (probably one half to two thirds) strains of *Pseudomonas;* and in the remainder of isolates, these drugs are either addictive or are indifferent (75, 76). Combined therapy might hopefully 1. provide optimal therapeutic ratios in vivo, particularly in immuno-suppressed patients, 2. decrease the chance that resistant variants would emerge either in the individual patient, or 3. be selected epidemiologically, and 4. decrease the chances of gentamicin toxicity by lowering the gentamicin dosage required to achieve "adequate" serum bactericidal activity. It is unlikely that all of these goals will be achieved by combination therapy. Despite combined therapy, superinfections occur with other resistant Gram-negative bacilli, and resistant *Pseudomonas* variants have emerged (67). Final resolution of data suggesting effective results with carbenicillin alone (65) compared with findings of more effective response with combined therapy when the two drugs are synergistic (77), must await further definition of the pharmacologic-microbiologic findings in such series, hopefully prospectively controlled. Nevertheless, statistically improved results (82% "clinical success") when synergism was demonstrated versus 53% when the drugs used were not synergistic (77) and the weight of present evidence seems to favor combined therapy at least for severe infections with *Pseudomonas* when the infecting strain is synergistically inhibited in vitro (77, 82, 83).

CLINICAL PHARMACOLOGY   Carbenicillin sodium is relatively unstable in acid pH and must be administered parenterally; it is approximately 50% protein bound and like penicillin G, is not a notably lipid-soluble compound, yet achieves reasonable tissue distribution. It is rapidly excreted in the urine, with most of the active drug recovered in the urine (Table 2). Following 0.5 g im doses, peak serum levels of 10–18 $\mu g/ml$ are achieved. Intravenous infusions of 4 or 5 g can be given, producing rapid peak serum levels of several hundred $\mu g/ml$, and with levels 1 hr later still at 200 $\mu g/ml$. This exceeds the MIC of the majority of strains of *Pseudomonas,* but because many isolates show MICs in the range of 64–256 μg/ml (Table 1), it is clear that for such strains only marginal therapeutic ratios would be achieved (Table 3) and would be maintained only for the first hr following the infusion.

The serum half-life of approximately 1 hr is slightly longer than penicillin or ampicillin. Thus, hepatic excretion and/or degradation of carbenicillin is slower than other penicillins. This is reflected also in longer half-lives in anuric patients (Table 7): 10–16 hours for carbenicillin compared with 3–4 hr for penicillin G and 8–9 hr for ampicillin. Primary hepatic failure also increases the serum half-life of carbenicillin up to 2 hr (78), but the severity of impairment in hepatic function was not correlated with the carbenicillin half-life (except in patients who also had impaired renal function). Kunin found the half-life of penicillin G was also markedly prolonged in patients with combined hepatic as well as renal failure (79). Probenecid delays renal secretion, elevating and prolonging the peak serum levels (80).

CARBENICILLIN INACTIVATION BY GENTAMICIN   In view of the recommended combination of carbenicillin plus gentamicin therapy for serious Gram-negative infection, the report of apparent inactivation of gentamicin by carbenicillin in vivo as well as in vitro (81) has raised continuing concern. Several investigators have negated the in vivo implications of the original report, and Riff & Jackson have summarized further in vitro and in vivo data (84–87). Carbenicillin and gentamicin interact when mixed in vitro resulting in mutual inactivation, with higher rates of inactivation at higher temperatures, at high ratios of carbenicillin:gentamicin, and in water solution compared with saline (with the least reaction in serum). In vivo, however, Jackson found inactivation only in patients in severe renal failure with the expected gentamicin half-life > 60 hours; the half-life of a dose of gentamicin was decreased to 24 hr by concomitant carbenicillin (87).

CLINICAL APPLICATIONS   Clinical applications of sodium carbenicillin have been reviewed (67). The primary use of carbenicillin is for serious *Pseudomonas* infection, either alone or in combination with gentamicin, including septicemia (64), severe burns (88), osteomyelitis (89), meningitis (90), urinary tract infections (91a), and pulmonary infections (91). Many patients who develop *Pseudomonas* infections, of course, have serious underlying disease, and evaluation of the response to antibiotic therapy is difficult, particularly in pulmonary infections. Nevertheless, despite the relatively high MICs of many strains of *Pseudomonas,* carbenicillin is the only available penicillin analog with significant activity against *Pseudomonas,* and the only other available agents are gentamicin with its potential for toxicity, and the polymyxins, which probably are of limited value in systemic treatment of serious tissue infection. Carbenicillin is the only "nontoxic" antibiotic with demonstrated reasonable clinical efficacy in serious *Pseudomonas* infection. Similarly, carbenicillin is the only alternative or adjunctive nontoxic drug available for treatment of serious infection due to nonmirabilis *Proteus* or due to occasional additional tetracycline, ampicillin, and cephalosporin-resistant Gram-negatives that are often nosocomial in origin.

Indanyl Carbenicillin

CLASSIFICATION AND ACTIVITY Indanyl carbenicillin is the indanyl ester of carbenicillin (Figure 1). Sodium carbenicillin is not absorbed after oral administration,
but the indanyl ester is stable at 37°C for 1 hr in gastric juice pH2, and as indicated
in Table 2, some 40% absorbed. Specific assay for the ester shows an early transient
peak in the serum at 30 min. Following absorption the ester is promptly cleaved by
serum and tissue esterases to yield the primary antibiotic carbenicillin plus free
indanol, and by 90 min the ester is no longer detectable in serum (92). The free
indanol is conjugated as glucuronide and sulfate esters and is excreted almost
completely in the urine (93). The indanyl ester is the most lipophilic of the penicillins
and is highly protein bound (94). It has intrinsic antimicrobial activity which is
similar to disodium carbenicillin for Gram-negatives, but which is significantly more
active against Gram-positive pathogens, apparently as the result of the modified
physical-chemical properties of the ester. Hydrolysis of the ester to carbenicillin
takes place over a period of hours in broth but occurs quite rapidly in vivo, hence
the actual activity in vivo is that of carbenicillin. The MIC and therapeutic ratio
values listed in Tables 1 & 3 thus are those assayed as carbenicillin, not as the
indanyl ester.

CLINICAL PHARMACOLOGY AND APPLICATIONS   Some 40% is absorbed orally from
0.5 g doses, producing serum levels in the range of 5–10 $\mu g/ml$ (102, 103). Higher
dosage and multiple dose schedules produced increased levels, up to doses of 16–26
g/day which produced nausea, some vomiting and diarrhea, which limited further
absorption. Serum levels reached 40 $\mu g/ml$ and urine levels up to 7000 $\mu g/ml$ on
the large oral doses (94). On dosage schedules tolerated by most patients, however,
the serum levels are not high enough to provide significant therapeutic ratios against
Gram-negative organisms (see Table 3), and effective levels are achieved only in the
urine. Indanyl carbenicillin therefore is indicated only for treatment of urinary tract
infections where the drug provides unique therapeutic advantage against those
organisms that are uniquely susceptible to carbenicillin among the "nontoxic" drugs
—namely against *Pseudomonas,* nonmirabilis *Proteus,* and a few other selected
enteric Gram-negative bacilli. The clinical efficacy of indanyl carbenicillin in treatment of urinary tract infection has been well documented (95–99). Cox has reviewed
the clinical-pharmacologic paradox, however, that confronts the clinician attempting to manage patients with *Pseudomonas* or "persistent" *Proteus* urinary tract
infections. Such patients too often have chronic renal disease and are already in renal
failure (creatinine clearance under 15 ml/min), such that urinary concentrations of
indanyl carbenicillin (or of other antibiotics) are too low to permit successful treatment (100, 101).

Ticarcillin

Ticarcillin (or α-carboxyl thienylmethyl-penicillin, Figure 1) is a semisynthetic
penicillin that is unstable in acid solution and must be administered parenterally.
The spectrum of organisms inhibited and the mechanisms and degree of activity are
similar to sodium carbenicillin, with therapeutic utility also because of its activity

specifically against *Pseudomonas,* nonmirabilis *Proteus* species, and selected other Gram-negative bacilli usually resistant to other antibiotics except gentamicin or kanamycin. It is also synergistically active with gentamicin.

Early studies of ticarcillin show two potential advantages over carbenicillin sodium. First, its in vitro activity against a variety of organisms, but particularly against *Pseudomonas,* is slightly greater than carbenicillin (104–106). Secondly, it shows slightly advantageous pharmacologic characteristics in that serum levels are slightly higher and serum half-life slightly longer (107–109). These differences (see Tables 1 and 2) are therefore sufficient to produce a theoretically slight advantage in Therapeutic Ratio compared with carbenicillin sodium, as summarized in Table 3. Data from clinical applications of this compound have not yet been published.

CEPHALOSPORINS

An expanding series of semisynthetic cephalosporins have been produced from cephalosporin C, one of the three natural products originally derived from a strain of *Cephalosporium acremonium,* the other two antibiotics being cephalosporin N and a steroid antibiotic similar to fusidic acid. The 7-amino-cephalosporanic acid nucleus of course is related closely in structure to the penicillin nucleus, but has a fused dihydrothiazine instead of a fused thiazolidine betalactam ring (110). Production of 7-amino-cephalosporanic acid from cephalosporin C (5, 6) permitted evolution of a large number of derivatives with varying physical, biological, and antimicrobial properties. This group has been reviewed (111–115). We will comment on the "older" cephalosporins as a base for comparison with "newer" cephalosporins.

Cephalothin and Cephaloridine

Sodium cephalothin (thiophene-acetamido-cephalosporanic acid, Figure 2) was the first derivative marketed, and cephaloridine (with two side chains added, thienyl- and pyridylmethyl) soon followed. The cephalosporins antibacterial activity is via mechanisms similar to the penicillins interference with cell-wall synthesis and is also usually bactericidal. Cephalothin and cephaloridine have similar spectra of antimicrobial activity, including good activity against Gram-positive cocci and bacilli and against a broad (but not complete) spectrum of Gram-negative organisms. Important exceptions, such as *Pseudomonas* and *Enterobacter* species, are often resistant by virtue of production of β-lactamase (or "cephalosporinases") with varying substrate affinities and specificities (116–121).

Gram-negative β-lactamases can be inhibited or inactivated by binding if simultaneously exposed to a penicillinase-resistant penicillin such as cloxacillin (122, 123). Combined therapy with such a combination (e.g. cloxacillin plus ampicillin, or cloxacillin plus cephaloridine) has been accomplished in vivo (124–126) as well as in vitro, but this approach now is clinically useful or necessary only rarely, especially with the availability of carbenicillin.

Resistance to staphylococcal penicillinase is a major advantage of the antimicrobial activity of the cephalosporins. Cephalothin is highly resistant to hydrolysis by staphylococcal penicillinase. Cephaloridine is sufficiently less resistant than ceph-alothin to penicillinase that use of cephaloridine for staphylococcal endocarditis has been questioned (116a). However, the predominant clinical experience has been favorable, including therapy of serious staphylococcal disease (115).

Table 4 summarizes the antibacterial activity of cephalothin and cephaloridine as well as the newer analogs. There is considerable variation in modes and ranges of MICs reported from various laboratories, depending upon methodology, inoculum size, strain selection, etc. This is particularly relevant in comparing data for many of the Gram-negative organisms for which a change in inoculum size may shift MIC endpoints twofold to eightfold and produce markedly different interpretation of susceptibility, as implied in the "Therapeutic Ratio" estimated in Table 6. For example, a three-dilution, methodology-induced variation in MIC endpoint of a *Streptococcus viridans* to cephalothin from 0.01 to 0.08 μg/ml need not raise therapeutic concern because of the high therapeutic ratio even at an MIC of 0.08 (Table 6); the therapeutic ratio for cephalothin in an *E. coli* tissue infection on the other hand is marginal at best (Table 6) and a three-dilution shift in MIC endpoint, from 2 to 16 μg/ml, might carry different implications concerning the susceptibility of that strain to therapy. This in part explains the variations reported in "percent susceptible" of various Gram-negative organisms to the various cephalosporins. Standardization of methodology and of interpretive standards for susceptibility testing is in need of improvement (see below).

Selected clinical-pharmacologic characteristics of cephalothin and cephaloridine are summarized in Table 5. Neither is significantly absorbed orally. Cephaloridine produces twice the serum levels of equivalent dosage of cephalothin, and the clear-ance of cephaloridine is slower, with a half-life of 1 hr compared with one-half hr for cephalothin. Therapeutic levels thus may be present in serum for only a brief period if cephalothin is given at 6 hr intervals. Both drugs are excreted in the urine in high concentrations.

Cephalothin is a weakly ionized salt, with a pK of about 2.8 similar to the pencillins, and a large component of the renal clearance of cephalothin is via tubular secretion. Cephaloridine is a zwitterion, relatively nonpolar, and renal clearance is equivalent to the glomerular filtration rate. Therefore, probenecid markedly delays urinary secretion of cephalothin, producing higher, more prolonged serum levels, whereas cephaloridine clearance is either unaffected (113) or only slightly delayed (111) by probenecid. Although cephalothin is 50–65% protein bound compared with only 25% for cephaloridine, and although neither is highly lipid soluble, both drugs appear in tissues and body fluids (114) and show 18 and 16 L/1.73 m² volumes of distribution, respectively (117a). CSF levels are poor, however, particularly for cephalothin (118a) and, while pneumococcal meningitis has been successfully treated with cephaloridine, cephalothin and cephaloridine have failed to clear meningococcal meningitis adequately despite in vitro susceptibility of the organism (119a).

Successful clinical application of cephalothin and cephaloridine have been exten-sive and comprise infection in most organ systems and with virtually all susceptible pathogens. Meningitis, particularly meningococcal, is an exception already men-tioned. Septicemia or serious tissue infection, aside from pyelonephritis, due to

Table 4 Antibacterial activity of representative cephalosporin antibiotics

Bacterial Species	Cephalothin MIC Mode (Range) (µg/ml)	Prop. "Resist."[a] (%)	Cephaloridine MIC Mode (Range) (µg/ml)	Prop. "Resist."[a] (%)	Cefazolin MIC Mode (Range) (µg/ml)	Prop. "Resist."[a] (%)	Cefoxitin MIC Mode (Range) (µg/ml)	Prop. "Resist."[a] (%)	Cephaloglycine MIC Mode (Range) (µg/ml)	Prop. "Resist."[a] (%)	Cephalexin MIC Mode (Range) (µg/ml)	Prop. "Resist."[a] (%)
Strep. pneumoniae	0.1(0.02-0.4)	(0)	0.03(0.01-0.2)	(0)	(0.1-0.3)	(0)	3		0.1(0.05-0.8)		2(0.1-12)	(1)[b]
Strep. pyogenes (A)	0.12(0.05-0.5)	(0)	0.01(0.002-0.1)	(0)	(0.1-0.3)	(0)	<0.8		0.2(0.05-2)		0.6(0.2-6)	(1)
Staph. aureus (Non-Pase)	0.1 (0.08-0.8)	(0)	0.1 (0.04-1)	(0)	0.1(0.06-2)	(0)	3		1.6(0.2-8)		2-6(0.5-16)	(1)
Staph. aureus (Pase)	0.2 (0.06-2)	(0)	0.5 (0.06-8)	(0)	0.3(0.06-8)	(0)	3		3(0.5-8)		2-9(0.5-16)	(1)
Enterococci	24(8-32)	(100)	16(4-32)	(100)	32(15-50)	(100)			50(16-128)		100(32-256)	(100)
N. gonorrhoeae	(0.25-3)	(1)	1.5	(1)	1(0.1->50)	(1)					3(0.1-6.3)	(1)
H. influenzae	(2-8)	(1)	(4-16)	(1)	(2-12)	(1)					>100(12.5->100)	(100)
E. coli	4(2-128)	(15a)	2(1-256)	(15a)	2(1-256)	(5a)	3(1-25)	(5a)	1(0.5-12.5)		4(1-32)	
Salmonella	(1.5-12)		(3-12)		2(1-6.25)						5(4-50)	(20a)
Proteus mirabilis	2(0.5-12)	(10)	2(1-25)	(15)	1(0.5-5)	(5)	1(0.5-6)	(0)	3(1-25)		8(4-50)	
Proteus other	(32->256)	(100)	(64->256)	(100)	50(2.5-100)	(60a)	6(3-25)	(10)	16->256		>100(25->100)	(100)
K. pneumoniae	4(1-8->256)	(15a)	4(1-8->256)	(15a)	2(1-8->256)	(15a)	3(0.8->256)	(10a)	1(0.25-4->256)	(10a)	12(1->100)	(30a)
Enterobacter	>100(2->256)	(90a)	>100(2->256)	(90a)	>100(2->256)	(80a)	50(2->256)	(75a)	>256		>100(50->100)	(100a)
Pseudomonas	>256		>256		>256		>256				>256	

a "Resistant" to serum concentrations of drug achieved with "normal" dosage. Proportion may vary markedly depending on strain selection, nosocomial origin, and testing methodology including inoculum size.

b 1 = Many strains intermediate in susceptibility.

Table 5 Clinical-pharmacologic characteristics of selected cephalosporin antibiotics

Drug	Proportion of Oral Dose Absorbed (%)	Apparent Volume of Distribution (L/1.73 M²)	Protein-Bound (%)	Route of Admin.	Maximum Serum Level 0.5 g Dose Mode or Range (µg/ml)	Serum Half-Life (hr)	Renal Clearance / Creatinine Clearance (Ratio)	Recovery in Urine (% of Dose)
Cephalothin (CT)	2	18	50-80	im iv	6-11 30-40 (18[a])	0.8 0.5[a]	2.4[a]	50-75 50-65
Cephapirin	–		44-50	im iv-inf.	8 30	0.8 0.5		65
Cephacetrile (CCT)	–		38	im iv-inf.	12[b] 35[b] (16–28[a])	1.3[a]	2.2[a]	88
Cephaloridine (CR)	5	16	20-35	im iv	18-22 60 (25[a])	1.1-1.5 1.1[a]	1.0[a]	60-90 85[a]
Cefazolin (CZ)	–	10	74-86	im iv-inf.	40 120	1.8 1.8[a]		70-80 96[a]
Cephaloglycine	20-30		15	oral	2-4.5	2		8-25
Cephalexin (CX)	80+	15	12-15	oral im iv-inf.	10-18 8-10 40 (27[a])	0.6-1.2 0.9 (0.6-0.9)[a]	1.7[a]	70-100 96[a]
Cephradine	95		15	oral	9-13	0.8		98
Cefoxitin				im iv-inf.	11 47	0.8		78

[a]Data following continuous iv infusion to achieve steady state (CT and CX = 0.5 g/hr; CR = 0.25 g/hr; CCT = 0.4-0.5 g/hr).
[b]Estimated by extrapolation from levels after 1 g doses.

Table 6 Estimated minimum therapeutic ratios for cephalosporin antibiotics against common pathogens

Drug	Route of Admin. of 0.5 g Dose	Ratio (minimum peak serum level[a]/MIC[b])									
		Str. pn.	Str. A	St. aur. (Pase)	St. aur. (N-Pase)	Enteroc.	E. coli[c]	Klebs.[c]	Enterob.[c]	Pr. mirab.[c]	Prot. other[c]
Cephalothin	im	15	12	3	10	0.2	1	0.5	0	1.5	0.2
	iv-inf.	50	40	10	20	1	2.5	2.5	0	2	1
Cephapirin	im	30	25	3	10		0.7	0.8	0	1	0.2
	iv-inf.	100	75	10	20		2	2.5	0	3	1
Cephacetrile	im		12	2	5	0.5	4	1		1	
	iv-inf.		35	6	15	1.5	12	3		3	
Cephaloridine	im	100	200	2.5	20	1	5	2	0	5	0.2
	iv-inf.	300	600	8	60	3	15	6	0	15	1
Cefazolin	im	120	120	5	20	1	10	5	0	10	1
	iv-inf.	400	400	40	60	3	30	15	0	30	2
Cephaloglycine	oral	2.5	1	0.3	0.3	0.04	1	0.5	0.04	1	0.1
Cephalexin	oral	1	1.5	0.7	0.7	0.1	1	0.7	0	1	0
	im	1	1.5	0.7	0.7	0.1	1	0.7	0	1	0
	iv-inf.	4	6	2	2	0.5	4	3	0	3	0
Cephradine	oral	1	1.5	0.7	0.7	0.1	0.7	0.4	0	1	0
Cefoxitin	im	3	20	3	3		2	2	0.2	5	1
	iv-inf.	12	80	12	12		8	8	0.8	20	4

[a] Minimum value from reported range of peak serum levels, unadjusted for duration of level, volume of distribution, etc.

[b] MIC - Minimum inhibitory concentration - (Maximum of range of MICs for species or strains considered "susceptible" to therapy, unadjusted for protein-binding, tissue diffusion, etc.; used in deriving the ratio estimate.)

[c] Higher dosage would achieve higher ratios with some strains but a variable proportion are quite resistant and would not be amenable to any therapy. Others are inhibited at high levels such as achieved in urine.

Gram-negative bacilli such as *E. coli* or *Klebsiella* which appear susceptible to cephalosporins, show variable outcomes, only partly successful. Fatal or unsatisfactory outcome is usually caused by serious underlying or complicating disease. Nevertheless, caution is needed in interpretation of therapeutic results with serious tissue Gram-negative bacillary infection treated with cephalosporins, as well as penicillins, because of the narrow therapeutic margins for the cephalosoporins, even in those strains that are not highly resistant by virtue of cephalosporinase production. Use of large doses, when possible, improves the ratios, but many investigators prefer to employ kanamycin or gentamicin instead or along with the cephalosporin.

Significant renal toxicity has occurred in a small number of patients treated with large doses of cephaloridine (120a) and this drug induces renal lesions in animals, whereas little reaction is seen with cephalothin (121a). Cephaloridine dosage must, therefore, be limited to approximately 4 g per day and be adjusted downward in the presence of markedly impaired renal function (120a).

Primary allergic and hypersensitivity reactions occur with these drugs, just as with the penicillins. Immunologic cross-reactivity between the penicillins and the cephalosporins is demonstrable both clinically and experimentally (122a, 123a). However, cross-allergy is sufficiently incomplete that numerous patients with a history of allergy to penicillin have received cephalosporins without reaction; indeed, cephalothin or cephaloridine have been considered excellent drugs for treating serious Gram-positive coccal infections such as endocarditis in patients allergic to penicillin (124a). Nevertheless, the incidence of reaction to cephalothin or cephaloridine is higher in patients with than in those without a history of penicillin allergy (125a); therefore, caution is still advisable in evaluating indications and initiating therapy in such patients.

Cephalogycline

Cephaloglycine (α-amino-phenyl cephalosporanic acid) was the first marketed cephalosporin with marginal but clinically useful oral absorption. Protein binding is low. However, only some 10–25% is absorbed, and serum levels remain too low for effective systemic therapy (126a) (Tables 5, 6). It is only because of good renal clearance by both filtration and tubular secretion that urinary levels are adequate to treat urinary tract infections (127). A large portion of the drug is converted to the desacetyl derivative that is excreted in the urine. Cephaloglycine is somewhat unstable in vitro, particularly at neutral or slightly alkaline pH (128), explaining some of the variability in reported MICs and in bioassay of serum levels. The drug shows moderate activity against a spectrum of Gram-positive cocci and Gram-negative bacilli similar to that of cephalothin. Activity in experimental infection is higher than predicted from the low serum activity, suggesting that the desacetyl product might show some intrinsic additive antibacterial activity in vivo (128). Clinical application of cephaloglycine has been limited to treatment of urinary tract infection, but it now has limited use even for this indication in view of the later development of cephalexin and cephradine, and the availability of other drugs that also show better serum and tissue activity.

Cephalexin

Cephalexin (7-α-amino-α-phenylacetamido-3-methylcephemcarboxylic acid) is minimally protein bound, acid stable and well absorbed (80% or better) following oral administration. Virtually all of the absorbed drug is recovered in the urine in unchanged, active form (129). Serum half-life from steady-state iv administration is 0.6–0.9 hr, intermediate between cephalothin and cephaloridine (130). Renal clearance includes some tubular secretion as well as filtration (130); probenecid will therefore enhance the duration of serum levels.

There has been considerable variation in the ranges of MICs for cephalexin reported by various investigators. For example, Braun et al reported median MICs for penicillinase-producing *Staph. aureus* of 12.5 μg/ml (131), whereas other laboratories report siginificantly lower modes and ranges (126–130, 132–134). Differing methodology again undoubtedly accounts for these differences. Oral cephalexin in fact has produced good clinical responses even in staphylococcal septicemia (135). Furthermore, efficacy equivalent to that of penicillin V has been demonstrated in controlled trials of streptococcal pharyngitis therapy (136, 137), despite higher MICs of streptococci to cephalexin. These clinical experiences suggest that even relatively low therapeutic ratios, if coupled with at least fair tissue distribution, as has been demonstrated for cephalexin (138) and reasonable drug distribution volumes equivalent to those of cephalothin and cephaloridine (130), can produce adequate response. It is clear, however, that regardless of the exact MIC values, cephalexin is comparatively less active than penicillin G or V, cephalothin, or cephaloridine against streptococci, pneumococci, and penicillin-sensitive staphylococci, and less active than nafcillin, the isoxazolyl penicillin, cephalothin, or cephaloridine against penicillinase-producing *Staph. aureus* (126–134). Therefore, it is doubtful that cephalexin should be recommended as standard therapy for serious staphylococcal infection.

Against "susceptible" Gram-negative bacilli the activity of cephalexin is often less than that of cephalothin or cephaloridine, but usually in the same range (Table 4). Levels in the urine are high and usually adequate to achieve satisfactory clinical response against organisms with reasonably low MICs. Even in renal failure, adequate levels of cephalexin are usually achieved in the urine for treatment of urinary tract infections. Clark noted that in 17 of 49 patients being treated for urinary tract infection, bacteriuria did not clear (139)—this was not a controlled study but represented a higher failure than anticipated in that patient group. A variety of other Gram-negative infections have been successfully treated with cephalexin usually in uncontrolled studies (e.g. 140, 141).

Cephradine

CLASSIFICATION AND ANTIMICROBIAL ACTIVITY   Cephradine is 7-amino-cyclohexadienyl-acetamido-(cephalosporanic acid) with structure, activity, and pharmacology very similar to cephalexin. It is acid stable and shows low protein binding. Antibacterial spectrum and relative activity are also similar to that of cephalexin.

Against pneumococci, streptococci, and *Staph. aureus* cephradine, as well as cephalexin, has moderately high activity but less than cephalothin or cephaloridine. Against noncephalosporinase-producing Gram-negative bacilli its activity, as cephalexin, is only moderate, with many strains of *E. coli, Proteus mirabilis* and *Klebsiella* inhibited by 3 to 12 μg/ml but with a number of strains slightly (e.g. one dilution) more susceptible to cephalexin (142). Bactericidal activity is relatively good, with usually only one dilution separating inhibitory and bactericidal endpoints (142).

CLINICAL PHARMACOLOGY AND CLINICAL APPLICATION   Like cephalexin, cephradine is well absorbed orally; serum levels ranged from 9–13 μg/ml but were a little lower than recorded for cephalexin. During treatment even of Gram-negative infections, serum inhibitory titers were usually at least 1:2 on 2–3 g dosage per day provided the MIC of the pathogen was <3 μg/ml. The serum half-life (0.8 hr) is similar to that of cephalexin, and high levels of active drug appear in the urine. Few studies of clinical efficacy have yet appeared, but available uncontrolled data indicates that, just as for cephalexin, a variety of respiratory, soft tissue, wound and urinary tract infections due to Gram-positive and Gram-negative pathogens should respond to treatment (143). Uncontrolled cephradine therapy in treatment of *Salmonella* and *Shigella* gastroenteritis was difficult to evaluate (144) as would be expected. Super-infections occurred (142), again as anticipated following therapy with any broad-spectrum antibiotic. There is no indication to date that side effects or toxicity will differ from those from cephalexin. Cephradine appears equivalent clinically to cephalexin, but if any minor theoretical difference is notable, it is that the combination of slightly lower serum levels and slightly higher MIC values for some enteric organisms may produce some slightly lower estimated therapeutic ratios (Table 6).

Cephapirin

CLASSIFICATION AND ANTIBACTERIAL ACTIVITY   Cephapirin (7-pyridylthioacetamid-cephalosporonate) is a semisynthetic cephalosporin that is similar to cephalothin in activity, phamacology, and application. It is only slightly less serum bound (44–50% compared with 65% for cephalothin), and is not orally absorbed but is stable for 8 hr at room temperature in standard iv fluids. Antibacterial activity against pneumococci and Group A streptococci is excellent, in the range 0.01 to 0.06 μg/ml, and is two- to fourfold more active than cephalothin (145–147). Resistance to *Staph.* penicillinase is excellent, and activity against *Staph. aureus* is comparable to that of cephalothin. Against Gram-negative bacilli, cephapirin shows moderate activity, comparable to that of cephalothin, but where minor twofold differences have been noted such as with *E. coli, Klebsiella,* and *Proteus mirabilis,* the differences favored cephalothin (145, 146). Like cephalothin the drug is not active against *Enterobacter,* nonmirabilis *Proteus, Enterococci,* or *Pseudomonas. H. influenzae* is only moderately susceptible to cephalosporins, and Khan (148) noted failure of cephapirin to clear the organism from pulmonary infections in children.

CLINICAL PHARMACOLOGY AND CLINICAL APPLICATION   Serum levels of cephapirin following iv and im administration are comparable to cephalothin (Table 4), and the drug is rapidly cleared, serum T ½ 0.5–0.8 hr, with high urinary level, as with cephalothin (149, 150). A number of early reports have shown satisfactory clinical response in treatment of a similar spectrum of serious infections due to Gram-positive coccal and Gram-negative organisms as expected for cephalothin. Inadequate information is yet available to establish any differences in reaction rates [e.g. eosinophilia noted by Gordon (145)]. However, less pain upon im injection has been noted compared with cephalothin (146), and two prospective controlled studies recorded less phlebitis from iv cephapirin than from cephalothin (151, 152).

Cefazolin

CLASSIFICATION AND ANTIMICROBIAL ACTIVITY   Cefazolin is a semisynthetic cephalosporin that differs from cephalothin and cephaloridine in that it has both a tetrazolylacetyl side chain at the amino linkage and a methyl-thiadiozolyl-thiomethyl group at R_2, the 3-position of the 7-aminocephalosporanic acid (Figure 2). Cefazolin is some 75% protein bound, similar to cephalothin but considerably higher than cephaloridine. Antibacterial activity against streptococci, pneumococci, and staphylococci is excellent, approximately the same as cephalothin, severalfold more active than cephalexin, but two- or fourfold less active than cephaloridine. With α strep. and *Staph. epidermidis* from patients with endocarditis, Quinn (153) found cefazolin less active than cephalothin or cephaloridine, whereas cefazolin was comparable to the other compounds in activity against *Staph. aureus.*

Activity of cefazolin against susceptible Gram-negative pathogens, although variable, as with other cephalosporins, is usually similar or somewhat greater than the activity of cephalothin and cephaloridine, although in one series (154) cefazolin did not inhibit heavy inocula of proteus mirabilis. *Pseudomonas* are quite resistant, and cefazolin shows little activity against other *Proteus, Enterobacter,* and enterococci. Studies of cephalosporinase activity from several specific hospital-isolated strains of Gram-negative bacilli indicated that cefazolin was the most labile of the cephalosporins studied (119). Further experience is needed to determine the degree of variability in cephalosporinases from a wider sampling of strains in different locations and their stability and reproducibility, especially in view of their transmissibility by episomal R-factors (116–121).

CLINICAL PHARMACOLOGY   Cefazolin shows several marked differences in pharmacokinetics compared with cephalothin and cephaloridine (Table 5), (154, 155, 161, 162). A number of studies have demonstrated the highest serum levels following im injection of cefazolin compared with any of the cephalosporins, approximately twice as high as cephaloridine and four times the levels of cephalothin. Experimental renal toxicity is minimal (163). Plasma and renal clearance is much slower than most of the other cephalosporins, with a serum half-life of 1.8 hr determined following continuous infusion to achieve a steady-state baseline (155). Cephanone is the only cephalosporin with a longer half-life (2.5 hr). The apparent pharmacologic advantages of high serum levels and longer half-life may theoreti-

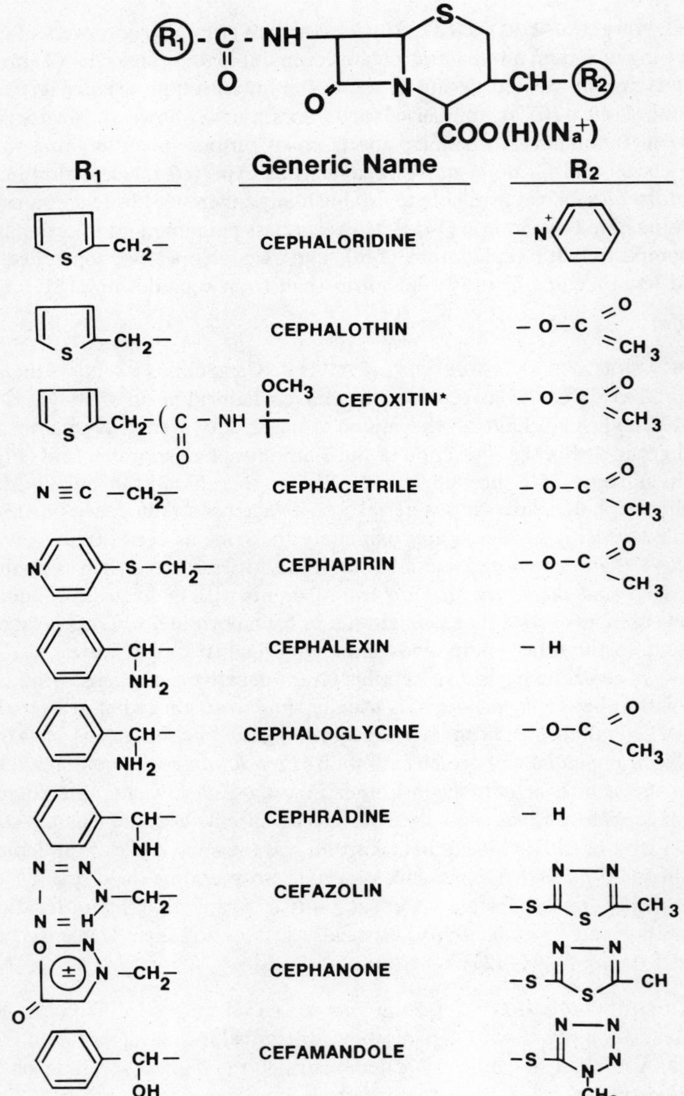

Figure 2 Structure of cephalothin and representative newer cephalosporin antibiotics
 * = Derivative of cephamycin series of naturally occurring 7-methoxylated cephalosporin antibiotics.

cally be contradicted in clinical application by the higher protein binding of cefazolin and the smaller volume of distribution. It is possible that cephaloridine or cephalexin, with low protein binding and larger volumes of distribution, may have greater concentrations of free drug available in tissue fluids. This possibility is not borne out by animal studies showing high levels of cefazolin in bile and in other tissues (156, 157). It is not known whether these apparently paradoxical findings can be extrapolated to humans. Cefazolin is not transported into uninflamed meninges (154), but is found in the inflamed synovial fluid, and to a lesser extent is excreted in bile (154).

CLINICAL APPLICATIONS   Limited studies have demonstrated effective therapy by cefazolin for urinary tract infections, a variety of respiratory infections including notably one bacteremic *H. influenzae* infection, skin and soft-tissue infections, and bone and joint infections (154, 158–161). Several of these patients were bacteremic, and the cure of a number of cases of endocarditis (153) would further substantiate that cefazolin is established as an effective agent against susceptible organisms. Thorough evaluation of the results to be expected as a sole agent in treatment of Gram-negative bacillary septicemia will require much additional data.

Cephacetrile

CLASSIFICATION AND ANTIMICROBIAL ACTIVITY   Cephacetrile, (7-cyan-acetamido-cephalosporanic acid, Figure 2), is a semisynthetic cephalosporin that is not absorbed orally and resembles cephaloridine in protein binding. Knusel recorded 38% protein binding for cephacetrile, compared with 35% for cephaloridine and 62% for cephalothin (164). Cephacetrile resembles cephalothin and cephaloridine in spectrum and degree of antibacterial activity, with median MICs against *Staph. aureus* slightly higher than cephalothin or cephaloridine, although cephalothin was more resistant than the other two drugs to in vitro hydrolysis against penicillinase produced by two specific strains (165). Methicillin-resistant strains of *Staph. aureus* showed resistance to cephacetrile, as to cephalothin and cephaloridine (164, 165). Cephalothin gave more stable endpoints to changing inoculum size of *Staph. aureus* strains. Against both cephalosporinase and noncephalosporinase-producing strains of *E. coli,* inoculum size strongly influenced the MIC endpoints for cephacetrile, cephalothin, and cephaloridine. Overall distribution of *E. coli* MICs for cephacetrile was intemmediate between the other two drugs, with a modal MIC of approximately 3 μg/ml. *Proteus* species showed a similar distribution for all three drugs, with modal values approximately 6–10 μg/ml for cephacetrile being slightly higher. Enterococci were only moderately sensitive, with Knusel's endpoints of $\sim$ 3 μg/ml intermediate between cephalothin and cephaloridine (164).

CLINICAL PHARMACOLOGY   Cephacetrile must be administered parenterally, producing serum levels of 20–25 μg/ml after *1* g doses. Serum half-life ranges from 0.5 to 0.6 hr following single rapid iv infusions, up to 1.3 hr for calculated $T_{1/2}$ after continuous iv infusions to achieve steady-state conditions (166). Most of the active drug is recovered in urine (approximately 88%), and calculation of renal/creatinine clearances gave a ratio of 2.2, similar to the 2.4 ratio for cephalothin, indicating significant tubular secretion (166). Little drug was found in human bile following single doses (167). Severe renal failure increased serum half-life to 24 hr (166), Table 7.

Detailed studies in dogs revealed no nephrotoxicity for cephaloridine or cephacetrile, even with concomitant furosemide (168). Both cephaloridine and cephacetrile showed significant levels in renal lymph when plasma concentration was high, but cephacetrile was much lower at low plasma levels (168). Overall, the data indicates that cephacetrile should be a comparably effective drug to cephaloridine and cephalothin, with comparable therapeutic ratios (see Table 6).

CLINICAL APPLICATIONS   Clinical results in uncontrolled evaluation of treatment of 27 patients comprising soft tissue infections, respiratory infections, and urinary tract infections suggest comparable results to those anticipated for cephalothin or other cephalosporins (169). Hodges et al found no renal toxicity, but did encounter phlebitis, some pain on injection, eosinophilia, and benign thrombocytosis [which Olef (170) has reported during convalescence from infection.] Transient benign direct Coombs positivity was also noted, as previously seen with cephalothin and cephaloridine (171, 172).

Cefoxitin

CLASSIFICATION AND ANTIBACTERIAL ACTIVITY   The cephamycins are a series of natural occurring 7-methoxylated cephalosporin antibiotics originally derived from strains of *Streptomyces* (173). From among cephamycins A, B, and C, cephamycin C showed greater resistance to specific β-lactamases and greater activity primarily against Gram-negative organisms. Synthetic modification of cephamycin C was aimed at enhancing the Gram-positive spectrum, while retaining β-lactamase resi-

Table 7 Effect of severe renal failure on clearance of penicillins and cephalosporins

	Serum Half-Life (Hours)	
Drug	Normal Subjects	Patients in Severe Renal Failure (Anuric or Creatinine Clearance under 5 ml/min)
Penicillin G	0.4-0.6	3-4
Ampicillin	0.6-1	8-12
Carbenicillin	1.0	10-16
Cephalothin	0.5-0.8	3
Cephaloridine	1.1-1.5	8-24
Cephacetrile	1.3	24
Cefazolin	1.8	25-45
Cephalexin	1.7	20-30

tance and Gram-negative activity. Cefoxitin is 7-α-methoxyl, 7-thienyl-acetamido cephalosporanic acid (see Figure 2). It is more active than cephalothin against Gram-negative bacilli. Cefoxitin particularly shows unique activity among the cephalosporins in that it inhibits *Serratia* at 6–50 μg/ml and *Proteus morgagni* at 3–12 μg/ml, two species that are usually resistant to cephalothin. Cefoxitin is also two- to fourfold more active than cephalothin against Gram-negative bacilli such as *E. coli* and *Klebsiella*. Only a minor portion of *Enterobacter* strains are inhibited, and all *Pseudomonas* are resistant. Activity against Gram-positive cocci is distinctly less than cephalothin or cephaloridine but still should be adequate for effective therapy. In summary, cefoxitin shows a unique antibacterial spectrum advantage in its activity against *Serratia* and *Proteus morgagni;* its somewhat improved activity against other Gram-negative bacilli is also of interest and will require clinical evaluation (174–177).

CLINICAL PHAMACOLOGY   (Table 5). Serum levels following 0.5 g doses im and iv reach an average of 11 and 47 μg/ml respectively, in the same range as cephalothin and cephacetrile, but not as high as cephaloridine or cefazolin. Serum and urinary clearance is rapid, with a serum half-life of 0.8 hr, similar to cephalothin, cephapirin, and im cephalexin. Renal excretion is via both glomerular filtration and tubular secretion (178–180).

COMMENT—SELECTED PROBLEMS

Inactivation of Cephalosporins and Penicillins by β-Lactamases

β-Lactamases produced by different bacterial species show different chemical properties, substrate specificities, etc, and these characteristics are relevant in determining resistance to penicillins and cephalosporins (116–123). For example, Jackson (119) recently reported starch-gel electrophoretic study of six cephalosporins, grouped by side-chain structure, as test substrates for β-lactamases extracted from hospital strains of *Klebsiella, Enterobacter, E. coli* and *Pseudomonas,* both penicillin-induced and noninduced. Variable specificities were confirmed. Cephalosporinase from a *Klebsiella* strain degraded cephaloridine at the least rate and cefazolin some 11 times greater, with cephacetrile and cephalothin intermediate, but avidity and activity of the *Klebsiella* enzyme were greatest for penicillin. In contrast, an *Enterobacter* strain produced enzyme that was a much more active cephalosporinase than penicillinase. Jackson's and Fraher's findings further suggest that resistance may relate better to avidity of enzyme for drug, than to substrate reaction velocity (119, 123). The penicillin-induced *Pseudomonas* β-lactamases exhibited high avidity and activity for both penicillins and cephalosporins.

Jackson's findings indicated that against the *Klebsiella* enzyme, the side-group diazole (cephanone) was more stable than the tetra-azole group, (cefazolin) in the R-1 position (Figure 2). Against *Enterobacter* β-lactamase, the cyano group at R-1 (cephacetrile, Figure 2) was the most stable, but against the *Klebsiella* enzyme, the R-1 thiophene group in cephalordine and cephalothin was more stable than the cyano-(cephacetrile) group (119). Further development of semisynthetic cephalosporin and penicillin antibiotics of course are being aided by such studies relating natural inactivating enzyme avidities and kinetics to specific chemical side-chain moieties (116–121).

Standardization and Interpretation of Antimicrobial Susceptibility Testing

In the past, various procedures have been used in clinical microbiology laboratories for routine susceptibility testing of antimicrobial agents, and often the disc-diffusion methods have not been well controlled. Shortcuts in technique such as lack of standardization of inoculum size and failure to measure the size of the zone of inhibition have led to errors and inconsistencies. Misleading information has also resulted from testing of inappropriate drugs and testing of organisms that are not rapid-growing pathogens or organisms for which susceptibility tests do not assist and may even confuse clinical management. The US Food and Drug Administration has now officially required that antibiotic discs include a package insert describing standard methodology, either the "Kirby-Bauer" method (181), or standardized modifications (182), as recommended by the National Committee for Clinical Laboratory Standards. Improved standardization of microbiologic methodology used even in research laboratories engaged in clinical-pharmacologic investigation of newer antibiotics would also help avoid the significant discrepancies in data reported from different centers. Adoption of standard reference antibiotic testing methods, as recommended by the Report of an International Collaborative Study (183), would result in less conflicting microbiologic data, facilitate coordinated evaluation of new agents, and assist in deriving standards for interpretation.

Once standardization of procedures has been achieved in clinical laboratories, further revisions are needed in deriving more appropriate standards for interpretation of susceptibility testing results. Present guidelines (181) divide the ranges of MICs estimated from the disc test into three categories: Sensitive, Intermediate, and Resistant. This interpretation is partly misleading in that the Sensitive category is extremely broad, e.g. placing a Sensitive staphylococcus with an MIC to cephalothin of 0.1 μg/ml in the same interpretive category as an *E. coli* which is a hundredfold less susceptible, with a cephalothin MIC of 10–15 μg/ml. For the *E. coli,* this MIC can be exceeded with a reasonable average Therapeutic Ratio of 5 or 10 or more only in the urine, with low, "standard" doses, or else requiring high doses for achieving adequate serum levels for treatment of tissue infection (see Table 6). Much more directly relevant would be the adoption of four interpretive categories (183): (*a*) highly sensitive (*b*) moderately sensitive (*c*) slightly sensitive, and (*d*) completely resistant. With these guidelines, testing, for example, of a *Klebsiella* from a urinary tract infection with an MIC to cephalothin of 32 μg/ml could quite appropriately be evaluated as group *c* or slightly sensitive, implying that with normal dosage it would be amenable to inhibition only by the high levels achieved in the urine.

Evaluation of Antibiotics—Role of Tissue Levels

The pharmacologic findings reviewed in sections A and B and the summary data in Tables 1–7 rely heavily on pharmacologic kinetics of blood levels. Probably of greater physiologic importance may be the levels actually attained and maintained in the infected tissue, with the blood levels of indirect importance. The pharmacokinetics of delivery of antibacterial agents into tissue or interstitial fluid is complex, and must take into account more information than merely protein binding and serum and urine level kinetics. For newer antibiotics, further data should be derived concerning more detailed aspects of lipid solubility, ionization constants, and membrane transport in order to compare effective tissue levels. For example, lipid solubility and tissue diffusion of the penicillins and cephalosporins, most of which are weakly ionized, is generally only moderate in the absence of inflammation (184), whereas higher tissue levels should be achieved with lipid soluble drugs such as the tetracyclines, chloramphenicol, or erythromycin. Experimental models for sampling of skin, tissue fluid, or lympatics in man or animals give somewhat variable results, with different sampling systems showing differing time-diffusion kinetics and serum/tissue concentration ratios, and variable correlation with protein binding. Furthermore, the relationship of such experimental systems to natural infection is unsettled and clinical confirmation is needed. For example, Calnan's perforated plastic cylinders produce "physiologic" tissue fluid (188, 189), but the integrity of blood supply has been questioned (191). Further studies of methods for measuring tissue diffusion in relation to clinical pharmocology and clinical effectiveness of antibiotics would aid in evaluation of newer agents (185–187, 190).

Literature Cited

1. Sheehan, J. 1957. *Ann. NY Acad. Sci.* 145:216
2. Sheehan, J., Henery-Logan, K. 1957. *J. Am. Chem. Soc.* 79:1262
3. Bachelor, F. et al 1959. *Nature* 183:257
4. Huang, H., English, A., Seto, T., Shull, G., Sobin, B. 1960. *J. Am. Chem. Soc.* 82:3790
5. Loder, B., Newton, G., Abraham, E. 1961. *Biochem. J.* 79:408
6. Morin, R., Jackson, B., Flynn, E., Roeske, R. 1962. *J. Am. Chem. Soc.* 84:3400
7. Barber, M., Waterworth, P. 1964. *Brit. Med. J.* 2:344
8. Simon, H. 1965. *Antimicrob. Ag. Chemother.* 1964, p. 280
9. Rosenblatt, J., Kind, A., Brodie, J., Kirby, W. 1968. *Arch. Int. Med.* 121:345
10. Gilbert, D., Sanford, J. 1970. *Med. Clin. N. Am.* 54:1113
11. Marcy, S., Klein, J. 1970. *Med. Clin. N. Am.* 54:1127
12. Sutherland, R., Croydon, E., Rolinson, G. 1970. *Brit. Med. J.* 4:455
13. Weinstein, L., Lerner, P., Chew, W. 1964. *N. Engl. J. Med.* 271:525
14. Lerner P., Smith, H., Weinstein, L. 1967. *Ann. NY Acad. Sci.* 145:310

15. Stamey, T., Govan, D., Palmer, J. 1965. *Medicine* 44:1
16. Jordan, M., De Maine, J., Kirby, W. 1971. *Antimicrob. Ag. Chemother.* 10:438
16a. Wick, W. E., Preston, D. A. 1972. *Antimicrob. Ag. Chemother.* 1:221
16b. Meyers, B. R., Hirschman, S. Z., Nicholas, P. 1972. *Antimicrob. Ag. Chemother.* 2:250
17. Dittert, L., Griffen, W., LaPiana, J., Shainfeld, F., Doluisio, J. 1970. *Antimicrob. Ag. Chemother.* 1969. p. 42
18. Bear, D., Turck, M., Petersdorf, R. 1970. *Med. Clin. N. Am.* 54:1145
19. Rolinson, G., Stevens, S. 1961. *Brit. Med. J.* 2:191
20. Klein, J., Finland, M., Wilcox, C. 1963. *Am. J. Med. Sci.* 245:544
21. Cole, M., Kenig, M., Hewitt, V. 1973. *Antimicrob. Ag. Chemother.* 3:463
22. Sutherland, R., Robinson, O. 1967. *Brit. Med. J.* 2:804
23. Tuano, S., Johnson, L., Brodie, J., Kirby, W. 1966. *N. Engl. J. Med.* 275:635
24. Thrupp, L. et al 1966. *Antimicrob. Ag. Chemother.* 1965. p. 206
25. Kirby, W., Kind, A. 1967. *Ann. NY Acad. Sci.* 145:291

26. Smith, M., Sandstrom, S., Hoffpauir, C. 1967. *Ann. NY Acad. Sci.* 145:502
27. Louria, D., Schultz, M. 1967. *Ann. NY Acad. Sci.* 145:387
28. Chawla, V., Chandra, R., Bhujwala, R., Ghai, O. 1970. *J. Pediat.* 77:471
29. Kaye, D., Rocha, H., Eyckmans, L., Prata, A., Hook, E. 1967. *Ann. NY Acad. Sci.* 145:423
30. Knudsen, E. 1970. *Proc. Symp. Aspects of Infection, Auckland, Sydney, and Melbourne*, p. 115
31. Shapiro, S., Slone, D., Siskind, V., Lewis, G., Jick, H. 1969. *Lancet* 2:969
32. Jaffe, I. 1970. *Lancet* 1:24
33. Pullen, H., Wright, N., Murdoch, J. 1967. *Lancet* 2:1176
34. Bierman, W., Pierson, W., Zeitz, S., Hoffren, L., Van Arsdel, P. 1972. *J. Am. Med. Assoc.* 220:1098
35. Sutherland, R., Rolinson, G. 1971. *Antimicrob. Ag. Chemother. 1970.* p. 411
36. Neu, H., Winshell, E. 1971. *Antimicrob. Ag. Chemother. 1970.* p. 407
37. Bodey, G., Nance, J. 1972. *Antimicrob. Ag. Chemother.* 1:358
38. Neu, H., Winshell, E. 1971. *Antimicrob. Ag. Chemother. 1970.* p. 423
39. Croydon, E., Sutherland, R. 1971. *Antimicrob. Ag. Chemother. 1970.* p. 427
40. Acred, P., Hunter, P., Mizen, L., Rolinson, G. 1971. *Antimicrob. Ag. Chemother. 1970.* p. 416
41. Gordon, R., Regamey, C., Kirby, W. 1972. *Antimicrob. Ag. Chemother* 1: 504
42. Sutherland, R., Croydon, E., Rolinson, G. 1972. *Brit. Med. J.* 3:13
43. Handsfield, H., Clark, H., Wallace, J., Holmes, K., Turck, M. 1973. *Antimicrob. Ag. Chemother.* 3:262
44. Middleton, F., Poretz, D., Duma, R. 1973. *Antimicrob. Ag. Chemother.* 4:25
45. Harding, J., Lees, L. 1973. *Practitioner* 209:363
46. Basch, H., Erickson, R., Gadebusch, H. 1971. *Infect. Immun.* 4:44
47. Dolfin, J. et al 1971. *J. Med. Chem.* 14:117
48. Beck, J., Hubscher, J., Caloza, D. 1971. *Curr. Ther. Res.* 13:530
49. Alora, B., Estrada, F., Lansing, S. 1972. *Curr. Ther. Res.* 14:358
50. Brogden, R., Avery, G. 1972. *Drugs* 3:314
51. Michel, M., Van Waardhuizen, J., Kerrebijn, K. 1973. *Chemotherapy* 18:77
52. Tuneval, C., Frisk, A. 1968. *Antimicrob. Ag. Chemother. 1967.* p. 573
53. Sjoberg, B., Ekstrom, B., Forsgren, U. 1968. *Antimicrob. Ag. Chemother.* 1967, p. 560
54. Hansson, E., Magni, L., Wahlquist, S. 1968. *Antimicrob. Ag. Chemother. 1967.* p. 568
55. Wasz-Hockert, D., Nummi, S., Voupala, S., Jarvinen, P. 1970. *Scand. J. Infec. Dis.* 2:125
56. Lithander, A., Lithander, B. 1968. *Antimicrob. Ag. Chemother. 1967.* p. 578
57. Kerrebijn, K., Michel, H., Masurel, N., Van Waardhuizen, J. 1972. *Chemotherapy* 17:416
58. Rosenman, S., Weber, L., Owen, G., Warren, G. 1968. *Antimicrob. Ag. Chemother. 1967,* p. 590
59. Alburn, H., Clark, R., Fletcher, H., Grant, N. 1968. *Antimicrob. Ag. Chemother. 1967.* p. 586
60. Hopper, M., Yurchenco, J., Warren, G. 1968. *Antimicrob. Ag. Chemother. 1967.* p. 597
61. Yurchenco, J., Hopper, M., Warren, G. 1968. *Antimicrob. Ag. Chemother. 1967.* p. 602
62. Christensen, H., Jones, J. 1962. *J. Biol. Chem.* 237:1203
63. Stillerman, M., Isenberg, H. 1971. *Antimicrob. Ag. Chemother. 1970.* p. 270
64. Eickhoff, T., Marks, M. 1970. *J. Infec. Dis.* 122 (Suppl):84
65. Bodey, G., Whitecar, T., Middleman, E., Rodriguez, V. 1971. *J. Am. Med. Assoc.* 281:62
66. Shapera, R., Matsen, J. 1971. *Postgrad. Med.* 49:120
67. Hewitt, W., Winters, R. 1973. *J. Infec. Dis.* 127 (Suppl.):120
68. Rolinson, G., Sutherland, R. 1968. *Antimicrob. Ag. Chemother. 1967.* p. 609
69. Bodey, G., Terrell, M. 1968. *J. Bacteriol.* 95:1587
70. English, A. 1969. *Antimicrob. Ag. Chemother. 1968.* p. 482
71. Smith, C., Finland, M. 1968. *Appl. Microbiol.* 16:1753
72. Rosdahl, V. 1971. *Chemotherapy* 16:18
73. Lowbury, E., Kidson, A., Lilly, H., Ayliffe, G., 1969. *Lancet* 2: 448
74. Bell, S., Smith, D. 1969. *Lancet* 1:753
75. Smith, C., Wilfert, J., Dans, P., Kurrus, T., Finland, M. 1970. *J. Infect. Dis.* 122 (Suppl.):14
76. Phair, J., Watanakunakorn, C., Ban-

nister, T. 1968. *Appl. Microbiol* 16:1753
77. Klastersky, J., Cappel, R., Daneau, D. 1972. *Antimicrob. Ag. Chemother.* 2: 470
78. Hoffman, T., Bullock, W. 1970. *Ann. Intern. Med.* 73:165
79. Kunin, C. 1966. *Clin. Pharmacol. Ther.* 7:166
80. Standiford, H., Kind, A., Kirby, W. 1969. *Antimicrob. Ag. Chemother. 1968.* p. 286
81. McLaughlin, J., Reeves, D. 1971. *Lancet* 1:261
82. Andriole, V. 1971. *J. Infec. Dis.* 124:46
83. Somme, J., Jawetz, E. 1969. *Appl. Microbiol.* 17:893
84. Eykyn, S., Phillips, I., Ridley, M. 1971. *Lancet* 1:545
85. Levison, M., Kaye, D. 1971. *Lancet* 2:45
86. Noone, P., Pattison, J. 1971. *Lancet* 2:575
87. Riff, L., Jackson, G. 1972. *Arch. Intern. Med.* 130:887
88. Curreri, P., Lindberg, R., Pruitt, B. 1970. *J. Infec. Dis.* 122 (Suppl.):40
89. Nelson, J. 1970. *J. Infec. Dis.* 122 (Suppl.):48
90. Richardson, A., Spittle, C., James, K., Robinson, O. 1968. *Postgrad. Med. J.* 44:844
91. Pines, A., Raafat, H., Siddiqui, G., Greenfield, J. 1970. *Brit. Med. J.* 1:663
91a. Turck, M., Silverblatt, F., Clark, H., Holmes, K. 1970. *J. Infec. Dis* 122 (Suppl.):29
92. Knirsch, A., Hobbs, D., Korst, J. 1973. *J. Infec. Dis.* 127 (Suppl.):105
93. Hobbs, D. C. 1972. *Antimicrob. Ag. Chemother.* 2:272
94. Butler, K., English, A., Knirsch, A., Korst, J. 1971. *Del. Med. J.* 43:366
95. Bailey, R., Koutsaimanis, K. 1972. *Brit. J. Urol.* 44:235
96. Turck, M. 1973. *J. Infec. Dis.* 127 (Suppl.):137
97. Ries, K. et al 1973. *J. Infec. Dis.* 127 (Suppl.):148
98. Baker, D., Andriole, V. 1973. *J. Infec. Dis.* 127 (Suppl.):136
99. Wallace, J. et al 1971. *Antimicrob. Ag. Chemother. 1970.* p. 223
100. Westenfelder, M., Madsen, P. 1973. *J. Infec. Dis.* 127 (Suppl.):154
101. Cox, C. 1973. *J. Infec. Dis.* 127 (Suppl.):157
102. Bran, J., Karl, D., Kaye, D. 1971. *Clin. Pharmacol. Ther.* 12:525

103. Fabre, J., Burgy, C., Rudhardt, M., Herrera, A. 1972. *Chemotherapy* 17: 334
104. Bodey, G., Deerhake, B. 1971. *Appl. Microbiol.* 21:61
105. Sutherland, R., Burnett, J., Rolinson, G. 1971. *Antimicrob. Ag. Chemother. 1970.* p. 390
106. Acred, P., Hunter, P., Mizen, L., Rolinson, G. 1971. *Antimicrob. Ag. Chemother. 1970.* p. 396
107. Sutherland, R., Wise, P. 1971. *Antimicrob. Ag. Chemother. 1970.* p. 402
108. Klastersky, J., Daneau, D. 1972. *Curr. Ther. Res.* 14:503
109. Rodriquez, V., Inagaki, J., Bodey, G. 1973. *Antimicrob. Ag. Chemother.* 4:31
110. Abraham, E., Newton, G. 1961. *Biochem. J.* 79:377
111. Saslaw, S. 1970. *Med. Clin. N. Am.* 54:1217
112. Kayser, F. Feb. 1971. *Postgrad. Med. J. Suppl.* 47:14
113. Klein, J., Eickhoff, T., Tilles, J., Finland, M. 1964. *Am. J. Med. Sci.* 248: 640
114. Griffith, R., Black, H. 1971. *Postgrad. Med. J. Suppl.* 47:32
115. Smith, I. Feb. 1971. *Postgrad. Med. J. Suppl.* 47:78
116. Ayliffe, R. 1965. *J. Gen. Microbiol.* 40:119
116a. Rountree, P., Bullen, M. 1967. *Brit. Med. J.* 2:373
117. Sabath, L., Jago, M., Abraham, E. 1965. *Biochem. J.* 96:739
117a. Kirby, W., DeMaine, J., Serrill, W. Feb. 1971. *Postgrad. Med. J. Suppl.* 47:41
118. Jack, G., Richmond, M. 1970. *J. Gen. Microbiol.* 61:43
118a. Murdoch, J., Speirs, C., Geddes, A., Wallace, E. 1964. *Brit. Med. J.* 2:1238
119. Jackson, G., Lolans, V., Gallegos, B. Presentation to Symposium on Cefazolin, Miami, 1973. *J. Infec. Dis.* In press
119a. Brown, J., Mathies, A., Ivler, D., Warren, S., Leedom, J. 1970. *Antimicrob. Ag. Chemother. 1969.* p. 432
120. Neu, H. 1971. *Antimicrob. Ag. Chemother. 1970.* p. 534
120a. Benner, E. J. *J. Infect. Dis.* 122:104
121. Goldner, M., Glass, D., Fleming, P. 1968. *Can. J. Microbiol.* 14:139
121a. Silverblatt, F., Turck, M., Bulger, R. 1970. *J. Infec. Dis.* 122:33
122. Acred, P., Sutherland, R. 1967. *Antimicrob. Agents Chemother. 1966.* p. 53

122a. Petz, L. D. Feb. 1971. *Postgrad. Med. J. Suppl.* 47:64

123. Fraher, M., Jawetz, E. 1968. *Antimicrob. Ag. Chemother. 1967.* p. 711

123a. Fass, R., Perkins, R., Saslaw, S. 1970. *J. Am. Med. Assoc.* 213:121

124. Sabath, L., Gerstein, D., Leaf, C., Finland, M. 1970. *Clin. Pharm. Ther.* 11: 161

124a. Apicella, M., Perkins, R., Saslaw, S. 1966. *N. Engl. J. Med.* 274:1002

125. Sabath, L., Elder, H., McCall, C., Finland, M. 1967. *N. Eng. J. Med.* 277: 232

125a. Merrill, S., David, A., Smolens, B., Finegold, S. 1966. *Ann. Intern. Med.* 64:1

126. McKee, W., Turck, M. 1967. *Antimicrob. Ag. Chemother. 1967.* p. 705

126a. Pitt, J., Siasoco, R., Kaplan, K., Weinstein, L. 1968. *Antimicrob. Ag. Chemother.* 1967. p. 630

127. Ronald, A., Turck, M. 1967. *Antimicrob. Ag. Chemother. 1968.* p. 82

128. Wick, W. 1967. *Appl. Microbiol.* 15: 765

129. DeMaine, J., Kirby, W. 1971. *Antimicrob. Ag. Chemother. 1970.* p. 190

130. Kirby, W., DeMaine, J., Serrill, W. Feb. 1971. *Postgrad. Med. J. Suppl.* 47:41

131. Braun, P., Tillotson, J., Wilcox, C., Finland, M. 1968. *Appl. Microbiol.* 16:1684

132. Perkins, R., Carlisle, H., Saslaw, S. 1968. *Am. J. Med. Sci.* 256:122

133. Thornhill, T., Levison, M., Johnson, W. 1969. *Appl. Microbiol.* 17:457

134. Kayser, F. Feb. 1971. *Postgrad. Med. J. Suppl.* 47:14

135. Kind, A., Kestle, D., Standiford, H., Kirby, W. 1968. *Antimicrob. Ag. Chemother. 1967.* p. 361

136. Stillerman, M., Isenberg, H. 1971. *Antimicrob. Ag. Chemother. 1970.* p. 270

137. Disney, F., Breese, B., Green, J., Talpey, W., Tobin, J. Feb. 1971. *Postgrad. Med. J. Suppl.* 47:47

138. Orsolini, P. 1970. *Postgrad. Med. J. Suppl.* 46:13

139. Clark, H., Turck, M. 1969. *Antimicrob. Ag. Chemother. 1968.* p. 296

140. Levison, M., Johnson, W., Thornhill, T., Kaye, D. 1969. *J. Am. Med. Assoc.* 209:1331

141. Fass, R., Perkins, R., Saslaw, S. 1970. *Am. J. Med. Sci.* 259:187

142. Klastersky, J., Daneau, D., Weerts, D. 1973. *Chemotherapy* 18:191

143. Limson, B., Siasoco, R., Dial, F. 1972. *Curr. Ther. Res.* 14:101

144. Landa, L. 1972. *Curr. Ther. Res.* 14: 496

145. Gordon, R., Barrett, F., Clark, D., Yow, M. 1971. *Curr. Ther. Res* 13:398

146. Bodner, S., Koenig, M. 1972. *Am. J. Med. Sci.* 263:43

147. Axelrod, J., Meyers, B., Hirschman, S. 1971. *Appl. Microbiol.* 22:904

148. Khan, A., Pryles, C. 1973. *Curr. Ther. Res.* 15:198

149. Bran, J., Levison, M., Kaye, D. 1972. *Antimicrob. Ag. Chemother.* 1:35

150. Axelrod, J., Meyers, B., Hirschman, S. 1972. *J. Clin. Pharmacol.* 12:84

151. Lane, A., Taggart, J., Iles, R. 1972. *Antimicrob. Ag. Chemother.* 2:234

152. Inagaki, J., Bodey, G. 1973. *Curr. Ther. Res.* 15:37

153. Quinn, E. et al. Presentation to Symposium on Cefazolin, Miami, 1973. *J. Infec. Dis.* In press

154. Reller, L., Karney, W., Beaty, H., Holmes, K., Turck, M. 1973. *Antimicrob. Ag. Chemother.* 3:488

155. Kirby, W., Regamey, C. Presentation to Symposium on Cefazolin, Miami, 1973. *J. Infec. Dis.* In press

156. Ishiyama, S. et al 1971. *Antimicrob. Ag. Chemother. 1970.* p. 476

157. Nishida, M. et al 1970. *Antimicrob. Agents Chemother. 1969.* p. 236

158. Gold, J., McKee, J., Ziv, D. Presentation to Symposium on Cefazolin, Miami, 1973. *J. Infec. Dis.* In press

159. Cox, C. Presentation to Symposium on Cefazolin, Miami, 1973. *J. Infec. Dis.* In press

160. Pickering, L. et al. Presentation to Symposium on Cefazolin, Miami, 1973. *J. Infec. Dis.* In press

161. Phair, J., Carleton, J., Tan, J. 1972. *Antimicrob. Ag. Chemother.* 2:329

162. De Schepper, P., Harvengt, C., Vranckx, C., Boon, B., Lamy, F. 1973. *J. Clin. Pharmacol.* p. 83

163. Silverblatt, F., Harrison, W., Turck, M. Presentation to Symposium on Cefazolin, Miami, 1973. *J. Infect. Dis.* In press

164. Knusel, F., Konopka, E., Gelzer, J., Rosselet, A. 1971. *Antimicrob. Ag. Chemother. 1970.* p. 140

165. Russell, A. 1972. *Antimicrob. Ag. Chemother.* 2:255

166. Nissinson, A., Levin, N., Parker, R. 1972. *Clin. Pharmacol. Ther.* 13:887

167. Brogard, J., Dorner, P., LaVillaureix, J. 1973. *Antimicrob. Ag. Chemother.* 3:19

168. Naber, K., Madsen, P. 1973. *Antimicrob. Ag. Chemother.* 3:81

169. Hodges, G., Scholand, J., Perkins, R. 1973. *Antimicrob. Ag. Chemother.* 3: 228
170. Olef, I. 1936. *Arch. Intern. Med.* 57: 1163
171. Gralnick, H., Wright, L., McGinniss, M. 1967. *J. Am. Med. Assoc,* 199:725
172. Molthan, L., Reidenberg, M., Eichman, M. 1967. *N. Eng. J. Med.* 277: 123
173. Stapley, E. et al 1972. *Antimicrob. Ag. Chemother.* 2:122
174. Miller, T., Goegelman, R., Weston, R., Putter, I., Wolf, F. 1972. *Antimicrob. Ag. Chemother.* 2:132
175. Miller, A., Celozzi, E., Pelak, B., Stapley, E., Hendlin, D. 1972. *Antimicrob. Ag. Chemother.* 2:281
176. Miller, A. et al 1972. *Antimicrob. Ag. Chemother.* 2:287
177. Wallick, H., Hendlin, D. Sept. 1972. Presentation to 12th Intersci. Conf. Antimicrob. Agents Chemother.
178. Brumfitt, W., Kosmides, J., Hamilton-Miller, J., Gilchrist, J. 1973. *Abstr. Intersci. Conf. Antimicrob. Ag. Chemother., 13th*
179. Goodwin, C., Raftery, E., Skeggs, H., Till, A., Martin, C. 1973. *Abstr. Intersci. Conf. Antimicrob. Ag. Chemother., 13th*
180. Sonneville, P., Kartodirdjo, R., Skeggs, H., Till, A. E., Martin, C. M. 1973. *Abstr. Intersci. Conf. Antimicrob. Ag. Chemother., 13th*
181. Bauer, A. W., Kirby, W., Sherris, J. 1966. *Am. J. Clin. Pathol.* 45:493
182. Barry, A., Garcia, F., Thrupp, L. 1970. *Am. J. Clin. Pathol.* 53:149
183. Ericsson, H., Sherris, J. 1971. *Acta Pathol. Microbiol. Scand., Sect B, Suppl.* 217
184. Kunin, C. 1970. *Proc. Int. Congr. Nephrol.* 4th Stockholm 1969, 3:342 New York: Karger
185. Cockett, A., Moore, R., Roberts, A. 1967. *Invest. Urol.* 5:250
186. Raeburn, J. 1971. *J. Clin. Pathol.* 24: 633
187. Tan, J., Trott, A., Phair, J., Watanakunakorn, C. 1972. *J. Infec. Dis.* 126:492
188. Calnan, J. S., Pflug, J., Chisholm, G., Taylor, L. 1972. *Proc. Roy. Soc. Med.* 65:715
189. Chisholm, G., Waterworth, P., Calnan, J., Garrod, L. 1973. *Brit. Med. J.* 1:569
190. Waterman, N., Kastan, L. 1972. *Arch. Surg.* 105:192
191. Dawes, G. 1973. *Brit. Med. J.* 1:798

ANTIVIRAL AGENTS ❖6603

Jeremiah G. Tilles

California College of Medicine, University of California at Irvine, Irvine, California

With the recent unraveling of many of the biophysical, biological, and biochemical properties of the viruses that infect man, a groundswell of enthusiasm has gathered in anticipation of an era of viral chemotherapy. Because an impressive amount of time and money has already been devoted to the development of antiviral agents, it is appropriate, at this time, to evaluate the progress that has occurred. To do so, it is helpful and perhaps essential to consider, first, the problems that must be overcome by a successful antiviral agent and a few fundamental concepts about viruses. Therefore, this report begins with an enumeration of serious problems peculiar to the field of viral chemotherapy and continues with a short description of the general structure and classification of viruses, the sites of action of various antiviral agents in the viral replicative cycle, and finally a consideration of the structure, action, pharmacology, toxicology, and clinical efficacy of each of the candidate antiviral agents.

PROBLEMS

The first and most challenging problem is the concomitant toxicity to mammalian cells usually displayed by chemotherapeutic agents effective against viruses. Underlying the problem is the fact that a virus is an obligate intracellular parasite that must use the metabolic pathways of host cells. In contrast, a bacterium has enzymes and subcellular particles that have evolved separately from the mammalian counterparts and therefore are sufficiently different in a variety of ways to be susceptible to specific attack. Thus, while the ratio of the minimal toxic dose to the minimal therapeutic dose, or chemotherapeutic index, is high for approved antibacterial agents, it is generally quite low for the antiviral agents. There are at least two situations in which the use of a drug with a low chemotherapeutic index is morally justified: one, if it is to be used for a life-threatening illness having no other specific treatment, and, two, if it is to be used for an isolated problem accessible to therapy by local administration. It is therefore not surprising that, to date, most clinical

469

evaluations of antiviral agents have been confined to these two clinical situations (1–4).

The second problem is the frequent occurrence of what in bacteriology is termed the *inoculum* effect and in virology might better be termed the *multiplicity* (number of infectious particles per cell) effect. As applied to viruses, it describes the situation in which an antiviral agent is effective against virus in low concentration (low inoculum or multiplicity if being tested in vitro) but much less effective against virus in high concentration (high inoculum or multiplicity). Most antiviral agents display this multiplicity effect with the result that they are not very effective against symptomatic disease because of the high concentrations of virus present at that time. However, such drugs may still be useful as chemoprophylactic agents if used during the incubation period when virus is in low concentration. In fact, the two antiviral agents with the highest chemotherapeutic indices, amantadine and methisazone, suffer from the multiplicity effect in vitro (5, 6) and are therefore of questionable usefulness as therapeutic agents (7, 8) but nevertheless are of significant utility for chemoprophylaxis (9, 10).

The third problem is the difficulty in evaluating the efficacy of a drug to be used for a mild disease of short duration. For a disease that is so benign a question may appropriately be asked as to the necessity for any chemotherapeutic agent. The answer, of course, is that a specific therapeutic agent would be useful either for the rare occasion when the disease is quite severe or, more important, when an ordinary form of the disease occurs in a debilitated individual. To evaluate the utility of a chemotherapeutic agent in the usual presentation of mild disease is very difficult. By the time an individual is sick enough from his symptoms to seek medical attention, this type of viral illness may no longer be associated with viral replication, or the replication may be greatly reduced. Even if replication is still occurring, it may be that the viral illness will be over within 24 or 48 hr. Under such circumstances, if a drug were available that could reduce by 50% the symptomatology and duration of illness, it would be very difficult to prove, in fact, that the drug could do it. The magnitude of the challenge becomes apparent when it is realized that to solve the problem one must be able to quantify a number of subjective symptoms. We are only just beginning to understand which parameters are useful in making such an evaluation.

The fourth problem for viral chemotherapy is the emergence of drug resistant viruses. The history of drug resistant bacteria, following the use of antibiotics, has been well documented (11). In the case of antiviral agents, it has already been demonstrated that drug resistance tends to develop both in vitro and in vivo (12). Fortunately, drug resistance has not yet become a significant problem with the candidate antiviral agents, although this is most likely due to the discretion exercised in the use of agents with low chemotherapeutic indices.

To recapitulate, the four obstacles in the pathway of a candidate antiviral agent are as follows: 1. toxicity to mammalian cells resulting in a low chemotherapeutic index; 2. a multiplicity effect resulting in poor utility against virus in high concentration; 3. the difficulty in demonstrating clinical efficacy against mild disease; and 4. the emergence of drug resistant virus.

GENERAL STRUCTURE AND CLASSIFICATION OF VIRUSES

It can be seen schematically in Figure 1 that the virus particle has an inner nucleo-protein core that is either DNA (*b*) or RNA (*a*) in type. With respect to the viruses known to infect animals, the DNA viruses all have double stranded DNA, while the RNA viruses usually contain single stranded RNA. (Exceptions include the reoviruses and colorado tick fever virus.) It is also schematically shown in Figure 1 that around the inner core of a virus particle there is usually a protein coat (*c*) which may or may not have an external lipid membrane (*d*). It is thus convenient to classify the major groups of viruses according to their nucleic acid type and the presence or absence of a lipid membrane or envelope (Table 1).

SITES OF ACTION OF ANTIVIRAL AGENTS

Before indicating the sites of action of the antiviral agents, it will be necessary to consider first the normal viral replicative cycle. The replicative cycle for an RNA virus is shown schematically in Figure 2. Initially, the particle attaches to the cell membrane by physical forces in the process known as attachment, *1*. In some cases attachment is a highly specific reaction occurring only with cells having very specific receptors in the cell membrane (13, 14). In such circumstances, those cells lacking the specific receptors cannot be infected by that particular virus. The second step is the penetration of the cell membrane by the virus in a process sometimes called viropexis, *2*. Often this step consists of invagination by the cell membrane with pinocytosis of the virus particle. Step *3* is known as uncoating and consists of an opening up of the particle's protein coat with subsequent release of its nucleic acid into the cytoplasm of the cell. In the simplest viral replicative cycles, the viral RNA (input RNA) acts as RNA.

In the process known as translation, *4*, polyribosomes form when ribosomes attach to the virus RNA and begin to translate the nucleic acid sequence into proteins. One protein will be a "turn-down" protein which will be capable of turning down the host cell's own RNA and protein synthesis. Other proteins will usually include a RNA-dependent RNA-polymerase as well as the structural proteins required for the mature virus particle. With many RNA viruses, the RNA-dependent RNA-polymerase is coded for on the viral message as described. With some viruses (15, 16) this particular enzyme is part of the mature virus particle. In other words, one of the structural proteins in the mature virus can function as an RNA-dependent RNA-polymerase. In such a case, once the virus particle enters a cell, the functional protein can separate from the particle and carry out its function without requiring prior synthesis of viral specific proteins.

In the next step of the viral replicative cycle, *5*, the RNA-dependent RNA-polymerase, regardless of whether it was synthesized in the cell or brought in preformed, will find a strand of input viral RNA and begin to synthesize a complementary strand (mirror image) to the input RNA. With completion of the complementary strand, the double stranded structure realized is known as the replicative form, *6*. The replicative form serves as template for viral RNA production. For

Table 1 Human virus families

Membrane	RNA	DNA
+	myxovirus	herpesvirus
+	paramyxovirus	poxvirus
+	rhabdovirus	
+	togavirus	
−	picornavirus	adenovirus
−	reovirus	papovavirus

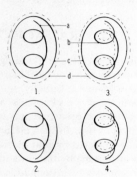

Figure 1 General structure of the animal viruses. Both RNA viruses, *1* and *2*, and DNA viruses, *3* and *4*, are depicted in this scheme. Each virus particle has a protein coat, *c*, and an inner nucleoprotein core containing either RNA, *a*, or DNA, *b*. Certain viruses have an external lipid membrane, *d*.

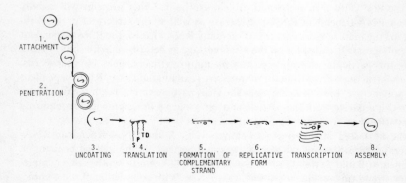

Figure 2 Replicative cycle of an RNA virus, described in text.

transcription, 7, the same RNA-dependent RNA-polymerase or perhaps a second polymerase (which should rightfully be called a replicase) reads the replicative form with the production of new single stranded RNA that is identical with the input RNA. This new RNA can go back and serve as message for more protein synthesis, can be used to produce templates for production of more RNA, or can be incorporated into mature virus. The next step, 8, is assembly of the new RNA, 7, and the new structural protein, 4, into mature virus. The mature virus is subsequently released from the cell.

One of the candidate chemotherapeutic agents against RNA viruses, amantadine, acts in the replicative cycle at step 2, penetration. Thus amantadine prevents the penetration of some RNA membrane viruses into cells (17). Neutralizing antibody has also been shown to prevent the penetration of cells by virus (13). The substance known as interferon is believed to have at least two sites of action. Evidence has been presented that step 4, translation, is effected such that ribosomes from interferon-treated cells become attenuated and no longer read viral RNA message, although they continue to read the host cell RNA message (18). Another site of action by interferon can be demonstrated against those particular viruses that bring into the cell a preformed RNA-dependent RNA-polymerase. In the latter situation interferon has been reported to inhibit the function of this enzyme and thereby block replication of new RNA (19, 20). Thus interferon can, at the present time, be shown to interfere with transcription for certain viruses and with translation for others. A substance known as isoprinosine has not been completely evaluated, but it is believed to work on ribosomes like interferon, i.e. attenuate ribosomes so they no longer function with viral messenger RNA. Guanidine (a chemical with a particularly low chemotherapeutic index and associated with too rapid a development of drug resistant virus to be of use in vivo) affects transcription, 7, by inhibiting the initiation of new strands of RNA (21). Thus, antiviral agents effective against the RNA viruses in vitro include the following: amantadine and antibody, which prevent the penetration of virus particles into the cell; interferon, which can work both on translation by affecting ribosomes and on transcription by inhibiting the RNA-dependent RNA-polymerase; isoprinosine, believed to work on ribosomes like interferon; and guanidine, which will inhibit the initiation of RNA strands during transcription.

The replicative cycle of a DNA virus is shown schematically in Figure 3. The first three steps, attachment, penetration, and uncoating, are analogous to the similar steps in the RNA virus replicative cycle just considered. However, in subsequent steps, there is a marked difference between the two replicative cycles. Even among the DNA viruses there are differences in replicative cycles. The cycle here depicted is for vaccinia virus, which at the present time is the one most completely understood. Vaccinia has been shown to bring into the cell a preformed polymerase which, in this case, is a DNA-dependent RNA-polymerase or transcriptase, P_1. Thus as the vaccinia DNA becomes uncoated, the enzyme begins to transcribe a viral RNA message from the double-stranded DNA, 4. This "early message" is relatively small with a sedimentation coefficient of 12S. When ribosomes begin to read the message, there is formation of an early polyribosome structure. In step 5, there is translation of the message to proteins that include the "early enzymes" such as a DNA-dependent DNA-polymerase or replicase, thymidine kinase, and DNase. It is evident that the enzymes translated from early message are those necessary to produce

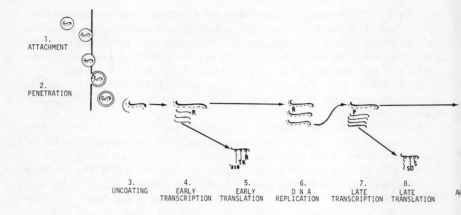

Figure 3   Replicative cycle of a DNA virus, described in text.

DNA. Hence the replication of DNA can occur as depicted in step *6.* The new DNA formed is called daughter DNA and is also capable of being transcribed. Thus in step *7,* late transcription occurs in which daughter DNA is transcribed to late mRNA (sedimentation coefficient of approximately 20S). In step *8,* late translation takes place on polyribosomes formed from the late message. Among the proteins formed are the structural protein that will go into the mature virus particles and another protein called "switch-off" protein. The latter protein appears to switch off the early message and is associated with a disintegration of the early polyribosomes. Finally, assembly occurs in step *9,* with the new DNA and structural protein brought together on a newly formed membrane (22). Ultimately, the mature virus particle is released from the cell.

The antiviral agents considered to have an effect on both RNA and DNA viruses, interferon and isoprinosine, are believed to have an action on early translation as already indicated. In addition, interferon can inhibit transcription of viruses which bring in a preformed polymerase. Thus interferon's inhibition of early transcription (step *4*) has been demonstrated with vaccinia virus which brings in a DNA-dependent RNA-polymerase, or transcriptase (23). The inhibitors of DNA production, 5-iodo-2'-deoxyuridine (IDU), cytosine arabinoside (AraC), and adenine arabinoside (AraA), all act on DNA replication in step *6.* The substances known as thiosemicarbazones act on late translation in step *8.* They may act on the switch-off protein so that it becomes less specific and switches off not only early message but also late message. In any case, there is disintegration of both early and late polyribosomes. Rifampin appears to work on assembly or, more accurately, immediately prior to assembly in step *9.* Rifampin apparently inhibits the cleavage of a protein precursor that otherwise is cleaved at the time of assembly into smaller polypeptides required for the assembly of the virus core (24). It is apparent that in considering antiviral activity against DNA viruses there are currently substances that in vitro will block each step in the replicative cycle. Thus, early transcription is blocked by interferon; early translation, by interferon and isoprinosine; DNA replication, by

IDU, AraC, and AraA; late translation, by methisazone; and assembly, by rifampin. The extent to which these in vitro activities can be translated to efficacy in man will become apparent shortly.

CANDIDATE ANTIVIRAL AGENTS

Before taking up the specific antiviral agents, it will be helpful to consider the three phases of drug evaluation as they apply to viral chemotherapy. Phase one is the preclinical phase. In this phase a prospective antiviral agent is evaluated both in cell culture and in animal models for antiviral activity and toxicity. Human experimentation begins with phase two, which is concerned with the pharmacology of the drug in man. Information concerning tolerable dosage and general toxicology is expected from this phase. With an agent having a very low chemotherapeutic index, the phase two studies can only be morally justified in patients having severe or potentially fatal disease. However, unless such studies have been appropriately set up to also determine clinical efficacy, documentation of clinical utility is neither derived nor expected from these investigations. It is the rightful objective of a phase three study, i.e. the formal therapeutic trial, to determine clinical efficacy. Because of the variable nature of the clinical course in the vast majority of virus diseases, virologists are convinced that clinical efficacy can only be demonstrated by double-blind controlled studies: netiher the patient nor the investigator knows whether the medication given is the drug being evaluated or its placebo. A rare exception to this requirement might occur with a drug being evaluated, for example, against symptomatic rabies, which is considered to be 100% fatal with the presently available modes of treatment.

There are many chemical and biological substances that have some antiviral effects in cell culture and even in laboratory animals but do not show sufficient potency and/or freedom from toxicity to be considered likely candidates to leave phase one for human studies. A much smaller number of antiviral agents have received phase two evaluation for toxicology and dosage in man, although most of these studies were not controlled in a manner that would document efficacy. There are a handful of antiviral agents that have received phase three evaluation with double-blind controlled studies. The candidate antiviral agents to be considered below are those that have either already made phase three or have good reason from the phase two studies to be seriously considered for phase three.

Amantadine.

The structure for 1-adamantanamine hydrochloride (amantadine) is given in *1* of Figure 4. This uniquely symmetrical primary amine has a pK_a of 9.0 and therefore exists as an ammonium ion at physiological pH. In cell culture, amantadine and certain other ammonium salts will prevent the penetration into cells of several RNA membrane viruses: myxoviruses (types A and C influenza), a paramyoxovirus (Sendai virus), and a togavirus (rubella) (17, 25–27). Unfortunately, the multiplicity effect is usually significant. In addition there is considerable variation in susceptibility among strains believed to be similar, except for minor differences in their outer membranes. Strains of influenza A_2 virus are clearly the most susceptible, and in mice the drug has been shown to have both prophylactic and therapeutic activity against such strains (25, 26, 28, 29).

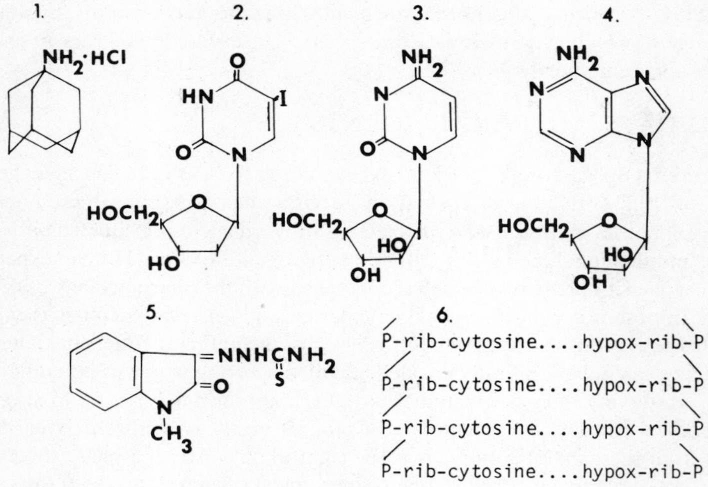

Figure 4 Chemical structure of candidate antiviral agents.   Represented are the structures of amantadine *1*, idoxuridine *2*, cytosine arabinoside *3*, adenine arabinoside *4*, methisazone *5*, and poly I · poly C *6*.

Human studies have revealed that amantadine administered by the oral route is absorbed slowly but probably completely, has a long half-life, and is almost entirely recoverable in the urine (30, Table 2). With a dose of 100 mg, twice daily, gastrointestinal upset and transitory central nervous system phenomena are noted in 1–2% of patients (31, 32). In one study, when the drug was given over a one year period for treatment of Parkinson's disease, the only additional adverse effects were livedo reticularis and mild ankle edema (33).

Early double-blind efficacy studies demonstrated that amantadine prophylaxis would significantly reduce the clinical and/or serological attack rate of either naturally acquired (34–37) or intranasally administered (38) Asian strain influenza A_2 virus. Further double-blind studies were carried out in student volunteers when the Hong Kong strain of influenza A_2 virus became prevalent. At least 50% protection was again found when amantadine was used in prophylaxis against natural infection (9) or against challenge with intranasally administered virus (39) (Table 3). Thus, it is evident that amantadine is effective as a chemoprophylactic agent against sensitive strains of influenza A_2 virus. However, there is no evidence that it is more effective than a vaccine containing the appropriate antigen. Therefore, in years when an appropriate vaccine is available, it would appear reasonable to immunize, rather than chemoprophylax, those debilitated individuals whom the Public Health Service recommends protecting against influenza (40). A different practice must be recommended for years when the prevalent virus is an antigenic variant of influenza A_2, for which a vaccine has not yet been prepared. In this case, it would appear prudent, during the epidemic period, to chemoprophylax with amantadine those individuals

Table 2 Clinical pharmacology of antiviral agents

	mol wt	pK	Route	Single Dose (mg)	Peak Time (hr)	Serum Concen (µg/ml)	$T_{1/2}$ (hr)	Renal Clearance[a] (xGFR)	Elimination Urine (%)	Metab (%)	(CSF) (Serum)	References
Amantadine	151	9.0	po	100.	1-4	0.2	15.	5.	86	—	—	30
Idoxuridine	354	8.25	iv	80/Kg 2 hr[b] 24 hr	during during	80.0 ≤2.5[c]	0.5	0.5	20	80	0.02[d]	56-58 49
AraC	246	4.5	iv	10/Kg 24 hr	during	0.5	0.2	0.6	8	76	0.4	67
AraA	271		iv	15/Kg 12 hr	during	—	1.5	1.0	49	—	0.5	75
Methisazone	238		po	200/Kg	6.	20.	2.7	—	—	—	—	85
Interferon	23,000		iv	8×10^5 u[e] 12 hr	during	—	ca 12.[a]	<0.1	—	>95[a]	—	100, 103, 104
Poly I · Poly C			iv	x 1/m²	during	—	<0.5[a]	—	—	>95[a]	—	100, 112

[a] author's estimate.
[b] infusion interval.
[c] µg (0.4 m).
[d] in the dog.
[e] units.

who require protection, provided the strain has been shown to be in fact sensitive to amantadine (41).

The efficacy of amantadine in the treatment of influenza has also been investigated with double-blind studies. In these investigations, a major problem has been the already discussed difficulty of demonstrating the influence of chemotherapy on a relatively benign viral disease of short duration. Although the studies appear to show a tendency for symptoms to be less severe and recovery to be earlier with amantadine, a significant difference (when compared with placebo) has been difficult to document. One objective parameter which has been easily quantitated is the interval of temperature elevation. In studies of natural outbreaks with either the Asian (42–44) or Hong Kong (7, 45) strain of influenza A_2 virus, the average interval of fever following initiation of treatment has been found to be significantly shortened by intervention with amantadine (Table 4). Whether aspirin will reduce the febrile period and other symptomatology as much or more is not known. An appropriately designed study comparing aspirin with amantadine is indicated at the present time. An important question is whether amantadine should be used for cases of influenza associated with pneumonia, particularly those pneumonias that occur in debilitated individuals. Although superinfecting bacterial pneumonia is a well-recognized complication of influenza, the importance of an underlying viral pneumonia should not be overlooked. In fact, 20–25% of the lungs from patients dying with influenza and pneumonia grow out influenza virus but no bacteria (46, 47). Therefore, it is important to find out if amantadine can 1. prevent the development of viral pneumonia in patients with influenza and/or 2. decrease the mortality of patients who contract influenza pneumonia.

Idoxuridine

5-Indo-2'-deoxyuridine (idoxuridine, IDU) has been the most thoroughly evaluated of the halogenated pyrimidine nucleosides. The contribution of the iodo group at the 5-position (*2* in Figure 4) makes this molecule a halogenated analog of thymidine. Although IDU appears to inhibit many of the enzymes used in the synthesis of DNA, its important action is considered to be its incorporation into a bogus DNA (48). IDU has been shown in cell culture to be consistently effective against the following human pathogens: herpesvirus hominis types 1 and 2 (49), cytomegalovirus (also a herpesvirus, 50), and vaccinia, a poxvirus (51). Its effect against varicella-zoster (a herpesvirus) has been equivocal (52, 53). Although IDU is found in animal studies to be consistently effective against corneal infections with either herpesvirus hominis (1) or vaccinia (54), its efficacy against systemic viral infection in animals is much less convincing (55).

In man, idoxuridine is rapidly metabolized to iodouracil and iodide giving a serum half-life of about 30 min (56) and resulting in only 20% of the intravenously administered dose appearing in the urine as active compound (Table 2) (57). To maintain the presence of active IDU, continuous intravenous infusions over as long as 24 hr have been used in the past. However, recent work indicates that such infusions result in serum levels no greater than 2.5 μg/0.4 ml (49). It has therefore been recommended that the daily dose be divided into 1 hr infusions given every

Table 3 Chemoprophylaxis with amantadine against infection with influenza A_2/Hong Kong

Transmission (Ref.)	No.	Serological Infection (%)		Clinical Infection (%)	
Induced (39)					
Amantadine	17	24		35	
Placebo	16	88		82	
Protection			73%[a]		57%[a]
Natural (9)					
Amantadine	192	14.1		11	
Placebo	199	29.6		26	
Protection			52%[a]		58%[a]

[a] [(Percentage of Placebo − percentage of Amantadine) ÷ percentage of Placebo] x 100.

Table 4 Treatment of naturally acquired influenza A_2 infection: effect of amantadine on febrile interval

Population (Ref.)	AMANTADINE		PLACEBO		p VALUE
	No.	Mean Interval (Hr $T > 99°$)	No.	Mean Interval (Hr $T > 99°$)	
ASIAN STRAIN					
Prison (44)[a]					
Texas #1	23	40.9	20	66.4	0.01
Texas #2	17	26.3	17	59.9	0.01
Maryland	12	46.7	13	69.3	ns
Prison (42)	20	23[b]	39	45[b]	0.01
Home for aged (43)	13	37	15	75	0.05
HONG KONG STRAIN					
Family practice (45)	72	46.6	81	75.1	0.01
Prison (7)	13	44.5	16	71.3	0.05

[a] Double-blind, placebo controlled studies in which patients with serologically proven influenza were treated within 48 hr of the onset of symptoms; the mean febrile interval following initiation of treatment was statistically analyzed.

[b] Interval with $T > 100°$.

12 hr (49). Studies in the dog indicate that even with intravenous doses adequate to give good serum levels, no significant quantities of IDU reach the cerebral spinal fluid in the absence of meningeal inflammation (58).

Toxicity from IDU is a direct result of its action on cells having rapid turnover. Thus the effect on muscosal cells of the gastrointestinal tract may be manifest by anorexia and stomatitis; the effect on bone marrow, by leukopenia, anemia, and thrombocytopenia; and the effect on epidermal tissues, by alopecia and loss of nails (57). The severity of the toxic effects varies with the total 5 day dose, the daily dose, and the rate of administration of individual infusions (59). With continuous infusion of the recommended dose, the nadir of marrow depression can be found 5 to 18 days after the onset of therapy (3). Thrombocytopenia and hemorrhage should be expected in those patients who have received a total dose greater than 20 g (3).

Numerous anecdotal studies have purported to demonstrate the efficacy of IDU in the treatment of either local or systemic infection with viruses of the herpesvirus and poxvirus families. However, efficacy has been definitely demonstrated only for epithelial keratitis due to herpesvirus hominis. Double-blind studies have shown that 0.1% IDU or placebo administered locally (at 1 hr intervals during the day and 2 hr intervals at night) will, on the average, result in healing of the corneas in 72% or 24% of the cases, respectively (60). It is generally recognized that IDU is ineffective for corneal stromal lesions associated with herpesvirus hominis infection, and its efficacy for herpetic skin lesions remains controversial (61, 62).

The efficacy of IDU for systemic viral infection has not been established, in part because the natural history of the disease under study has frequently been unknown; in part because the dose and schedule of administration of IDU has varied among investigators with the optimal schedule still unclear; and in part because suitable controls have always been lacking. The disease that has received most attention is herpesvirus hominis encephalitis. The largest individual study shows no difference in mortality (33%) when patients given IDU are compared with untreated patients cared for in neighboring hospitals (3). Evidence given for the occurrence of significantly fewer neurologic residua in the treated patients would have been convincing if control patients had been used in a double-blind fashion. Clearly, a double-blind controlled evaluation of IDU for herpes encephalitis is vitally needed; fortunately one is now in progress. If it should later become apparent that IDU is not effective for systemic viral disease of man, this information would be understandable in view of the past difficulty in showing efficacy for IDU against systemic infection in animals. It is of interest that for herpetic keratitis, the effective topical dose (given on 20 occasions/24 hr) has a concentration of 1000 μg/ml, which is at least 12 times the maximal level of IDU reached in the serum, when the recommended total daily systemic dose for herpes encephalitis is rapidly infused over 2 hr (56).

Cytosine Arabinoside

The structure of cytosine arabinoside, 1-β-D-arabinofuranosyl cytosine (araC), is given in 3 of Figure 4. The molecule differs chemically from cytidine by having arabinose instead of ribose for its sugar moiety which, in fact, merely makes the 2'-hydroxyl *trans* instead of *cis* to the 3'-hydroxyl. Because the sugar then lacks a

2'-*cis*-hydroxyl, it is handled by enzymes as deoxyribose. Thus, araC is really an analog for cytosine deoxyribose or deoxycytidine. As the di- and triphosphorylated derivatives, araC competes with the similar forms of deoxycytidine for enzymes such as DNA polymerase used in the production of DNA. In cell culture, araC has activity against human viruses of the herpesvirus family as well as the poxvirus, vaccinia, and the rhabdovirus, rabies (63). With experimental infections in animals, topical activity has been found for herpesvirus hominis and vaccinia keratitis (64, 65), but efficacy against systemic viral infection has not yet been documented (66).

In man, intravenously infused araC is rapidly deaminated to 1-β-D-arabinofuranosyl uracil (araU), which lacks antiviral activity. Therefore, araC has a serum half-life of only 12 min and only 8% of the active compound is recovered in urine (Table 2, 67). For this reason araC is usually given as a continuous infusion. Deamination is much slower in the spinal fluid where araC has been found at a concentration equal to 40% of the steady state serum level (67). AraC resembles IDU with dose- and schedule-related toxicities resulting from its action against rapidly dividing cells in the bone marrow and gastrointestinal mucosa (68). In addition araC, even in low dosage, has a profound immunosuppressive effect resulting in a reduced response to the induction of cellular immunity (established cellular immunity persists) and a depression of both primary and anamnestic antibody response (69).

There have been a number of enthusiastic but anecdotal reports concerning the use of araC in the treatment of infection with varicella-zoster, herpesvirus hominis, or cytomegalovirus in immunosuppressed or nonimmunosuppressed individuals. However, the clinical efficacy of araC for any viral infection of man remained unclear until recently, when the results of a double-blind placebo controlled study finally became available (70). Not only did this study fail to show any efficacy for araC in the treatment of varicella-zoster infections, but it also clearly defined a group of lymphoma patients who did poorer with araC than placebo, presumably because of the immunosuppressive activity of araC. Such results again focus on the strict necessity for further double-blind studies in order to establish the clinical efficacy of araC for any viral infection of man.

Adenine Arabinoside

The most promising of the arabinosyl nucleosides at the present time is adenine arabinoside, 1-β-D-arabinofuranosyl adenine (araA), which differs from araC by having a purine base, adenine, rather than a pyrimidine base, cytosine (*4* in Figure 4). Because the 2'-carbon lacks a *cis*-hydroxyl group, araA is an analog of deoxyadenosine. As the triphosphate it presumably competes with deoxyadenosine triphosphate for enzymes such as DNA polymerase used in the synthesis of DNA. With human viruses in cell culture, araA is quite active against herpesvirus hominis, varicella-zoster, cytomegalovirus, and vaccinia (71, 72). In experimental animals, araA has been found effective both topically for herpesvirus hominis keratitis (72) and systemically for encephalitis due to vaccinia or herpesvirus hominis type 1 or 2 (73).

In man, araA is first quickly deaminated to 1-β-D-arabinofuranosyl hypoxanthine (araHx), which has comparable activity against viruses in vivo (74). The further metabolism of araHx to inactive products is comparatively slow. As a result, the potency of araA has a serum half-life of 90 min and appears in the urine in 49% of the administered dose (Table 2, 75). The concentration of araA in the cerebral spinal fluid has been reported to be 50% of the simultaneous serum level. Based on the results of phase two studies, it is currently recommended that araA, for systemic use, be given as a continuous infusion over 12 hr. Although the relevant studies in man are not published in detail, it appears that the expected marrow depression is mild with the dosages being evaluated (76). There is a transient elevation of serum glutamic oxaloacetic transaminase, and a preliminary report showed a significant increase in leukocyte chromosome breakage (77). Thus far, there has been no evidence of immunosuppression by araA.

The clinical efficacy of topical araA has been demonstrated in a double-blind study in which araA ointment, 33 mg/ml (three to five times per day) was found to be as effective as the standard IDU ointment, 5 mg/ml, for herpesvirus hominis epithelial keratitis (2). From patients included in phase two studies, there is also evidence suggestive of a favorable response in systemic infection with herpesvirus hominis, varicella-zoster, vaccinia, or cytomegalovirus. However, all of these latter experiences are anecdotal. To determine the true clinical efficacy of araA for systemic viral infection, a multihospital double-blind placebo controlled study is presently being carried out. There is optimism that araA may prove to be more efficacious than araC for the following reasons: araA has successfully been used to treat systemic infection in animals; araHx, its deamination product, is also active; araA does not immunosuppress; and the marrow depression from araA is not severe.

Methisazone

Methisazone, N-methylisatin-3-thiosemicarbazone (*5* in Figure 4), is considered the best candidate antiviral agent of several N-substituted analogs of isatin-3-thiosemicarbazone (isatin) (78). The analogs lose antiviral activity when substitution is made on either the side chain or the aromatic ring, or if the sulfur of the side chain is replaced by oxygen. As already indicated, the action of the thiosemicarbazones occurs late in the viral replicative cycle and, at least for vaccinia virus, is at the level of translation from late mRNA, resulting in disintegration of both early and late polyribosomes (79). In cell culture, methisazone and its analogs are known to have activity against vaccinia and the other human poxviruses, varicilla-zoster virus, and adenoviruses (80, 81). Surprisingly, activity has also been reported for several human RNA viruses (82). In experimental encephalitis in mice, methisazone has been found effective against vaccinia, alastrim, and variola major viruses (83, 84).

Methisazone has too low a solubility to be given as a solution (in the concentrations needed for man or large animals) and therefore is recommended only by the oral route as a micronized preparation in sucrose syrup (78). Although its clinical efficacy has been widely studied, there is still very little information available on the absorption, distribution, and elimination of methisazone in man (Table 2). From the scant number of patients studied, it appears that the peak serum level occurs at about 6 hr and that the serum half-life is approximately 2.7 hr (85). The only important side effect of methisazone is vomiting, which has been reported in 11–66% of subjects taking the drug, usually about 4 to 6 hr after ingestion (10, 86, 87). Vomiting may have significantly interfered with the clinical evaluation of methisazone in that patients who vomited, retained an unknown proportion of the medication, knew they had not received placebo, and may have elected to omit further doses.

A major thrust in the efforts to establish the clinical utility of methisazone has been to determine its efficacy in the chemoprophylaxis of smallpox. In countries where smallpox is endemic, close contacts of index cases have been given methisazone in doses ranging from 3–6 g per day for 1–4 days. Control contacts, picked in alternating of random fashion, have been given either no drug or placebo (10, 86–88). It is evident from the summary of these studies in Table 5 that the evidence for the efficacy of methisazone is based on the first two studies. However, despite dealing with impressive numbers of contacts, these studies were unfortunately not designed with double-blind placebo controls. Because in each of the studies the group treated with methisazone had a lower incidence of smallpox than the respective control group, it is likely that methisazone did have a chemoprophylactic effect. It is important that this speculation finally be verified by a double-blind study with sufficient numbers of cases. In countries that have discontinued routine smallpox immunization, e.g. the United States, the nonimmunized population now has an increased vulnerability to smallpox (note study 3, which used contacts lacking previous immunization). Contacts of a case introduced from an endemic area, would be expected to benefit greatly if an effective chemoprophylactic agent could be added to primary immunization given after exposure.

Although a number of reports describe the use of methisazone therapeutically, its efficacy as a chemotherapeutic agent has yet to be extablished. A controlled study of its use in the treatment of smallpox failed to show significant effect (8). Unfortunately, reports of its successful use in the therapy of serious dermal complications

Table 5 Methisazone: chemoprophylaxis for smallpox contacts

Study	Double-Blind Design	Total No. Contacts		Clinical Disease		p value
		Methisazone	Control	Methisazone	Control	
				(%)	(%)	
1. Bauer (86)	No	2610	2560	0.69	3.99	0.001
2. do Valle[a] (87)	No	384	520	2.1	8.1	0.05
3. Rao[b] (88)	Yes	17	20	11.8	40.	ns
4. Heiner (10)	a. No	156	157	1.9	5.	ns
	b. Yes	106	103	3.7	4.8	ns

[a]Epidemic of alastrim.

[b]Contacts lacked previous immunization.

of vaccinia immunization, i.e. eczema vaccinatum and vaccinia gangrenosa, have all been anecdotal in nature (78, 89, 90). In light of the rising number of individuals with depressed cellular immunity, the time is ripe for a good double-blind study to determine the efficacy of methisazone as an adjunct to vaccinia immune globulin in the treatment of the serious vaccinial infections that occur in such individuals.

Interferon

Interferon is a proteinacious substance, released from cells during viral infection and under certain other circumstances, that has the capacity to convey on other cells a resistance to challenge with virus. Since interferon has been identified in both man and the lower animals during natural infection with virus, it is considered likely to be an important natural defense mechanism (91, 92). In addition, there is widespread anticipation of eventual fulfillment of a therapeutic potential for the interferon system, i.e. the use of exogenous interferon itself or an inducer of endogenous interferon, to prevent or treat viral disease in man.

Human interferon has never been fully purified, but has been found to behave chemically like a glycoprotein (93). Viral-induced human interferon has several molecular species that may be multiples of a predominant dimer form having a molecular weight of 23,000 and an isoelectric point of 5.6 (94, 95). The antiviral activity of interferon is still under investigation but is known to require the production of a second protein (96). Evidence has been presented that the resulting antiviral action can either attenuate ribosomes so they will no longer read viral RNA (18) or inhibit the activity of those RNA dependent polymerases brought into the cell by a virus (19, 20). In cell culture, interferon produced by cells of human or other animal origin has been shown to protect cells of the same or phylogenetically related species against a great variety of RNA and DNA viruses (97). Against experimental local or systemic viral infection in animals, interferon from the same or related species has also been found to be protective (98, 99).

Because the methods of producing large quantities of human interferon are only now being developed, and because full purification of interferon has still not been perfected, clinical studies in man have been quite limited, and the pharmacology of human interferon remains largely unknown. From the rate of disappearance of serum interferon after induction with a synthetic polymer, the serum half-life of human interferon can be estimated at less than 12 hr (100). It is also known that human interferon given intravenously to a rabbit has a serum half-life in the rabbit of about 73 min (101). Because serum, urine, saliva, spinal fluid, bile, and feces each have been shown capable of inactivating human interferon in vitro, it is likely that the fate of natural human interferon in vivo is almost entirely accounted for by metabolic degradation (102, 103). Partially purified human viral-induced leukocyte interferon has been associated with fever and chills when given intravenously to terminal cancer patients (104). However, these effects are considered secondary to leukocyte incompatability, and sufficiently pure human interferon would presumably have no toxicities because it is a native metabolite.

The same factors that have held up the pharmacological evaluation of interferon have made the determination of its clinical efficacy all but impossible. Several volunteer studies, using highly purified interferon for prophylaxis against local infection, are currently under way. The best study so far reported a double-blind investigation using a total of 14 million units of interferon per volunteer. The interferon was given locally by nasal spray in multiple doses beginning 24 hr prior to innoculation of rhinovirus 4 (105). A significant decrease in both severe symptoms and frequency of virus-shedding was found. Although the therapy was far from being practical, at least the ability of exogenous human interferon to prophylactically attenuate a local viral infection was clearly established. For systemic viral disease, clinical trials to determine the efficacy of prophylactic or therapeutic exogenous human interferon, unfortunately, must await both a perfection in the purification of interferon and further development in the logistics of its production.

Polyriboinosinic Acid and Polyribocytidylic Acid

Because of the still unresolved problems in establishing a practical use for interferon itself, attention has turned to the various nonviral inducers of interferon as alternative means for prophylactic or therapeutic intervention. The best studied nonviral inducer of interferon is polyriboinosinic acid • polyribocytidylic acid (poly I•poly C, Figure 4–6). Poly I•poly C is the equal molar complex of the synthetic homopolymers of the nucleotides, inosinic acid, and cytidylic acid. By X-ray diffraction study, sedimentation coefficient, ultraviolet absorption, and melting point determination, poly I•poly C is a double stranded helical complex of the two homopolymers (106, 107). In low concentration poly I•poly C will protect cells in culture from challenge with virus. In higher concentrations the complex with both protect the cells and release assayable interferon into the medium (108). The mechanism by which interferon is induced is not fully worked out, although it is known to require derepression of the host cell genome with host directed protein synthesis (109) and may accomplish this without entering the cell (110). When given to a variety of animals by topical or parenteral administration, poly I•poly C is associated with a rapid rise in interferon levels and definite protection against local or systemic viral infection, respectively (111).

Studies with human plasma in vitro have shown it capable of almost completely inactivating poly I•poly C within 1 hr, presumably through circulating nucleases (112). It is likely therefore that in man metabolism accounts for the elimination of almost all of the administered dose. Biologically, it is found in man that parenteral poly I•poly C leads to a hyporeactive state lasting several days during which additional injections will not induce further interferon (100) [animal studies have indicated that protection against virus is not present during such a hyporeactive state (113)]. Unfortunately, the intravenous administration of poly I•poly C in a dose of 2.5 mg/m² to man is associated with increased fibrin split monomers, a prolongation of thrombin time, and fever; even with a dose of 1.0 mg/m², there is a detectable increase in fibrin split monomers. In dosage low enough to avoid toxicity there is no detectable interferon in the serum (114).

A double-blind study of topical poly I•poly C (1000 μg/ml) has shown it to be as effective as topical IDU (0.2%) for the treatment of superficial herpetic keratitis (115). Another double-blind study using nasal drops of poly I•poly C both prophylactically and therapeutically has shown it to induce only minimal amounts of nasal interferon and to be associated with a small reduction in the severity of respiratory symptoms [following innoculation of either rhinovirus 13 or the Hong Kong strain of Influenza A_2 (116)]. As already noted, phase two studies have demonstrated that intravenous poly I•poly C is rapidly degraded and toxic and in addition has a tendency to produce a hyporeactive state. Further trials to determine its clinical efficacy via parenteral routes of administration have not been attempted.

Conclusion

It is evident that a monumental amount of hard work has been devoted to establishing practical viral chemotherapy. Nevertheless, it is quite clear that clinical efficacy has been established in a very few circumstances (Table 6). Clearly, there is a place for the topical use of antiviral agents in the treatment of herpetic keratitis, but at the present time there is no systemic viral disease for which we have a proven means of chemotherapy. It is encouraging that the use of amantadine and methisazone in the prophylaxis of influenza A_2 and smallpox, respectively, has been accepted. Hopefully, there will be a day soon when the problems peculiar to the field of viral chemotherapy will be effectively overcome and a proven treatment for systemic viral diseases will be at hand.

Table 6   Established clinical efficacy of antiviral agents

	TOPICAL		SYSTEMIC	
	Prophylaxis	Therapy	Prophylaxis	Therapy
Amantadine			+	
IDU		+		
AraC				
AraA		+		
Methisazone			+	
Interferon	+[a]			
Poly I-Poly C	+[a]	+		

[a] Protection against challenge inoculation but without adequate field trial against natural infection.

Literature Cited

1. Kaufman, H. E. 1962. *Proc. Soc. Exp. Biol. Med.* 109:251–52
2. Pavan-Langston, D., Dohlman, C. H. 1972. *Am. J. Ophthalmol.* 74:81–88
3. Nolan, D. C., Lauter, C. B., Lerner, A. M. 1973. *Ann. Intern. Med.* 78:243–46
4. Juel-Jensen, B. E. 1970. *Brit. Med. J.* 2:154–55
5. Saben, A. B. 1967. *J. Am. Med. Assoc.* 200:943–50
6. Bauer, D. J., Sadler, P. W. 1961. *Nature* 190:1167–69
7. Knight, V., Fedson, D., Baldini, J., Douglas, R. G., Couch, R. B. 1970. *Infect. Immunity* 1:200–4
8. Rao, A. R. Quoted by Bauer, D. J. 1972. In *Int. Encycl. Pharmacol. Ther. Vol. 1, Chemotherapy of Viral Diseases,* ed. D. J. Bauer, Sect. 61, p. 79

9. Oker-Blom, N. et al 1970. *Brit. Med. J.* 3:676–78
10. Heiner, G. G. et al 1971. *Am. J. Epidemiol.* 94:435–49
11. Finland, M., Jones, W. F. Jr., Barnes, M. W. 1959. *J. Am. Med. Assoc.* 170: 2188–97
12. Jawetz, E., Coleman, V. R., Dawson, C. R., Thygeson, P. 1970. *Ann. NY Acad. Sci.* 173:Article 1, 282–91
13. Holland, J. J., Hoyer, B. H. 1962. *Cold Spring Harbor Symp. Quant. Biol.* 27: 101–11
14. DeSomer, P., Prinzie, A., Schonne, E. 1959. *Nature* 184:652–53
15. Baltimore, D., Huang, A. S., Stampfer, M. 1970. *Proc. Nat. Acad. Sci. USA* 66:572–76
16. Huang, A. S., Baltimore, D. 1970. *Bacteriol. Proc.,* 215
17. Hoffmann, C. E., Neumayer, E. M., Haff R. F., Goldsby, R. A. 1965. *Bacteriol.* 90:623–28
18. Marcus, P. I., Salb, J. M. 1966. *Virology* 30:502–16
19. Marcus, P. I., Engelhardt, D. L., Hunt, J. M., Sekellick, M. J. 1971. *Science* 174:593–98
20. Manders, E. K., Tilles, J. G., Huang, A. S. 1972. *Virology* 49:573–81
21. Caligiuri, L. A., Tamm, I. 1970. *Ann. NY Acad. Sci.* 173:Article 1, 420–26
22. Dales, S., Mosbach, E. H. 1968. *Virology* 35:564
23. Bialy, H. S., Colby C. 1972. *J. Virol.* 9:286–89
24. Katz, E., Moss, B. 1970. *Proc. Nat. Acad. Sci. USA* 66:677–84
25. Davies, W. L. et al 1964. *Science* 144:862–63
26. Maassab, H. F., Cochran, K. W. 1964. *Science* 145:1443–44
27. Oxford, J. S., Schild, G. C. 1967. *Brit. J. Exp. Pathol.* 48:235–43
28. Grunert, R. R., McGahen, J. W., Davies, W. L. 1965. *Virology* 26:262–69
29. McGahen, J. W., Hoffmann, C. E. 1968. *Proc. Soc. Exp. Biol. Med.* 129:678–81
30. Bleidner, W. E., Harman, J. B., Hewes, W. E., Lynes, T. E., Hermann E. C. 1965. *J. Pharmacol. Exp. Ther.* 150: 484–90
31. Peckinpaugh, R. O. et al 1970. *Ann. NY Acad. Sci.* 173:Article 1, 62–73
32. AMA Council on Drugs. 1967. Evaluation of a new antiviral agent—amantadine hydrochloride. *J. Am. Med. Assoc.* 201:114–15
33. Parkes, J. D. et al 1971. *Lancet* i:1083–87

34. Finklea, J. F., Hennessy, A. V., Davenport, F. M. 1967. *Am. J. Epidemiol.* 85:403–12
35. Quilligan, J. J. Jr., Hirayama, M., Baernstein, H. D. Jr. 1966. *J. of Pediat.* 69:572–75
36. Wendel, H. A., Snyder, M. T., Pell, S. 1966. *Clin. Pharmacol. Ther.* 7:38–43
37. Galbraith, A. W., Oxford, J. S., Schild, G. C., Watson, G. I. 1969. *Lancet* ii:1026–28
38. Togo, Y., Hornick, R. B., Dawkins, A. T. 1968. *J. Am. Med. Assoc.* 203: 1089–94
39. Smorodintsev, A. A. et al 1970. *J. Am. Med. Assoc.* 213:1448–54
40. Public Health Service Advisory Committee on Immunization Practices. 1972. *Morbidity and Mortality Weekly Rep.* 21:No. 25 Suppl., 10–11
41. Tilles, J. G. 1971. *N. Engl. J. Med.* 285:1260–61
42. Wingfield, W. L., Pollack, D., Grunert, R. R. 1969. *N. Engl. J. Med.* 281: 579–84
43. Walters, H. E., Paulshock, M. 1970. *Mo. Med.* 67:176–79
44. Togo, Y. et al 1970. *J. Am. Med. Assoc.* 211:1149–56
45. Galbraith, A. W., Oxford, J. S., Schild, G. C., Potter, C. W., Watson, G. I. 1971. *Lancet* ii:113–15
46. Hers, J. F. Ph., Mulder, J. 1961. *Am. Rev. Resp. Dis.* 83:No. 2 Suppl., 84–94
47. Rogers, D. E. *Am. Rev. Resp. Dis.* 83:No. 2 Suppl. 61–63
48. Goz, B., Prusoff, W. H. 1970. *Ann. Rev. Pharmacol.* 10:143–70
49. Lerner, A. M., Bailey, E. J. 1972. *J. Clin. Invest.* 51:45–49
50. Sidwell, R. W., Arnett, G., Brockman, R. W. 1970. *Ann. NY Acad. Sci.* 173: 592–602
51. Loddo, B., Muntoni, S., Ferrari, W. 1963. *Nature* 198:510
52. Rapp, R., Vanderslice, D. 1964. *Virology* 22:321–30
53. Rawls, W. E., Cohen, R. A., Herrman, E. C. 1964. *Proc. Soc. Exp. Biol. Med.* 115:123–27
54. Kaufman, H. E. 1963. *Perspect. Virol.* 3:90–103
55. Tomlinson, A. H., MacCallum, F. O. 1970. *Ann. NY Acad. Sci.* 173:Article 1, 20–28
56. Calabresi, P., Creasey, W. A., Prusoff, W. H., Welch, A. D. 1963. *Cancer Res.* 23:583–92
57. Calabresi, P. et al 1961. *Cancer Res.* 21:550–59

58. Clarkson, D. R., Oppelt, W. W., Byvoet, P. 1967. *J. Pharmacol. Exp. Ther.* 157:581–88
59. Calabresi, P. 1963. *Cancer Res.* 23:1260–67
60. Leopold, I. H. 1965. *Ann. NY Acad. Sci.* 130:Article 1, 181–91
61. Kibrick, S., Katz, A. S. 1970. *Ann. NY Acad. Sci.* 173:Article 1, 83–89
62. Juel-Jensen, B. E., MacCallum, F. O. 1965. *Brit. Med. J.* 1:901
63. Campbell, J. B., Maes, R. F., Wiktor, T. J., Koprowski, H. 1968. *Virology* 34:701–8
64. Underwood, G. E. 1962. *Proc. Soc. Exp. Biol. Med.* 111:660–64
65. Underwood, G. E. 1964. *Int. Congr. Chemother. Proc., 3rd,* 1:858–60
66. Sidwell, R. W., Dixon, G. J., Sellers, S. M., Schabel, F. M. 1968. *Appl. Microbiol.* 16:370–92
67. Ho, D. H. W., Frei, E. III. 1971. *Clin. Pharmacol. Ther.* 12:944–54
68. Talley, R. W., O'Bryan, R. M., Tucker, W. G., Loo, R. V. 1967. *Cancer* 20:809–16
69. Mitchell, M. S., Wade, M. E., De Conti, R. C., Bertino, J. R., Calabresi, P. 1969. *Ann. Intern. Med.* 70:535–47
70. Stevens, D. A., Jordan, G. W., Waddell, T. R., Merigan, T. C. *N. Engl. J. Med.* In press
71. De Rudder, J., Privat De Garilhe, M. 1966. *Antimicrob. Ag. Chemother. 1965.,* 578–84
72. Schabel, F. M. Jr. 1968. *Chemotherapy* 13:321–38
73. Sloan, B. J., Miller, F. A., McLean, I. W. Jr. 1973. *Antimicrob. Ag. Chemother.* 3:74–80
74. Sloan, B. J., Miller, F. A., Ehrlich, J., McLean, I. W., Machamer, H. E. 1969. *Antimicrob. Ag. Chemother. 1968,* 161–71
75. Ch'ien, L. T., Glazko, A. J., Buchanan, R. A., Alford, C. A. 1971. *Program Abstr. Intersci. Conf. Antimicrob. Ag. Chemother., 11th,* p. 47
76. Ch'ien, L. T., Schabel, F. M. Jr., Alford C. A. Jr. *Selective Inhibitors of Viral Function,* ed. W. A. Carter. In press
77. Wilkerson, S., Finely, S. C., Finely, W. H., Ch'ien, L. T. 1973. *Clin. Res.* 21:52
78. Bauer, D. J. 1972. *Int. Encyclopedia Pharmacol. Therapeut.* Vol. 1, *Chemotherapy of Viral Diseases,* ed. D. J. Bauer, Sect. 61
79. Woodson, B., Joklik, W. K. 1965. *Proc. Nat. Acad. Sci. USA* 54:946–53
80. Caunt, A. *Int. Congr. Chemother., 5th, Vienna, 1967,* 4:313–17
81. Bauer, D. J., Apostolov, K. 1966. *Science* 154:796–97
82. Bauer, D. J., Apostolov, K., Selway, J. W. T. 1970. *Ann. NY Acad. Sci.* 173:Article 1, 314–19
83. Bauer, D. J., Sadler, P. W. 1960. *Brit. J. Pharmacol. Chemother.* 15:101–10
84. Bauer, D. J., Dumbell, K. R., Fox-Hulme, P., Sadler, P. W. 1962. *Bull. WHO* 26:727–32
85. Kempe, C. H., Rodgerson, D., Sieber, O. F. Jr. 1965. *Lancet* i:824–25
86. Bauer, D. J., St. Vincent, L., Kempe, C. H., Young, P. A., Downie, A. W. 1969. *Am. J. Epidemiol.* 90:130–45
87. do Valle, L. A. R., de Melo, P. R., de Gomes, L. F., Proenca, L. M. 1965. *Lancet* ii:976–78
88. Rao, A. R., Jacobs, E. S. Kamalakski, S., Bradbury S., Swamy, A. 1969. *Indian J. Med. Res.* 57:477–83
89. Bauer, D. J. 1965. *Ann. NY Acad. Sci.* Article 130, 110–17
90. Kempe, C. H., Fulgeniti, V., Sieber, O. *Int. Congr. Chemother., 5th, Vienna, 1967,* Abstr. Pt. 2, 1234
91. Baron, S. 1967. *Interferons* pp. 268–93
92. Wheelock, E. F., Sibley, W. A. 1964. *Lancet* ii:382–85
93. Cesario, T. C., Tilles, J. G. Presented at the Interscience Conference on Antimicrobial Agents and Chemotherapy, 13th, Washington DC, September 1973
94. Carter, W. A. 1970. *Proc. Nat. Acad. Sci. USA* 67:620–28
95. Cesario, T. C., Tilles, J. G. Manuscript in preparation
96. Taylor, J. 1964. *Biochem. Biophys. Res. Commun.* 14:447
97. Ho, M. 1962. *Engl. J. Med.* 226:1258–64
98. Finter, N. B. 1966. *Interferons* pp. 232–67
99. Finter, N. B. 1967. *J. Gen. Virol.* 1:395–97
100. Hill, D. A. et al 1971. *Perspectives Virol.* 7:198–222
101. Cantell, K., Pyhala, L. 1973. Personal communication
102. Casario, T. C., Tilles, J. G. 1973. *J. Infec. Dis.* 127:311–14
103. Cesario, T. C., Mandell, A., Tilles, J. G. *Proc. Soc. Exp. Biol. Med.* In press
104. Falcoff, E., Falcoff, R., Fournier, F., Chany, C., Gallot, B. 1966. *Ann. Inst. Pasteur Paris* 3:562–84
105. Merigan, T. C., Reed, S. E., Hall, T. S., Tyrell, D. A. J. 1973. *Lancet* i:563–67
106. Field, A. K., Tytell, A. A., Lampson, G. P., Hilleman, M. R. 1967. *Proc. Nat. Acad. Sci. USA* 58:1004–10

107. Rich, A., Watson, J. D. 1954 *Proc. Nat. Acad. Sci. USA* 40:759
108. Field, A. K., Tytell, A. A., Lampson, G. P., Hilleman, M. R. 1967. *Proc. Nat. Acad. Sci., USA* 58:1004
109. Falcoff, E., Perez-Bercoff, R. 1969. *Biochim. Biophys. Acta.* 174:108–16
110. Taylor-Papadimitriou, J., Kallos, J. 1973. *Nature New Biol.* 245:143–44
111. Nemes, M. M., Tytell, A. A., Lampson, G. P., Field, A. K., Hilleman, M. R. 1969. *Proc. Soc. Exp. Biol. Med.* 132: 776–83

112. Norlund, J. J., Wolff, S. M., Levy, H. B. 1970. *Proc. Soc. Exp. Biol. Med.* 133: 439–40
113. De Clercq, E. 1971. *Proc. Soc. Exp. Biol. Med.* 141:340–45
114. De Vita, V. et al 1970. *Proc. Am. Soc. Cancer Res.* 11:21
115. Guerra, R., Frezzotti, R., Bonanni, R., Dianzani, F., Rita, G. 1970. *Ann. NY Acad. Sci.* 173:Article 1, 823–30
116. Hill, D. A. et al 1972. *J. Am. Med. Assoc.* 219:1179–84

REGULATION OF BIOSYNTHESIS OF CATECHOLAMINES AND SEROTONIN IN THE CNS

❖6604

E. Costa and J. L. Meek
Laboratory of Preclinical Pharmacology, National Institute of Mental Health, Saint Elizabeths Hospital, Washington DC

INTRODUCTION

Brain contains several aralkylamines of considerable functional importance: norepinephrine (NE), dopamine (DA), and serotonin (5-hydroxytryptamine, 5HT). Their importance lies in an involvement in the exchange of information between two neurons where they function as neurotransmitters.

The overall process of neurotransmission and its changing frequency in different types of neurons can be studied either by recording the electrical activity of neurons or by examining the dynamics of the release of neurotransmitters. Because it is not possible to study the amount of neurotransmitter that reaches the receptors except in artificial conditions, the overall amount of neurotransmitter in the tissue is all that can be measured. The amount present extraneuronally is small in comparison with the amount of neurotransmitter present intraneuronally, so what is measured is largely intraneuronal. Additionally, some of the neurotransmitter molecules that are synthesized intraneuronally are destroyed before they can reach the receptor sites. The turnover rate in vivo of a neurotransmitter is a useful measure of the utilization rate of transmitter molecules as it may reflect the rate of synaptic transactions. The methods and the assumptions involved in measuring turnover and the limitations necessary in interpreting the results of turnover studies have been reviewed (1–3).

The rate of biosynthesis of neurotransmitters in the CNS is subject to alterations by many factors, but the nervous system is able to control this rate in response to varying demands. The object of this review is to bring into focus the molecular nature of the various processes involved in the regulation of the biosynthesis of catecholamines and serotonin. We review sites of physiological control that have emerged during the last few years and stress the information important in the study of the mode of action of drugs on the CNS.

491

The rate of aralkylamine biosynthesis in any part of the CNS reflects the local equilibrium among small molecules and macromolecules—the biosynthetic enzymes, their cofactors, substrates, products, inhibitors, and activators. Each of these molecules is itself subject to an equilibrium between renovation and disappearance. In different areas, the factors affecting these equilibria are functionally different due to the peculiar nature of the neuron. In the perikarya, enzyme molecules are renovated by de novo synthesis; in nerve terminals, however, the renovation of enzyme molecules depends on transport from the perikarya. Thus, in the former site, the regulation of one half of the equilibrium depends on the control of DNA transcription and RNA translation, while in the terminals, introduction of new enzyme molecules involves axoplasmic flow and transport which are as yet poorly understood. At steady state, the rate of enzyme degradation balances that of synthesis. Again, the processes involved in the two sites are different: in perikarya, the axoplasmic flow is probably the major process causing disappearance of enzyme molecules, whereas in the nerve terminals, destruction is caused by proteolysis or elimination by exocytosis. Because the nature of enzyme degradation in nerve terminals is still poorly understood, the role it may play in the regulation of transmitter biosynthesis is currently unknown.

Portions of our topic have been considered at recent symposia (4–6). Recent reviews have summarized other aspects of catecholamine and serotonin research including biochemistry of the catecholamines (7), regulation of catecholamine turnover in the periphery (8, 9), structure and function of synaptic vesicles (10), pteridine cofactors (11), biogenic amines and mental disorders (12–14), axonal transport (15), LSD and serotonin (16), drugs affecting biogenic amines (17), and amine uptake mechanisms (18).

HYDROXYLATION OF TRYPTOPHAN AND TYROSINE

Tryptophan and tyrosine are the amino acids that function as precursors in the biosynthesis of indolealkylamines and catecholamines respectively. The first step in the biosynthesis of these two amines involves ring hydroxylation by two mixed function oxygenases, tyrosine hydroxylase (EC 1.10.3.1) and tryptophan hydroxylase (EC 1.99.1.4). Although these two enzymes are themselves similar, the possibilities for regulation differ in the two types of neurons. For example, there is not enough tryptophan in brain to saturate tryptophan hydroxylase, while tyrosine hydroxylase is saturated with tyrosine. In addition, tryptophan hydroxylase is not inhibited by high concentrations of 5-hydroxytryptophan or 5HT, whereas tyrosine hydroxylase is inhibited by NE ($10^{-4}M$) (19). To understand the phenomena involved in the regulation of these two enzymes better we discuss the hydroxylation step from the standpoint of cofactor requirements, end-product inhibition, and the possibility of allosteric changes in conformation.

Pterin Cofactors

Pterins are necessary cofactors for hydroxylation (11, 19–21), but the exact chemical structure of the natural cofactor in brain is not certain. Most of the studies on the kinetic constants of tryptophan hydroxylase have been made with the synthetic cofactor, 6,7-dimethyltetrahydropterin (DMPH$_4$) (22). When these constants are compared with those obtained with tetrahydrobiopterin (BH$_4$), the probable natural cofactor, it is clear that many of the inferences made concerning the regulation of tryptophan hydroxylase in vivo do not hold. For instance, the K_m of this enzyme using DMPH$_4$ as a cofactor is 290 μM (22), a finding which supports the view that enzyme in vivo is not saturated by tryptophan since its concentration in brain is about 50 μM. However, the K_m for tryptophan measured using BH$_4$ is 50 μM (22). Analogous differences have been reported measuring the K_m for O$_2$ with DMPH$_4$ (20%) and with BH$_4$ (2.5%) (22). The K_m values obtained with the probable natural cofactor for tryptophan and O$_2$ are therefore similar to the concentrations of these substrates in vivo. These data are consistent with the magnitude of increase in hydroxylation which is obtained by loading animals with tryptophan or subjecting them to hyperbaric oxygen. It has been suggested that most enzymes operate in vivo with substrates at a concentration approximately similar to the K_m (23).

Assuming that BH$_4$ or a pterin with similar biological properties is the natural cofactor, the pterin can function in hydroxylation only in the reduced form. Dihydropteridine reductase which has been isolated and purified from liver homogenates (24) can maintain the cofactor in the reduced state. This enzyme is also present in high concentrations in liver, kidney, brain, and adrenal medulla. This reductase might be regulatory for the hydroxylation of tyrosine and tryptophan (25, 26) but such a possibility is not substantiated by the available data (24). It would seem that the amount of reduced BH$_4$ rather than the enzyme could perform a regulatory function. The concentration of BH$_4$ in adrenal is 10 μM (20) and in brain is estimated to be 0.75 μg/g (3 μM if evenly distributed) (27). Inferences as to regulatory potential for the biosynthesis of NE, DA, and 5HT in brain are premature until we know more about the regional and cellular distribution of BH$_4$. Nonetheless, we can speculate that the BH$_4$ concentrations may be limiting in some circumstances because the K_m of adrenal tyrosine hydroxylase is 20 μM (19) and that of brain tryptophan hydroxylase is 31 μM (22). The value of such speculation for catecholamine biosynthesis is further supported if one considers that the catechol products of tyrosine hydroxylase inhibit their own formation by competing with the pterin cofactor. If the pterin were to be in concentrations below the K_m, its potential as a regulatory mechanism would be enhanced. In addition, conformational changes of tyrosine hydroxylase (28–30) have been described and these are associated with changes of K_i values for the catecholamines, increasing the possibility of a physiological regulation by this mechanism.

The cofactors for dopamine-β-hydroxylase are ascorbic acid and copper. Ascorbic acid is probably not limiting in norepinephrine synthesis because the apparent K_m for ascorbate with the adrenal enzyme (0.9 mM) (31) is less than or similar to the reported content of ascorbate in adrenal and brain (32). Before the discovery of the noradrenergic pathways in the brain, histochemical evidence (33) suggested that there might be high ascorbic acid concentrations in the cells of the locus coeruleus and in the hypothalamus, areas rich in NE. Although it would be tempting to speculate that cells containing dopamine-β-hydroxylase are rich in ascorbic acid, it might be that the silver stain used to detect ascorbic acid was actually being reduced by NE. Peripherally injected ^{14}C-ascorbic acid does not concentrate in brain in areas with high concentrations of NE (34).

pO_2

Molecular oxygen is required for hydroxylation of tyrosine, tryptophan, and DA. The K_m of tryptophan hydroxylase from rabbit brain for oxygen is approximately 2.5%, which is a concentration in the order of magnitude of those reported in brain (22), although pO_2 varies in different brain parts. When rats inhale 100% O_2, the pO_2 in various areas approximately doubles (35, 36). Under these conditions, the turnover rate of brain 5HT and cathecholamines increases (37, 38). Anoxia produces a decrease in the hydroxylation of tryptophan in vivo; this parallels the fall in arterial pO_2 (39). Tyrosine hydroxylase is also not saturated with oxygen (40), and breathing a concentration of oxygen lower than normal decreases the hydroxylation of tyrosine in vivo (39). Dopamine-β-hydroxylase is apparently also not saturated at normal pO_2 (41). Although changes in pO_2 may alter the rate of amine formation, oxygen is not likely to play a physiological role in regulating the catecholamine turnover rate. However, it would be desirable to know whether conformational changes in these hydroxylases alter the K_m for O_2 before ruling out changes in pO_2 as a physiological control mechanism for hydroxylation.

Allosteric and Other Conformational Changes of Hydroxylases

It is well established that nerve stimulation can increase the synthesis of catecholamines by a mechanism which is too rapid to be caused by de novo synthesis of tyrosine hydroxylase (8, 9). Part of the increased catecholamine synthesis might be related to a decrease in end-product inhibition, but Weiner and colleagues have concluded that additional factors may be operating (42). The conformation of tyrosine hydroxylase (and its activity) might vary with nerve firing rate, due to changes in the ionic environment or binding to membranes.

Potassium and sulfate ions can stimulate tyrosine hydroxylase activity in vitro. Sulfate ions in high concentrations (30) appear to interact with the enzyme molecules, but the high concentrations involved indicate that the effect is probably devoid of physiological importance. The activation by potassium (43) is probably not via direct interaction with the enzyme molecules, because it occurs only in slices, and thus requires the integrity of nerve endings. Potassium might affect tyrosine hydroxylase by interacting with nerve ending constitutents such as membranes, but the action is probably related to the release of catecholamines and the resulting decrease in end-product inhibition.

Tyrosine hydroxylase appears to occur partially free and partially bound to membranes (28, 44). The enzyme molecules are presumed to have the same amino acid sequence because the fraction that is bound depends on the homogenization conditions (28, 45). However, the conformations of the two forms are probably different because their catalytic properties are not identical. According to Kuczenski & Mandell (28), the membrane bound form of tyrosine hydroxylase, compared with the soluble form exhibits a smaller apparent K_m for DMPH$_4$ and a lower K_i for dopamine. They suggested that the membrane binding of the enzyme has an important regulatory value in synaptic function. The kinetic parameters of the soluble enzyme become like those of the particulate form if heparin is added: it lowers the K_m for DMPH$_4$, decreases the K_i for dopamine and increases the apparent V_{max} of the enzyme (28, 30). Heparin is not an important constituent of the brain, but other sulfated mucopolysaccharides are components of cellular and synaptic membranes. This activation occurs only in the presence of tris buffer at certain pHs and has not yet been achieved with preparations of naturally occurring brain membranes.

The ratio of the particulate form to the soluble form is smaller in areas rich in aminergic cell bodies. This finding supports the possibility that the apparent two forms of subcellular localization are real. In adrenal chromaffin cells, tyrosine hydroxylase was thought to occur primarily in a bound form (46, 47). Recent work suggests that the adrenal enzyme is mainly free and that the apparent particulate nature was due to an aggregation of enzyme molecules (48, 49). This question is still controversial (50).

Whether or not the adrenal enzyme is particulate, it may be that the activity of the brain enzyme can be modified by a shift in location from a free to a bound form. It is quite possible that the control mechanisms operating in the brain differ from the adrenal where end-product inhibition and enzyme induction are more likely to be important.

The ratio in brain of free to bound tyrosine hydroxylase can be changed by pharmacological manipulations. A single dose of methamphetamine (2.5 mg/kg) produced a slight but significant shift in localization of tyrosine hydroxylase from the soluble to the particulate form (51). A similar effect was seen after reserpine and α-methyltyrosine. However, imipramine, foot shock, and/or electroconvulsive shock (all of which increase the turnover rate of brain NE) failed to increase the activity of tyrosine hydroxylase (51).

In our laboratory, Drs. Zivkovic and Guidotti have found that free, but not bound striatal tyrosine hydroxylase activity is doubled within 30 min after injection of small doses of tranquilizers of the phenothiazine or butyrophenone type. These compounds are dopamine receptor blockers, and increase the firing rate of dopaminergic neurons, probably via a neuronal feedback loop (see below). The effect on tyrosine hydroxylase can be reversed by apomorphine, which stimulates dopamine receptors and slows the firing rate of the dopaminergic neurons. These changes in tyrosine hydroxylase activity were observed in the dopaminergic neurons of the striatum, but did not occur in the noradrenergic neurons of the hypothalamus.

The occurrence of two forms of tryptophan hydroxylase in brain and their varying regional distribution have been discussed by Knapp & Mandell (52–55). Homogenizing tissues with isotonic sucrose, they found that the enzyme of brain stem (cell bodies) is soluble, whereas that of other parts of brain is particle bound because it is associated with synaptosomes (the particle bound tyrosine hydroxylase discussed above occurs even after lysis of the synaptosomes). This tryptophan hydroxylase is not activated by the synthetic cofactor (DMPH$_4$), because the cofactor cannot penetrate the synaptosomal membrane (56). After chronic morphine administration, Knapp & Mandell have described an increase in tryptophan hydroxylase activity compensatory to an initial inhibitory action. The question of whether two forms of tryptophan hydroxylase exist in vivo and their regulatory significance deserves further investigation.

The best direct evidence that allosteric effects alter the conformation of one of the mixed function oxygenases acting upon an amino acid comes from studies of liver phenylalanine hydroxylase, which shares with tyrosine hydroxylase many kinetic properties, cofactor requirements, and antigenic nature (57). Lysolecithin, a detergent-like lipid, reversibly stimulates phenylalanine hydroxylase activity and causes a conformational change of the enzyme which results in exposing a SH group (58). A similar stimulation of brain tyrosine hydroxylase (59) occurs with the synthetic detergent Triton X-100, although the enzyme was not purified enough to study directly a conformational change. When solubilized hydroxylases from brain or adrenal medulla are treated with proteolytic enzymes, the enzyme's molecular weight is reduced (29, 44, 50, 58, 60) but the catalytic activity tends to increase (29, 58). The increased activity is associated with a decreased K_m for substrate and cofactor. These findings support the possibility that if depolymerization occurs in vivo it may produce significant increases in enzyme activity.

End-product Inhibition

Tyrosine hydroxylase can be inhibited in vitro by its end-product 3,4-dihydroxyphenylalanine (Dopa) or by its metabolites DA and NE (46). DA is more active than NE in competing with the pteridine cofactor for tyrosine hydroxylase (28, 46). The first demonstration that feedback inhibition may be important in the control of tyrosine hydroxylation in vivo came from studies with monoamine oxidase inhibitors (MAO) (61–64). Pargyline causes a decrease in the rate of NE and DA biosynthesis in the CNS and peripheral tissues. In the CNS, the DA and NE concentrations increase rapidly and the turnover rate is decreased within 1 or 2 hr after the injection of paragyline. This increase in concentration of catecholamines could inhibit tyrosine hydroxylase by competition with cofactors. However, the possibility cannot be ruled out that pargyline slows down the rate of catecholamine synthesis by slowing the firing rate of catecholamine neurons, or by other actions associated with MAO inhibitors.

The importance of endproduct inhibition in the regulation of peripheral catecholamine biosynthesis can be documented in heart. Here, due to the slow synthesis rate of catecholamines, they accumulate more slowly after inhibition of MAO (65). It is therefore possible to show that the time course of reduction of the rate of catecholamine biosynthesis parallels the accumulation rate of catecholamines and not the concentration of the MAO inhibitor in tissues.

If tyrosine hydroxylase is located outside the granules, then only the extragranular pool of Dopa and catecholamines can function in the physiological control of catecholamine biosynthesis by end-product inhibition. While the extragranular pool may be large after MAO inhibition, approximate estimates of pool sizes can be made. In the dopaminergic terminals of the striatum, the total dopamine concentration has been calculated to be at least 10^{-2} M (66). Since the K_i of striatal tyrosine hydroxylase for inhibition by dopamine is less than $10^{-4}M$ (28), significant inhibition would occur if only 1% of the dopamine were extragranular. The estimate of the K_i for dopamine is made with saturating concentrations of cofactor. If the cofactor is limiting, the inhibition would occur at even lower concentrations.

In noradrenergic terminals of spinal cord, the NE concentration is also calculated to be greater than 10^{-2} M. Because the DA concentration in various tissues may be 12–18% (67) that of NE, the total concentration of DA in the terminals might be 10^{-3} M. The distribution of DA in NE terminals is not established, but significant amounts are likely to occur free. Since DA is a more effective feedback inhibitor than NE, the possibility that DA operates in the feedback control of NE biosynthesis cannot be disregarded (68). The availability of specific MAO inhibitors which cause DA but not NE to increase, makes it possible to test this hypothesis (69).

Despite the difficulty of providing conclusive evidence on the physiological role of feedback control by product inhibition, the possibility that such control contributes to noradrenergic regulation should be investigated further.

Tryptophan hydroxylase is not inhibited in vitro by high concentrations of 5HTP, 5-hydroxyindole acetic acid (5HIAA) or 5HT. The enzyme is inhibited by catecholamines, but such inhibition is probably only important under artificial conditions such as after treatment of animals with large doses of Dopa. The turnover rate of brain 5HT is the same whether measured when the concentration of brain 5HT is normal or when it is increased threefold by MAO inhibition (70). In experiments with labeled tryptophan, the rate of synthesis of 5HT was measured in vivo without considering the change with time of the specific activity of the precursor and product (71). It was concluded that the 5HT synthesis could be controlled by end-product inhibition. Because the validity of these experiments has been questioned on technical grounds (72) the issues involved are still unsettled.

LONG-TERM INCREASES IN ENZYME ACTIVITIES IN MONOAMINERGIC CELLS

Persistent increases of impulse traffic in noradrenergic or dopaminergic cells or in the afferents to chromaffin cells bring about an increase of tyrosine hydroxylase (73) and dopamine-β-hydroxylase activities of tissue homogenates (74). Perhaps, this increase is due to enzyme induction (an increased synthesis of enzyme molecules) because it can be blocked by inhibition of protein synthesis (75, 76). The increase in the adrenal enzyme is described as trans-synaptically induced, a term seldom applied to the CNS. However, in both cases the delayed long-term increases in enzyme activity probably arise from long-term increases of firing rate (CNS) or rate of stimulation (chromaffin cells) and require the presence of an intact afferent system. These long-term increases have been best studied in the adrenal; less information is available for sympathetic ganglia and brain. The peripheral systems will be considered first to provide a framework for discussion of the data available for the brain.

Adrenal Medulla

Studies from this laboratory (77–82) have suggested that the increase of tyrosine hydroxylase activity in adrenal medulla involves the following sequence of events: 1. stimulation of nicotinic receptors, 2. increase of the concentration ratio of 3',5'-adenosine monophosphate (cAMP) to 3',5'-guanosine monophosphate (cGMP), 3. elaboration of the stimulus and 4. increase of enzyme activity.

1. Stimulation of nicotinic receptors: In the adrenal medulla, catecholamine secretion from chromaffin cells is elicited by cholinergic stimuli acting via nicotinic receptors (83). Exposure to 4°C for 1 hr or injection of a cholinomimetic (carbamylcholine or mecholine) can increase the activity of tyrosine hydroxylase after a latency of about 12 to 16 hr. Denervation of adrenals prevents the increase of tyrosine hydroxylase activity elicited by cold exposure but not that following the injection of the two cholinomimetics. Pretreatment with mecamylamine or hexamethonium (nicotinic blockers) prevents the increase of tyrosine hydroxylase activity elicited by either type of stimulus.

2. Increase of cAMP/cGMP concentration ratio: Exposure of rats to 4°C for 60 min or the injection of nicotinic stimulants causes an increase of the cAMP/cGMP concentration ratio which persists for about 2 hr even when the rats are exposed to cold for several hours. Denervation of the adrenal gland fails to change their phosphodiesterase activity or the concentration of cAMP but reduces the activity of cyclic nucleotide synthesizing enzymes and the concentrations of cGMP. If slices of adrenal medulla are incubated with carbamylcholine ($5 \times 10^{-5} M$), cAMP tends to accumulate in these slices at a rate faster than that of slices incubated without the nicotinic receptor stimulant. Chromaffin cells contain high concentrations of cAMP (about 40 pmol/mg protein) (78, 84, 85) and possess a very high adenylcyclase activity (39 pmol/mg protein/min). Cold exposure or the injection of nicotinic receptor stimulants (86) increases the catecholamine output from medulla and other peripheral stores. However, the concentration of cAMP in the adrenal medulla is not affected by drugs that increase circulating catecholamines but do not stimulate adrenal nicotinic receptors. The increase of medullary cAMP can therefore be dissociated from the release of catecholamine from adrenal medulla, but not from conditions that cause long-term increase of tyrosine hydroxylase activity. The report by Kvetnansky and colleagues (87) that the injection of dibutyryl cAMP restores the activity of tyrosine hydroxylase which had been reduced by hypophysectomy supports this relationship. Recent studies have shown that acetylcholine can cause accumulation of cGMP in heart, brain, vas deferens, and intestine; this effect is inhibited by atropine (88–91). Actually, Lee et al (90) recently suggested that excitation of muscarinic receptors increases the cGMP/cAMP concentration ratio in target cells whereas adrenergic receptor stimulation should increase the cAMP/cGMP concentration ratio in these cells. Because carbamylcholine injections increase the cAMP/cGMP concentration ratio in the adrenal medulla, this change is not exclusively elicited by adrenergic stimulation. Perhaps, we should refrain from explaining excitation of specific receptors in terms of changes of cyclic

nucleotide concentration ratios until we understand the location where cyclic nucleotides accumulate in response to receptor stimulation.

The view that a sustained increase of cAMP is an important signal in eliciting an increase of tyrosine hydroxylase activity in the adrenal medulla has been challenged (92). Thoenen et al (92) made 100 g rats swim in a water bath at 15°C for 7 to 10 min, and repeated this stress six times in 2 hr. This procedure caused a delayed and prolonged increase of medullary tyrosine hydroxylase although cAMP concentrations in this tissue were not increased at the end of each swimming stress. These authors (92) concluded that an increase of cAMP concentration did not necessarily precede trans-synaptic induction of tyrosine hydroxylase activity. However, we (80) found that swimming stress at 15°C in 100 g rats caused a decrease in body temperature of about 17°C which lasted more than 40 min. In adrenal medulla, the increase of cAMP/cGMP concentration ratio occurs only after the body temperature has returned to normal. Thus, swimming stress experiments do not negate the concept that in adrenal medulla an increase of cAMP/cGMP concentration ratio precedes the increase of tyrosine hydroxylase activity elicited trans-synaptically.

3. Elaboration of the stimulus: As mentioned previously, the increase of cAMP/cGMP concentration ratios occurs several hours before the long-term increase of tyrosine hydroxylase activity. There is no information yet on the phenomena involved in the elaboration of the message brought about in the chromaffin cells by the increase of cAMP/cGMP concentration ratios. Although we know from the work of Axelrod and colleagues (76) that the control of protein concentration is involved, we have no data to suggest whether it is at the transcription or at the translation level, or whether there is an increase in the synthesis rate of tyrosine hydroxylase or a reduction of its catabolism. The only information available is that a blockade of the nicotinic receptor during the elaboration of the stimulus fails to impair the increase of tyrosine hydroxylase activity (80).

4. Increase of enzyme activity: The term enzyme induction implies either an increased synthesis rate of enzyme molecules or an increase in the number of molecules from whatever cause. The latter use is more common, because unless the number of molecules can be estimated immunologically (93), it is difficult to determine the exact cause of long-term increases in enzyme activity. The concentration of an enzyme in a neuron depends on the balance of two processes: synthesis which occurs in the cell body and breakdown which can occur anywhere in the neuron. In the chromaffin cell, these sites are much closer together. In discussing activity of tyrosine hydroxylase in adrenal medulla one should keep in mind that there is a certain degree of functional alternation among cells of this tissue and that a masking or an unmasking of enzyme activity could be associated to this functional alternation. If this were the case, it would seem quite unusual that the mechanisms involved in this chemistry have a time constant of several hours. Another consideration concerns the possible hyperplasia or hypertrophy of the tissue. In chromaffin tissue, hyperplasia is probably a process of limited importance in the genesis of increases of tyrosine hydroxylase enzyme molecules. An increase in the number of cells is also not a cause for increased amounts of enzyme in brain, because adrenergic

neurons in brain stop dividing early in life. Noradrenergic terminals in brain can sprout in response to injury (94), but there is no evidence that sprouting is a mechanism involved in the long-term increase of enzyme activity elicited trans-synaptically.

Sympathetic Ganglia

Thoenen (95) first reported that exposure to 4°C for 48 hr increases tyrosine hydroxylase activity in sympathetic ganglia. Similar studies were extended to dopamine-β-hydroxylase. Hanbauer et al (96) have analyzed whether a sequence of events, similar to that reported for adrenal medulla is operative in the increase of tyrosine hydroxylase activity of rat cervical sympathetic ganglia elicited by cold exposure. Normally, rats require long-lasting exposure to cold before one can detect an increase of tyrosine hydroxylase activity in their ganglia. But, if the rats are demedulated at least 3 weeks prior to the experiment, then an exposure to 4°C for only 4 hr is sufficient to elicit an increase of tyrosine hydroxylase activity 48 hr later. Decentralization or pretreatment with mecamylamine or hexamethonium abolishes the delayed increase of tyrosine hydroxylase. However, if hexamethonium or mecamylamine are injected, after the stimulus, they fail to inhibit the increase of tyrosine hydroxylase activity (96). In ganglia of demedullated rats there is an increase of cAMP concentration and a decrease of cGMP concentration during the stimulus application (Hanbauer & Guidotti, unpublished). The increase of the cAMP/cGMP concentration ratios persists for the duration of the stimulus application (exposure to 4°C). Treatment with hexamethonium before exposure to cold prevents the increase of cAMP/cGMP concentration ratios as well as the delayed increase of tyrosine hydroxylase activity.

Pretreatment with atropine before or after the stimulus application fails to change the increase of tyrosine hydroxylase activity elicited by exposure to 4°C. In contrast, decentralization performed before or at various times after the cold exposure prevents the delayed increase of tyrosine hydroxylase activity in the ganglia. In addition, the injection of carbamylcholine to rats with unilateral decentralization of the superior cervical ganglion fails to elicit an increase of cAMP/cGMP concentration ratios or a delayed long-term increase of tyrosine hydroxylase activity in either ganglion. It is therefore apparent that in rats exposed to 4°C the correlation between the early increase of cAMP/cGMP concentration ratios and the delayed long-term increase of tyrosine hydroxylase activity which appears to be valid in the adrenal medulla might not be extrapolated to the sympathetic ganglia. This is not surprising because the cell population of adrenal medulla is rather uniform functionally and morphologically whereas the cells of sympathetic ganglia differ in both respects. The cyclic nucleotides in ganglia could be localized in presynaptic cholinergic endings, noradrenergic neurons, small intensely fluorescent cells and in a variety of supporting cells.

Central Nervous System

The delayed increase in long-term activity of brain tyrosine hydroxylase (95) and tryptophan hydroxylase differ significantly from those seen in the adrenal: the magnitude of the change is much less, and the delay is longer. Moreover, the interpretation of brain tyrosine hydroxylase increases is complicated, because in several brain areas both dopaminergic and noradrenergic neurons are present. In the brain, another factor which must be considered is that the enzyme is synthesized in cell bodies and must be moved a considerable distance to the nerve terminals by axonal transport. Thus, in brain there is a considerable lag between onset of increased protein synthesis and any increase in enzyme in the nerve terminals (97–99) (especially in large species); whereas in the adrenal, the only lag is the time interval needed for protein synthesis.

The tyrosine hydroxylase activity of several brain areas is increased 2 to 8 days after reserpine or cold exposure, but the extent of the increase is rather small (73, 95, 97, 100). In caudate, the extent of this increase is greater, but occurs within a few hours after the injection of reserpine or within 30 min after phenothiazines. Zivkovic and Guidotti have shown that protein synthesis inhibition does not affect this enzyme increase, suggesting that a mechanism different from the long-term increase of enzyme activity is involved. Repeated convulsive shocks increase brain tyrosine hydroxylase activity after 7 days (101) while phenothiazine-neuroleptics decrease it (97). Attempts at correlating the long term-delayed increase of tyrosine hydroxylase and the increase of cAMP/cGMP concentration ratios is impractical because the two nucleotides are present in a variety of other neurons present in the same brain areas and in numerous supporting cells.

There are conflicting reports as to whether morphine increases tryptophan hydroxylase activity (102–104). When the studies were conducted distinguishing between tryptophan hydroxylase in cell bodies and nerve endings, chronic morphine administration produced an immediate decrease (53) and a long-term increase of tryptophan hydroxylase in areas rich in serotonergic nerve endings, but it did not change enzyme activity in an area containing cell bodies. Short-term treatment with lithium chloride stimulates the uptake of tryptophan and its conversion to serotonin by synaptosomes (54). Cell body tryptophan hydroxylase activity is reduced at 5 days of treatment even if the uptake of tryptophan is increased. After 10 days of lithium treatment, the tryptophan hydroxylase activity in the nerve endings is decreased while the tryptophan uptake remains increased. The delay in the transfer of the alteration from cell bodies to nerve terminals corresponds in time to the axoplasmic transport for tryptophan hydroxylase (105). Lysergic acid diethylamide (LSD) is reported to decrease tryptophan hydroxylase activity (99). The mechanism is unknown but LSD, which is possibly a 5HT agonist at postsynaptic receptors, decreases the firing rate of serotonergic neurons.

Bilateral adrenalectomy reduces the tryptophan hydroxylase activity and the turnover rate of 5HT in the midbrain (106). The adrenocortical function plays a role in regulating tryptophan hydroxylase activity, and many drug effects appear to be mediated by adrenocortical secretion. Reserpine in high doses (5 mg/kg ip)(99) causes an increase of midbrain tryptophan hydroxylase activity beginning 10–14 hr after the injection. This increase reaches a plateau between 36 and 48 hr after the injection of the drug. The increase extends to the serotonergic endings after a latency time compatible with the axoplasmic transport of the enzyme. Inhibition of protein synthesis by injection of cycloheximide into the cerebral vertricles abolishes the reserpine-induced long-term delayed increase of tryptophan hydroxylase activity. The increase of enzyme activity elicted by reserpine appears to involve the increased secretion of corticosteroids elicited by this drug. Pargyline prevents this action of reserpine, possibly by inhibiting the increase of plasma corticosteroids (99). Forebrain tryptophan hydroxylase is increased 4 hr after an injection of reserpine, presumably via a different mechanism (107).

In conclusion, various drugs can elicit a delayed long-term increase in tyrosine or tryptophan hydroxylase activity in the CNS, possibly via mechanisms that are similar to those seen in the periphery. In general, the long-term responses require prolonged and drastic treatment. Perhaps, because the brain has greater plasticity and the neurons have complex patterns of innervation, enzyme induction may be less important as a control mechanism. The functional significance of the long-term increase of hydroxylase activity remains to be established.

FEEDBACK CONTROL OF MONOAMINE SYNTHESIS VIA A NEURONAL LOOP

In brain, the short-term control of monoamine synthesis involves feedback control of the firing rate of monoaminergic neurons, which is linked in some unknown way to the regulation of monoamine synthesis rate. The neuronal feedback can be illustrated by the increase in turnover rate of dopamine in the striatum, which is elicited by many blockers of dopaminergic receptors, including chlorpromazine (108–110). Carlsson & Lindqvist (111) proposed the following explanation: chlorpromazine blocks the dopamine receptors in the striatum, thus altering the firing rate of the postsynaptic neurons. These neurons via collaterals or a series of interneurons increase the firing rate of the dopaminergic neurons, thus causing an increased release of dopamine in attempt to overcome the receptor inhibition caused by the phenothiazine. The resulting changes in striatal tyrosine hydroxylase activity might be explained by a decreased end-product inhibition, or by a change of the K_m of the enzyme for the pteridine cofactor.

There is now a considerable body of evidence consistent with this model not only for dopaminergic neurons, but also for serotonergic and noradrenergic neurons (112–115). Direct evidence for drug-induced changes in firing rate of aminergic neurons has been made possible by extracellular recordings of the cell bodies of serotonergic neurons in the raphe, of the dopaminergic neurons in the substantia nigra, and of the noradrenergic neurons in the locus coereleus (113–115). These electrophysiological experiments confirm that phenothiazines increase the firing rate of dopaminergic neurons. Monoamine oxidase inhibitors, which raise the transmitter amine's concentrations by blocking their destruction, decrease the firing rate of serotonergic and dopaminergic neurons, and decrease the synthesis of norepinephrine. LSD, which is claimed to be a serotonergic agonist (116), slows the firing rate of serotonergic neurons and decreases the turnover of 5HT. Apomorphine, which stimulates dopamine receptors, slows the firing rate of dopaminergic neurons and slows dopamine synthesis (114). Carlsson and co-workers have attempted to alter directly the firing rate of aminergic neurons by axotomy and have then studied the "in vivo activity" of tyrosine and tryptophan hydroxylase (117). They measured the accumulation of Dopa and 5HTP induced by a decarboxylase inhibitor. The results with the different amines and in the different areas of the CNS do not form a consistent picture: spinal transection markedly slows the accumulation of 5HTP in the caudal half of the spinal cord suggesting that axotomy decreased amine turnover. In contrast, brain transection rostral to the cell bodies in mesencephalon does not alter the rate of Dopa accumulation in noradrenergic neurons, or that of 5HTP in serotonergic axons and endings in the forebrain. A still different effect was seen in the dopaminergic system: cerebral hemisection increases the Dopa accumulation in striatum and causes a rapid rise in DA (118).

The negligible effect of axotomy on 5HTP and Dopa accumulation in the cerebral hemispheres cannot be readily explained because of a number of uncontrolled factors involved in these experiments. When measuring Dopa, in the forebrain one includes Dopa measurements in dopaminergic and noradrenergic neurons, and this discrepancy is reflected in diminishing the specificity of this estimation.

A model can be proposed to explain these effects, based on a hypothetical system of interneurons and presynaptic receptors (114, 119). It suggests that the dopaminergic neurons have presynaptic inhibitory dopamine receptors on their terminals (Figure 1a). Activation of these receptors inhibits the release and synthesis of dopamine. When the axons are cut, impulse flow stops, and due to a decrease in stimulation of the inhibitory receptor, synthesis of dopamine increases. Serotonergic neurons in the cord might not have serotonin presynaptic receptors, but they might be controlled presynaptically through either a collateral of the target cell or an interneuron. These can be activated by other synaptic inputs but inhibit presynaptically the serotonergic neuron (Figure 1b). When the serotonergic neuron is cut by spinal section at the midthoracic level, the collateral is not cut, the postsynaptic cell continues to fire by virtue of its innervation by other neurons, and synthesis and release of 5HT is inhibited. A similar situation may exist in noradrenergic and serotonergic endings in the forebrain, but transection is much closer to the terminals and also involves the collaterals mediating the feedback. Alternately, the feedback loop in the brain extends to the aminergic cell body and is cut by the hemisection. In either case, whether or not the postsynaptic cell fires, there would be no inhibition of release or synthesis, because there is no input to the terminals.

The following evidence is consistent with this model:

1. Presynaptic receptors exist in the CNS and have been shown in the peripheral adrenergic system. Presynaptic inhibition in the CNS has been reviewed (120, 121). The best studied case involves the primary afferent terminals (which innervate motor neurons) and are innervated by terminals of another system. This second system makes axo-axonal synapses on the primary afferent terminals. Stimulation of the second system depolarizes the primary afferent terminals, blocking action potentials, and inhibiting release of transmitter. In the peripheral nervous system there is evidence for prejunctional α-adrenergic (122, 123) and muscarinic receptors (124), both of which can affect NE release.

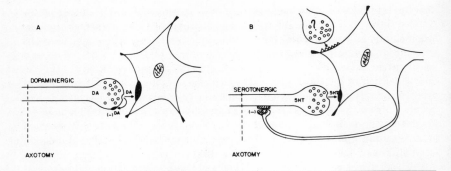

Figure 1 Model illustrating possible feedback loops in (*A*) dopaminergic terminals of the striatum, and (*B*) serotonergic terminals in the spinal cord. Dopamine via a presynaptic receptor inhibits its own synthesis and release. The inhibition is removed by axotomy. Serotonin inhibits its own synthesis via a collateral from the post-synaptic neuron. The inhibition continues or is increased after axotomy.

2. Dopamine receptor stimulators can decrease DA synthesis in striatal slices. This effect is seen both when the compounds are given in vivo, or added in vitro at 10^{-6} *M* concentrations (125). This effect is not seen in homogenates, and the compounds do not affect tyrosine hydroxylase directly at this concentration. The slices are probably too small to allow an extensive feedback system, and the post-synaptic cell might not be able to respond to apomorphine stimulation even if feedback were possible. The situation in slices is not completely clear because the apomorphine effect is blocked by haloperidol when it is given in vivo but not in vitro. Tyrosine hydroxylase in slices is increased by dibutyryl cyclic AMP (125) while release of norepinephrine is enhanced (126), but it is not clear whether receptors are involved.

3. Apomorphine injections reduce the amine accumulation seen in the striatum after cerebral hemisection (118), and apomorphine antagonizes the increase in enzyme activity elicited by injection of haloperidol.

PRECURSOR CONCENTRATIONS

Serotonin is the only one of the three putative neurotransmitters considered in this review whose synthesis can be accelerated by injections of its precursor, tryptophan. It is believed that tryptophan hydroxylation may function as a rate limiting step in 5HT formation, because its maximum velocity is lower than that of the aromatic decarboxylase which controls the successive step. Because the amount of tryptophan present in brain does not saturate the enzyme, the tryptophan concentration in brain determines the rate of 5HT formation. If an enzyme is saturated, that is the substrate concentrations present at the catalytic sites are at least several times the K_m, then small modifications in the substrate concentration will not affect the rate of reaction. It is well known that administration of tryptophan, or withholding it from the diet will increase, and decrease, respectively the concentration of 5HT in brain (127–131). In contrast, loading rats with tyrosine increases brain tyrosine, but does not affect the concentrations of the catecholamines in brain (132). In vitro, very high tyrosine concentrations can inhibit catechol formation (50) but this effect has not been observed in vivo (132).

Early work with tryptophan hydroxylase in vitro (133) showed that the K_m for tryptophan using a synthetic cofactor (DMPH$_4$) was 300 μM. This K_m is high compared with the concentration of tryptophan in brain (approximately 30 μM). Jequier et al (133) therefore suggested that "the enzyme may not be fully saturated with substrate normally, and that the overall rate of serotonin synthesis may be partially dependendent upon availability of tryptophan." It has since appeared that the K_m of tryptophan hydroxylase is much lower (50 μM) when BH$_4$ is used as a cofactor (22). This K_m value appears to be consistent (22) with data from experiments with tryptophan loading. A dose of 50 mg/kg ip, tryptophan causes the brain tryptophan concentration to be about 100 μM (threefold normal), and the brain serotonin concentration doubles (134). Larger doses of tryptophan increase the brain tryptophan content proportionately, but produce no further appreciable increase in brain 5HT. Grahame-Smith (135) noted a similar effect, but found that the maximum rise in 5HT occurred with a dose of 120 mg/kg tryptophan which produced a brain tryptophan concentration of approximately 350 μM. Thus, serotonin formation in vivo is maximal when the brain tryptophan concentration rises by 3–6 times (reaching 3–6 times the K_m of tryptophan hydroxylase measured in vitro with BH$_4$ as the cofactor). A similar conclusion was derived from estimates of the "in vivo activity" of tryptophan hydroxylase (117). Therefore, it appears that tryptophan hydroxylase is not saturated in vivo and that by changing the brain tryptophan concentrations it is possible to control the rates of 5HT synthesis and accumulation.

A major current controversy concerns whether drugs and physiological variables that affect 5HT synthesis do so by means of an effect on brain tryptophan concentrations. Tagliamonte et al (136–140) have shown that there are many drugs that produce parallel changes in brain tryptophan and brain 5HT turnover rate. (In these studies and most of the others to be discussed, changes in brain 5HT turnover rate are inferred from changes in steady-state 5HIAA concentrations). They showed that amphetamine, lithium salts, dibutyryl cyclic AMP, reserpine, 40°C environment, and electroconvulsive shock increase brain 5HT turnover rate and also increase the concentration of tryptophan in brain. In contrast, p-chlorophenylalanine, which slowly inhibits tryptophan hydroxylase and promptly lowers brain tryptophan, decreases 5HT turnover (136, 137) when only brain tryptophan is lowered. They therefore suggested that changes in the serotonin turnover produced by these drugs might be secondary to their effects on brain tryptophan concentrations. Although in many cases plasma tryptophan was increased when brain tryptophan rose, there was not a complete correlation. Brain tryptophan is, of course, derived from plasma, and after a tryptophan load the concentrations in brain and plasma are directly proportional to each other (135). However, tryptophan requires a transport mechanism to pass the blood brain barrier, and so factors that affect this uptake can alter the distribution between plasma and brain which is normally 4–6:1.

Fernstrom & Wurtman have examined in detail factors that affect brain and plasma tryptophan concentrations. Plasma tryptophan is subject to diurnal variations (21 μg/ml at noon; 32 μg/ml at midnight), due to variations in diet corticosteroid levels and the activity of hepatic catabolizing enzymes (134, 141). Intraperitoneal doses of tryptophan which change plasma tryptophan concentrations by an extent smaller than the circadian variation also produce a significant rise in brain 5HT content (134). However, a rise in plasma tryptophan does not increase brain tryptophan if high concentrations of other amino acids are present to inhibit tryptophan uptake completely. Oldendorf (142) has studied penetration into brain of tryptophan that was injected into the carotid artery. The amino acids that inhibited this process were tyrosine, phenylalanine, histidine, leucine, isoleucine, valine, and methionine. Excess phenylalanine is known to decrease brain 5HT, either when present in the diet (130) or given acutely (143, 144), or in phenylketonuria (145, 146) due to an enzymatic defect. A diet low in tryptophan leads to a decrease in brain tryptophan and 5HT (130, 147). A diet rich in carbohydrates increases brain tryptophan and 5HT, apparently because insulin is released causing plasma trytophan to rise (148–150).

Tryptophan is one of the few amino acids that is bound to plasma albumin. The ratio of bound to free (20:1) (151) or 2:1 (152) can be altered by agents that compete for binding sites including nonesterified fatty acids and salicylates (153). Curzon and co-workers suggest that the tryptophan that actually influences 5HT turnover is that which is free in the plasma (151). They showed that food deprivation and immobilization stress increase brain tryptophan, 5HT turnover, and free tryptophan in plasma, while total plasma tryptophan remained constant. Administration of nonesterified fatty acids or of heparin (which increases plasma nonesterified fatty acids) can also release tryptophan bound to plasma (154), but it hasn't yet been shown that these treatments increase brain 5HT turnover rate.

TRYPTOPHAN CONCENTRATIONS AND SEROTONERGIC FUNCTION

All of these studies show that brain 5HT and 5HIAA concentrations correlate fairly well with brain tryptophan and with free and total tryptophan in plasma. However, the correlations are not perfect. There are conditions when brain or plasma tryptophan levels (free or total) are high, while 5HT and/or 5HIAA concentrations are below normal, and vice versa (150, 155–157). This incomplete correlation means that there are other parameters that can control brain 5HT synthesis, but they do not necessarily negate the possibility that control of 5HT synthesis via brain tryptophan concentrations is operative. A major unanswered question is the functional consequences of the increase of brain 5HT synthesis brought about by increases in tryptophan brain concentrations. It seems unlikely that a neurotransmitter such as 5HT, which is possibly involved in sleep, sexual activity, motor behavior, and emotional states, would be subject to functional control by dietary composition and so on, although the firing rate of raphe neurons is affected by tryptophan loading (115). Changes in blood tryptophan may be read out by the brain in a yet unknown way (148), but it also seems likely that the diverse brain functions mediated by serotonergic neurons are not controlled by gross changes in plasma tryptophan concentration. Several authors have suggested that the amount of 5HT formed is in excess of the amount needed, and that this excess is not stored in vesicles, but is immediately degraded by monoamine oxidase (135, 158, 159). As evidence, Grahame-Smith (135) points out that animals receiving tryptophan display an increase of 5HT concentrations, but that motor behavior does not change. On the other hand, when the rats are treated with tryptophan and a monoamine oxidase inhibitor even when smaller amounts of 5HT are formed, motor behavior is strikingly increased, probably due to a spillover of "active" 5HT onto receptors. Welch has also suggested (159) that an excess of 5HT is formed and hypothesized that the activity of monoamine oxidase is modulated to control the amount of 5HT available for use. It is also possible that MAO activity is constant, but that access of the amines to the mitochondrial MAO is variable, depending, for example, upon the availability of vesicles for storage. Unfortunately, no method exists for measuring what fraction of the 5HT synthesized is eventually released into the synaptic cleft.

CONCLUSIONS

The synthesis of neurotransmitter amines in the CNS normally reflects the rate of impulse flow in aminergic neurons, but when drugs are administered such a relationship does not necessarily hold. A number of other factors can change amine synthesis rate. Neither the effects of psychotropic drugs on these rates, nor the normal control mechanisms can be understood until we have a deeper insight into the function of the various regulatory processes involved. It is now clear that control mechanisms involved are the concentration of pterin cofactors, end-product inhibition by the catecholamines, tryptophan concentration, activation of enzymes by allosteric changes, and long-term increases in enzyme activity. However, large gaps in our knowledge make it difficult to assess the importance of these variables.

For a clear understanding of these processes, we need to know the following: 1. The exact chemical structure of the cofactor present in brain with each of the hydroxylases, and the amount present in the reduced form in vivo; 2. whether or not the hydroxylases are saturated with cofactor in vivo, and whether a decrease in the K_m for the cofactor by allosteric changes increases enzyme activity; 3. whether the particulate and soluble forms of the hydroxylases represent functionally different but interconvertible forms.

Other possibilities can, in turn, be examined only when we begin to find answers to the questions formulated above. In this review we have discussed general mechanisms that control monoamine synthesis that might be possible sites for drug action. Many pharmacologically interesting compounds affect aminergic neurons by mechanisms of action which are completely unknown. For example, the benzodiazepines (minor tranquilizers) block the increase in NE turnover produced by stress, in doses devoid of any effect on amine turnover in normal animals (160, 161). One of the mechanisms discussed above might be directly affected by the benzodiazepines, but they might directly affect another system of neurons that in stress influence the noradrenergic neurons. It is apparent that much remains to be learned about the anatomical inputs to the monoaminergic neurons as well as their biochemistry.

At a recent symposium, "Frontiers in Catecholamine Research," many of the topics considered dealt with the questions discussed above. It appears that within the next few years, great strides will be made in our understanding of the functional complexity of the aminergic systems. In addition to our current knowledge of the anatomy of the aminergic pathways, we can hope to understand better their biochemical and neurophysiological nature and their significance in terms of behavior and psychiatry.

Literature Cited

1. Costa, E., Neff, N. H. 1970. *Handb. Neurochem.* 4:45–90
2. Costa, E. 1970. *Advan. Biochem. Psychopharmacol.* 2:169–204
3. Costa, E. 1972. *Proc. Int. Congr. Pharmacol., 5th, Basel, Switzerland* 4: 215–26
4. Cotten, M., Ed. 1972. *Pharmacol. Rev.,* Vol. 24 (2) (Proc. NY Heart Assoc. Symp. Regul. Catecholamine Metab. Sympathetic Nervous System)
5. Usdin, E., Snyder, S., Eds. *Frontiers in Catecholamine Research.* (Proc. Int. Catecholamine Symp., 3rd.) London: Pergamon. In press
6. Costa, E., Gessa, G. L., Sandler, M., Eds. 1974. *Advan. Biochem. Psychopharmacol.* Vols. 10, 11. In press (Proc. Int. Symp. 5-Hydroxytryptamine and other Indolealkylamines in Brain)
7. Molinoff, P. B., Axelrod, J. 1971. *Ann. Rev. Biochem.* 40:465–500
8. Weiner, N. 1970. *Ann. Rev. Pharmacol.* 10:273–90
9. Udenfriend, S., Dairman, W. 1970. *Advan. Enzyme Regul.* 9:1445–65
10. Geffen, L. B., Livett, B. G. 1971. *Physiol. Rev.* 51:98–157
11. Kaufman, S. 1967. *Ann. Rev. Biochem.* 36:171–81
12. Boulton, A. 1971. *Nature* 231:22–28
13. Chase, T. N., Murphy, D. L. 1973. *Ann. Rev. Pharmacol.* 13:181–97
14. Schildkraut, J. J. 1973. *Ann. Rev. Pharmacol.* 13:427–54
15. Dahlstrom, A. 1971. *Phil. Trans. Roy. Soc. London* 261B:325–58
16. Aghajanian, G. K. 1972. *Ann. Rev. Pharmacol.* 12:157–68
17. Creveling, C. R., Daly, J. W. 1971. *Med. Res. Ser. Monogr.* 5:355–411
18. Iversen, L. L. 1971. *Brit. J. Pharmacol.* 41:571–91
19. Nagatsu, T., Mizutani, K., Nagatsu, I., Matsura, S., Sugimoto, T. 1972. *Biochem. Pharmacol.* 21:1945–53
20. Lloyd, T., Weiner, N. 1971. *Mol. Pharmacol.* 7:569–80
21. Lovenberg, W., Jéquier, E., Sjoerdsma, A. 1967. *Science* 155:217–19
22. Friedman, P. A., Kappelman, A. H., Kaufman, S. 1972. *J. Biol. Chem.* 247: 4165–73
23. Cleland, W. W. 1967. *Ann. Rev. Biochem.* 36:77–112
24. Craine, J. E., Hall, E. S., Kaufman, S. 1972. *J. Biol. Chem.* 247:6082–91
25. Musacchio, J. M. 1969. *Biochem. Biophys. Acta* 191:485–87
26. Musacchio, J. M., D'Angelo, G. L., McQueen, C. A. 1971. *Proc. Nat. Acad. Sci. USA* 68:2087–91
27. Guroff, G., Rhoads, C. A., Abramowitz, A. 1967. *Anal. Biochem.* 21: 273–78
28. Kuczenski, R. T., Mandell, A. J. 1972. *J. Biol. Chem.* 247:3114–22
29. Kuczenski, R. T. 1973. *J. Biol. Chem.* 248:2261–65
30. Kuczenski, R. T., Mandell, A. J. 1972. *J. Neurochem.* 19:131–37
31. Foldes, A., Jeffrey, P. L., Preston, B. N., Austin, L. 1973. *J. Neurochem.* 20: 1431–32
32. Kirk, J. E. 1962. *Vitam. Horm. New York* 20:67–139
33. Shimizu, N., Matsunami, T., Onishi, S. 1960. *Nature* 186:479–80
34. Hammarström, L. 1966. *Acta Physiol. Scand.* 70:Suppl. 289,1–84
35. Cater, D. B., Garattini, S., Marina, F., Silver, I. A. 1961. *Proc. Roy. Soc. London* B155:136–57
36. Jamieson, D., Van Den Brenk, H. A. S. 1963. *J. Appl. Physiol.* 18:869–76
37. Diaz, P. M., Ngai, S. H., Costa, E. 1968. *Advan. Pharmacol.* 6B:75–92
38. Neff, N. H., Costa, E. 1967. *Fed. Proc.* 26:463
39. Davis, J. N., Carlsson, A. 1973. *J. Neurochem.* 20:913–15

40. Fisher, D. B., Kaufman, S. 1972. *J. Neurochem.* 19:1359–65
41. Goldstein, M., Joh, T. H., Garvey, T. 1968. *Biochemistry* 7:2724–30
42. Weiner, N., Cloutier, G., Bjur, R., Pfeffer, R. I. 1972. *Pharmacol. Rev.* 24:203–21
43. Harris, J. E., Roth, R. H. 1971. *Mol. Pharmacol.* 7:593–604
44. Nagatsu, T., Sudo, Y., Nagatsu, I. 1971. *J. Neurochem.* 18:2179–89
45. Coyle, J. T. 1972. *Biochem. Pharmacol.* 21:1935–44
46. Nagatsu, T., Levitt, M., Udenfriend, S. 1964. *J. Biol. Chem.* 239:2910–17
47. Petrack, B., Sheppy, F., Fetzer, V. 1968. *J. Biol. Chem.* 243:743–48
48. Laduron, P., Belpaire, F. 1968. *Biochem. Pharmacol.* 17:1127–40
49. Wurzburger, R. J., Musacchio, J. M. 1971. *J. Pharmacol. Exp. Ther.* 177: 155–68
50. Shiman, R., Akino, M., Kaufman, S. 1971. *J. Biol. Chem.* 246:1330–40
51. Mandell, A. J., Knapp, S., Kuczenski, R. T., Segal, D. S. 1972. *Biochem. Pharmacol.* 21:2737–50
52. Knapp, S., Mandell, A. J., 1972. *Life Sci.* 11:761–71
53. Knapp, S., Mandell, A. J. 1972. *Science* 177:1209–11
54. Knapp, S., Mandell, A. J. 1973. *Science* 180:645–47
55. Knapp, S., Mandell, A. J. *Serotonin and Behavior*, ed. J. Barchas. New York: Academic. In press
56. Grahame-Smith, D. G. 1967. *Biochem. J.* 105:351–60
57. Friedman, P. A., Lloyd, T., Kaufman, S. 1972. *Mol. Pharmacol.* 8:501–10
58. Fisher, D. B., Kaufman, S., 1973. *J. Biol. Chem.* 248:4345–53
59. Kuczenski, R. 1973. *J. Biol. Chem.* 248:5074–80
60. Musacchio, J. M., Wurzburger, R. J., D'Angelo, G. L. 1971. *Mol. Pharmacol.* 7:136–46
61. Carlsson, A., Lindqvist, M., Magnusson, T. 1960. *Adrenergic Mechanisms.* ed. J. R. Vane, G. E. W. Wolstenhome, M. O'Connor, 432–439. London: Churchill
62. Spector, S., Gordon, R., Sjoerdsma, A., Udenfriend, S. 1967. *Mol. Pharmacol.* 3:549–55
63. Neff, N. H., Costa, E. 1966. *Life Sci.* 5:951–59
64. Neff, N. H., Costa, E. 1968. *J. Pharmacol. Exp. Ther.* 160:40–47
65. Ngai, S. H., Neff, N. H., Costa, E. 1968. *Life Sci.* 7: Part II, 847–55
66. Andén, N. E., Fuxe, K., Hamberger, B., Hökfelt, T. 1966. *Acta. Physiol. Scand.* 67:306–12
67. Costa, E., et al 1972. *Pharmacol. Rev.* 24:167–90
68. Musacchio, J. M., McQueen, C. A., Craviso, G. L. 1973. *New Concepts in Neurotransmitter Regulation,* ed. A. J. Mandell, 69–88. New York: Plenum
69. Neff, N. H., Yang, H-T., Goridis, C. See Ref. 5
70. Lin, R. C., Neff, N. H., Ngai, S. H., Costa, E. 1969. *Life Sci.* 8:Pt.1, 1077–84
71. Macon, J. B., Sokoloff, L., Glowinski, J. 1971. *J. Neurochem.* 18:323–31
72. Millard, S. A., Costa, E., Gál, E. M. 1972. *Brain Res.* 40:545–51
73. Mueller, R. A., Thoenen, H., Axelrod, J. 1969. *J. Pharmacol. Exp. Ther.* 169: 74–79
74. Molinoff, P. B., Brimijoin, S., Axelrod, J. 1972. *J. Pharmacol. Exp. Ther.* 182: 116–29
75. Patrick. R. L., Kirshner, N. 1971. *Mol. Pharmacol.* 7:87–96
76. Axelrod, J. 1972. *Science* 173:598–606
77. Guidotti, A., Costa, E. 1973. *Science* 179:902–4
78. Guidotti, A., Zivkovic, B., Pfeiffer, R., Costa, E. 1973. *Naunyn Schmiedebergs Arch. Pharmakol. Exp. Pathol.* 278: 195–206
79. Costa, E., Guidotti, A., See Ref. 68, pp. 135–52
80. Guidotti, A., Mao, C. C., Costa, E. 1974. *Advan. Cytopharmacol.* 2: In press
81. Guidotti, A., Mao, C. C., Costa, E. See Ref. 5
82. Hanbauer, I., Kopin, I. J., Costa, E. *Naunyn Schmiedebergs Arch. Pharmakol. Exp. Pathol.* In press
83. Douglas, W. W., Rubin, R. P. 1961. *Nature* 192:1087–89
84. Paul, M. I., Kvetnansky, R., Cramer, H., Silbergeld, S., Kopin, I. J. 1971. *Endocrinology* 88:338–44
85. Serck-Hanssen, G., Christoffersen, T., Mørland, J., Osnes, J. B. 1972. *Eur. J. Pharmacol.* 19:297–300
86. Douglas, W. W. 1966. *Pharmacol. Rev.* 18:471–80
87. Kvetnansky, R., Gewirtz, G. P., Weise, V. K., Kopin, I. J. 1971. *Endocrinology* 89:50–55
88. George, W. J., Polson, J. B., O'Toole, A. G., Goldberg, N. D. 1970. *Proc. Nat. Acad. Sci. USA* 66:398–403
89. Ferrendelli, J. A., Steiner, A. L., McDougal, D. B., Kipnis, D. M. 1970.

Biochem. Biophys. Res. Commun. 41: 1061–67
90. Lee, T. P., Kuo, J. F., Greengard, P. 1972. *Proc. Nat. Acad. Sci. USA* 69: 3287–91
91. Schultz, G., Hardman, J. G., Davis, J. W., Schultz, K., Sutherland, E. W. 1972. *Fed. Proc.* 31:440
92. Thoenen, H., Otten, U., Oesch, F. See Ref. 5
93. Hartman, B. K., Udenfriend, S. 1972. *Pharmacol. Rev.* 24:311–30
94. Björklund, A., Katzman, R., Stenevi, U., West, K. 1971. *Brain Res.* 31:21–33
95. Thoenen, H. 1970. *Nature* 228:861–62
96. Hanbauer, I. See Ref. 5
97. Besson, M. J., Cheramy, A., Gauchy, C., Musacchio, J. 1973. *Eur. J. Pharmacol.* 22:181–86
98. Zivkovic, B., Guidotti, A., Costa, E. 1973. *Brain Res.* 57:522–26
99. Zivkovic, B., Guidotti, A., Costa, E. 1974. *Advan. Biochem. Psychopharmacol.* 10: In press
100. Segal, D. S., Sullivan, J. L., Kuczenski, R. T., Mandell, A. J. 1971. *Science* 173:847–49
101. Musacchio, J. M., Julou, L., Kety, S. S., Glowinski, J. 1969. *Proc. Nat. Acad. Sci. USA* 63:1117–19
102. Azmitia, E. C. 1970. *Life Sci.* 9: Pt. 1, 633–37
103. Fukui, K., Shiomi, H., Takagi, H. 1972. *Eur. J. Pharmacol.* 19:123–25
104. Schecter, P. J., Lovenberg, W., Sjoerdsma, A. 1972. *Biochem. Pharmacol.* 21:751–53
105. Meek, J. L., Neff, N. H. 1972. *J. Neurochem.* 19:1519–25
106. Azmitia, E. C., McEwen, B. S. 1969. *Science* 166:1274–76
107. Gál, E. M., Heater, R. D., Millard, S. A. 1968. *Proc. Soc. Exp. Biol. Med.* 128: 412–15
108. Andén, N. E., Corrodi, H., Fuxe, K., Ungerstedt, U. 1971. *Eur. J. Pharmacol.* 15:193–99
109. Neff, N. H., Costa, E. 1967. *Proc. Int. Symp. Antidepressant Drugs,* ed. S. Garattini, M. N. C. Dukes, 28–33. New York: Excerpta Med. Found. Ser. 122
110. Nybäck, H., Sedvall, G. 1971. *J. Pharm. Pharmacol.* 23:322–26
111. Carlsson, A., Lindqvist, M. 1963. *Acta. Pharmacol. Toxicol.* 20:140–44
112. Andén, N. E., Carlsson, A., Häggendal, A. J. 1969. *Ann. Rev. Pharmacol.* 9: 119–34
113. Aghajanian, G. K., Bunney, B. S., Kuhar, M. J. 1973. See Ref. 68, pp. 115–19
114. Aghajanian, G. K., Bunney, B. S. See Ref. 5
115. Aghajanian, G. K. 1972. *Fed. Proc.* 31:91–96
116. Andén, N. E., Corrodi, H., Fuxe, K., Hökfelt, T. 1968. *Brit. J. Pharmacol.* 34:1–7
117. Carlsson, A., Kehr, W., Lindqvist, M., Magnusson, T., Atack, C. V. 1972. *Pharmacol. Rev.* 24:371–84
118. Andén, N. E., Magnusson, T., Stock. G. 1973. *Naunyn. Schmiedebergs Arch. Pharmacol. Exp. Pathol.* 278:363–72
119. Andén, N. E. See Ref. 5
120. Eccles, J. C., Schmidt, R., Willis, W. D. 1963. *J. Physiol.* 168:500–30
121. Schmidt, R. F. 1971. *Ergeb. Physiol.* 63:21–101
122. Starke, K., Altmann, K. P. 1973. *Neuropharmacol.* 12:339–47
123. Enero, M. A., Langer, S. Z., Rothlin, R. P., Stefano, F. J. E. 1972. *Brit. J. Pharmacol.* 44:672–88
124. Loffelholz, K., Muscholl, E. 1969. *Naunyn Schmiedebergs Arch. Pharmacol. Exp. Pathol.* 265:1–15
125. Goldstein, M., Anagnoste, B., Shirron, C. 1973. *J. Pharm. Pharmacol.* 25: 348–51
126. Wooten, G. F., Thoa, N. B., Kopin, I. J., Axelrod, J. 1973. *Mol. Pharmacol.* 9:178–83
127. Moir, A. T. B., Eccleston, D. 1968. *J. Neurochem.* 15:1093–1108
128. Weber, L. J., Horita, A. 1965. *Biochem. Pharmacol.* 14:1141–49
129. Ashcroft, G. W., Eccleston, D., Crawford, T. B. B. 1965. *J. Neurochem.* 12: 483–92
130. Green, H., Greenberg, S. M., Erickson, R. W., Sawyer, J. L., Ellison, T. 1962. *J. Pharmacol. Exp. Ther.* 136:174–78
131. Hess, S. M., Doepfner, W. 1961. *Arch. Int. Pharmacodyn.* 134:89–99
132. Dairman, W. 1973. See Ref. 68, pp. 1–20
133. Jéquier, E., Lovenberg, W., Sjoerdsma, A. 1967. *Mol. Pharmacol.* 3:274–78
134. Fernstrom, J. D., Wurtman, R. J. 1971. *Science* 173:149–52
135. Grahame-Smith, D. G. 1971. *J. Neurochem.* 18:1053–66
136. Tagliamonte, A., Tagliamonte, P., Perez-Cruet, J., Gessa, G. L. 1971. *Nature New Biol.* 229:125–26
137. Tagliamonte, A., Tagliamonte, P., Perez-Cruet, J., Stern, S., Gessa, G. L. 1971. *J. Pharmacol. Exp. Ther.* 177: 475–80

138. Perez-Cruet, J., Tagliamonte, A., Tagliamonte, P., Gessa, G. L. 1971. *J. Pharmacol. Exp. Ther.* 178:325–30

139. Tagliamonte, A. et al 1971. *J. Neurochem.* 18:1191–96

140. Tagliamonte, A., Tagliamonte, P., DiChiara, G., Gessa, R., Gessa, G. L. 1972. *J. Neurochem.* 19:1509–12

141. Fernstrom, J. D., Larin, F., Wurtman, R. J. 1971. *Life Sci.* 10: Part 1, 813–19

142. Oldendorf, W. H. 1971. *Am. J. Physiol.* 221:1629–39

143. Yuwiler, A., Loutit, R. T. 1961. *Science* 134:831–32

144. McKean, C. M., Boggs, D. E., Peterson, N. A. 1968. *J. Neurochem.* 15:235–41

145. McKean, C. M. 1972. *Brain Res.* 47:469–76

146. Oldendorf, W. H. 1973. *Arch. Neurol.* 28:45–48

147. Fernstrom, J. D., Wurtman, R. J. 1971. *Nature New Biol.* 234:62–64

148. Fernstrom, J. D., Wurtman, R. J. 1971. *Science* 174: 1023–25

149. Fernstrom, J. D., Wurtman, R. J. 1972. *Metabolism* 21:337–42

150. Madras, B. K., Cohen, E. L., Munro, H. N., Wurtman, R. J. 1974. *Advan. Biochem. Psychopharmacol.* 10: In press

151. Knott, P. J., Curzon, G. 1972. *Nature* 239:452–53

152. Lipsett, D., Madras, B. K., Wurtman, R. J., Munro, H. N. 1973. *Life Sci.* 12:Pt. 2, 57–64

153. McArthur, J. N., Dawkins, P. D. 1969. *J. Pharm. Pharmacol.* 21:744–50

154. Curzon, G., Friedel, J., Knott, P. J. 1973. *Nature* 242:198–200

155. Korf, J., Van Praag, H. M., Sebens, J. B. 1972. *Brain Res.* 42:239–42

156. Bruinvels, J. 1972. *Eur. J. Pharmacol.* 20:231–37

157. Leonard, B. E., Shallice, S. A. 1972. *Neuropharmacology* 11:373–84

158. Moir, A. T. B. 1971. *Brit. J. Pharmacol.* 43:715–23

159. Welch, B. L., Welch, A. S. 1970. *Amphetamines and Related Compounds,* ed. E. Costa, S. Garattini, 415–445. New York: Raven

160. Corrodi, H., Fuxe, K., Lidbrink, P., Olson, L. 1971. *Brain Res.* 29:1–16

161. Doteuchi, M., Costa, E. 1973. *Neuropharmacology,* 1059–73

DRUGS OF ABUSE 1973:
TRENDS AND DEVELOPMENTS

❖6605

David E. Smith and Donald R. Wesson
University of California Medical Center, San Francisco, California,
West Coast Polydrug Abuse Treatment and Research Project, San Francisco, California

INTRODUCTION

The accelerated transience of social phenomena is one of the most distinguishing features of the past decade. Drug abuse has been no exception. Major drug abuse patterns shifted so rapidly that descriptive and phenomenological analyses frequently were no longer valid by the time they appeared in print. Treatment efforts generally lacked the flexibility necessary to adapt to rapid change and fragmented as swiftly as they had coalesced around quickly shifting priorities and sources of funding.

Social reaction to drug abuse also shifted. As drug abuse became an activity of middle and upper class youth in the mid-1960s, enthusiasm grew for treatment instead of for criminal prosecution. Drug treatment of heroin dependence, especially methadone maintenance, was enthusiastically endorsed as the major thrust of treatment and research efforts. Politically, drug abuse was practically synonymous with heroin use, and the number of methadone clinics throughout the country mushroomed. Education was hailed as preventative. Predictably, when education and treatment failed to produce an immediate halt to the heroin abuse phenomenon, social attitudes gradually shifted back to a hard-line prohibition approach, especially with regard to the heroin pusher.

In 1973 divergent sources indicate, however, that the incidence of *new* heroin cases is declining markedly, although multiple or polydrug abuse is increasing. While this decrease in heroin use may be thought initially to be the result of treatment, law enforcement or education, other explanations are equally plausible, for the choice of a particular drug is dependent on a number of variables. For example, it is rarely considered that as a drug becomes faddish with different socioeconomic or cultural groups there is a reservoir of individuals who are ready to try it as soon as it becomes available. These individuals constitute the first wave of users who may eventually become addicts. A second population is susceptible to using the drug as a result of peer pressure. After a time everyone who is willing to

513

use the drug already has tried it, and new users are made up primarily by youth who are just reaching the age where experimentation with drugs is possible. Graphically the result appears as below:

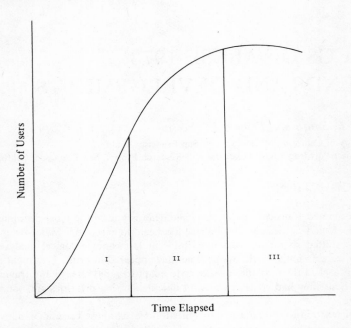

Figure 1 Phases of a drug "epidemic."

Phase I: New drug is introduced and receives enthusiastic acceptance. Tributes to the drug "high" spread through news media, underground press, and word of mouth. Individuals who will readily experiment with new drugs rush to get a supply.

Phase II: The number of new users begins to level off but continues to rise, because some new users succumb to peer pressure or become convinced of the drug's "safety."

Phase III: The total number of users of a particular drug levels off or begins to drop as drug users switch to other drugs, enter treatment, or die.

During the third phase the total number is increased by new youth who are reaching drug using age and decreased by individuals who enter treatment, die, or move to other drugs.

The shift from heroin to a variety of other drugs appears to be the dominant trend in the early 1970s. The differences that distinguish current use patterns from past ones are the wide variety of drugs used, the younger age at which drug use begins, and the worldwide communication and transportation systems that result in the rapid dissemination of drug-use patterns and fads throughout the world.

Some individuals believe that the motivation for drug use by preteens and adolescents also has changed. In the past, drug use by this group appeared to be motivated by sporadic efforts to prove they could handle "adult" pleasures or to "get even" with parents. Today's many youthful users seek the "high" or altered state of consciousness as an end in itself in addition to the traditional motivations of rebellion and response to peer group pressure.

The only constant about America's drug abuse scene is that it will change. The purpose of this chapter is to highlight some recent trends and developments in the major drug abuse groups.

THE GENERAL CENTRAL NERVOUS SYSTEM STIMULANTS

Amphetamines

Amphetamines are CNS stimulants that have been widely prescribed by physicians for almost 40 years for a variety of disorders including parkinsonism, depression, narcolepsy, asthma, the hyperkinetic syndrome of children, and obesity as well as to counteract the sedative effects of other drugs. Methylphenidate (Ritalin ®), a newer stimulant used medically for the same indications as amphetamines, has proven to have approximately the same abuse potential as dextroamphetamine.

METHYLPHENIDATE   AMPHETAMINE   METHAMPHETAMINE

The ability of amphetamines to relieve sleepiness and fatigue and to increase short-term performance has resulted in frequent nonmedically sanctioned use. As early as 1936, concern was expressed about the possible abuse potential of the amphetamines. A decade later, high-dose intravenous methamphetamine abuse in Japan reached epidemic proportions. The Japanese experience, however, did not receive widespread notice in this country, and in another ten years a similar abuse pattern began in the United States.

Because of the experience of Japan and the growing concern about abuse of many other psychoactive drugs, an awareness of the high abuse potential of amphetamines developed in this country. Amphetamines were the subject of Senate hearings in 1971 and 1972, focusing not only on high-dose intravenous use but also on the even more widespread oral misuse of physician prescribed amphetamines. The hearings were published in two volumes, *Amphetamine Legislation 1971* (1) and *Diet Pill (Amphetamine) Traffic, Abuse and Regulation* (2), which contain a wealth of material concerning the use and abuse of stimulants in the United States.

A clear trend is the development of increasing restrictions concerning the production and prescription of stimulants. The United States, for example, put federal control over stimulants in the same category as narcotics control and in 1972 reduced legitimate production of stimulants by 80%, with still further decreases in production in 1973.

Canada increased restrictions on amphetamine prescriptions and limited the use of these drugs to the treatment of narcolepsy, hyperkinetic disorders of children, mental retardation caused by minimal brain dysfunction, epilepsy, parkinsonism, and hypotensive states associatedwith anesthesia. Prescription of amphetamines for long-term weight control is not indicated according to recent FDA guidelines (3). A survey of 450 randomly selected US physicians (4), however, indicated that the majority of physicians felt that weight reduction was a legitimate indication for the use of appetite suppressants. Some county medical societies throughout the country asked their members to restrict voluntarily their prescription of amphetamines for weight control, and the debate over use vs misuse of legitimately prescribed amphetamines continues, although the high-dose intravenous abuse of black market synthesized amphetamine has declined significantly.

Cocaine

Cocaine, a general CNS stimulant which has gained recent greatly enhanced status, has emerged sporadically but did not achieve widespread use except in certain minority and artistic subcultures. In the late sixties, however, cocaine became a fad drug and re-emerged as a recreational drug among youth from all socioeconomic levels. The incidence of recreational cocaine use rose rapidly in 1970 and then increased at a slower rate until mid-1972. At present, cocaine is very much available to street drug buyers if they can afford its extravagant price. "Coke," "snow," "gold dust," "bernice," "the rich man's drug," or "the pimp's drug" (all slang terms for cocaine) can be bought on the street for $500 to $1500 an ounce or about $50 a gram.

Much of what is sold as cocaine is not cocaine. Cocaine is rarely pure and may be a mixture of various drugs. Depending on how a pusher chooses to adulterate his goods, the cocaine user can wind up snorting or shooting almost anything. Data from street drug analysis programs reveal that heroin, methamphetamine, or other local anesthetics such as procaine mixed with methamphetamine are often sold as cocaine. Samples that do contain cocaine frequently include only a small percentage of actual cocaine with the larger portion being another white, powdery substance such as lactose. The chief danger to the user is that he cannot calculate the amount of cocaine he is using or even be sure of the quality or purity of the drug he is taking.

Cocaine can be either snorted or injected. Snorting consists of sharply inhaling cocaine power through one nostril while holding the other closed. The material usually is chopped up into a fine powder with a razor blade, arranged into thin lines or columns and then sniffed. Thus a user may say, "I just snorted two lines of coke." Silver straws, expensive coke spoons, or a rolled one hundred dollar bill often are used as symbols of affluence when snorting cocaine.

The user experiences 15 to 20 minutes of pleasurable exhilaration and euphoria. In spite of subjective interpretation the pharmacological effects are almost identical with those produced by the amphetamines. Typically, "cokeheads" talk a lot and feel energetic and self-confident until the tensed, "wired" high of cocaine is replaced by nervousness and depression which can last for hours or days. Irritability, loss of temperature sensations, and tightening of muscles often accompany cocaine's post-reactive depressive state. This depression is in such marked contrast to the previous pleasurable sensations that heavy users will continue to sniff or inject cocaine every ten minutes or so for several hours to avoid the onset of depressive symptoms.

A second method of maintaining the euphoria produced by cocaine is to administer it in combination with a longer lasting euphoriant such as heroin. (Mixtures of cocaine and heroin often are sold in the street as "speedballs.")

Cocaine is also a popular drug among methadone maintenance clients, because cocaine will exert its powerful stimulant actions even in the presence of opiates.

The properties of the cocaine high are indeed appealing to the pleasure seeker, but the hazards inherent in chronic high-dose cocaine use make the drug equally dangerous. In addition to the dangers inherent in acute toxicity, a frequent side effect of heavy cocaine snorting is damage to the nasal membranes produced by intense vasoconstriction. After only a few months on the drug the cartilage separating the nasal passages may have necrosed.

Chronic use in the pursuit of maintaining a constant euphoric state increases the severity of cocaine's stimulant effects. After a few days the pleasurable effects give way to an intense anxiety state with gross paranoid features including auditory and visual hallucinations similar to an amphetamine psychosis.

Low-dose, chronic use of cocaine is not typical of American usage patterns, but such use is common in Peru where coca leaves are chewed by Andean Indians as a social ritual and mild stimulant, much as coffee drinking is enjoyed in the United States. Members of the upper socioeconomic classes in Peru make a tea from coca leaves. The pattern of chewing coca leaves or using them to make tea by Andean inhabitants involves only small doses of cocaine. Leaves of the coca plant contain only 0.6 to 1.8% cocaine, the rest of the coca ingredients being harmless alkaloids. This use parallels the use of caffeine in America and most individuals can use cocaine in this manner on a regular basis for months or years and experience no serious adverse effects.

Although psychological dependence on cocaine does occur, it is controversial whether or not cocaine produces true physical dependence. If deprived of his drug the cokehead will not experience the withdrawal symptoms seen with heroin or barbiturate addicts, but the compulsion to continue cocaine use is strong because of the severe depression accompanying abstinence.

Acute toxicity can occur from either snorting or intravenous use. The individual quickly becomes restless, garrulous, anxious, and confused. Pulse rate increases, and respiration becomes irregular. Nausea, vomiting, and abdominal pains occur frequently. Convulsions may then appear with the patient eventually lapsing into coma and death resulting from respiratory or cardiac arrest.

THE CENTRAL NERVOUS SYSTEM DEPRESSANTS

Methaqualone

The short-acting barbiturates constitute a major and growing drug abuse problem. In addition, nonbarbiturate sedative hypnotics such as methaqualone (available from US drug manufacturers under the brand names of Quaalude®, Sopor®, Optimil®, and Parest®) became a fad drug of abuse in 1972–1973. Methaqualone was introduced to the American medical market in 1965 for the treatment of insomnia and anxiety. Heavy advertising in medical journals by pharmaceutical manufacturers and promotion by drug salesmen emphasized that methaqualone was a *nonbarbiturate* hypnotic with low abuse potential and only rare incidence of physical dependence. Methaqualone has become widely prescribed by physicians, in great part because of their belief that it is a sedative-hypnotic with none of the abuse potential of short-acting barbiturates.

Inevitably, methaqualone was tried by those individuals looking for a better high. Knowledge of the drug spread throughout the country, helped along by publicity in the news media which reported the alarming increase in its use among youth nationwide and by articles that extolled the qualities of methaqualone intoxication. A new drug epidemic occurred throughout the country. By all indications it has reached the third phase (see Figure 1).

Basically, intoxication with methaqualone is similar to intoxication with barbiturates or alcohol and subjects the individual to the same risks: death by overdose, accidents due to confusion and impaired motor coordination, and escalating drug involvement to the point of addiction. Like barbiturate tolerance, tolerance to the intoxicating effects of methaqualone develops more rapidly than does tolerance to the lethal dose. Death has occurred with the ingestion of as little as 8 grams in a nontolerant individual. Overdose with methaqualone produces coma, muscle spasm, convulsions, and hemorrhaging due to interference with blood coagulation. Withdrawal from methaqualone dependence carries approximately the same risk as withdrawal from the short-acting barbiturates. The patterns of nonprescribed use of methaqualone are similar to those of oral barbiturates. Methaqualone is sometimes taken in combination with wine, a practice known as "luding out." This is especially hazardous, however, as methaqualone has a compounding effect when taken with alcohol, making the simultaneous effect of both drugs particularly likely to result in overdose.

Methaqualone has gained special favor with individuals who are patients in methadone maintenance programs because of the "additive high" the drug combination produces. In addition, street mythology holds that methaqualone is difficult to detect in urine samples containing methadone. This is not the case, however. The myth most likely started when methadone maintenance patients discovered that they could use methaqualone without its being detected in their urine samples. Methaqualone use most probably escaped detection in methadone maintenance programs because it was not one of the drugs routinely looked for in the urine samples required by methadone programs to monitor drug use and not because of any technical difficulties of detection. With the widespread publicity given to the abuse of methaqualone, this drug is now being added to the "urine screen" in many methadone programs.

Recently evidence appeared that diversion of pure methaqualone from manufacturers is occurring before it is made into tablets or capsules. Sidney Schnoll reported finding two samples of orange capsules sold as "mandrakes" (a street name for the British product, Mandrax®, which contains methaqualone and diphenhydramine, an antihistamine) containing over 200 mg of pure methaqualone hydrochloride without filler (5). This finding appears to indicate that *bulk* methaqualone is now being diverted from legitimate manufacturing sources.

With only minimal knowledge of the past history of methaqualone, the current pattern of abuse in this country could have been anticipated. Methaqualone was available as an over-the-counter drug in Japan (under the trade name of Hyminal ®) in 1960 and was widely abused by youth in that country.

During 1963 to 1966 a survey of drug addicts in mental hospitals in Japan found 176 out of 411 (42.8%) to be addicted to methaqualone. The primary reason for hospital admission was violent behavior associated with methaqualone abuse. Withdrawal convulsions occurred in 7% of the methaqualone addicts, and 9% developed delirium symptoms (Kato, 6).

Nonetheless, when methaqualone was introduced into the American market in 1965, advertising claimed low abuse potential for the drug, and controls over its manufacture, distribution, and prescription were minimal. This naiveté could be understood had the same pattern not occurred previously. In 1954 glutethimide (Doriden®) and in 1955 ethchlorvynol (Placidyl®) were initially acclaimed to be effective nonbarbiturate hypnotics free from some of the disadvantages of the barbiturates and without addictive potential. The drugs were widely prescribed, but gradually reports of fatal overdoses and addiction appeared in the literature. Controlled clinical studies found the drugs to be comparable to barbiturates in adverse reactions as well as efficacy. The consensus subsequently developed that the drugs were typical central nervous system depressants with no special advantages over the barbiturates.

Whether methaqualone could produce physical dependence was not determined prior to its being marketed in Japan, Germany, England, and the United States. Although physical dependence can be easily studied in laboratory animals, the ability of methaqualone to produce physical dependence was determined primarily by the study of patients who abused the drug.

In a letter to the Editor of the March 12, 1966, *British Medical Journal* (7), Dr. J. S. Madden of the Addiction Unit of Moston Hospital, Chester, England, mentioned four individuals who increased their use of methaqualone far beyond the usual prescribed levels. The *Medical Letter* (8), a bulletin which independently evaluates drugs and therapeutic information for physicians, in citing Dr. Madden in its April 22, 1966 issue indicated that he had reported four cases of physical dependence upon methaqualone. This was erroneous, as Dr. Madden had specifically written: ". . . not having had the opportunity to observe the patients when methaqualone was removed from them, I cannot objectively confirm or deny the presence of an abstinence syndrome" (7).

Gustav J. Martin, Director of Research of William H. Rorer, Inc. (the first pharmaceutical manufacturer to market methaqualone in the US), pointed out the *Medical Letter's* error in a letter to the Editor of the *British Medical Journal* on July 9, 1966 (9). Martin concluded: "This is an unfortunate lapse, and one which, by misinformation, indicts without justification a relatively safe and effective sedative-hypnotic."

The following year Drs. Robin B. Lockhart Ewart and Robin G. Priest, also writing in the *British Medical Journal* (10), reported a clear case of physical dependence upon methaqualone in a 47 year old man who was allegedly taking nine grams of methaqualone daily. One evening the man was found unconscious and his supply of methaqualone was taken from him. By the next evening he was ". . . restless and confused, and complained of seeing strangers in the dark corners of the room." The following day he was admitted to a hospital where he was reported to be anxious, restless, and having frightening visual hallucinations. He was reported to be in delirium with obvious tremor.

Subsequently other case reports have appeared in both the British and American literature. In 1969, the report of the Japanese experience with methaqualone appeared in the *International Journal of the Addictions* (Kato, 11). Research conducted recently at the Help Free Clinic in Philadelphia and the Haight-Ashbury Free Clinic in San Francisco have documented the high abuse potential and dependency producing properties of methaqualone as well as its cross-tolerance with the short-acting barbiturates.

In 1973 the *Second Report of the National Commission on Marihuana and Drug Abuse* (12) concluded: "The risk potential of methaqualone is roughly equivalent to that of the short-acting barbiturates." Although the Commission did not recommend placing Schedule II controls over any of the barbiturates it did recommend such controls for methaqualone:

Since unlike the barbiturates, methaqualone does not have large-scale medical uses, and does present a significant problem of misuse, it should be placed in Schedule II, along with the amphetamines (13).

Probably no short-acting hypnotic will be free of abuse potential. There is little doubt that those drugs improve the quality of life for some individuals who experience difficulty in adjusting their sleep cycle. Given the abuse experience of the past decade, however, the current competitive Madison Avenue marketing practices of drug manufacturers for sedative-hypnotics can at best be termed irresponsible.

Literature Cited

1. Subcommittee to Investigate Juvenile Delinquency. 1971. *Amphetamine Legislation 1971.* Hearings before the Subcommittee to Investigate Juvenile Delinquency of the Committee on the Judiciary, United States Senate, 92nd Congress, First Session, July 15 and 16, 1971. Washington DC: GPO. 1039 pp.
2. Subcommittee to Investigate Juvenile Delinquency 1972. *Diet Pill (Amphetamines) Traffic, Abuse and Regulation.* Hearings before the Subcommittee to Investigate Juvenile Delinquency of the Committee on the Judiciary, United States Senate, 92nd Congress, First Session, February 7, 1972. Washington DC: GPO. 749 pp.
3. *Med. Trib.* February 7, 1973. 14(5):3
4. Lasagna, L. July 2, 1973. *J. Am. Med. Assoc.* 225(1):44–48

5. Schnoll, S. H., Fiskin, R. Fall 1972. *J. Psychedelic Drugs* 5(1):79–80
6. Kato, M. December 1969. *Int. J. Addict.* 4(4):591–621
7. Madden, J. S. March 12, 1966. *Brit. Med. J.* 1:676
8. *Med. Lett.* April 22, 1966. 8(190):29–30
9. Martin, G. J. July 9, 1966. *Brit. Med. J.* 2:114
10. Ewart, R. B. L., Priest, R. G. July 8, 1967. *Brit. Med. J.* 3:92–93
11. Kato, M. December 1969. *Int. J. Addict.* 4(4):591–621
12. National Commission on Marihuana and Drug Abuse. March 1973. *Drug Use in America: Problem in Perspective. Second Report of the National Commission on Marihuana and Drug Abuse.* Washington DC: GPO. 481 pp.
13. See Ref. 12, p. 446

REVIEW OF REVIEWS[1] ❖6606

Chauncey D. Leake
University of California School of Medicine, San Francisco, California

Reviews of pharmacological interest continue to increase in number and in significance. Often they are the most satisfactory way by which busy members of the health professions can keep up with the flood of new information on drugs and their mechanisms of action, their metabolism, and their toxicity.

It is important, then, for reviewers of pharmacological reports to write clearly and concisely, so that members of the health professions may readily comprehend what verifiable information about drugs is now available. In-group jargon is an unfortunate affectation. Reviewers of pharmacological information would be wise to avoid it. Reviewing of scientific information, like any other literary effort, is a fine art, and it deserves to be cultivated as such.

Annual Review of Pharmacology affords the easiest and least expensive way of keeping abreast of the vast accumulation of information on drugs which occurs each year. The surveys in it indicate the broad-ranging scope of the science, covering as they do the ever growing information on the interaction of chemical compounds with living material from macromolecules such as genes and viruses, through subcellular units, cells, organs and tissues, individuals, and societies, to ecological complexes.

Pharmacology is now important not merely for the practice of medicine, but for all the health professions and services, as well as for agriculture, agronomy, economics, engineering, environmental control, law, criminology, sociology, and politics. Competent reviews of pharmacological information remain the most satisfactory way by which concerned people can keep abreast of it all.

GENERAL

Methodology is arousing increasing interest among pharmacologists. Chignell edits 14 reviews on physical methods used in pharmacology ranging from fluorescence spectroscopy to heat-burst microcalorimetry, and including electron spin resonance,

[1]This review was completed July 1, 1973, for material available at that time. References are cited at the end of the chapter, by author, without numbering. Names are arranged alphabetically for convenience.

521

nuclear magnetic resonance, X-ray diffraction, and mass spectrometry. Clarke edits data books on isolation and identification techniques with toxicological information on over a thousand drugs, with 450 infrared spectra for a variety of complex compounds. Florey offers analytical profiles of drug substances. Schwartz edits 18 reviews on current methods of studying nerve and nerve-muscle preparations, the use of microelectrodes, and techniques for examining contractile proteins, microsomal enzyme systems, and myocardial metabolism.

Controversies over methods used in clinical pharmacology and drug development are reviewed in discussions edited by Palmer. The psychiatric complications of commonly used drugs (including placebos) are surveyed in twelve reports edited by Shader. Using 167 references, Yesair, Bullock & Coffey review the pharmaco-dynamics of drug interactions, cautioning against multiple drug use. A helpful survey of fetal pharmacology is edited by Boreus. This includes considerations of drug distribution by placenta, fetal vascular shunts, fetal drug metabolism, and equilibration.

Biographical sketches of great pharmacologists are ever of interest. Fishman tells about Henry Dale (1875–1968) and acetylcholine. Golikov gives an account of S. V. Anichkov and his pupils at the Institute of Experimental Medicine in Leningrad. Raffel gives a well-deserved account of Windsor Cutting (1907–1972).

SOCIAL PHARMACOLOGY

The social implications of psychotropic drugs are well discussed by Berger. The social aspects of alcoholism are well reviewed by Kissen & Begleiter in the fourth volume of their comprehensive treatise on the biology of alcoholism. Milner considers the effects of various drugs on drivers of automobiles, with much on alcoholic beverages.

Drug abuse screening programs are outlined by Kaistha, with details on field tests and social implications. Siargh, Miller & Lab edit two volumes of reviews on drug addiction, the first dealing with pharmacological mechanisms and the second covering sociolegal aspects. Stewart surveys drug abuse in industry, with emphasis on prevention. Mills & Brawley review the psychopharmacology of *Cannabis sativa.*

McCawley, Hart & Crowe recommend a national advisory review committee to aid clinical investigators of drugs. Moxley, Yingling & Edwards offer reasons for the review of over-the-counter drugs by the Food and Drug Administration. Maronde and colleagues report on prescription data processing for the control of drug abuse.

Matties concludes that drug influences on teaching and memory are mostly inhibitory. Vesell reviews environmental and genetic factors affecting human drug responses. Wolff & Wasserman call for study of potential hazards of nitrates, nitrites, and nitrosamines added to foods.

ABSORPTION, FATE, AND ELIMINATION

In a couple of his neat "Vignettes in Nuclear Medicine," Brucer gives a sharp critique of pitfalls in estimating gut absorption by radioactive preparations. Cooksley & Powell review hepatic enzymes in regard to biotransformation of drugs, including induction and inhibition, and effects of liver disease. Hartiala reviews the metabolism of hormones and related drugs by the gut. Hausch points out quantitative relations between lipophilic properties of a drug and its metabolism. O'Reilly reviews the pharmacokinetics of drug metabolism. Wagner concludes that bioavailability, or rapid absorption, is a large factor in the therapeutic activity of drugs.

Several reviews refer to the absorption, fate, and elimination of specific drugs. Thus Christensen surveys the biological fate of decamethonium, while Juchau & Horita review, with 85 references, the biotransformations of hydrazine derivatives. Hirom and colleagues review molecular weight and chemical structure as factors in the biliary excretion of sulphonamides. Kimrich reviews coupling between sodium and sugar transport in the small bowel. Ling & Ochsenfeld survey the control of cooperative absorption of solutes and water in body cells by hormones, drugs, and metabolic products. Massry & Coburn review the hormonal control of renal excretion of calcium and magnesium. Sullivan reviews oxygen transport in mammals.

ANTISEPTICS AND CHEMOTHERAPY

Finland reviews studies on antibacterial drugs. Lucey introduces a symposium on use of hexachlorophene as an antiseptic in nurseries, in which it was agreed that it controls staphylococcal infections, with hazards not significant relative to its value. Pittin carefully reviews mechanisms of bacterial resistance to antibiotics. Raab surveys "Natamycin" (pimaricin) as a broad spectrum antifungal antibiotic of effectiveness and safety. Thompson & Werbel offer a comprehensive review of useful antimalarial drugs, emphasizing chemistry, effects on parasites, and effects on hosts.

AUTONOMIC NERVOUS SYSTEM

Bell offers a full review, with 856 references, of autonomic nervous control of reproduction, emphasizing circulatory factors influencing both male and female functions. Blaschko & Muscholl edit 20 reviews of various aspects of catecholamine pharmacology. With 582 references, Burnstock well reviews purinergic nerves, with much relating to adenosine triphosphate formation, release, and inactivation. New vistas, some 33 of them, on monoamine oxidases are edited by Costa & Sandler. Cotten edits 17 reviews of catecholamine metabolism in the sympathetic nervous system.

In a review, with 393 references, on drug action on adipose tissue, Fain gives evidence for adrenergic receptors on fat cells, with catecholamines as stimulators of lipolysis, activators of adenylate cyclase, and stimulators of cyclic AMP accumulation, with many drugs from amytal to xanthines affecting these actions. Harrison edits eight reviews of the circulatory effects and clinical uses of β-adrenergic blocking drugs. Wong & Schreiber review the metabolism (by oxidative deamination) of β-adrenergic blocking agents. Odell moderated a symposium on clinical aspects of catecholamines. With 102 references, Smith reviewed subcellular localization of noradrenaline in sympathetic neurons. Higgins, Vatner & Braunwald, with 328 references, reviewed the parasympathetic control of hearts, detailing mechanisms of action of acetylcholine in relation to catecholamine release and sympathetic modulation, with adrenergic activity in right ventricles and cholinergic in left.

CENTRAL NERVOUS SYSTEM

Anesthesia

With physicochemical data from Veda and colleagues on firefly enzymes, Eyring updates the reversible protein denaturation theory of anesthesia of Claude Bernard (1814–1878). In reviewing neurophysiological effects of general anesthetics, Clark & Rosner find that fluorine adds to the central nervous system irritability of general anesthetics. Dundee, Forrester & Simpson chaired sections in a conference on a steroid intravenous anesthetic agent, althesin, dealing with laboratory and clinical pharmacology, and with clinical experiences. Metabolic aspects of halothane-liver relations are reviewed by Dykes and associates, while Ross & Cardell survey the effects of halothane on the ultrastructure of rat liver cells. With 67 references, Seeman offers a comprehensive review of the responses of membranes to anesthetics and CNS depressants. Especially interesting are sections on membrane expansion and fluidization.

Tricyclic Antidepressants

Blackwell and associates review dose-response relations between the anticholinergic action of tricyclic antidepressants and mood. Fournier surveys poisoning due to tricyclic antidepressants, while Lambert reviews their many undesirable side effects, and Pichot covers the criteria for the evaluation of their effects in humans. Simon reviews preclinical studies on them, while Tillement analyzes their pharmacokinetics. Schmutz offers a general review of their actions and uses.

General

Burns opened a symposium on L-dopa in parkinsonism, while Malitz edited 9 essays on its behavioral effects. Furchgott edited 3 keen reviews on effects of drugs, chiefly stimulants, on behavior. A new antidepressant, butriptyline HCl, was the subject of a symposium opened by Lippman, while Spencer opened one on oxypertine, another anti-anxiety agent. Van Praag introduced a symposium on amphetamine derivatives.

Chemical modulation of brain function is the subject of a volume of 20 essays edited by Sabelli and dedicated to J. E. P. Toman.

The clinical pharmacology of sleep is critically reviewed by Freeman with respect to drugs. Barbitals and alcohol decrease the percentage of rapid-eye-movement (REM) sleep, but they lose this effect on repeated use. King also reviews the pharmacology of REM sleep. Kissin & Begleiter conclude their four-volume treatise on the biology of alcoholism: the first covers biochemistry; the second physiology and behavior; the third, clinical pathology; and the fourth, social biology. De Feudis reviews the actions of lithium on cerebral carbohydrate metabolism: it increases glycogen in brains. Bowden & Maddux discuss various aspects of methadone maintenance.

Diamond, Bates & Levine review the pharmacology of drugs used in treating migraine. Kosterlitz and Villareal edit 20 essays on the agonist and antagonist action of narcotic and analgesic drugs. Brogden, Speight & Avery offer a review of the pharmacology, therapeutic efficacy and dependence liability of pentazocine, a useful analgesic. Woodbury, Penry & Schmidt edit 59 essays on anti-epileptic drugs.

CARDIOVASCULAR, RESPIRATORY, BLOOD, AND RENAL

Beal reviews the pathophysiology and clinicopharmacological aspects of hematinics, especially iron, Vitamin B_{12}, and folic acid preparations. Edwards edits 12 reviews of drugs affecting kidney function and metabolism. Ehrlich & Stivala survey the chemistry and pharmacology of heparin. With 452 references, Fisher well reviews the pharmacology, biogensis, and production control of erythropoietin. Horowitz analyses the mechanism of action and clinical use of nitroglycerin.

With 796 references, Kones offers a comprehensive survey of molecular and ionic factors of altered myocardial contractility. Digitaloids are specific inhibitors of sarcolemnae, while Na- and K-activated ATP are concerned with active pumping of these ions. Ngai edits a well documented symposium of eight reviews on the pharmacology of oxygen, with special references to anesthesia. Tong reviews the clinical pharmacology of aminophylline.

ALIMENTARY AND NUTRITIONAL

Fidanza reviews the physiological actions of pantothenic acid, while Perri does likewise for Vitamin B_{12}. Gershberg analyzes the drug treatment of obesity. The regulation of Vitamin D metabolism and function is reviewed by Omdahl & De Lucca. Rindi surveys the physiological actions of thiamin, while Wasserman & Taylor review the metabolic roles of Vitamins D, E, and K.

HORMONES

Prostaglandins are now making it in a big way. Bergström edits the 110 reviews of the Vienna conference on this family of lipid acids and their wide activity. Hinman reviews recent aspects of their biochemistry. Kumar & Solomon analyze their significance in cutaneous biology. Lee reviews the interrelations between renal prostaglandins and blood pressure regulation. The Alza conference on prostaglandins, with 22 reviews, was edited by Ramwell & Pharris. This emphasized their significance in cellular biology. Southern edited reviews on the clinical applications of prostaglandin pharmacology to human reproduction from menstrual regulation to pregnancy termination.

Beroza & Knipling, in reviewing sex-attractant pheromones, conclude that they can be used to trap, or to prevent male gypsy moths from finding mates, and thus aid in control. Feldman, Funder & Edelman review subcellular mechanisms in the action of adrenal steriods. The influence of ergot alkaloids on pituitary prolactin is reviewed by Floss, Cassady & Robben. The clinical pharmacology of gastroenteric hormones is reviewed by Grossman. The mechanisms of action of female sex hormones are summarized by Jensen & DeSombre. Shafrir edits the Jerusalem Symposium on the 50th anniversary of insulin. Sutherland's Nobel Lecture details, with 74 references, the mechanism of hormone action and the discovery of adenosine-3, 5-monophosphate.

TOXICITY

Baker edits important Berlin session on toxicological problems of drug combinations, including modification of absorption, distribution, and metabolism. With 241 references, Bischoff reviews biocompatibility and toxicology of organic polymers used as tissue adhesives, prostheses, artificial organs, food packaging, and cookware. All are carcinogenic in rodents. Slater proposes tissue injury by free-radicle lipid peroxidation, with the self-destructive role of microsomal electron transport chain. Teratogenic drug screening procedures are reviewed by Tuchmann-Duplessis.

Metals

Angle edits 12 reviews of poisoning with iron compounds, usually hepatotoxicity from overload. Dales summarizes the neurotoxicity of alkyl mercury compounds. Felton and associates edit UCLA conference on poisoning with lead, mercury, and their compounds. With 130 references, Haley reviews pediatric and adult lead poisoning. Oehme surveys the mechanisms of heavy metal toxicities. Okamoto & Gunther edit a symposium on organic selenium and tellurium compounds, with much on toxicity, metabolism, and carcinogenesis. The hazards of lithium therapy during pregnancy are emphasized by Schou and associates. Vallee & Ulmer review the biochemical effects of cadmium, lead, and mercury, and their compounds. The relation of metals, ligands, and cancer is reviewed by Williams.

Organic Compounds

Bedford & Robinson review the alkylating properties of organophosphates. Daly, Jerina & Witkop survey the metabolism, toxicity, and carcinogenicity of arene oxides. Fukuto analyzes the metabolic toxicity of some 13 carbamate insecticides. With 78 references, Habermann reviews the pharmacotoxicity of the peptides, phospholipases, and hyaluronidases of bee and wasp venoms. Mellitin has 26 amino acid hydrophobic units with hydrophillic side chains and a molecular weight of 2840. James reviews oxalate toxicosis. Kadis, Ciegler & Ajl edit 11 reviews of fungal toxins including coumarins and various phytopathogenic toxins. Kao well reviews tetrodotoxin and saxitoxin, and their significance in excitation phenomena. Kryzhanovsky reviews the mechanism of action of tetanus toxin, with its effects on synaptic processes. Lehr describes sulfonamide vasculitis. Shinozuka and associates review acute liver cell injury from D-galactosamine. Oxygen toxicity is reviewed by Winter & Smith.

ODDS AND ENDINGS

Bektemirov & Bektemirova review artificial interferon inducers. Guth & Bobbin survey the effects of drugs on peripheral auditory processes. Johne & Groger describe naturally occurring acridine derivatives. Pfeifer reviews new papaverine alkaloids. With 69 references, Plotnikoff gives a review of the performance of pemoline, which may be useful in brain dysfunction in hyperkinetic children. Shader edits 12 reviews of the psychiatric complications of common drugs from digitalis to placebos. Speight & Avery review the pharmacology of "pizotifen" and its efficacy in treating vascular headaches. Weisburger, with 519 references, comprehensively reviews the pharmacology, toxicology, and pathological properties of hydroxylamines and hydroxamic acids, which play a role in immunological and allergic reactions and mutagenicity.

IN PROSPECT

Reviews of pharmacological information continue to increase in number and significance. Many, however, are buried in symposium or "recent advance" volumes. Publishers of such items would seem to have an obligation to assure that the contents of such review volumes would receive conventional indexing.

Literature Cited

Angle, C. R., Ed. 1971. *Clin. Toxicol.* 4: 525–643
Baker, S. B. de C., Ed. 1972. *Toxicological Problems of Drug Combinations.* Amsterdam: Excerpta Medica. 352 pp.
Beal, R. W. 1971. *Drugs* 2:190–206
Bedford, C. T., Robinson, J. 1972. *Xenobiotica* 2:307–38
Bektemirov, T. A., Bektemirova, M. S. 1973. *Vop. Virusol.* 2:131–41
Bell, C. 1972. *Pharmacol. Rev.* 24:657–736
Berger, F. 1972. *Advan. Pharmacol. Chemotherap.* 10:105–18
Bergström, S., Ed. 1973. *International Conference on Prostaglandins.* Oxford: Pergamon. 903 pp.
Beroza, M., Knipling, E. F. 1972. *Science* 179:19–27
Bischoff, F. 1972. *Clin. Chem.* 18:869–94
Blackwell, B., Lipkin, J. O., Meyer, J. H., Kuzma, R., Boulter, W. V. 1972. *Psychopharmacology* 25:205–62
Blaschko, H., Muscholl, E., Eds. 1972. *Catecholamines.* Berlin: Springer. 1050 pp.
Boreus, L. O., Ed. 1972. *Fetal Pharmacology.* New York: Raven. 465 pp.
Bowden, C. L., Maddux, J. F. 1972. *Am. J. Psychiat.* 129:435–46
Brogden, R. N., Speight, T. M., Avery, G. S. 1973. *Drugs* 5:6–91

Brucer, M. 1972. *Vign. Nucl. Med.* No. 63, 64
Burns, J. J. 1972. *Neurology* 22: No. 5, Pt. 2. 101 pp.
Burnstock, G. 1972. *Pharmacol. Rev.* 24: 509–81
Chignell, C. F. 1972. *Methods in Pharmacology,* Vol. 2: *Physical Methods.* New York: Appleton. 499 pp.
Christensen, C. B. 1972. *Acta Pharmacol. Toxicol.* 31: Suppl. 3. 62 pp.
Clark, D. L., Rosner, B. S. 1973. *Anesthiology* 38:564–82
Clarke, E. G. C., Ed. 1972. *Isolation and Identification of Drugs in Pharmaceuticals, Body Fluids, and Post-mortem Material.* Philadelphia: Rittenhouse. 896 pp.
Cooksley, W. G. E., Powell, L. W. 1971. *Drugs* 2:177–89
Costa, E., Sandler, M., Eds. 1972. *Monamine Oxidases,* New York: Raven. 464 pp.
Cotten, M. de V., Ed. 1972. *Regulation of Catecholamine Metabolism, Pharmacol. Rev.* 24:163–434
Dales, L. G. 1972. *Am. J. Med.* 53:219–32
Daly, J. W., Jerina, D. M., Witkop, B. 1972. *Experientia* 28:1129–48
De Feudis, F. V. 1973. *Res. Com. Chem. Pathol. Pharmacol.* 5:789–96

Diamond, S., Bates, B. J., Levine, H. W. 1972. *Headache* 12:37–44

Dundee, J. W., Forrester, A. C., Simpson, B. R. J. 1972. *Post-Grad. Med. J.* 48: Suppl. 1. 140 pp.

Dykes, M. H. M., Gilbert, J. P., Schur, P. H., Cohen, E. N. 1972. *Can. J. Surg.* 15:217–38

Edwards, K. D. G. Ed. 1972. *Drugs Affecting Kidney Function Metabolism.* Basel: Karger. 552 pp.

Ehrlich, J., Stivala, S. S. 1973. *J. Pharm. Sci.* 62:517–44

Eyring, H., Woodbury, J. W., D'Arrigo, J. S. 1973. *Anesthesiology* 38:415–24

Fain, J. N. 1973. *Pharmacol. Rev.* 25:67–118

Feldman, D., Funder, J. W., Edelman, I. S. 1972. *Am. J. Med.* 53:545–60

Felton, J. S., Kahn, E., Salick, B., Van Nattle, F. C., Whitehouse, M. W. 1972. *Ann. Intern. Med.* 76:779–801

Fidanza, A. 1971. *Acta Vitaminol. Enzymol.* 25:135–44

Finland, M. 1972. *Clin. Pharmacol. Ther.* 13:469–511

Fisher, J. W. 1972. *Pharmacol. Rev.* 24:459–508

Fishman, M. C. 1972. *Yale J. Biol. Med.* 45:104–19

Florey, K. 1972. *Analytical Profiles of Drug Substances,* New York: Academic. 492 pp.

Floss, H. G., Cassady, J. M., Robben, J. E. 1973. *J. Pharmaceut. Sci.* 62:699–714

Fournier, E. 1973. *Therapie* 28:307–320

Freeman, F. R. 1972. *Phys. Drug Man.* 3: 98–108

Fukuto, T. R. 1972. *Drug Metab. Rev.* 1: 117–51

Furchgott, E., Ed. 1971. *Pharmacological and Biophysical Agents and Behavior,* New York: Academic. 402 pp.

Gershberg, H. 1972. *Post-Grad. Med.* 51: 135–43

Golikov, S. N. 1972. *Farmakol. Toksikol.* 35:517–28

Grossman, M. I. 1972. *Scand. J. Gastroenterol.* 7:97–105

Guth, P. S., Bobbin, R. P. 1971. *Advan. Pharmacol. Chemother.* 9:93–130

Habermann, E. 1972. *Science* 177:314–22

Haley, T. J. 1971. *Clin. Toxicol.* 4:11–29

Harrison, D. C., Ed. 1972. *Circulatory Effects and Clinical Uses of Beta-Adrenergic Blocking Drugs* Amsterdam: Excerpta Medica. 160 pp.

Hartiala, K. 1973. *Physiol. Rev.* 53:496–523

Hausch, C. 1972. *Drug Metab. Rev.* 1:1–14

Higgins, C. B., Vatner, S. F., Braunwald, E. 1973. *Pharmacol. Rev.* 25:119–55

Hinman, J. W. 1972. *Ann. Rev. Biochem.* 41:161–78

Hirom, P. C., Millburn, P., Smith, R. L., Williams, R. T. 1972. *Xenobiotica* 2:205–15

Horowitz, L. D. 1973. *Post-Grad. Med.* 53: 167–75

James, L. F. 1972. *Clin. Toxicol.* 5:231–44

Jensen, E. V., DeSombre, E. R. 1972. *Ann. Rev. Biochem.* 41:203–30

Johne, S., Groger, D. 1972. *Die Pharmacol.* 27:195–208

Juchau, M. R., Horita, A. 1972. *Drug Metab. Rev. 1:71–100*

Kadis, S., Ciegler, A., Ajl, S. G. 1972. *Fungal Toxins* New York: Academic. 426 pp.

Kaistha, K. K. 1972. *J. Pharmaceut. Sci.* 61: 655–79

Kao, C. Y. 1966. *Pharmacol. Rev.* 18:998–1049

Kimrich, G. A. 1973. *Biochim. Biophys. Acta* 300:31–79

King, C. D. 1971. *Advan. Pharmacol. Chemother.* 9:1–91

Kissin, B., Begleiter, H. 1972. *Biology of Alcoholism.* New York: Plenum. 4 Vols. 630, 552, 580, 540 pp.

Kones, R. J. 1973. *Res. Com. Chem. Pathol. Pharmacol.* 5: Suppl. 1. 84 pp.

Kosterlitz, H. W., Villareal, J. E., Eds. 1972. *Agonist and Antagonist Actions of Narcotic Analgesic Drugs.* Baltimore: Univ. Park Press. 300 pp.

Kryzhanovsky, G. N. 1973. *Arch. Pharmakol.* 276:247–70

Kumar, R., Solomon, L. M. 1972. *Arch. Dermatol.* 106:101–11

Lambert, P. A. 1973. *Thérapie* 28:269–306

Lee, J. B. 1972. *Am. J. Med. Sci.* 263:334–46

Lehr, D. 1972. *J. Clin. Pharmacol.* 12: 181–90

Ling, G. N., Ochsenfeld, M. M. 1973. *Ann. NY Acad. Sci.* 204:325–37

Lippman, W. 1971. *J. Med.* 2:250–349

Lucey, J. F. 1973. *Pediatrics* 51:329–435

Malitz, S. 1972. *L-Dopa and Behavior.* New York: Raven. 144 pp.

Maronde, R. F., Seibert, S., Katzoff, J., Silverman, M. 1973. *Calif. Med.* 117:22–28

Massry, S. G., Coburn, J. W. 1973. *Nephron* 10:66–112

Matties, G. 1972. *Farmakol. Toksikol.* 35: 259–66

McCawley, E. L., Hart, H. C., Crowe, A. W. 1972. *Clin. Pharmacol. Therap.* 13:299–306

Mills, L., Brawley, P. 1972. *Agents Actions* 2:201–15

Milner, G. 1971. *Drugs and Driving.* Basel: Karger. 135 pp.

Moxley, J. H., Yingling, G. L., Edwards, C. C. 1973. *Fed. Proc.* 32:1435–37

Ngai, S. H., Ed. 1972. *Anesthesiology* 37: 99–260

Odell, N. D. 1972. *Calif. Med.* 117:32–62

Oehme, F. W. 1972. *Clin. Toxicol.* 5:151–68

Okamoto, Y., Gunther, W. H. H., Eds. 1972. *Ann. NY Acad. Sci.* 192:1–225

Omdahl, J. L., De Lucca, H. F. 1973. *Physiol. Rev.* 53:327–72

O'Reilly, W. J. 1972. *Can. J. Pharmaceut. Sci.* 7:66–77

Palmer, R. F., Ed. 1972. *Controversies in Clinical Pharmacology and Drug Development.* Mt. Kisco, NY: Futura. 218 pp.

Perri, G. 1971. *Acta Vitaminol. Enzymol.* 25:100–21

Pfeifer, S. 1971. *Die Pharm.* 26:328–41

Pichot, P. 1973. *Therapy* 28:225–34

Pittin, J. S. 1972. *Ergeb. Physiol. Biol. Chem. Pharmakol.* 65:15–93

Plotnikoff, N. 1971. *Texas Rep. Biol. Med.* 29:467–79

Raab, W. P. 1972. *Natamycin (Pimaricin).* Stuttart: Thieme. 142 pp.

Raffel, S. 1973. *Ann. Rev. Pharmacol.* 13:1–4

Ramwell, P. W., Pharriss, B. B., Eds. 1972. *Prostaglandins in Cellular Biology.* New York: Plenum. 526 pp.

Rindi, G. 1971. *Acta Vitaminol. Enzymol.* 25:81–100

Ross, W. T., Cardell, R. R. 1972. *Am. J. Anat.* 135:5–23

Sabelli, H. C., Ed. 1973. *Chemical Modulation of Brain Function,* New York: Raven. 338 pp.

Schmutz, J. 1973. *Pharmaceut. Acta Helv.* 48:117–32

Schou, M., et al. 1973. *Brit. Med. J.* 2:135–39

Schwartz, A., Ed. 1971. *Methods in Pharmacology,* Vol. 1. New York: Appleton. 500 pp.

Seeman, P. 1972. *Pharmacol. Rev.* 24:583–656

Shader, R. I., Ed. 1972. *Psychiatric Complications of Medical Drugs.* New York: Raven. 345 pp.

Shafrir, E., Ed. 1972. *Israel J. Med. Sci.* 8:175–495

Shinozuka, H., Farber, J. L., Konishi, Y., Anukarahanonta, T. 1973. *Fed. Proc.* 32:1516–26

Siargh, J. M., Miller, L. H., Lab, H., Eds. 1972. *Drug Addiction.* New York: Futura. 2 Vols. 288, 244 pp.

Simon, P. 1973. *Thérapie* 28:209–24

Slater, T. F. 1972. *Free Radical Mechanisms in Tissue Injury.* London. Pion. 296 pp.

Smith, A. D. 1972. *Pharmacol. Rev.* 24:435–58

Southern, E. M., Ed. 1972. *Prostaglandins: Clinical Applications in Human Reproduction.* Mt. Kisco, NY: Futura. 576 pp.

Speight, T. M., Avery, G. S. 1972. *Drugs* 3:159–203

Spencer, P. S. J. 1972. *Post-Grad. Med. J.* 48:7–56

Stewart, W. W. 1972. *Drug Abuse in Industry.* Mt. Kisco, NY: Futura. 276 pp.

Sullivan, S. F. 1972. *Anesthesiology* 37:140–47

Sutherland, E. W. 1972. *Science* 177:401–08

Thompson, P. E., Werbel, L. M. 1972. *Antimalarial Agents: Chemistry and Pharmacology.* New York: Academic. 422 pp.

Tillement, J. P. 1973. *Thérapie* 28:249–68

Tong, T. G. 1973. *Drug Intell. Clin. Pharm.* 7:156–67

Tuchmann-Duplessis, H. 1972. *Teratology.* 5:271–301

Veda, I., Kavoraya, H. 1973. *Anesthiology.* 38:425–36

Vallee, B. L., Ulmer, D. D. 1972. *Ann. Rev. Biochem.* 41:91–128

Van Praag, H. M. 1972. *Psychiat. Neurol.* 75:163–234

Vesell, E. S. 1972. *Fed.Proc.* 31:1253–69

Wagner, J. G. 1973. *Drug Intell. Clin. Pharm.* 7:168–76

Wasserman, R. H., Taylor, A. N. 1972. *Ann. Rev. Biochem.* 41:179–202

Williams, D. R. 1972. *Chem. Rev.* 72:203–14

Winter, P. M., Smith, G. 1972. *Anesthesiology.* 37:210–41

Wolff, I. A., Wasserman, A. E. 1972. *Science* 177:15–19

Wong, K. W.,Schreiber, C. C. 1972. *Drug Metab. Rev.* 1:101–16

Woodbury, D. M., Penry, J. K., Schmidt, R. P., Eds. 1972. *Antiepileptic Drugs.* New York: Raven. 536 pp.

Yesair, D. W., Bullock, F. J., Coffey, J.J. 1972. *Drug Metab. Rev.* 1:35–70

REPRINTS

The conspicuous number aligned in the margin with the title of each article in this volume is a key for use in ordering reprints.

Available reprints are priced at the uniform rate of $1 each postpaid. Payment must accompany orders less than $10. A discount of 20% will be given on orders of 20 or more. For orders of 200 or more, any Annual Reviews article will be specially printed.

The sale of reprints of articles published in the Reviews has been expanded in the belief that reprints as individual copies, as sets covering stated topics, and in quantity for classroom use will have a special appeal to students and teachers.

AUTHOR INDEX

A

Abayang, N., 369
Abbasi, K. M., 121
Abbott, A. H. A., 37
Abdallah, M., 428
Abdel Razek, S., 428
Abernathy, J. R., 428
Abernathy, R. S., 38
Abildgaard, U., 426
Abood, L. G., 246
Abraham, E. P., 435, 449, 450, 457, 461, 462
Abraham, G. E., 414, 415
Abramowitz, A., 493
Abrams, A., 312
Abrams, R., 165
Abrams, W. B., 94, 95
Abramsky, O., 101
Aceves, J., 78, 79
Acker, L., 139, 150
Ackermann, E., 223, 224
Acred, P., 441, 442, 449, 461
Adachi, F., 376
Adam, R., 427
Adams, F. W., 292
Adams, J. H., 426
Adams, P. W., 429
Adamson, R. H., 172, 173, 223, 234, 235
Adamsons, K., 211
Adelmann, J., 81
Adir, J., 41
Adlercreutz, H., 427
Aftergood, L., 198
Aggeler, P. M., 42, 259
Aghajanian, G. K., 492, 502, 503, 506
Agieva, A. K., 356
Agin, D., 333
Agre, K., 167, 168
Aguiar, A. J., 40
Agulian, S. K., 77
Agurell, S., 221
Ahmed, V., 241
Ahrén, K., 395, 399, 407
Aiken, J. W., 59, 70
Ailion, J., 390, 393
Aiman, R., 121
Ainardi, V. R., 299
Aird, R. B., 245
Aitken, J. R., 294
Ajabor, L. N., 427
Ajl, S. B., 526
Ajo, D., 327
Akert, K., 407
Akino, M., 495, 496, 505
Akita, H., 103

Aladjem, S., 212
Alauddin, M., 20
Alberici, M., 11
Albert, O., 20
Albom, J. J., 139, 150
Alburn, H. E., 445
Alden, H. S., 150
Aldinger, S. M., 298
Alegnani, W. C., 43, 266
Alexander, M. K., 426
Alexanderson, B., 257
Alexandrov, V. A., 192, 193, 196, 198
Alfin-Slater, R. B., 198
Alford, C. A. Jr., 477, 482
Algeri, E. J., 264
Allen, J. C., 80
ALLEN, J. L., 47-55; 51, 52
Allen, J. R., 139, 146, 152
Allen, R. C., 328
Allinger, N. L., 332
Allmark, M. G., 130, 131, 133
Allport, N. L., 37
Almond, C. H., 221
Alora, B., 443
Althaus, J. R., 281
Althoff, J., 197
Altmann, K. P., 503
Alvares, A. P., 224
Alving, R. E., 319
Amador, L. V., 101
Ambani, L. M., 100, 102
Ambaye, R., 165
Ambrus, C. M., 426
Ambrus, J. L., 426
Amenomori, Y., 397
Ames, A. III, 241
Amin, A. H., 121
Anagnoste, B., 101, 504
Anand, N., 121, 122
Andén, N. E., 92, 93, 98, 101, 497, 502-4
Anders, M. W., 267, 274, 276, 283
Andersen, B. Z., 83
Andersen, C. J., 133
Andersen, O., 81
Andersen, S. A., 260
Anderson, D. W., 295, 297
Anderson, J., 54, 264
Anderson, J. L., 300
Anderson, N. C., 347
Anderson, R. S., 291
Anderson, W. B., 30
Andersson, M., 139, 150, 381

Andolset, L., 426
Andrade e Silva, J., 319
Andrea, F. P., 188
Andreasen, P. B., 260
Andrews, P. R., 324, 334
Andrianova, M. M., 130
Andriole, V., 446, 448
Angeletti, R. H., 382
Anggard, E., 57, 64
Angle, C. R., 526
Ankermann, H., 85, 226
Annenkov, G. A., 356
Ansel, R. D., 94, 96
Anton, S. M., 394, 395
Antoniades, H. N., 365
Anton-Tay, F., 394, 395
Antun, F., 10
Anukarahanonta, T., 526
Apelo, R., 430
Apfelderfer, B. Z., 327
Apicella, M., 449, 454
Aponte, G. E., 82
Apostolov, K., 482
Appleman, M. M., 24, 26, 27
April, S. P., 307
Aramaki, Y., 170
Arbit, J., 96
Arcadi, J. A., 362
Arcamone, F., 159
Archer, R. A., 332
Arcos, J. C., 320
Arena, E., 159, 161
Areskog, N. H., 240
Argus, M. F., 320
Arias, I. M., 234
Ariëns, E. J., 42, 325, 326
Arimura, A., 389, 402, 407
Armitage, P., 93, 99
Armstrong, D. T., 70
Armstrong, K. J., 367
Armstrong, P. D., 326
Arnault, L. T., 130
Arnett, G., 478
Arnold, K., 41
Aronow, L., 36
Aronson, A. L., 85
Arora, C. K., 117
Arora, R. B., 117
Arora, S., 68
Arquilla, E. R., 382
Arrata, W. S. M., 429
Arscott, G. H., 292
Arthes, F. G., 425
Artuson, G., 240
Arvela, P., 224
Arvidsson, J., 94
Arya, P. C., 120, 122
Asatiani, V. S., 356

531

Edman, K. A. P. , 347
Edrada, L. S. , 227
Edwards, C. C. , 522
Edwards, K. D. G. , 525
Egan, R. S. , 329
Egbert, A. , 298
Eggena, P. , 83
Eggleton, M. G. , 78
Ehrich, J. , 80
Ehringer, H. , 92, 93
Ehrlich, E. N. , 79
Ehrlich, J. , 525
Ehrnebo, M. , 221
Eichelbaum, M. , 275, 284
Eichman, M. F. , 460
Eickhoff, T. C. , 445, 447, 449, 450
Eigler, J. , 78, 79
Eisalo, A. , 427, 429
Eisen, M. J. , 42
Ekbladh, L. , 67
Eklund, H. W. , 312
Eknoyan, G. , 80, 81
Ekstein, D. M. , 343
Ekstrom, B. , 443, 444
El-Allowy, R. M. M. , 366
Eldefrawi, A. T. , 310
Eldefrawi, M. E. , 310, 311
Elder, H. , 449
Eldridge, R. , 105
Elford, H. , 165
Elgee, N. J. , 424, 429
Elger, W. , 208
Elion, G. , 163
Elison, C. , 267
Elizondo, R. S. , 78
el Jack, M. H. , 291
Elkin, H. , 428
Elliott, H. W. , 267
Ellison, A. C. , 207
Ellison, R. R. , 163
Ellison, T. , 505, 506
Ellsworth, H. S. , 430
Elmadjian, F. , 361
Elmqvist, S. , 308
Elshove, J. , 207, 208
Elson, P. M. , 390
Elstein, M. , 427
Embry, R. , 49
Emmens, C. W. , 421, 422
Emmer, M. , 30
Emminger, A. , 197
Enderson, J. H. , 297, 298
Endo, H. , 273
Endo, S. , 241
Enero, M. A. , 503
Engel, D. J. C. , 329
Engel, J. , 98
Engelbreth-Holm, J. , 134
Engelhardt, D. L. , 474, 484
Engelund, A. , 425, 426
England, A. C. , 96, 99
English, A. , 435, 445, 448
Enomoto, Y. , 78
Enoyan, G. , 75

Entman, M. L. , 351
Epps, J. E. , 259, 260
Epstein, F. H. , 81
Erickson, R. , 442, 443
Erickson, R. P. , 228
Erickson, R. W. , 505, 506
Ericson, L. E. , 405
Ericsson, A. L. , 99
Ericsson, H. , 462
Ericsson, J. L. E. , 76, 214, 223
Ericsson, L. E. , 77
Eriksson, M. , 219, 231
Erlanger, B. F. , 283
Erlichman, J. , 23
Ernst, A. M. , 101, 397
Esmann, V. , 376
Estrada, F. , 443
Etchart, M. , 423
Euker, J. S. , 396
Evans, D. A. , 257, 259
Evans, I. A. , 197
Evans, J. S. , 161
Evans, K. , 208
Evans, R. J. , 292
Everett, G. M. , 101
Everett, J. W. , 401
Ewart, R. B. L. , 520
Exton, J. H. , 26, 373-77
Eyckmans, L. , 438
Eyring, H. , 320, 524

F

Fabiani, A. , 192-94
Fabiani, J. M. , 97
Fabre, J. , 448
Fabro, S. , 207, 223
Fagerhol, M. K. , 426
Fahn, S. , 105
Fain, J. N. , 368, 376, 379, 523
Fairbairn, A. S. , 425
Fairburn, B. , 425
Fairley, K. F. , 162
Fairweather, F. , 421
Fairweather, F. A. , 131
Falbriard, J. G. , 28
Falch, D. , 43
Falchuk, K. , 83
Falck, B. , 246
Falcoff, E. , 477, 484, 485
Falcoff, R. , 477, 484
Faleski, E. J. , 291
Falkson, G. , 170
Falkson, H. , 170
Fambrough, D. M. , 311
Fancher, O. E. , 144, 145
FANELLI, G. M. JR. , 356-62
Fanestil, D. D. , 84
Fantel, A. G. , 213, 224
Farber, E. , 285
Farber, J. L. , 526
Faresi, R. V. , 26

Farinas, B. R. , 348-50
Farkas, M. , 328
Farmer, M. , 131
Farnebo, L. O. , 103
Fass, R. , 449, 454, 455, 461
Faurbye, A. , 92
Fawcett, C. P. , 395, 396, 401
Fechner, R. E. , 430
Feder, N. , 241, 242
Fedrick, J. , 207
Fedson, D. , 470, 478, 479
Fehling, C. , 101
Feinstein, M. B. , 347
Fekete, M. , 393
Feldberg, W. , 64, 67, 68, 119, 240
Feldman, D. , 525
Feldman, J. G. , 430
Feldman, J. M. , 392, 399, 405
Feldman, S. , 40, 42
Feldmann, J. , 402
Feldner, M. A. , 357
Felici, M. , 402, 403
Felig, P. , 370
Feller, D. R. , 281
Felton, J. S. , 526
Feltz, P. , 105
Feng, H. , 43
Fenstermacher, J. D. , 241
Fenyvesi, T. , 267
Ferguson, D. R. , 79
Ferguson, F. G. , 356, 357
Ferguson, J. , 281
Ferguson, N. E. , 84
Ferin, M. , 414
Fermaglich, J. , 95
Fernández-Alonso, J. I. , 320, 323, 324
Ferni, G. , 159, 161
Fernstrom, J. D. , 506, 507
Ferrari, G. , 246
Ferrari, W. , 478
FERREIRA, S. H. , 57-73; 57-59, 63-68, 70
Ferrendelli, J. A. , 26, 498
Ferrier, W. R. , 40
Fetzer, V. , 495
Feuer, G. , 226, 336
Fex, S. , 313
Fichardt, T. , 170
Fichter, E. G. , 227
Fichter, G. , 223
Fidanza, A. , 525
Fieber, M. M. , 177
Field, A K. , 485
Field, E. O. , 170
Fieschi, C. , 99
Fike, W. W. , 265
Filho, J. A. , 423
Filshie, G. , 67
Fimognari, G. M. , 84

SUBJECT INDEX

Ether
on pituitary function, 403
Ethinamate
concentration/effect of, 264
Ethinyl estradiol
in cancer chemotherapy,
161, 166
effect on menstrual cycle,
416-17
oral contraceptive use of,
420
structure of, 419
Ethyl biscoumacetate
distribution of, 255
Ethyl ether
concentration/effect of,
264
1-Ethyl-4-(isopropylidenehy-
drazine-1H-pyrazolo-3,
4)-pyridine-5-carboxylic
acid ethyl ester (SO-
20009)
on phosphodiesterases, 28
3-Ethyl-8-methyl-1,3,8-tri-
azabicycle(4,4,0)decan-
2-one
antifilarial activity of, 121
Ethylnitrosourea (ENU)
carcinogenesis by, 192-
94
α-Ethyltryptamine
on pituitary function, 390
Ethynodiol diacetate
oral contraceptive use of,
420
Ewing's sarcoma
chemotherapy of, 158, 160,
165
EX 10-029
see 11-(3-Dimethylaminopro-
pylidene)-5-methyl-5,6-
dihydromorphanthridine
dicyclohexylsulfamate
Excitation-secretion coupling
calcium in, 309
Excretion
neonatal, 235
Extracellular fluid (ECF)
and permeability of blood-
brain barrier, 239-41

F

Fat cells
prostaglandins in, 70
FD&C colors
toxicology of
Blue No. 1, 128-29, 135
Blue No. 2, 129, 133,
135
Green No. 1, 128-29
Green No. 2, 128-29
Green No. 3, 128-29, 135
Orange No. 1, 128, 130-
31
Orange No. 2, 131
Red No. 1, 130-31

Red No. 2, 130-31,
135
Red No. 3, 133, 135
Red No. 4, 130-31, 135
Red No. 32, 128, 131-
32
Violet No. 1, 128-29, 135
Yellow No. 3, 132, 134
Yellow No. 4, 128, 132-
33, 134
Yellow No. 5, 133, 135
Yellow No. 6, 130-31, 133,
135
Fenamates
mode of action of, 67
Fetal pharmacology
review of, 522
Fetus
drug disposition in, 219-
26
fetal drug biotransforma-
tion, 223-26
transplacental drug move-
ment, 220-21
in utero drug distribution,
221-23
tumors in, 185, 197, 200
Fever
role of prostaglandins in,
67-68
Firefly enzymes
and anesthesia, 524
Fishes
drug movement across gills
of, 47-55
as experimental animals,
47-48
renal pharmacology, 76-78,
82
Flavonoids
anti-inflammatory activity
of, 121
Floridzine
renal effects of, 82
Flufenamic acid
mode of action of, 60
N-2-Fluorenylacetamide (AAF)
carcinogenic studies of,
188, 191
Fluorindomethacin
mode of action of, 58
Fluorine
in anesthesia, 524
N-4-(4'-Fluorobiphenyl)acet-
amide
carcinogenesis by, 188,
192
Fluorouracil
in cancer chemotherapy,
161, 163, 176-77
Fluoroxene
toxicity of, 283
Fluoxymesterone
in cancer chemotherapy,
161, 166
Folic acid antagonists
teratogenicity of, 206-7

Follicle stimulating hormone
(FSH)
hypothalamic drug effects
on pituitary release of,
395, 398-402
catecholaminergic input in,
398-400
cholinergic, 401-2
serotonergic, 400-1
in normal menstruation,
413-18
Folpet
teratogenicity of, 206
Food
effect on drug absorption,
41
Food colors
toxicology of, 127-37
introduction, 128
key to chemical names,
127
miscellaneous colors,
133
natural food colors, 134
oil-soluble azo colors,
131-33
sulfonated naphthalene azo
colors, 130-31
summary of present status
of, 135
triphenylmethane colors,
128-29
Frog
renal pharmacology of, 76-
79
Fungal toxins
review of, 526
Furadroxyl
toxicity of, 281
Furans
antifertility studies of,
122
Furosemide
comparative studies of, 78-
79
renal effects of, 80-82, 85
toxicity of, 277, 285
Fusaric acid
in akinesia, 98

G

D-Galactosamine
liver cell injury from,
526
Galago crassicaudatus
renal uric acid transport in,
356
Generic drugs
bioavailability differences
in, 42
Genetics
transcription or translation
cAMP role in, 30-31
Genistein
estrogenic activity of, 189-
90

CUMULATIVE INDEXES

CONTRIBUTING AUTHORS VOLUMES 10-14

CHAPTER TITLES VOLUMES 10-14

594   CHAPTER TITLES